PHARMACODYNAMICS AND PATIENT CARE

PHARMACODYNAMICS AND PATIENT CARE

MARJORIE P. JOHNS, R.N., B.S., M.S.
Associate Professor and Coordinator, Baccalaureate Program
Medical-Surgical Nursing, College of Nursing,
Northeastern University, Boston, Massachusetts

With 62 illustrations

THE C. V. MOSBY COMPANY

Saint Louis / 1974

Copyright © 1974 by The C. V. Mosby Company

All rights reserved. No part of this book may be reproduced in any manner without written permission of the publisher.

Printed in the United States of America

Distributed in Great Britain by Henry Kimpton, London

Library of Congress Cataloging in Publication Data

Johns, Marjorie P   1922-
   Pharmacodynamics and patient care.

  1. Pharmacology. I. Title. [DNLM: 1. Drug therapy—Nursing texts. 2. Nursing care. 3. Pharmacology—Nursing texts. QV4 J65p 1974]
RM125.J63   615′.7   73-8617
ISBN 0-8016-2528-9

To my husband
    GEORGE
and my children
    GEORGE, JEFFREY, and KATHLEEN

whose love, optimism, vision, and enthusiasm
    have made many wondrous things possible

PREFACE

Proliferation of knowledge in pharmacology has produced an awesome amount of information about the source, structure, function, actions, and interactions of drugs. To add to the dilemma, social problems with drug use and abuse and legislative controls of drug distribution have become part of the overall designation of pharmacology content for professionals. Knowledge of differing aspects of pharmacology is used by pharmacologists, physicians, legislators, and nurses. The text delineates the content about drugs nurses must know so that they can participate as informed professionals in planning patient care.

The nurse's role in health maintenance requires knowledge of the contribution drugs make to prevention and control of disease processes. In many instances, drug therapy is an integral part of patient care, and nursing measures can improve the effectiveness of the pharmacotherapeutic plan.

The framework of the book grew out of an interest in providing a relevant approach to learning information about drugs that the nurse can use as a base in planning patient care. The text follows a consistent pattern for presentation of functional problems, drug effect on biochemical or physiologic processes, and guidelines for nursing measures indicated by those pharmacodynamic effects. The approach provides a framework for study of drugs that allows maximum use of previously acquired knowledge of physiologic processes and nursing concepts.

Drugs are presented in the context of their principal use for control of functional problems. Using patient problems as the conceptual framework has allowed single in-depth presentation of drugs and decreased the amount of repetition required when drugs are grouped by chemical structure or body system effect.

The chapters have been assembled in units that represent commonalities of patient problems, and each chapter within the units is planned as an independent module. The plan allows correlation of content with presentation of nursing course content. Drug groupings reflect commonalities of action at particular effector sites, and the unique actions of individual drugs in the groupings are included.

Content about the pharmacodynamic effect of drugs has been drawn from the best evidence available from research in the fields of physiology, biochemistry, and pharmacology, and drugs included are those with known therapeutic effectiveness. Change is constant; therefore the content is presented as a base line for study of drugs in the hope that it will provide a guide for consideration of new drugs with comparable pharmacodynamic effects.

I am grateful to Dean Juanita O. Long for her continued interest in the project and for the time release arranged during the crucial days of final manuscript preparation. I am grateful to the faculty of the College of Pharmacy and the College of Nursing at Northeastern University, who generously shared ideas and materials with me. The enthusiasm and suggestions of students in the nursing program have been a continued source of stimulation and assistance in preparing the manuscript.

I am deeply grateful to Marita Bitans, whose fine illustrations of physiologic and pharmacodynamic concepts clarify content within the text. The suggestions for format contributed by Barbara Doten, who typed the many pages of the material, helped make final preparation of the manuscript a reality.

Marjorie P. Johns

CONTENTS

1 / Drug therapy, 1

UNIT ONE
DRUGS USED TO CONTROL INFECTION AND INFLAMMATION

2 / Invading bacteria, 15

3 / Fungus and parasite invasion, 44

4 / Immune and allergic responses, 58

UNIT TWO
DRUGS USED TO CONTROL EXCRETION OF FLUID, METABOLIC WASTES, AND TOXICANTS

5 / Pulmonary ventilation, 83

6 / Fluid balance, 94

7 / Tissue toxicants and debris, 108

8 / Enteric elimination, 121

9 / Emesis, 128

10 / Gastric acidity and intestinal motility, 135

UNIT THREE
DRUGS USED TO CONTROL HEMODYNAMICS

11 / Cardiac output, 147

12 / Cardiac arrhythmias, 156

13 / Vascular tone, 164

x   Contents

14 / Vascular constriction, 171

15 / Blood coagulation, 182

16 / Red blood cell deficiency, 191

UNIT FOUR
DRUGS USED TO CONTROL ACTIVITY AND PAIN

17 / Emotional responses, 199

18 / Cerebrocortical activity, 213

19 / Skeletal muscle contraction, 224

20 / Sleep patterns, 230

21 / Anesthesia, 239

22 / Pain, 244

UNIT FIVE
DRUGS USED TO CONTROL ANABOLIC-CATABOLIC BALANCE

23 / Malnutrition, 257

24 / Metabolic activity, 264

25 / Glucose assimilation, 271

UNIT SIX
DRUGS USED TO CONTROL REPRODUCTION AND FERTILITY

26 / Cell proliferation, 283

27 / Gonadal function and fertility, 295

PHARMACODYNAMICS AND PATIENT CARE

1

Drug therapy

Clinical drug trials
Legal regulation of drug distribution
    Official drug standards
    F.D.A. controls
    Narcotic regulations
Dose-response relationships
Pharmacodynamics
    Absorption
    Distribution
    Cumulative effects
    Adverse effects
    Responses of individuals
    Drug interactions
Patient care
    Drug administration routes

Modern drug therapy is a culmination of historic experience and extensive research that has made hundreds of drugs and combinations of drugs available for use. The frequency with which drugs are employed and the availability of information about drugs in the news media have had a positive effect on public interest in drugs. The patient receiving agents for control of a particular problem usually expects to be involved in the plan of therapy. He may be the best resource person for definition of the action of drugs he is taking, and he may provide clues that help in identification of problems before they are obvious by objective tests. His knowledge of personal physiologic patterns and responses can be used to evaluate the effectiveness of the therapeutic plan.

Physician, pharmacist, and nurse each have a particular area of expertise and interest to bring to planning and evaluating the patient's drug regimen. Working together, team members can outline plans to protect the patient's resources, support the action of the drug being given, and make optimal use of restored function effected by the drug.

Participation in planning requires knowledge of the patient's physiologic problem, the predictable pharmacodynamic effect of the drug, and the contribution drug therapy will make to the total plan for the patient. It is possible to define the probable biochemical or physiologic effect of drugs used for therapy, but those pharmacodynamic effects must be considered with an understanding that drug action is subject to variations in individual responses to drugs.

Clinical pharmacology involves the pharmacist in a role that is a modern expansion of his traditional function. The multiplicity of drugs and the potential for chemical interactions make it useful to have clinical and community consultants with special knowledge of the properties of pharmaceuticals. The pharmacist is becoming more consistently involved in clinical evaluation of patient care plans. In large urban areas, pharmacists also are active participants in poison control centers that provide round-the-clock telephone contact for community members.

CLINICAL DRUG TRIALS

Each new drug or drug combination is subjected to extensive trials on animals before findings are submitted to the federal Food and Drug Administration (F.D.A.) of the Department of Health, Education, and Welfare for approval of selective use in clinical trials. Each planned study has clearly defined statements of purpose, limits, and criteria for cessation of patient participation in the study.

Specifically identified staff retain control of drug use in the agency where the study is conducted. To assure objectivity and validity of the findings, a double-blind approach is required. Neither researchers nor patients know whether the particular tablet or liquid is the drug or the placebo. Containers are marked with coded numbers, and administration schedules for both experimental and control group are comparable.

Each patient is informed of the purpose of the trials, and participation during the study period is planned after his written consent is obtained. Assignment of patients to a particular group is done by random placement from a sample of individuals with the problem being studied. The code assignment is "broken" only when a patient is removed from the study; otherwise the code remains secure until the trial period is completed.

Meticulous attention to details during study periods produces copious amounts of data related to drug reactions, and F.D.A. clearance of the drug depends on the findings of the study. When the drug is released, the particular therapeutic use is specified, and use of the drug for a different purpose requires additional clinical trials.

Generic or nonproprietary names are assigned to drugs before they are released. The name does not necessarily reflect the chemical composition of the drug. Drug manufacturers may register a particular name (proprietary, or trade, name) for a generic drug when it is prepared in their laboratories.

In a clinical agency, drugs are purchased on a competitive basis, but the drug purchased from a manufacturer under its trade name is the same generic drug prescribed by the physician. Use of the generic or nonproprietary name in practice identifies the common properties of a drug produced under varying trade names. The language is difficult, but the attempt to establish a common terminology and frame of reference makes the effort to learn the language worthwhile.

Clinical drug trials provide base-line information that is expanded each time a health team member identifies and records an observation of drug effect or adverse effect. It is probable that there are data recorded over many years on records stored in agencies throughout the world. The increasing use of computers for tabulating observations should provide retrievable data that can be used in the future to identify patterns and configurations in patients' reactions to particular drugs.

Whenever a patient is receiving a drug, the nurse's observations of drug effect are important to evaluation of the progress of his drug regimen. As the most consistently available observers, nurses can make a meaningful contribution to drug research.

LEGAL REGULATION OF DRUG DISTRIBUTION

Widely publicized information about false claims for drug effect in the advertising of major drug companies and withdrawal of some commonly used drugs from the market have increased public consciousness of the activity of the F.D.A. The authority for the F.D.A. action is the federal Food, Drug, and Cosmetic Act enacted in 1938. The aim of the legislation is protection of public health. Amendments to the law in recent years (1952 and 1962) have led to more stringent requirements for labeling and advertising by manufacturers.

Official drug standards

The United States Pharmacopeia (U.S.P.) and *The National Formulary* (N.F.) are the two books that provide the official drug standards in the United States. The U.S.P. provides comprehensive information about drugs, and compounds manufacturered are required to conform to the official standards for each ingredient. An additional criterion is that labeling of drugs include the quantity of each ingredient of the compound.

The N.F. provides inclusive information about formulas for drug mixtures and, like the U.S.P., it is an official standard and guide for drugs produced by manufacturers. Each ingredient of a mixture is required to conform to N.F. standards or to indicate the specific differences (i.e., addition of flavoring).

F.D.A. controls

The law places any drug used for treatment of disease or intended to affect the structure or function of the body under F.D.A. control. The law requires that drugs possess the properties, purity, and quality stated on labels and in information published about the drugs. Extensive tests of drugs and studies of their therapeutic value are conducted by the F.D.A.

Regulations for labeling of drugs are prescribed in the official publications, and any deviation from the official standards for designated drugs must be indicated clearly on labels and in published information about the drugs. Labels must provide warnings about situations in which the drug may be hazardous to health. When preparations contain any narcotic, or hypnotic habit-forming substance, or derivatives with similar properties, the label must include a warning that the drug may be habit-forming. Listing of pathologic conditions in which the drug may be hazardous or a clearly indicated warning against the use of the drug for children when such use is contraindicated is required by law.

The F.D.A. applies the regulations to all traffic in drugs, but the actions taken are subject to petition by researchers or professionals in the medical field. A few years ago the F.D.A. removed from the market the monoamine oxidase inhibitor tranylcypromine sulfate (Parnate). Physicians using the drug were aware of the life-threatening episodes that could be precipitated when patients ingested tyramine-containing foods during drug use, (i.e., aged cheese) but the drug was considered a valuable antidepressant. The physicians' petition for release of the drug led to its availability for use under carefully controlled conditions in which the patient was under continual supervision.

Narcotic regulations

Distribution of narcotics in the United States is controlled primarily by federal regulations, but states and cities also have laws that control distribution and sale of narcotics. Federal standards of purity and the regulation of sales and dispensing of opium and coca leaves (alphaprodine, levorphanol, marihuana, meperidine, methadone, and nalorphine) originated with the enactment of the *Harrison Narcotic Act of 1914*. Amendments to the law have been made in the intervening years, and the most recent controls of narcotics and their synthetic derivatives are implemented under the *Federal Controlled Substances Act of 1970*. Regulations require that physicians or other dispensers of the drugs be registered with the Collector of Internal Revenue in the district.

Any agent holding narcotics provided by the dispenser (i.e., pharmacist) is charged with responsibility for consistent tabulation of the amount of drug on hand and the clear identification of individuals to whom the narcotics are administered. In clinical agencies two nurses count the on-hand narcotics at regularly scheduled intervals during the 24-hour period. The count of narcotics in the locked cabinet is compared with the signed statement of administration by nurses on the unit, and the count sheet is then signed by the two nurses. Although systems vary in details, the method used for signing a narcotic sheet before administration of the drug and comparing the count before and after removal of the dosage is a required procedure to assure that all drugs provided by the registered dispenser are accounted for within the agency.

DOSAGE-RESPONSE RELATIONSHIPS

The amount of the drug prescribed is intended to maintain a therapeutic level of drug action for the individual patient. The minimum and maximum dosage levels within the range of safe use of drugs have been culled from the literature and appear in tables in subsequent chapters. The prescribed dosage for a particular patient may be at or above the minimum level or below the maximum level, and only in selected rare circumstances when a life-threatening situation exists will the dosage exceed the maximal level.

Maximum drug levels reflect the *therapeutic index* (TI) of the drugs. The therapeutic index is based on trials in animals and humans to ascertain the lethal and therapeutic dosage levels. The dosage that is lethal in 50% of animals is designated as LD_{50}, and the dosage that is effective for 50% of humans is designated as

ED_{50}. The therapeutic index is obtained by the following formula:

$$TI = \frac{LD_{50}}{ED_{50}}$$

Many drugs have a high therapeutic index and consequently the concern with toxic and lethal effects is negligible, but drugs with a low therapeutic index make it necessary to supervise the patient's progress continually. For example, antineoplastic drugs have a low therapeutic index, and the patient usually receives the drugs while in the hospital. Regularly scheduled observations and blood tests are planned to follow the effects of the drugs on normal body tissues as well as their effect on malignant tissue.

The therapeutic index guides the physician in the selection of dosage for the patient's particular problem. The amount of drug necessary to produce an action or reaction varies in individuals; therefore careful observation of the patient is necessary at initiation of drug therapy and periodically during long-term use of drugs.

Physical condition, age, and body size of the patient are considered by the physician in selection of drug dosage. Immaturity of hepatic and renal systems in the newborn and the possibility of some deterioration of the same organs in elderly or debilitated patients affect the amounts of drug that can be utilized; therefore specific dosage adjustment is planned.

Body size and weight are important determinants of the tolerable dosage, since the distribution of drug in the body depends on the relationship of drug to tissue mass. Calculations based on body weight are done on the basis of actual weight. If the patient has a large amount of tissue fluid or if he is obese, the dosage is based on ideal weight. The therapeutic range for adult dosage can be used as a guide for calculation of the probable dosage for children (Table 1-1).

Comparison of the individual adult patient's dosage against the therapeutic range appearing in tables throughout the text provides a guide to the margin of safety during drug therapy. Many metabolic factors have an effect on decreasing the amount of leeway, and continual assessment of the relationship of dosage to physiologic changes is necessary throughout the period of therapy.

PHARMACODYNAMICS

Pharmacotherapeutics is the term employed to describe the use of drugs for prevention and treatment of disease. *Pharmacodynamics* describes the biochemical and physiologic effects of drugs and their mechanisms of action. Pharmacodynamics includes the absorption, distribution, biotransformation, and excretion of drugs.* Pharmacotherapeutic plans for treatment of disease often include prescriptions for several drugs, and knowledge of the pharmacodynamic effect of each of the drugs is important in planning for implementation of the pharmacotherapeutic plan. Throughout the text

Table 1-1. Determination of children's doses from adult doses on the basis of body surface area*

Age	Weight† (kg.)	(lb.)	Surface area† ($M.^2$)	Fraction of adult dose‡
Birth	2.0	4.4	0.15	0.09
	3.4	7.4	0.21	0.12
3 weeks	4.0	8.8	0.25	0.14
3 months	5.7	12.5	0.29	0.17
6 months	7.4	16	0.36	0.21
9 months	9.1	20	0.44	0.25
1 year	10	22	0.46	0.27
1½ years	11	25	0.50	0.29
2 years	12	27	0.54	0.31
3 years	14	31	0.60	0.35
4 years	16	36	0.68	0.39
5 years	19	41	0.73	0.42
6 years	21	47	0.82	0.47
7 years	24	53	0.90	0.52
8 years	27	59	0.97	0.56
9 years	29	65	1.05	0.61
10 years	32	71	1.12	0.65
11 years	36	78	1.20	0.70
12 years	39	86	1.28	0.74

*From Done, Alan K.: Drugs for children. In Modell, Walter, editor: Drugs of choice 1972-1973, St. Louis, 1972, The C. V. Mosby Co., p. 55.
†Approximate average for age.
‡ Based on adult surface area of 1.73 $M.^2$

*Fingl, Edward, and Woodbury, Dixon M.: General principles. In Goodman, Louis S., and Gilman, Arthur, editors: The pharmacological basis of therapeutics, ed. 4, New York, 1970, The Macmillan Co., p. 2.

the pharmacodynamic effect and interactions of drugs are presented in the context of functional problems. In some patient situations several functional problems may coexist, and the drugs used for control of each of the problems contribute to the overall plan of therapy.

Drugs are prescribed for particular planned effect on target tissues, but there is seldom a purely specific drug–target tissue relationship. Patient care includes plans for observations of the pharmacodynamic effects on target tissues and concurrent effects on other body processes. Drugs produce no original physiologic effects, but they modify physiologic activity. Drugs can replace, interrupt, or potentiate physiologic processes.

Absorption

The route of administration of drugs is a primary factor affecting the onset of drug action. Drugs administered by any route must reach the circulating fluids to be disseminated to widely distributed target tissues.

There are drugs administered orally for their action in the gastrointestinal tract, but most oral agents are given to provide a systemic effect. Absorption of drugs from the digestive tract is dependent on their solubility, and drugs highly soluble in lipids are most readily moved across the lipid-containing cells of the gastrointestinal mucosa.

Ionization of the drug or its products is also an important factor in the rate of movement into circulating fluids and passage across cell membranes. Highly ionized compounds are repelled by cell membranes and are slowly absorbed. Weak acids (i.e., acetylsalicylic acid) move rapidly across the membrane of the gastrointestinal tract because the drugs are not ionized in stomach acids.

The rate of absorption of drugs from intramuscular or subcutaneous injection sites is dependent on the blood supply and rate of blood flow from the tissues. Extensive accumulation of fluids (edema) increases the distance between the pool of injected drug and the capillaries; therefore alternate injection sites are used to assure absorption of drugs when tissues are edematous (i.e., gluteal edema). The intravenous route is employed as an alternate method of providing drugs for systemic action when the rate of blood flow from peripheral tissues is decreased (i.e., in shock).

Distribution

Drugs that enter the bloodstream may remain free in the serum, or they may become bound to plasma proteins. Circulating fluids gradually move the drugs toward receptor sites where they accomplish their primary action. Receptors in varying tissues have an attraction for particular compounds, and drugs are chemical compounds with some specificity for selected receptors. The blood supply of the receptor sites and the rate of diffusion of the drug from the capillary bed affect the onset of drug action. The intensity of response is dependent on the concentration of the drug at the receptor sites, and the duration of drug action is dependent on the rate at which the drug is metabolized or excreted.

Protein binding. Many drugs are bound to plasma proteins, and the tenacity of protein binding affects the rate of delivery to receptor sites. Protein binding allows delivery of quantities of the drug to receptor sites, and sustained peak levels of the drug are maintained by liberation of the loosely bound drug when tissue levels are lowered by metabolism or excretion of the drug.

Tenacious protein binding affects the movement of drugs into tissues and into body fluids (i.e., cerebrospinal fluid), and it affects renal clearance of the bound drug. The protein-bound drug remains in the capillary blood at the glomerular filtration site. The normal capillary membrane presents a barrier to passage of the protein, but the free drug or its metabolites pass through the glomerular capillary membrane. At renal tubule cells the bound drug is detached from the protein, and the drug is secreted into the tubular urine.

Blood-brain barrier. The barrier to movement of some drugs into brain tissue is known to exist, but components of the hypothetical blood-brain barrier are not clearly defined. Characteristics of the capillary membranes in central nervous system tissues present a barrier to passage of many drugs. The capillaries are enveloped in *glial cells* that resist passage of many substances, but the glial cells allow movement of lipid-soluble substances (i.e., barbiturates, general anesthetics). When the meninges are inflamed, the integrity of the barrier is lessened, and many drugs (i.e., antibiotics) that cannot pass through the normal membrane readily cross the hypothetical blood-brain barrier.

Placental barrier. A primary concern when drugs are administered to young women of child-bearing years or to women in the first trimester of pregnancy is the possibility that some drugs may pass the placental barrier and effect the development of the fetus during the early stages of rapid cell growth. *Teratogenic drugs* affect the biosynthesis of protein or alter metabolism during the early weeks of development of the fetus.

The placental barrier protects the developing fetus against many toxic drugs. Enzymatic pathways for metabolizing drugs are not developed at a level allowing breakdown of drugs. Precautions against administration of drugs that pass the placental barrier are necessary throughout pregnancy because enzyme systems are deficient into the neonatal period. Obstetricians warn patients against taking drugs while they are pregnant. The patient is told to report emerging problems so that drugs can be prescribed. The practice is aimed at decreasing the possibility that any drug with teratogenic or toxic effects on the fetus will be taken by the pregnant woman.

Throughout pregnancy the placental barrier consists of the villi sheath (syncytium) and villi stroma, which substances must traverse to reach the fetal capillary bed. In the first 20 weeks of pregnancy, villi have an additional double covering of cell layers, and the added protection resists passage of many substances that may later move across the placental barrier. The villi and adjacent structures constitute a barrier to selected substances, but the structures are vitally involved throughout pregnancy in active and passive transfer of substances to the developing fetus in quantities required for growth and metabolism.

One of the objectives of drug studies in animals is to identify those drugs that have teratogenic effects. Many drugs have been tested, and those with teratogenic effects are clearly identified in all literature describing the actions of the drugs.

Drugs that pass the placental barrier have a pharmacodynamic effect on the fetus. An example is seen in drug addiction of newborn infants whose mothers are heroin addicts.

Cumulative effects

The metabolic fate and route of excretion are important to maintenance of therapeutic levels of drug in the body. Although drugs may be metabolized by other tissues, the liver is the chief organ for breakdown of drugs. The *microsomal liver enzyme system* alters most substances that enter the liver sinusoids. Drug alteration by acetylation, conjugation, hydroxylation, or oxidation changes the pharmacodynamic activity of the drugs, and in many instances the end product is an inactive metabolite. Metabolic alterations include conversion of lipid-soluble substances to water-soluble particles, and the process has a positive effect on readiness of the metabolite for renal excretion. After the drug is metabolized, the breakdown products are liberated into the bloodstream or into the biliary tract to be excreted with urine or feces.

Hepatic dysfunction can interfere with metabolism of the drug, and the retained agent can cause an excess blood level of the drug if administration is continued within the normal therapeutic range. Retention of unchanged drug or active metabolites is possible with renal dysfunction, as most drugs are excreted in the urine.

Cumulative levels constitute overdosage, and the patient will show the same symptoms as those present when the maximum therapeutic level has been exceeded. Monitoring of liver and kidney function is important when drugs having a high cumulative potential are used (i.e., digitalis). Hepatic and renal function as well as serum drug levels are evaluated frequently when the patient is hospitalized for intensive therapy with potent drugs.

Adverse effects

Any pharmacodynamic event other than the intended action of the drug is an adverse reaction. The complexity of actions and interactions of drugs can be simplified by viewing adverse effects in the context of *problems related to the primary action* of the drug and *problems unrelated to the primary action* of the drug. Within the category of problems related to the primary action of the drug are toxic effects that are pathologic extensions of the planned therapeutic action of the drug. For example, digitalis may be prescribed for its effect on the cardiac conduction pathway and myocardial tissue that slows conduction and strengthens cardiac contraction. Excessive slowing of cardiac action would be a pathologic extension of the planned therapeutic effect.

Problems unrelated to the primary action of the drug may result from the action of the drug on body systems other than the target tissues to produce adverse effects. For example, nausea that occurs with high blood levels of digitalis is unrelated to the primary action of the drug. Nausea occurs secondary to digitalis action at the chemoreceptor trigger zone in the medulla.

Studying drugs in groupings related to their primary pharmacodynamic action makes it easier to understand adverse effects occurring as pathologic extensions of the primary action. Pharmacologic grouping of drugs by commonalities of chemical composition within the pharmacodynamic groupings makes it possible to categorize many of the effects that are unrelated to the primary action because the chemical structure of many drugs precipitates the problems.

Drugs may occasionally be used to control adverse effects that are unrelated to the primary action of the drug being employed for therapy. For example, administration of antacids is a routine part of the therapeutic plan for patients receiving glucocorticoids. The cortical hormones may be used for their primary action in control of an inflammatory response, but they also cause gastric hyperacidity. Concurrent administration of gastric antacids decreases the ulcerogenic potential of the glucocorticoids.

Allergic or hypersensitivity responses are an important group of adverse effects occurring during drug therapy. The physiologic problems of allergy and pharmacodynamic agents used to control the responses are presented in Chapter 4.

Responses of individuals

There are variations in the natural responses of individuals to drugs. Natural variations are nebulous and unpredictable. A therapeutic dosage may elicit a different response in two individuals of similar age and body size. For example, a hypnotic drug may cause one individual to sleep for 10 hours and be groggy for a major part of the following morning, whereas the second individual may sleep only 3 hours after receiving the same dosage.

Individual variation in responses occurs in a relatively normal distribution within the population. Approximately 90% of the individuals given a comparable amount of a drug will respond in a similar manner. The foregoing example of two individuals receiving the same hypnotic drug to induce sleep represents the extremes on the distribution curve of responses. Five percent of the population is extremely sensitive, and 5% of the population is equally insensitive to the same dosage of drug that produces a given response in 90% of the population.

Acquired tolerances to drugs usually occur when a drug has been used by the patient for a long period of time. The patient on long-term therapy gradually finds he is not receiving the same therapeutic effect that previously was enjoyed when he took the drug. Acquired tolerances may result from several causes (i.e., alteration of metabolism, excretion, or change in sensitivity of organ systems). When tolerance occurs, the patient needs increased dosage to achieve the same effect attained during the initial phase of therapy. Interruption of the drug regimen for a short time may make it possible to reinstitute therapy with the same drug dosage.

Idiosyncrasies in responses to drugs may be seen as unexplainable responses. Idiosyncrasies are highly individual, and the recipient of the drug acts in an unusual way when given a drug not generally producing the response. For example, when phenobarbital is given to the individual for its sleep-inducing effect, the individual may become hyperactive and talkative and show no evidence of sleepiness.

Drug interactions

Within the body, drugs may interact to antagonize or enhance the action of other drugs. The pharmacodynamic and physiologic factors that contribute to drug interactions are the subject of intensive analysis and research at the present time.

Foods may interact with drugs to adversely affect the therapeutic plan. For example, when the patient is receiving a monoamine oxidase inhibitor, a hypertensive state may be precipitated by eating aged cheese. The tyramine-containing food provides a precursor to norepinephrine when monamine oxidase is not available to inactivate the amine, and widespread vasoconstriction ensues.

Drug antagonism. Antagonistic actions between drugs may occur at local tissue sites (i.e., receptor antagonism), or they may be more generalized antagonistic effects on physiologic processes, resulting in an alteration of metabolism, distribution, excretion, or plasma protein binding of either drug. For example, when a drug is being used for its effect on smooth muscles of arteries to cause vasoconstriction and a pain-relieving drug with smooth muscle–relaxant properties is prescribed, one drug may negate the effect of the other. The physician should be consulted if pain relief is needed. He may prescribe an alternate drug to assure continued effect of the vasopressor.

The interaction of narcotics and narcotic antagonists provides an example of drug antagonism at receptor sites. Narcotics act at receptor sites in the medullary centers to cause respiratory depression. Administration of narcotic antagonists (levallorphan tartrate, nalorphine hydrochloride, or naloxone) for treatment of acute narcotic-induced respiratory depression reverses the effects of the narcotic at the center by competing for receptor sites. The narcotic antagonists have a strong affinity for the receptors, and they block narcotic attachment. Absence of narcotic at the receptors reestablishes the sensitivity of the centers to carbon dioxide stimuli, and the rate and depth of respirations improves.

Alterations in drug metabolism affect the level of circulating drug, and one of the vital areas for drug metabolism is the liver. Antihistamines, chloral hydrate, and phenobarbital act as stimulants of the microsomal liver enzyme system, and metabolism of some drugs is accelerated when they are administered concurrent with the enzyme system stimulants. For example, patients receiving oral anticoagulants may require a given amount of the anticoagulant to maintain a therapeutic prothrombin level while they are receiving phenobarbital concurrently. When the phenobarbital is discontinued, less anticoagulant is required to maintain the therapeutic level, and the anticoagulant dosage must be decreased. Prior to definition of the acceleration of metabolism occurring with phenobarbital, patients maintained undetected elevated prothrombin levels after phenobarbital was discontinued, and hemorrhage was an outcome of the situation.

Oral anticoagulant (i.e., warfarin sodium) usually is bound loosely to plasma proteins, but drugs that compete for the protein-binding sites (i.e., phenylbutazone) prevent anticoagulant protein binding, and the drug remains free. Elevation of the prothrombin level above the therapeutic range may occur when antagonistic drugs are introduced into the anticoagulant regimen.

Drug action summation. Drugs may, by their combined or concurrent actions, increase the therapeutic effect, or they may increase the incidence of adverse effects. *Synergism, addition,* and *potentiation* are mechanisms leading to summation.

Synergism is the term used to describe the interaction of drugs at common receptor sites that alters metabolism or excretion. The synergistic action of the two drugs may provide more than twice the effect possible when either drug is used alone.

Addition is the term used to describe the action of two drugs at different receptor sites that produces an effect twice that possible when either drug is used alone. For example, diuretics are often used in combination to improve or accelerate the removal of tissue fluid. Each of the drugs may act at a different site in the renal tubule to prevent the reabsorption of sodium ions, and the net result is an increased output of sodium and water.

Potentiation is the term used to describe

drugs that have a greater effect when used in combination than when either agent is used alone. Although alcohol is not used routinely for therapeutic purposes, the action of alcohol in potentiation of the action of central nervous system depressants is an important example of the effect of two central nervous system depressants used concurrently. Ingestion of alcohol while taking a sedative can cause drowsiness that endangers the safety of the individual while doing tasks requiring alertness or while driving a motor vehicle. Under the foregoing circumstances, a single highball may provide enough alcohol to cause uncontrollable drowsiness.

Knowledge of drug interactions is proliferating at a rapid pace. Information about specific drug interactions is included within the text where the individual drugs and their pharmacodynamic actions are presented.

PATIENT CARE

When the patient is responsible for self-administration of drugs, safety in use is increased if he understands the reason the drug is being employed, the predictable effect of the drug, and the adverse effects that may occur. Careful planning and scheduling of drug use is necessary to assure that the scheduled dosage is consistently taken. It is possible, with careful modification of terms, to explain to the patient the relationship of the drug to the physiologic problem for which he is being treated. Information should be specific to the particular pharmacotherapeutic plan established for him, and samples of the drugs should be attached to a card with a statement of drug effect and problems he should report to the physician.

Schedules for follow-up care, refilling of his prescription, and a specific guide for recording dosage taken are discussed with the patient. One of the chief problems of self-administration is omitting one or more doses of the drug and taking double the amount to correct the deficit at a later time. Detailed planning with the patient may lessen the problem.

The patient should assume responsibility for his medication when possible. When the patient is unable or unwilling to assume responsibility for the therapeutic plan, the individual responsible for his care also should be instructed. It is important to pre-plan the presentation of data to assure inclusiveness of the information and to provide opportunity for clarification of points that are unclear. An important aspect of pre-planning is the preparation for discussion of adverse effects. Lists of specific problems may be confusing and frightening to the patient, but careful wording of the presentation and use of realistic concise examples of problems makes the discussion less threatening. A written list of adverse effects provides a ready reference when problems arise in the posthospital situation.

It is estimated that more than 50% of the patients with chronic health problems fail to follow the prescribed pharmacotherapeutic plan when they are independently responsible for their care. The nurse responsible for planning and supervising health maintenance can play a vital role in reducing the noncompliance percentage by personalized instruction concerning the relationship of drug action to the patient's health status.

Participation as an informed member of the health team can be stimulating and challenging. The pharmacotherapeutic plan is an integral part of each plan of therapy. The more frequently opportunities are used to discuss the pharmacotherapeutic program, the greater the pool of knowledge than can be contributed to each patient's overall plan for health maintenance.

Drug administration routes

The increasing use of unit dosage or prepackaged drugs in hospitals has decreased the confusing process of preparing drugs for large numbers of patients, but neither computerization nor prepackaging will entirely remove responsibility for administration of medications in hospital or home situations in the near future. The expense of individually packaged drugs will probably remain prohibitive for home use; therefore the nurse (and the patient) must have some basic information about commonly used preparations.

The drug dosage and route of administration are prescribed by the physician. When the patient is unable to take oral medication because of nausea or vomiting, the problem is discussed with the physician to determine whether the plan for administration should be revised. A similar conference is indicated when the patient's tolerance of oral liquids and foods suggests that the oral rather than the prescribed parenteral route should be used.

Ease of administration makes pills, tablets, or capsules the most desirable drug forms, but local factors affect absorption and decomposition of oral agents. Acidity of the stomach contents and the action of enzymes in the duodenum inactive protein compounds; therefore alternate routes must be used for hormones and other protein drugs.

Many drugs are irritating to the gastric mucosa, and nausea or other gastrointestinal disturbances occur during therapy. Administration of irritating agents with food or an antacid may decrease nausea, but the effect of foods on drug absorption or decomposition must be considered. Drugs that are irritating to the gastric mucosa are sometimes available as an *enteric-coated tablet* (E.C.T.) that prevents liberation of the irritating agent until the drug reaches the intestine. Aspirin is an example of a drug that is available with an antacid, or buffer, and as an enteric-coated tablet. Aspirin, like some other commonly used drugs, is also available in suppository form for rectal administration to patients unable to take oral tablets.

In addition to the frequently encountered forms of drugs for oral use (pills, tablets, capsules), many drugs are available in liquid forms (solutions, syrups, elixirs, emulsions) that facilitate administration to children and adults who have difficulty swallowing solid forms of the drug. Crushing of tablets and mixing with pureed fruit is a common method of administering solid forms, but the patient may receive insufficient dosage if he refuses some of the prepared formulation.

There are specific factors to be considered when each of the liquid preparations is used. For example, syrups (i.e., cough syrups) provide glucose; therefore they are not administered to diabetic patients unless the calculation of glucose content is related to their problems with glucose assimilation and considered in their dietary restriction.

Elixirs, tinctures, or fluidextracts contain alcohol and are not administered to alcoholics on a voluntary or therapeutic abstinence program. Most alcoholics on planned abstinence will examine and refuse any oral liquid containing alcohol, but inadvertent administration may trigger an insatiable thirst for alcohol that defeats the patient's efforts to abstain. Alcohol-containing medications administered to a patient on disulfiram for abstinence therapy will cause violent vomiting and may precipitate circulatory collapse.

Suspensions must be shaken vigorously to assure that the drug content of the suspension is evenly distributed. When the suspension is properly shaken, the first patient to receive a prescribed dose receives the same amount of the drug as the last patient when the amount of suspension administered is the same.

Sublingual or buccal tablets provide drug effect without awaiting the slower process of absorption from the gastrointestinal tract. The highly vascular surface of the oral mucosa allows rapid movement of dissolved drug into the venous circulation. For example, a nitroglycerin tablet placed under the tongue provides a vasodilator effect on coronary arteries within 2 minutes. An additional benefit of the sublingual or buccal route is that direct absorption into the circulation circumvents the enzymatic destruction of the drug in the stomach or intestine. Hormone tablets (i.e., progesterone) placed in the buccal pouch provide rapid action of the protein substance that would be destroyed by proteolytic enzymes in the gastrointestinal tract.

Intramuscular or subcutaneous administration may be prescribed when the patient is unable to take drugs by mouth, although the specific properties of many drugs requires that they only be administered parenterally. Injection of drugs into the tissues may be desirable to provide prompt drug effect, but the parenteral route also allows use of retardants for gradual release of the drug component of the preparation.

Materials added to drugs to modify absorption rate or decrease pain at the injection site make them inappropriate for use by alternate routes. For example, procaine added to an intramuscular preparation to decrease pain at the injection site limits its use to the intramuscular route, and it cannot be employed for intravenous administration.

Colloids, oils, metals, or vasoconstrictors are some of the additives to intramuscular preparations that retard absorption. The additives allow the drug to remain in local tissues for slow release from the depot site over a long period of time. Delayed absorption decreases the need for frequent administration while assuring the availability of a needed pharmacotherapeutic agent. For example, addition of protamine and zinc to insulin for injection increases the action time of the vital hormone from 6 to 24 hours, and a comparable increase in action time is obtained by addition of globin zinc to insulin. Package inserts and the labels on vials are useful sources of information about parenteral drugs and their diluents, routes of administration, and incompatability with other drugs and diluents.

Parenteral drug administration often requires calculation of fractional dosage. It is expected that the calculation of a divided dosage done by one nurse will be checked by another nurse before the drug is administered. Frequent need for calculation of divided dosage in care of children has led to establishment of criteria that are rigidly adhered to by nurses preparing the drugs. When insulin, digitalis, or narcotics are prepared, both the calculation of dosage and the amount of drug actually prepared for administration are checked by a second nurse before the drug is given to a child.

Alternation of administration sites lessens the patient's discomfort when frequent subcutaneous or intramuscular injections are necessary. Absorption of drug from the injection site is dependent on venous circulation from the area, and in patients with fluid accumulation in tissues (i.e., gluteal edema) it is necessary to use the upper extremities for injections. It is important to review anatomic landmarks (i.e., routes of nerves, arteries, and veins) when unfamiliar sites are used for injection. It is a challenge to find sites for injection in patients with extensive burns, but drugs that are prescribed must be given. Nurses caring for patients with burns often keep graphic records of sites and plans for rotation of injections within available sites.

Intravenous administration is frequently planned for the multiple drugs required by the acutely ill patient. Various types of needles are used for administration, but when the infusion is planned over a prolonged period of time, an intravenous catheter is generally used to provide stability within the vein.

In addition to calibration of the amount of drug being administered during intravenous infusion, the site of injection is examined periodically for evidence of tissue fluid and tenderness. Extravasation of fluid into tissues or phlebitis may necessitate removal of the needle or catheter and insertion at another intravenous site. Routines for changing infusion sites are usually established in the agency (i.e., every 3 days), and on interim days the dressing around the catheter may be changed. Application of antibiotic ointments around the insertion site are also a planned part of site care. Using a ball-point pen to record the date of insertion on the tape around the catheter assures attention to the routine time for change of the catheter.

Care in preparation of accurate dosage is essential when drugs are administered by all routes. There is some protection provided for correction of drug error when the preparation is administered by the oral route because an emetic, lavage, or an antidote may be administered to delay absorption of the drug. Administration of a drug that causes a toxic or allergic reaction may be delayed by application of ice or a tourniquet when the drug is administered intramuscularly or subcutaneously into an extremity. Intravenous administration disseminates the drug throughout the body, and attempts to slow or halt drug effect requires use of drugs that neutralize or inactivate the drug before it becomes sequestered in tissues.

In addition to oral and parenteral use of drugs, the nurse often administers drugs to topical areas (i.e., skin, mucous membranes, or eyes). Drugs contained in ointments, lotions, and creams applied topically may be absorbed into the systemic circulation. In addition to the local effects, it is necessary to consider the effect of the components (i.e., cortisone) systematically and plan observations for general effects.

Ingredients of the topical compound should be clearly identified. When there is insufficient information about the effect of particular components of the material, the physician should be consulted before applying the drug.

Each of the foregoing considerations is an important aspect of drug administration, and the patient who is responsible for self-administration should be informed of the factors appropriate to his use of drugs. An ideal method of defining whether the patient clearly understands directions for taking his prescribed drugs is to provide opportunity for him to take the drugs while he is being supervised, and the practice is being used consistently in patient-teaching programs.

REFERENCES

Aaron, Harold: Drugs: some adverse interactions, American Journal of Nursing **66**:1545, 1966.

Abels, David J.: Basic concepts of topical therapy, Modern Medicine **39**:77, 1971.

Done, Alan K.: The subtle overdose, Emergency Medicine **4**:134, 1972.

Goodman, Louis S., and Gilman, Arthur, editors: The pharmacological basis of therapeutics, ed. 4, New York, 1970, The Macmillan Co.

Goth, Andres: Medical pharmacology, ed. 6, St. Louis, 1972, The C. V. Mosby Co.

Hayes, Marsden H.: Pharmacists need nurses, nurses need pharmacists, patients need both, American Journal of Nursing **72**:723, 1972.

Hecht, Amy B.: Self-medication, inaccuracy, and what can be done about it, Nursing Outlook **18**:30, 1970.

Hussar, Daniel A.: Drug interactions by the hundreds! How can you possibly remember them all? Nursing '72 **2**:4, 1972.

Leary, Jean A., Vessella, Dolores M., and Yeaw, Evelyn M.: Self-administered medications, American Journal of Nursing **71**:1193, 1971.

Levine, Myra: Breaking through the medications mystique, American Journal of Nursing **70**:799, 1970.

Neely, Elizabeth, and Patrick, Maxine L.: Problems of aged persons taking medications at home, Nursing Research **17**:52, 1968.

UNIT ONE
DRUGS USED TO CONTROL INFECTION AND INFLAMMATION

2 Invading bacteria

3 Fungus and parasite invasion

4 Immune and allergic responses

2

Invading bacteria

Bacterial infection
    Entrance barriers
    Internal barriers
    Infectious process
    Initial defense mechanisms
    Secondary defense mechanisms
    Neutrophil response
    Macrophage activity
    Antibody formation
    Response assessment
    Microorganism characteristics
    Receptive hosts
    Pharmacodynamics
Specific drug groups
    Antibiotics
    Chemotherapeutics
    Kidney-specific drugs
    Mycobacterium-specific drugs
    Patient care

BACTERIAL INFECTION

Infection represents a disruption in the harmonious relationship between host, agent, and environment necessary to health maintenance. Control of an infection is dependent on the effectiveness of body defenses that provide barriers to intrusion and propagation of pathogens. The number, virulence, and distribution of the microorganisms invading body tissues affect the magnitude of the physiologic responses and the supportive measures necessary to control the invaders.

Entrance barriers

Primary barriers to bacterial invasion protect man against the numerous microorganisms in the environment that cause disease in humans. The intact skin protects the external surface of the body against intrusion of bacteria. Pathogens that enter body orifices encounter environmental conditions that threaten their survival. For example, pathogens entering the nose or throat may travel to the gastrointestinal tract, where they are exposed to the acid content of the stomach and proteolytic enzymes of the intestinal tract. Only bacteria with thick resistant cell walls (i.e., *Mycobacterium*) or bacterial toxins with a complex protein structure (i.e., *Clostridium botulinum*) survive in the presence of destructive digestive juices. Destruction also awaits many of the bacteria entering the respiratory passages. Mucus entraps bacteria entering the airway, and the lysozyme content of the secretions causes dissolution of many bacterial invaders.

Serum globulins provide natural barriers to microorganism travel into internal tissues. Circulating proteins (i.e., properdin) and globulins containing lipoprotein (i.e., complement) act together to enzymatically destroy some of the viruses and bacteria that move through the intestinal wall to extraintestinal tissues. Activity of properdin and complement provides a natural barrier that confines viruses and gram-negative bacteria in the intestinal lumen.

Internal barriers

The size of bacteria prevents their passage through intact capillary walls, and so they leave tissue sites via the lymphatic system. Lymphocytes engulf and digest (phagocytize) bacteria as they move slowly through the lymphatic channels. Phagocytosis continues in the lymph nodes, and the collection of bacteria and bacterial debris distends the lymph nodes. Microorganisms may survive travel through the lymphatic network, enter the thoracic duct, and move into the arterial blood.

Blood-borne bacteria are continually exposed to filtration and phagocytic activity as arterial blood enters the splenic red pulp and venous sinuses and the hepatic Kupffer cells. When blood passes through the bone marrow, phagocytes destroy the fine particles of many bacterial toxins that survive other internal barriers.

Infectious process

The site of attack influences whether local or general body responses are involved in resisting invasion by pathogenic bacteria. For example, a colony of bacteria in a hair follicle may elicit a response in a small circumscribed area. Natural rupture of encased material or incision by sterile needle puncture allows expulsion of contents to the surface. Removal of debris and cleansing of the site may terminate the problem. Comparable sequestered bacterial colonies may develop in internal tissues. Physiologic defense mechanisms are actively involved in attempts to confine bacterial invaders to areas at the initial assault site.

Microorganisms that find a route into the body interior may obtain a foothold for pathogenic activity that requires a sustained physiologic response. Metabolic work is increased, and body reserves are mobilized to supply white blood cells, oxygen, and nutrients in a protracted effort to control the invasion of pathogens.

Initial defense mechanisms

Pathogen intrusion into body tissues elicits a series of physiologic responses directed at isolating or destroying the invaders. Within minutes, tissue histocytes change into mast cells to entrap the invading pathogens. Concurrent release of *necrosin* and *leukocytosis-promoting factor* by pathogen-damaged cells initiates a sequence of physiologic protective mechanisms.

Necrosin increases the permeability of capillaries, and fluid, fibrinogen, and other proteins leak into the tissue spaces. The union of necrosin and fibrinogen causes clotting of tissue fluids that walls off the area and prevents movement of fluid and pathogens from the attack site. Tissue proteins osmotically attract fluid from capillaries, and distention of tissue ensues. Local inflammation increases as distended mast cells rupture and release additional vasoactive substances (heparin, histamine) at the tissue site. Extravasation of fluid into tissues is potentiated by the action of histamine on capillary and venule membranes. Attachment of histamine to venule walls causes constriction with consequent increase of capillary pressure, which in turn causes outward movement of fluid from the permeable capillary membrane.

Secondary defense mechanisms

The sequence of events occurring as initial defense mechanisms is so closely followed by a secondary response of additional mechanisms that to separate the phases of each response is difficult. The initial phase is followed by activation of plasma protein constituents (i.e., bradykinin, complement) that reinforce primary defense activity at the tissue level.

Accumulation of plasma in tissues contributes to the liberation of bradykinin from plasma proteins. Cleavage of bradykininogen yields bradykinin, and the polypeptide acts on the vasculature to cause vasodilation and capillary permeability. In addition to the effect on the vasculature, which is comparable to the effect of histamine, bradykinin causes pain by irritation of denuded nerve endings.

The activity of immune complexes (antigen-antibody reactions) or the presence of bacterial polysaccharides provides the factors leading to release of the enzymatic components of the complement system of plasma proteins. Complement components cause vascular permeability, but their chief contributions to body defenses are the chemotactic attraction of polymorphonuclear leukocytes to invasion sites and the facilitation of bacterial phagocytosis.

Neutrophil response

Leukocytosis-promoting factor released from damaged cells travels in the blood to bone marrow sites of leukocyte storage, and additional neutrophils are liberated in response to the stimulating factor. Neutrophil travel toward the invasion site is accelerated by the chemotactic attraction of complement components at the site of damaged tissues. Pathogens that are ingested by neutrophils are destroyed by the proteolytic enzymes and bactericidal agents (lysozyme, phagocytin) of the cytoplasmic substance. Complement components adhere to the outer membranes of bacteria, and their presence facilitates phagocytosis. When neutrophils become distended with bacterial debris, they burst and spew their contents into the area.

Macrophage activity

Slow-moving monocytes and lymphocytes arriving at the scene swell and become macrophages. Dead tissues and foreign protein provide the electropositive chemotactic force that continually attracts electronegative phagocytes to the site. Macrophages ingest pathogens, neutrophil debris, and enzymes from the area. Amino acids and sugars from the rubble are utilized by the macrophages for their metabolic processes during the invasion response period. Proteolytic enzymes, lipases, and bactericidal agents in the macrocyte cytoplasm inactivate or destroy most of the pathogens ingested. Some pathogens may remain in the cytoplasm and travel with the macrophage to tissues in other parts of the body.

Antibody formation

Termination of an infectious process by therapeutic intervention or completion of phagocytic destruction allows the macrophages remaining at the site to return to their tissues of origin. Lymphocytes return to the lymphatic tissues, and monocytes return to varying areas of the reticuloendothelial system. The returning cells carry materials that institute antibody formation by the plasma cells of the reticuloendothelial tissues. The antibodies formed subsequent to pathogen invasion prompty respond to repeat invasion by the same antigenic substance. Elimination of a subsequent invasion is more readily accomplished when immunologically competent cells (antibodies) are available to control activity of the bacterial antigen.

Response assessment

The endogenous responses to pathogen invasion are reflected in the blood values (leukocyte count) of the patient, and they provide guides to changing physiologic events during therapy. High levels of neutrophils in blood samples (normal: 4500/mm.^{3}) reflect the release of the cells from storage during the acute phase of infection. The number of circulating monocytes and lymphocytes may be unchanged during the first 48 hours after invasion of the pathogens. Initial activity of the cells is dependent on the ability of circulating monocytes and lymphocytes to change characteristics and swell to the point at which each macrophage can ingest up to 100 bacteria. Continuation of the pathogen stimulus to physiologic responses causes production and release of leukocytes from reticuloendothelial tissues, and increased numbers of circulating monocytes (normal: 400/mm.^{3}) and lymphocytes (normal: 2100/mm.^{3}) are present in blood samples. Levels of monocytes may be consistently elevated when an infection persists for protracted periods of time. Elevation of the blood elements is thought to result from the continued activity of lymphocytes that become macrophages at the site of infection and change characteristics to become monocytes when they return to the circulating blood.

Gradual improvement in the patient's condition will be evident as a decrease in metabolic rate and an increase in strength and feeling of well-being. Improved tissue function, normal or near-normal levels of body temperature, and cardiac and respiratory rate usually correlate with a gradual return of leukocyte counts toward normal values.

Microorganism characteristics

Differences in biologic characteristics of microorganisms affect the course of the infectious process and plans for treatment. Staphylococci liberate lethal cellular toxins that accelerate the release of necrosin. The area of invasion is walled off rapidly, and the organisms may be confined to a relatively small circumscribed area near the entry site. Eradication of the organisms is hampered when internal tissues contain the pathogens. Staphylococci produce sequestered exudates that resist penetration by drugs in the circulating fluids bathing the area. Isolated microorganisms survive in human phagocytic cells where drugs do not penetrate, and the sheltered site allows staphylococci to remain quiescent for short periods and reinstitute an infectious process at a later time.

The virulence of pneumococci and streptococci is increased by their ability to penetrate tissues adjacent to the entry site. The pathogens liberate *hyaluronidase* to enzymatically break down the molecular structure of the hyaluronic acid structural component of connective tissue. By increasing tissue permeability, streptococci rapidly move from site to site as they multiply.

The same process for enzymatic destruction of hyaluronic acid is used therapeutically to increase the absorption of large amounts of fluids administered into subcutaneous tissues during hypodermoclysis. Injection of a commercial preparation of hyaluronidase (Alidase, Diffusin, Enzodase, Hyazyme, Infiltrase, Wydase) allows fluid to move through tissues in a manner comparable to that of bacteria after liberation of hyaluronidase.

The thick lipid membrane of mycobacterium may resist destruction by macrophage lipases, and the pathogen may be carried to tissues distal to the site of entry. Resting organisms may encapsulate and remain quiescent for long periods of time. The patient with tuberculosis or leprosy is considered to have an arrested disease process at termination of therapy, but he must be alert throughout his lifetime for emergence of activated pathogens released from encapsulated foci in tissues.

Receptive hosts

Many factors govern the physiologic response elicited by invading pathogens and the ability of the individual to abort the invasion. A minor infection may be a major catastrophe for a seriously ill or debilitated patient. Bacteria naturally inhabiting the human intestine (i.e., *Enterobacter aerogenes, Escherichia coli, Proteus vulgaris, Pseudomonas aeruginosa*) may appear as pathogens in wounds, burns, or body cavities in malnourished or debilitated patients. The organisms propagate with minimal interference from body immune responses, since they are natural substances in the intestine. Except for *Escherichia coli,* the pathogens are resistant to many anti-infective agents, and eradication is difficult.

Individual sensitivities affect the pathogenicity of bacteria. In some individuals the *hemolysin* liberated into the systemic circulation by group A beta-hemolytic streptococci in a localized area (i.e., oropharynx) may damage cardiac and renal tissue.

The intensity of treatment is directly related to the health status of the individual and the virulence of the organism isolated or identified. In all situations, systemic infection disrupts physiologic function and places on the body a metabolic burden that must be alleviated. Therapeutic plans include measures to support physiologic efforts to eradicate the infection by maintaining or improving the resources of the host.

Pharmacodynamics

Drug therapy is directed at removing pathogens from body reservoirs. The chief barrier to eradication of bacteria is the nearly impregnable cell wall of the microorganisms. Glucose components (glucosamine, muramic acid) are interdigitated with amino acids (diaminopimelic acid or lysine, glutamine, glycine) in a manner that makes the wall an impenetrable barrier. The cell wall actively transports supplies to the intracellular protoplasm, and it controls the entrance and removal of cellular materials. Internal processes of intracellular structures are comparable to those of all cells maintaining life processes, but cellular fluids are maintained at a hypertonic level in relation to circulating fluids. The hypertonic level is maintained by the active-transport mechanisms of the bacterial cell wall.

Pathogen vulnerability. Strong chemicals for annihilation of bacteria would be destructive to normal body cells. The only way to destroy bacteria without damage to body tissues is to attack during vulnerable phases of the reproduction cycle. Interruption of new cell wall building may be accomplished by drugs disrupting the synthesis of intermediates, polysaccharides, or glycopeptides. During reproduction, there is also an opportunity for drugs to act on the dividing cell by disrupting the synthesis of intracellular proteins. Streptomycin (and similar drugs) takes advantage of the opportunity to cause misreading of the genetic code. While messenger ribonucleic acid (mRNA) is assembling nucleotides, the drugs intercede to cause mRNA to incorrectly read the genetic construction code. The error causes a reproduction defect. Substitution of the drug for an essential nucleotide builds nonfunctional protein and leads to death of the bacterium.

The effectiveness of drugs is dependent on their availability when cells are in the active process of dividing. Because partial disruption of bacterial reproduction could lead to emergence of mutants, the drugs must also be available in quantities adequate to inactivate or destroy bacteria for as long as the number of descendants exceeds the body's ability to destroy them. There is some effector-site specificity, but all the drugs used as systemic anti-infective agents are involved in destroying the cell wall or interrupting the reproductive sequence within the cell.

Selectivity of drug effect is accomplished by capitalizing on the differences between pathogens and normal human cells. The cell wall of bacteria is constructed of materials unlike those of human cells, and many drugs have a selective effect on the constituents of the resistant bacterial envelope. Bacterial propagation proceeds at a rate much faster than that of human cells, and drugs can intercede to affect bacterial reproduction with minimal effect on normal cells.

Pathogen elimination. High concentrations of many of the anti-infective drugs would destroy most bacteria, but the dosage level would also destroy normal tissues. Some drugs (i.e., penicillin) are capable of destroying bacteria at low concentrations, and they are used for their *bactericidal effect.* Drugs that increase the permeability of the bacterial cell wall have a bactericidal effect because subsequent leaking of intracellular contents disrupts the osmotic gradient necessary to bacterial life processes. Bactericidal drugs are particularly useful for therapy of patients with acute, overwhelming, life-threatening infections.

Many drugs slow reproduction of bacteria, and their effect is described as *bacteriostatic.* Slowing of bacterial proliferation prevents extension of the infectious process, and natural physiologic defense mechanisms are required for phagocytic abolition of the bacteria. Consistent use of the drug at prescribed dosage intervals is necessary to prevent emergence of mutant organisms during therapy with bacteriostatic drugs. The physiologic status of the patient is an important factor in the success of therapy with bacteriostatic drugs, and measures that maintain or build the patient's physiologic resources are an integral part of the therapeutic plan.

Pathogen identification. Cultures obtained from infected tissues or their exudate are used to identify the offending pathogens and their susceptibility to inactivation or destruction by particular drugs. Cultures are obtained before initiation of anti-infective therapy to assure identification of the microorganism before drug inactivation of it occurs. There is individual variation in the ability of bacteria to survive in the presence of particular anti-infective drugs (Fig. 2-1). The shaded areas on the illustration indicate the gram-positive and gram-negative organisms that are consistently susceptible to anti-infective drug action. In addition to the illustrated microorganism susceptibility, there are some strains of bacteria that have a variable and less consistent susceptibility to the effects of the anti-infective agents.

Bacterial resistance. Bacterial resistance to a drug may be a natural characteristic of the organism, or it may be a manifestation of spontaneous mutation or adaption of the microorganism. Bacteria initially showing susceptibility to the effect of a particular drug may gradually become resistant to the drug during therapy. Bacterial resistance is suspected when the infectious process becomes less responsive and the patient's condition regresses. Susceptibility testing is repeated to determine whether bacterial resistance has occurred and to select an alternate drug for eradication of the pathogen.

Specific characteristics of organisms help them deter the destructive effects of drugs. Some bacteria produce enzymes (i.e., acylase,

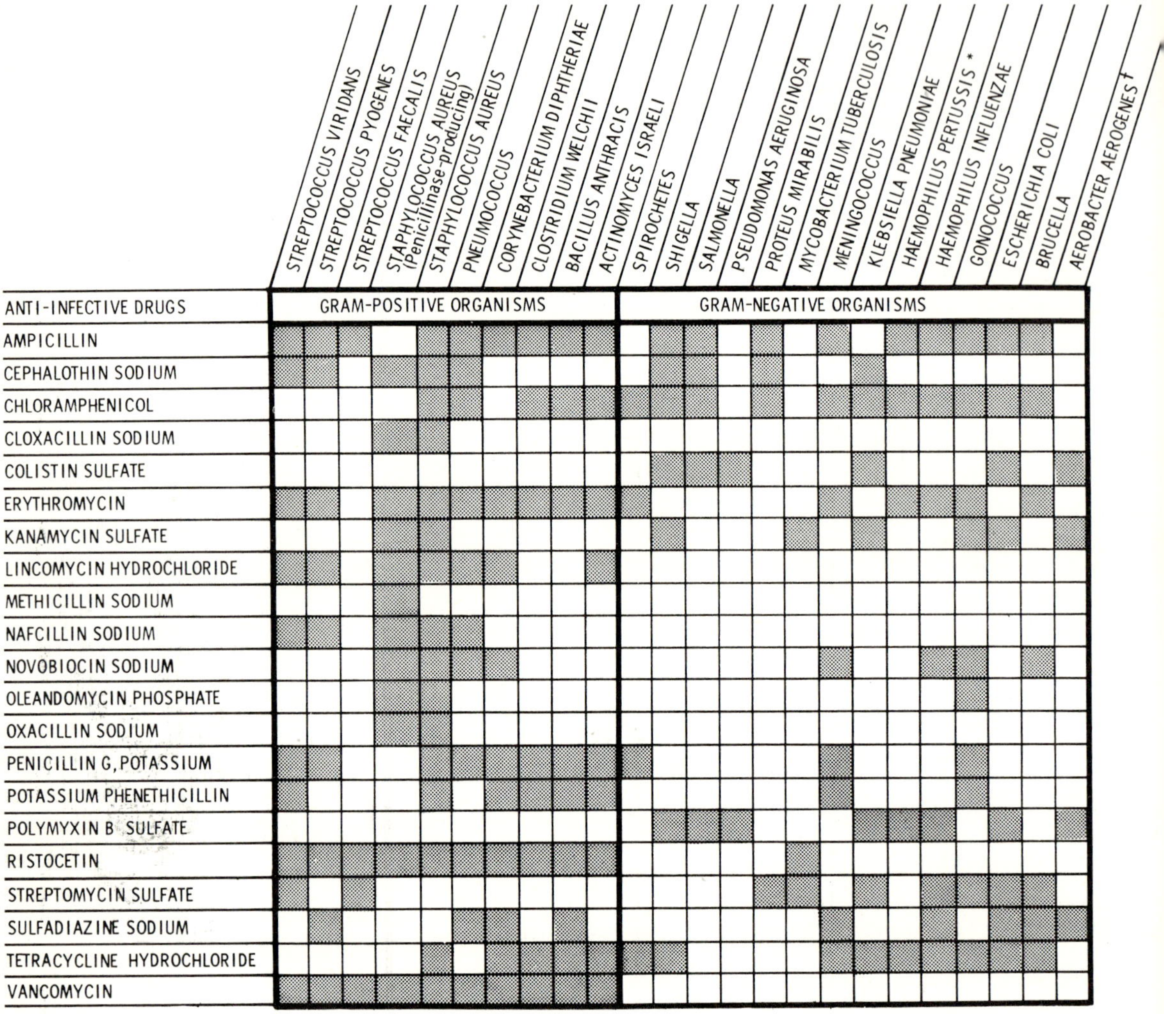

20 Drugs used to control infection and inflammation

Fig. 2-1. Microorganism susceptibility to anti-infective drug action. (See text.)

*Now called *Bordetella pertussis*.
†Now called *Enterobacter aerogenes*.

amidase) that inactivate or destroy pharmacologic agents. The enzymes may be drug-specific. For example, penicillinase strips penicillin of its therapeutic effect, and cephalosporinase inactivates cephalothin.

Pathogen-drug spectra. Drugs are described in terms of their spectrum of effect on pathogens. Fig. 2-1 shows a broad spectrum of gram-positive and gram-negative organisms that are susceptible to the action of some of the drugs. Ampicillin is an example of a drug that is described as a *broad-spectrum* anti-infective drug. Vancomycin effect is limited almost entirely to gram-positive organisms, and it represents a classification of drugs known as *narrow-spectrum* anti-infective agents. A drug may have a narrow spectrum but be highly effective in eradication of a particular organism, and so the drug is the agent of choice for control of the pathogen. Some of the drugs with a broad spectrum of effect (i.e., chloramphenicol) may be used selectively when other anti-infective agents are ineffective in control of a particular pathogen. The discriminating use of chloramphenicol is necessary because it frequently causes blood cell abnormalities during therapy.

Drug classification. Drugs used to affect systems within invading pathogens rather than host cells or tissues are described as *chemotherapeutic drugs*. Plans for use of the drugs in treatment of invading pathogens or cancer are described as *chemotherapy*.

Antibiotics represent a subclassification of pharmacologic agents used for control of pathogens. Antibiotic is the term designating a metabolic product of an organism that is used to destroy another organism. The drug may be derived entirely from a microorganism occurring in nature, or it may be a semisynthetic derivative produced by planned intervention during growth of the basic microorganism. Because penicillin is derived from fungi *(Penicillium notatum, Penicillium chrysogenum)*, it is described as an antibiotic. Penicillin represents a group of drugs known as *antibiotic chemotherapeutic* drugs.

Many descriptive terms specify the action or the pathogen target of drug therapy. Within this text the comprehensive term *anti-infective* is used to describe the drug action. The term appears in titles of tables throughout this chapter, for example, "anti-infective drugs: the penicillins." In subsequent chapters the pathogen target is used to identify the action of the drugs. The terms include "antimalarials," "amebicides," and "antifungals."

Prophylactic therapy. Anti-infective agents are used primarily to control existing infection, but they may be used to protect against the emergence of infection in selected situations. Prophylactic use may be planned for an individual whose medical history (i.e., rheumatic fever) indicates that subsequent pathogenic invasion would have a long-term detrimental effects on cardiac tissue. Prior to intestinal surgery, anti-infective drugs are used for short-term supression of the normal bacterial flora in an attempt to "sterilize" the bowel. The high incidence of infection in society would seem to indicate a need for widespread prophylactic use of anti-infective drugs, but knowledge of the potential for development of mutants, drug-resistant organisms, and allergic reactions has decreased appreciably the promiscuous prescription of anti-infective drugs.

Dosage range. Dosage of drugs for control of susceptible pathogens is dependent on the number of microorganisms or virulence of the infectious process as indicated by tissue cultures and the patient's clinical status. Within this chapter, tables indicating dosage ranges for anti-infective agents show minimal and maximal daily dosage for adults with infections. The minimal level is that necessary to effectively control invasion of microorganisms susceptible to the drug. Maximal dosage represents the highest level of the drug used for control of infection. The prescribed dosage for patients will be at or above the minimal dosage and at or below the maximal.

The site of invasion by pathogens enters into the physician's decision to use a particular dosage for control of the infection. The integrity of vital body processes may be adversely affected when major organ systems are infected by pathogens. For example, streptococci invading the endocardium initiate an infectious process that jeopardizes cardiac function. Massive doses of penicillin may be administered intravenously to abort the invasion. Intensive therapy is necessary to protect valvular integrity. Systemic infection caused by bacterial invasion and subsequent multiplication in the bloodstream (septicemia) also requires intensive therapy. At varying points on the continuum of infection designated as mild to severe bacterial invasion, the dosage of anti-infective drug is proportionately increased above the minimal inhibitory level required to control the activity of susceptible microorganisms.

Adverse effects. There are no innocuous anti-infective drugs. Use of the agents topically, orally, or parenterally carries with it the hazard of adverse effects unrelated to the action of the drug on the pathogen target. Multiple factors in the host-drug relationship influence the occurrence of adverse effects. Variation in the rate of absorption, distribution in tissues, rate of excretion, and individual characteristics of the drug influence the severity of adverse effects occurring during pharmacotherapy. The incidence of predictable adverse effects may be related to the patient's age, physical condition, metabolic rate, or extent of the infectious process. Drug dosage levels and duration of therapy are additional factors contributing to the emergence of problems. The factors that are individual to specific drug groups are presented with the description of drug action later in this chapter. Alterations of normal biologic flora, microorganism overgrowth, alternate pathogen emergence, and allergic reactions are potential problems during therapy with each of the anti-infective drugs.

Alteration of biologic flora. Orally administered anti-infective agents that are poorly absorbed from the intestinal tract are used for treatment of infections in the intestine. Long-term use may disrupt the natural symbiotic relationship between the large number of bacteria in the intestinal tract and the host. Some of the bacteria are involved in nitrogen cycling, and they have a vital role in the conversion of nitrogen to ammonia in the intestine before the organic compound enters the portal venous circulation on its way to the hepatic metabolic cycle. Intestinal bacteria also synthesize vitamin K that is used as a precursor to prothrombin formation at hepatic synthesis sites. Continued use of nonabsorbable anti-infective agents may alter the bacterial flora of the intestinal lumen and decrease the availability of products the bacteria contribute to physiologic processes.

Microorganism overgrowth. Anti-infective drugs, while accomplishing their purpose in destroying target organisms, may allow the emergence of other organisms and delay the recovery of the patient. Disruption of relationships between the normally nonpathogenic organisms in the body may allow overgrowth of yeast and fungi. The problem is relatively common when patients are receiving drugs for control of systemic infections. For example, the patient receiving an anti-infective drug may have an overgrowth of *Candida albicans* appearing as a white film on the tongue and buccal mucosa.

Overgrowth, or superinfection, occurs most frequently during therapy with broad-spectrum anti-infective drugs. The broad spectrum of effect on microorganisms increases the chances that suppression of normal flora will allow emergence of a single nonsusceptible component of the microflora. Unhampered by the natural competition of the usual companions in the area, the microflora gains prominence and causes infection.

Alternate pathogen emergence. Infections arising from the action of more than one organism (mixed infections) may cause emergence of alternate pathogens during therapy directed at eradication of a single component of the invaders. For example, the patient receiving an anti-infective drug (i.e., penicillin) for control of a penicillin-susceptible strain of staphylococci causing an infection may show an initial response to therapy. An interruption in his progress occurs as an alternate pathogen gains prominence. Culture of tissues or exudates may reveal the presence of a penicillinase-producing staphylococcal strain that has survived because of its ability to inactivate penicillin.

Assessment of status changes. A change in the patient's response to therapy necessitates exploration for contributing factors. Physical assessment may begin with the definition by the patient that there is something wrong or that he does not feel well. Physical assessment includes examination of body orifices for changes in tissues or secretions, stethoscopic examination of the chest for evidence of retained secretions, and tabulation of elimination patterns. Laboratory examination of stool and sputum specimens may provide evidence of pathogen emergence in the respiratory or intestinal tract. Interpretation of observations made by nursing and medical team members provides the base for modification of therapy directed at alleviation of the patient's problem.

Allergic reactions. Allergic reactions may occur during initial use of any of the anti-infective agents, but the incidence is highest when the drugs are employed for therapy for individuals with a history of allergic responses to pollens, foods, or drugs. Manifestations of allergic responses occur when antibodies respond to the introduction of the drug allergen during therapy. Drugs from protein sources (i.e., antibiotics) or chemical components attached to proteins institute the formation of antibodies during initial drug use, and subsequent therapy with the same drug or one that is structurally similar may precipitate an allergen-antibody response. Individuals who previously have experienced an allergic response during therapy with the drug may have a comparable response with subsequent provocative dosage of the same drug. It is noteworthy that sensitization increases allergic potential, but not all sensitized individuals have disruptive manifestations when the drug is employed subsequent to sensitization.

Allergen-antibody reactions and measures used for control of problems precipitated by provocative doses of the drugs are presented in Chapter 4. A brief outline of the chief drug-induced reactions is included here to provide a base for consideration of precautions and observations when planning care for the patient who is receiving anti-infective drugs.

Dissemination of parenterally administered drug causes generalized responses, but allergic responses may occur when drugs are administered by any route. The allergic response continues as long as the drug remains in the body to stimulate an antibody response. Depot forms of anti-infective agents present problems, since the drug may be released slowly from sequestered sites after the initial allergic response has subsided. *Anaphylaxis, urticaria,* or *angioedema* may occur as immediate responses when the allergen is given to an individual sensitized to the drug. *Serum sickness, fever, skin rash,* or *contact dermatitis* are manifestations occurring as delayed reactions to drugs. Each of the reactions may occur during therapy with anti-infective drugs.

Anaphylaxis. Anaphylaxis is a dramatic and life-threatening allergic response with systemic effects. Anaphylaxis occurs most frequently when an anti-infective drug is administered parenterally to an individual sensitized to the drug. In some sensitized individuals, drug administration promptly initiates an antibody response as the drug is distributed to tissues throughout the body. Histamine is released from mast cells in contact with the allergen-antibody reaction at extravascular sites. Histamine causes dilation of capillaries and constriction of venules at widely distributed tissue sites. Consequent permeability of capillaries and increased capillary pressure causes vascular fluid to leak into tissue spaces. The net effect of generalized fluid movement out of the vascular system is a decrease in circulating blood volume. A rapid fall in blood pressure (anaphylactic shock) may occur within minutes after administration of the drug. An additional component of the devastating response is the occurrence of histamine-induced bronchiole constriction. The patient may be dyspneic, or respiratory failure may be a consequence of extensive airway constriction.

Treatment consists of the prompt use of drugs (bronchodilator, antihistamine, or vasoconstrictor) and other resuscitative measures directed at returning the sequestered blood to the circulation and providing a patent airway. Death occurs in minutes if emergency measures are not available at the onset of anaphylaxis.

Urticaria. Urticaria is an immediate allergic response manifest as a widespread distribution of giant hives, or raised plateaus of tissue with whitish centers and deep pink borders, over the entire skin surface. Pruritus usually accompanies the skin lesions. Although the reaction site usually is limited to the skin surface, the reaction is believed to be the same allergen-antibody activity with histamine release that occurs with anaphylaxis. Discontinuance of drug administration removes the allergen stimulus. Urticaria may be relieved by an antihistamine and application of an antipruritic lotion to the eruptions on the body surface.

Angioedema. Angioedema may occur alone, or it may accompany urticaria as an extension of the same allergen-antibody-histamine response. Tissue fluid accumulations cause swelling of oral and respiratory tract mucosa and the soft tissues in the periorbital area. Progressive laryngeal edema may cause dyspnea or wheezing, and the patient may become increasingly apprehensive as he struggles to breathe. Because the tissue fluid collections are histamine induced, antihistamines are used to prevent extension of the edematous process.

Serum sickness. Serum sickness is an entity originally described as an allergic response to proteins in horse serum when individuals were inoculated with attenuated antibodies, or anti-

24 Drugs used to control infection and inflammation

toxins, produced in horses. A comparable symptom complex occurs when anti-infective drugs are administered. Manifestations of serum sickness occur 1 week or more after therapy is instituted. The time lapse is the interval during which the drug institutes formation of antibodies. As drug-specific antibodies are released into body fluids, the allergen remaining in the tissues reacts with the antibodies, and concurrent overt allergic reactions are evident. The patient may have generalized edema, dyspnea, joint pain, rash, and fever. Problems may persist after drug administration is discontinued, and the duration of the reaction is dependent on the period of time that the allergen remains in the body.

Other allergic reactions. Fever, skin rash, or contact dermatitis may occur during anti-infective drug therapy. The problems are less disruptive to the progress of the patient than the allergic responses previously described, and the extent of the reaction will influence the physician's decision to revise the therapeutic plan. When the planned course of therapy is near completion, the physician may continue use of the drug. Reevaluation of microorganism susceptibility to drugs may be planned to determine whether other drugs can be substituted for the offending drug allergen. Alternate drugs may be employed if the minimal therapeutic course for eradication of the microorganism will necessitate continuation of drug therapy for several days. There are instances when microorganism susceptibility to drug action is limited and eradication of an acute infection may require continued use of the allergen. Concurrent therapy is planned to relieve the discomfort of the patient (i.e., antihistamines, sedatives, antipyretics), and the patient's progress is observed for changes in the allergic response. Patients with allergic responses during drug therapy should be advised that future treatment with the drug may cause an allergic response.

SPECIFIC DRUG GROUPS

The physician considers the many variables in the host-parasite-drug relationship when selecting a pharmacotherapeutic plan for the patient. The success of the program is dependent on continual observations of the effect of the particular drug on the progress of the patient with an infectious process. The actions and adverse effects of each of the anti-infective agents will influence plans for patient care.

Antibiotics

Penicillins. Penicillin has been called the "wonder drug," and its bactericidal effect on organisms pathogenic to man seems to indicate that the title is appropriate. Introduction of the antibiotic derived from the fungus *Penicillium notatum* approximately thirty years ago brought with it spectacular changes in the course of diseases caused by bacteria.

All penicillins destroy bacteria by disrupting bacterial cell wall synthesis when new cells are forming. Penicillins interfere with the final stage of glycopeptide synthesis necessary for completion of the new cell wall. Transport mechanisms in the bacterial wall maintain a high intracellular osmotic pressure in the intact cell, and disruption of the wall by the antibiotic causes bacterial destruction by interfering with osmotic pressure maintenance within the cell.

There are structural differences between the natural and semisynthetic penicillins. Each of the semisynthetic forms of the antibiotic represents an addition to the basic 6-aminopenicillanic acid core of the natural penicillin.

Bacterial spectrum. Pathogen susceptibility varies from the limited effect of oxacillin sodium to the broad spectrum of ampicillin (Fig. 2-1). Penicillins are considered the drugs of choice for infections caused by staphylococcus. Penicillinase liberated by some *Staphylococcus aureus* inactivates ampicillin, carbenicillin disodium, hetacillin, and forms identified by the penicillin in the generic name (Table 2-1). Semisynthetic forms of penicillin that are resistant to penicillinase liberated by *Staphylococcus aureus* are cloxacillin sodium, dicloxacillin sodium, methicillin sodium, nafcillin sodium, and oxacillin sodium (Table 2-1). The development of semisynthetic forms that are lethal to enzyme-producing *Staphylococcus aureus* has widened the spectrum of penicillin-controlled staphylococcus infections.

Allergic reactions. Approximately 5% of the individuals receiving penicillin have some form

Table 2-1. Dosage range of anti-infective drugs: the penicillins

Nonproprietary name	Proprietary (trade) name	Daily adult dosage range	Nonproprietary name	Proprietary (trade) name	Daily adult dosage range
Ampicillin	Alpen, Amcill, Am-Pen, Ampi-CO, Amplin, Divercillin, Omnipen, Penbritin, Polycillin, Principen, Roampicillin, Supen, Tabocillin, Totacillin	Oral: 1-2 Gm. (÷4)	Oxacillin sodium	Prostaphlin, Resistopen	Oral: 2-6 Gm. (÷4-6) I.M.: 1-12 Gm. (÷4-6)
			Penicillin G, benzathine	Bicillin Permapen Isoject	Oral: 600,000-1 million U. (÷3-4) I.M.: Same
Ampicillin sodium	Alpen-N, Amcill-S, Omnipen-N, Penbritin-S, Polycillin-N, Principen-S, Totacillin-N	I.M.: 1-14 Gm. (÷6) I.V.: Same	Penicillin G, potassium	Cilloral penicillin, Dramcillin, Dropcillin, Orapen, Penalev, Penasoid, Pentids, Sugracillin	Oral: 1.2 million U. (÷3) I.M.: 1 million-12 million U. (÷6-12) I.V.: 1 million-100 million U.
Carbenicillin disodium	Geopen, Pyopen	I.M.: 1-8 Gm. (÷4) I.V.: 200-500 mg./kg.			
Cloxacillin sodium	Tegopen	Oral: 1-6 Gm. (÷4-6)	Penicillin G, procaine	Abbocillin, Crysticillin, Diurnalpenicillin, Duracillin, Wycillin	I.M.: 1 million-24 million U. (÷6-12)
Dicloxacillin sodium	Dynapen, Pathocil, Veracillin	Oral: 0.5-1 Gm. (÷4)			
Hetacillin	Versapen	Oral: 0.9-1.8 Gm. (÷4)	Penicillin O, potassium	Cer-O-Cillin	I.M.: 300,000-600,000 U. (÷6) I.V.: Same
Hetacillin potassium	Versapen-K	Oral: 0.9-1.8 Gm. (÷4) I.M.: Same I.V.: Same			
Methicillin sodium	Dimocillin-RT, Staphcillin	I.M.: 6-12 Gm. (÷4-6) I.V.: 4-30 Gm. (÷4-6)	Phenoxymethyl penicillin	Compocillin-V, Pen-Vee-L-A, V-Cillin	Oral: 0.375-3.75 Gm. (÷3-6)
			Potassium phenethicillin	Chemipen, Darcil, Dramcillin-S, Maxipen, Ro-Cillin, Semopen, Syncillin	Oral: 1-3 Gm. (÷4-6)
Nafcillin sodium	Unipen	Oral: 1.5-6 Gm. (÷4-6) I.M.: 2-4 Gm. (÷6) I.V.: 3-6 Gm. (÷6)	Potassium phenoxymethyl penicillin	Compocillin-VK, Ledercillin VK, Pen-Vee K, V-Cillin K	Oral: 0.5-1.2 Gm. (÷4)

of allergic reaction, and it is estimated that 15% of the American population have been sensitized to the drugs. The high percentage of reactions and sensitized individuals reflects the frequent and widespread use of penicillin for control of infections.

Allergic reactions occur more frequently when the drugs are administered parenterally, although they sometimes occur when penicillin is administered orally. Penicillin reactions are caused by the degradation products (i.e., penicilloyl poly-l-lysine). Sensitivity to any one form of penicillin is an indication of probable reaction to other forms of the drug, since all penicillins are built on the same basic 6-aminopenicillanic acid core. For example, a patient with known sensitivity to penicillin G is considered sensitized to other forms (i.e., ampicillin, oxacillin sodium) and should not receive the drugs.

In an effort to increase the predictability of allergic responses, penicillin metabolic products (penicilloyl poly-l-lysine and dia-mermeth) have been used for dermal-reaction testing of sensitivity to penicillin. Redness around the dermal site predicts a high probability of an allergic reaction to penicillin. Pretesting of individuals with a history of allergic reactions may decrease the incidence of drug-induced allergic reactions. Negative reactions in an individual known to have experienced an allergic reaction may allow penicillin use for therapy when susceptible pathogens cause acute illness.

Endogenous penicillin inactivation. Commercially available penicillinase (Neutrapen) has been employed to inactivate penicillin when a patient has a generalized allergic reaction. The drug acts exactly like the physiologic enzyme liberated by resistant bacteria. Penicillinase converts circulating penicillin to penicilloic acid that has neither antibiotic nor allergenic activity. From the patient's viewpoint, alleviation of the uncontrollable itching of the skin is a welcome relief during an urticarial reaction. For the patient with an anaphylactoid reaction, use of penicillinase may be lifesaving.

Penicillinase (800,000 units) is injected deep into the gluteal muscle, or it may be administered intravenously. Administration at the onset of an allergic reaction provides drug action in an hour, and the drug remains active in body fluids for 4 days. The drug has no effect on existing manifestations of the allergic response (i.e., hives), but it destroys the endogenous penicillin allergen. Although penicillinase is obtained from a microbe, *Bacillus cereus,* there is a low incidence of allergic reactions occurring with the use of the drug.

Adverse effects. Overgrowth of *Candida* and pseudomonas occurs during penicillin therapy. The principal sites of overgrowth are the respiratory and intestinal tracts. Periodic laboratory examination of stool and mucus helps in identification of alterations in the biologic flora. Varying gastrointestinal disturbances occur during therapy, but the onset of diarrhea may be an early warning of overgrowth of nonsusceptible bacteria.

Administration. Penicillins are widely distributed in body tissues, and the drugs penetrate collections of blood or pus to act on bacteria. Penicillins pass the placental barrier, and they enter the cerebrospinal fluid when the meninges are inflamed. Detoxification occurs in the liver, and small amounts of the drug appear in bile.

Serum binding affects the elimination of penicillin. For example, penicillin G is 46% to 58% bound to serum proteins, and the protein-bound drug does not pass through the glomerular capillaries. Renal tubular secretion rapidly moves penicillin into the tubular urine, and the mechanism can clear 560 to 1050 ml. of the drug per minute. Tubular secretion provides a mechanism for removal of 90% of penicillin G, and the remaining 10% is filtered through the glomerulus.

The tubular secretion sites are used by other drugs (i.e., salicylates, sulfonamides), and competition for transport sites may delay the elimination of penicillin. Probenecid (Benemid) is a sulfonamide derivative used therapeutically to slow the tubular secretion of penicillin. Lower penicillin dosage is needed when probenecid is administered. Oral administration of probenecid 30 minutes before intramuscular injection of penicillin can double the plasma levels of penicillin.

Administration of penicillin G leads to rapid, high serum levels of the drug. Addition of procaine to penicillin G slows absorption, but it increases the problems occurring during administration. Acute psychoses have been attributed to intravascular leak of procaine, and there have been sterile abscesses at tissue injection sites in infants and children.

Addition of benzathine to penicillin G has created a drug that has a long effective period. Administration of a single intramuscular dose of 1.2 million units of benzathine penicillin G provides therapeutic blood levels for 2 to 4 weeks. For example, intramuscular administration of benzathine penicillin G provides from the repository site penicillin that is bactericidal to *Treponema pallidum* organisms as they divide about every 33 hours in early syphilis. Blood levels with oral forms of the drug are slightly lower and less persistent.

Intravenous administration of most of the forms, except penicillin G, is accompanied by pain at the administration site, and thrombophlebitis may develop. Carbenicillin disodium is incompatible with many other intravenous solutions, and methicillin is degraded in the low pH of glucose solutions. The patient receiving methicillin must be observed carefully for evidence of nephrotoxicity (casts, albuminuria, and red blood cells in the urine) because a sensitivity-related nephritis has been reported.

Oral forms of penicillin provide peak blood levels of the drug in 1 to 2 hours. Penicillin G is commercially available as a buffered product that protects the drug against inactivation by gastric acids. Concurrent ingestion of food has little effect on phenoxymethyl penicillin, but the absorption of other forms of penicillin is delayed by the presence of food in the stomach. The drugs should be taken with water before meals or 2 to 3 hours after meals to assure maximum absorption.

Cephalosporins. The cephalosporins (Table 2-2) are structurally similiar to the penicillins, but there is enough difference between the two groups of drugs to make cephalosporins useful for patients who are allergic to penicillin. The mechanism of action is similar to that of penicillin. The drugs accomplish their bacterial effect by inhibiting glycopeptide synthesis in the final stage of bacterial cell wall synthesis.

Bacterial spectrum. The fairly broad spectrum of microbial susceptibility is somewhat limited by the sensitivity of cephalosporins to the action of cephalosporinase liberated by some gram-negative bacteria. The drugs have a wide range of clinical use for infection control. They have been employed for acutely ill patients prior to definition of the specific bacterial agent causing the infection. The drugs are administered before and after gastrointestinal surgery to suppress the diverse gram-positive and gram-negative organisms that emerge to initiate wound infections after surgery.

Adverse effects. Cephalosporins are widely distributed in body tissues. High concentrations of the antibiotic are achieved in the kidney when the drug is eliminated by glomerular filtration and tubular secretion. Large dosage increases the possibility of nephrotoxicity. Observation of the quantity and characteristics of the patient's urine (i.e., casts, cells, albumin) and the elimination rate of nitrogenous products is important during therapy. The drug and its metabolites may cause a false-positive reaction indicating glycosuria in tests done with cupric sulfate reagent (Benedict's qualitative reagent, Clinitest, Fehling's solution), but test tapes are not affected by the drug products.

Peak serum levels occur in about 1 hour. Food delays the absorption of oral forms, and solutions are unstable at alkaline pH ranges. In addition to the adverse effects occurring with use of all anti-infective agents, the cephalosporins occasionally cause dizziness, fatigue, and headache.

Erythromycins (and similar drugs). The varied forms of erythromycin (Table 2-3) have a fairly wide spectrum of bacteriostatic activity. They are classed pharmacologically as *macrolide* antibiotics. Other members of the pharmacologic group are oleandomycin phosphate and troleandomycin (Table 2-3). The pharmacodynamic effects of the macrolide antibiotics are similar to the effects of clindamycin hydrochloride and lincomycin hydrochloride (Table 2-3). The drugs act by competing for receptor sites on the ribosome unit to inhibit mRNA synthesis of protein necessary to bacterial reproduction.

Elimination route. The chief difference between this group of drugs and other anti-infective drugs is the excretion route. Drugs in the group are excreted chiefly in the bile rather

Table 2-2. Dosage range of anti-infective drugs: the cephalosporins

Nonproprietary name	Proprietary (trade) name	Daily adult dosage range
Cephalexin monohydrate	Keflex	Oral: 1 Gm. (÷4)
Cephaloglycin	Kafocin	Oral: 1-2 Gm. (÷4)
Cephaloridine	Loridine	I.M.: 0.5-3 Gm. (÷2-4)
		I.V.: Same
Cephalothin sodium	Keflin	I.V.: 40-80 mg./kg. (÷4-6)

Table 2-3. Dosage range of anti-infective drugs: the erythromycins (and similar drugs)

Nonproprietary name	Proprietary (trade) name	Daily adult dosage range
Clindamycin hydrochloride	Cleocin	Oral: 0.6-1.8 Gm. (÷4)
Erythromycin	E-Mycin, Erythrocin, Ilotycin	Oral: 1-4 Gm. (÷4)
Erythromycin estolate	Ilosone	Oral: 1-2 Gm. (÷4)
Erythromycin ethylsuccinate	Erythrocin, Pediamycin	Oral: 1-4 Gm. (÷4) I.M.: 200-600 mg. (÷2-6)
Erythromycin gluceptate	Ilotycin, I.V.	I.V.: 40-70 mg./kg. (÷4)
Erythromycin lactobionate	Erythrocin	I.V.: 1.5-4 Gm.
Erythromycin propionyl	Ilosone	Oral: 1-2 Gm. (÷4)
Erythromycin stearate	Erythrocin	Oral: 1-2 Gm. (÷4)
Lincomycin hydrochloride	Lincocin	Oral: 1.5-2 Gm. (÷3-4) I.M.: 0.6-1.2 Gm. (÷1-2) I.V.: 1.5-8 Gm. (÷2-3)
Oleandomycin phosphate	Matromycin	I.M.: 800 mg. (÷4) I.V.: 1-2 Gm. (÷2-4)
Troleandomycin	Cyclamycin, TAO	Oral: 1-2 Gm. (÷2-4)

than in the urine. Up to 90% of the drug is excreted in the bile and eliminated in the feces. The drugs are useful for treatment of susceptible bacterial infections in patients who have some renal dysfunction.

Adverse effects. Another characteristic shared by the drugs is a low incidence of the adverse effects that occur when other anti-infective drugs are administered. Gastrointestinal disturbances due to irritative effects of the drugs (nausea, vomiting, diarrhea, abdominal pain, stomatitis, black tongue) are relatively common problems during therapy. Patients also report a decreased tolerance to alcohol during the time they are taking erythromycin.

Administration. The intramuscular forms are irritating to tissues. Food delays absorption of orally administered forms; therefore administration before meals or 2 to 3 hours after meals is indicated. Some commercially available tablets are coated or buffered to protect the drug from degradation by gastric acids, and these tablets should be given with nonacid liquids.

Tetracyclines. The tetracyclines (Table 2-4) have a broad spectrum of microorganism susceptibility, but the drugs are used primarily for their bacteriostatic effect on gram-negative bacilli. The tetracyclines act by competing for receptor sites on the ribosome unit to inhibit mRNA synthesis of protein necessary to bacterial reproduction. Blocking the incorporation of amino acids required for protein synthesis prevents reproduction of the microorganisms, and body defenses eliminate the nonmultiplying bacteria. Drug therapy is continued beyond the time when overt evidence of infection subsides because continued therapy is necessary to assure elimination of remaining microorganisms. Because of structural similarities, individuals sensitive to one form of the anti-infective drug show sensitivity to other forms of it.

Adverse effects. Tetracycline's effectiveness against aerobic and anaerobic microbes alters the normal flora and allows overgrowth of highly resistant organisms. For example, gastroenteritis caused by enterotoxins elaborated by staphylococci necessitates immediate cessation of drug use. Appearance of liquid stools containing blood and the onset of fever provide early clues to the problem. Laboratory examination showing a high leukocyte content of the fecal material aids in differentiation between the nonbloody diarrhea of gastric irritation and staphylococcus-induced diarrhea. There have been fatalities resulting from sequelae of the staphylococcus gastroenteritis.

Tetracyclines have a hepatotoxic effect. The problem may be related to enterohepatic recycling of the drug that maintains high levels of tetracycline in the liver. Evidence of lethargy, anorexia, or changes in behavior (anxiety, depression) may precede the onset of jaundice. Careful observation of the patient may provide

Table 2-4. Dosage range of anti-infective drugs: the tetracyclines

Nonproprietary name	Proprietary (trade) name	Daily adult dosage range
Chlortetracycline hydrochloride	Aureomycin	Oral: 1-4 Gm. (÷4) I.V.: 0.5-2 Gm. (÷2-4)
Demeclocycline hydrochloride	Declomycin	Oral: 600 mg. (÷2-4)
Doxycycline hyclate	Vibramycin	Oral: 100-400 mg. (÷1-2)
Methacycline hydrochloride	Rondomycin	Oral: 600 mg. (÷2-4)
Minocycline hydrochloride	Minocin	Oral: 200-300 mg. (÷2)
Oxytetracycline hydrochloride	Terrabon, Terramycin	Oral: 1-4 Gm. (÷4) I.M.: 200-500 mg. (÷2-3) I.V.: 0.5-2 Gm. (÷2-4)
Rolitetracycline	Syntetrin, Velacycline	I.V.: 0.7-1.4 Gm. (÷2)
Tetracycline hydrochloride	Achromycin, Panmycin, Polycycline, Steclin, Sumycin, Tetrabon, Tetracyn, Tetrex	Oral: 1-4 Gm. (÷4) I.M.: 200-500 mg. (÷2-3) I.V.: 0.5-2 Gm. (÷2-4)

clues to an emerging problem. Children may eat poorly, withdraw, and cry easily for several days before jaundice appears. Tetracycline therapy is discontinued because hepatotoxicity progresses from fatty necrosis to fatal hepatic deterioration. A liver biopsy may be planned to confirm the diagnosis of drug-related hepatic damage when jaundice occurs.

The tetracyclines are widely distributed in body tissues. The drugs form a chemical union with calcium by mutual sharing of valence forces (chelation) that causes long-term deposition of the tetracycline at sites of active calcification in bones, teeth, and neoplastic tissues. Bone deposits may reduce the rate of bone growth in premature infants. The incidence of enamel hypoplasia and dental caries after the administration of the drug limits its usefulness for children under 8 years of age. Oxytetracycline seems to have less pronounced effect on bones and teeth. Crossing of the placental barrier may affect the calcification of bones and deciduous teeth in the fetus after the fourth month of gestation. The effect on teeth is seen as permanent brown or yellow pigmentation and enamel defects.

Tetracyclines are excreted in feces and urine. Large dosage of the drugs may block amino acid incorporation into body proteins in a manner comparable to the action of the drug on bacterial proteins, and the metabolism of the unused amino acids increases urea production. Serum and urinary levels of urea may be increased. Large intravenous dosage or the degradation products of outdated drug are nephrotoxic; therefore the quantity and characteristics of the urine are observed during therapy.

Patients taking the drug should avoid intense artificial ultraviolet light sources and sunlight. Exposure may lead to manifestations of the phototoxic reactions caused by the tetracyclines (i.e., exaggerated sunburn reactions and skin pigmentation). Phototoxic reactions have been reported most frequently during therapy with demeclocycline.

Administration. Intramuscular injections of tetracyclines are painful, as the drug is irritating to local tissues. Discomfort accompanying injection may be decreased by using a dry needle technique. After filling the syringe, the needle is changed. Use of a second needle avoids contact between drug adhering to the external surface of the needle used for withdrawal and tissues along the injection tract.

Tetracycline phosphate complex and minocycline hydrochloride may be given with milk or formula. Other oral forms are given before meals or 1 to 2 hours after meals because food interferes with absorption of the drug. Antacid administration is scheduled to avoid drug contact because aluminum, calcium, and magnesium content of antacids interferes with absorption of oral tetracyclines. In selected situa-

30 Drugs used to control infection and inflammation

tions the physician may prescribe the administration of the drug with food to decrease gastric irritation.

Formulations of tetracyclines for parenteral use contain ascorbic acid that is eliminated in the urine. Tests for glycosuria performed during or immediately after parenteral administration may be affected by the presence of ascorbic acid in the urine. A false-positive result may occur when a cupric sulfate reagent (Benedict's qualitative reagent, Clinitest) is used for testing, and a false-negative test may occur with use of glucose oxidase reagent (Clinistix, Tes-Tape).

Frequently used antibiotics. Many antibiotics (Table 2-5) frequently used for control of bacterial infections are structurally different, but they have a similar effect on bacteria. They accomplish their antibacterial effect by interfering with both cell wall and membrane synthesis during the reproduction of bacteria. The spectrum of bacterial susceptibility to the drugs varies considerably (Fig. 2-1), but there are many aspects of therapy with the antibiotics that affect planned observations of the patient.

Dosage limitations. The dosage level and the duration of therapy are carefully planned to provide maximal therapeutic effect and limit the high incidence of neurotoxicity and nephrotoxicity occurring as adverse effects when each of the drugs (Table 2-5) is administered parenterally. Prolonged administration, high dosage, or decreased renal clearance of the drugs may cause high serum levels, with subsequent neurotoxicity. The neural effects are seen as peripheral paresthesias (including circumoral or lingual paresthesias) and auditory or vestibular nerve injury. Damage to the auditory branch of the eighth cranial nerve causes loss of ability to hear high frequency sounds. Vestibular branch damage causes loss of equilibrium. Any evidence that the patient has a ringing sound in his ears (tinnitus), dizziness, or vertigo may be an indication of eighth cranial nerve damage. Neural damage can occur up to six months after therapy is terminated so that it is important for the patient to understand the necessity for consulting with his physician if any unusual problems arise.

The adverse neural effects are additive between these antibiotics and other drugs with properties causing ototoxicity. Retention of the drug increases the incidence of neurotoxicity. The drugs are excreted primarily by the kidneys, and renal dysfunction may cause elevated serum drug levels. Nephrotoxicity is related to the irritative effect of the drugs on renal tubules. High serum drug levels attained by large dosage of the drugs over long periods of time increase the incidence of nephrotoxicity. The patient's urine output is monitored carefully throughout drug use, and tabulation of fluid in-

Table 2-5. Dosage range of frequently used anti-infective drugs

Nonproprietary name	Proprietary (trade) name	Daily adult dosage range
Colistimethate sodium*	Coly-Mycin M	I.M.: 2.5-5 mg./kg. ($\div$2-4)
Colistin sulfate*	Coly-Mycin S	Oral: 3-5 mg./kg. ($\div$3)
Gentamicin sulfate†	Garamycin	I.M. 2-5 mg./kg. ($\div$3) I.V.: Same
Kanamycin sulfate†	Kantrex	I.M.: 10-15 mg./kg.
Neomycin sulfate†	Mycifradin	Oral: 30-60 mg./kg. ($\div$4) I.M.: 10-15 mg./kg. ($\div$4)
Paromomycin†	Humatin	Oral: 25-100 mg./kg.
Polymyxin B sulfate*	Aerosporin	Oral: 30-60 mg./kg. ($\div$4) I.M.: 1.5-2.5 mg./kg. ($\div$4)
Spectinomycin dihydrochloride†	Trobicin	I.M.: 2-4 Gm.
Streptomycin sulfate†	Strycin	Oral: 0.5-6 Gm. I.M.: 1-4 Gm. ($\div$2-4)
Vancomycin hydrochloride†	Vancocin	I.V.: 2-4 Gm. ($\div$4)

*Polymyxin group.
†Streptomycin group.

take is planned to assure adequate dilution of the drug in renal tubules.

Intestinal bacteria suppression. Colistin sulfate, kanamycin sulfate, neomycin sulfate, paromomycin, polymyxin B sulfate, and streptomycin sulfate are poorly absorbed from the intestine when administered orally. The drugs are frequently used for suppression of bacterial growth in the treatment of bacterial diarrhea and "sterilization" of the intestinal lumen prior to intestinal surgery.

Preoperative suppression of bacterial growth decreases the coliform bacteria liberated during manipulation of the intestine and has a positive effect on prevention of postoperative wound infections. The patient is often placed on a low-residue or elemental diet 3 to 5 days preoperatively, and anti-infective drug administration is started at least 48 hours prior to surgery. Control of bacterial growth in the intestine may include the use of oral anti-infectives administered when peristalsis resumes after surgery.

Therapeutic suppression of the intestinal microflora removes pathogens, but it also suppresses the activity of bacteria that contribute to nitrogen cycling by converting nitrogen to ammonia before it enters the hepatic metabolic cycle. Short-term therapy during the 3-day period prior to surgery may not have an adverse effect on nitrogen metabolism in the presence of adequate hepatic function. Suppression of intestinal bacteria that synthesize vitamin K adversely affects prothrombin production. Because maintenance of prothrombin levels is desirable prior to surgery, vitamin K is usually administered orally or parenterally during the preoperative period.

Streptomycin group. Streptomycin sulfate, gentamicin sulfate, kanamycin sulfate, neomycin sulfate, paromomycin, and spectinomycin dihydrochloride (Table 2-5) are classified pharmacologically as *aminoglycosides*. Degradation metabolites of the drugs are hydrolyzed to a comparable compound, and the drugs have a comparable bactericidal action.

The streptomycin-related drugs act on bacteria by increasing the permeability of the cell membrane and causing misreading of the genetic construction code. While mRNA is assembling nucleotides, the drugs intercede by substituting for an essential nucleotide, and the bacteria build nonfunctional protein.

Streptomycin sulfate is effective in control of several important gram-negative microorganisms (i.e., *Haemophilus influenzae, Neisseria gonorrhoeae, Escherichia coli, Proteus mirabilis, Mycobacterium tuberculosis*), but bacterial resistance occurs rapidly during therapy with streptomycin sulfate. Resistance of previously susceptible bacteria has occurred as early as 48 hours after initiation of therapy. Some bacteria become dependent on streptomycin sulfate for growth, and the drug becomes a necessary nutrient to the bacteria.

Streptomycin sulfate acts synergistically with penicillin, and the drugs have been used together for intensive therapy of acutely ill patients. The chief use of streptomycin sulfate is for the treatment of tuberculosis, and it is the prototype for antibiotics employed for tuberculosis control (i.e., capreomycin sulfate, cycloserine, rifampin, viomycin sulfate). When used at low dosage with isoniazid or aminosalicylic acid, bacterial resistance is slower to develop. Streptomycin sulfate is particularly useful in the intensive therapeutic period following the diagnosis of tuberculosis in acutely ill patients.

Streptomycin sulfate therapy causes some hearing loss in 4% to 15% of the patients receiving the drug daily for more than 1 week. The drug crosses the placental barrier, and irreversible hearing loss may occur in the fetus (i.e., when the pregnant woman is treated for tuberculosis).

Patients may complain of vertigo, ataxia, paresthesias, headache, or a sensation of muscle tension around the eyes after intramuscular injection of the drug. Exercise immediately following the injection seems to increase the incidence of the problems; therefore the patient may avert problems by resting for a short time after he receives the injection.

Neomycin sulfate is most frequently used for its antiseptic action in the intestine, and only 3% of the drug is absorbed after oral ingestion. Neomycin sulfate is used as an ingredient in topical ointments, and it is sometimes employed as a prophylactic application around insertion sites of tubes, catheters, or cardiac pacing wires to provide an antibiotic barrier to entrance of bacteria. Daily application of neomycin sulfate at sites of venous catheter insertion has decreased the incidence of infection from indwelling catheters. Neomycin sulfate is seldom administered parenterally because the risk of ototoxicity is high.

Gentamicin sulfate is used parenterally principally for serious infections caused by gram-negative bacteria (i.e., pseudomonas). Urinary excretion of the drug is nearly complete (86% to 100%) in 24 hours. When employed for treatment of urinary tract infections, alkalinization of the urine to pH 7.5 may increase the anti-infective activity up to thirty-two times that occurring at pH 5.5. The interval between doses may be lengthened by the physician after 2 days of therapy, as the drug tends to accumulate at that time.

Kanamycin sulfate is used for suppression of intestinal bacteria, and it is employed discriminately for treatment of systemic infections caused by *Staphylococcus aureus, Neisseria gonorrhoeae, Escherichia coli, Shigella,* or *Mycobacterium tuberculosis.* Therapy is usually discontinued after 7 days as a precaution against ototoxicity. Planned alternation of injection sites is necessary, since the drug tends to cause nodules in tissues.

Spectinomycin dihydrochloride is used principally for its bacteriostatic effect on *Neisseria gonorrhoeae.* Patients who have gonorrhea caused by strains resistant to penicillin therapy or who are allergic to penicillin may respond to therapy with spectinomycin dihydrochloride. The drug is administered deep into gluteal tissues, and the injection sites are rotated to decrease the discomfort caused by the irritative properties of the drug.

Vancomycin is used for its bactericidal effect on a wide range of gram-positive microorganisms. It is employed for treatment of infections that are resistant to other antibiotics. Limitations on usage are related to the high incidence of neurotoxicity, although modification of dosage and effective renal clearance decrease the neurotoxic effects.

Polymyxin group. Colistimethate sodium, colistin sulfate, and polymyxin B sulfate (Table 2-5) are antibiotics obtained from *Bacillus polymyxa,* and they have a comparable spectrum of susceptible gram-negative microorganisms (Fig. 2-1). The detergent-like effect of the drugs on the bacterial cell membrane increases membrane permeability, and consequent leakage of intracellular contents disrupts the intracellular osmotic gradient.

More than 60% of parenterally administered drug is removed by glomerular filtration within 24 hours. Urine production below 600 ml./24 hours is considered insufficient for removal of drug from the body. Retention of the drug increases the potential for neurotoxicity, and the drug prescription is usually discontinued when the urine output falls sharply.

Reserve antibiotics. Therapy with anti-infective drugs is planned after careful consideration of microorganism susceptibility, the status of the patient, and predictable problems or adverse effects known to occur with the particular drug. Anti-infective drugs producing a high incidence of adverse effects are used in situations in which the drugs are the only available agents showing microorganism susceptibility. The drugs may also be employed for therapy of acutely ill patients when the infection is life threatening and the blood or tissue cultures indicate the drug offers outstanding prospects for control of the pathogen.

Chloramphenicol. The broad antibiotic spectrum of chloramphenicol (Amphicol, Chloromycetin, Mychel) includes many of the gram-negative as well as some of the gram-positive bacteria. The drug blocks protein synthesis at the ribosomal binding sites for mRNA during the production of new bacteria. Chloramphenicol acts as an antimetabolite by substituting for the essential amino acid *phenylalanine* required for biosynthesis of protein in the cell, and the substitution leads to synthesis of an inactive complex. The toxic effects of chloramphenicol are partially attributable to concurrent antimetabolic action on normal body cells that also require the essential amino acid for protein construction.

Chloromycetin is widely distributed in body tissues, including pleural and cerebrospinal fluids. A small amount of the drug is excreted in the bile, but the chief excretory route is the kidney. In the nephron the drug is excreted by glomerular filtration, but the major portion (85% to 95%) is excreted by tubular secretion of the inactive metabolites. The primary metabolite is the glucuronic acid conjugate. Premature and newborn infants have deficient mechanisms for renal and hepatic glucuronide conjugation, and use of the drug would cause prolonged plasma levels of it. Chloramphenicol is seldom used for therapy of infants or adults with hepatic dysfunction because decreased metabolization of the drug causes a gray syndrome. The typical sequence of events related to the fatal syndrome include feeding disturbances, abdominal distention, pallid cyanosis, vasomotor collapse, ashen gray color, and death.

In addition to the adverse effects occurring with use of all anti-infective drugs, chloramphenicol may cause suppression of bone marrow (aplastic anemia, leukopenia, thrombocytopenia) with long-term use at high dosage. The incidence is greatest in patients with a high rate of bone marrow proliferation (i.e., children, premenopausal women). Some red blood cell maturation arrest is almost always seen during therapy. Bone marrow depression may be fatal, but experience with the drug and knowledge of the potential for occurrence of hypoplasia of bone marrow has led to discrimination in use of the drug.

During therapy with chloramphenicol, patients complain of a persistent bitter taste and dryness of the mouth. There have been some reports of neuritis, coolness, and weakness of the legs. Adverse central nervous system effects may be seen as headache, confusion, or mental depression. Gastrointestinal disturbances are fairly common and include nausea, vomiting, diarrhea, and abdominal pain. The daily dosage range of the oral form (chloramphenicol) and the drug for intravenous administration (chloramphenicol sodium succinate) is 50 to 100 mg., divided into 4 doses.

Novobiocin sodium. Novobiocin sodium (Albamycin, Cathomycin) has a spectrum of microorganism susceptibility that includes gram-positive microorganisms (staphylococcus, pneumococcus, and corynebacterium) and the gram-negative *Haemophilus,* meningococcus, gonococcus, and brucella. The chief problems occurring during therapy are bone marrow depression, intrahepatic biliary obstruction with jaundice, and allergic reactions. Drug forms are available for administration of the drug orally or parenterally, and the daily dosage range is the same by either route (1 Gm., divided into 2 to 4 doses).

Ristocetin. Ristocetin (Spontin) has a spectrum of effect that includes all the important gram-positive microorganisms and *Mycobacterium tuberculosis* (Fig. 2-1). Use of ristocetin is limited by the high incidence of blood dyscrasias occurring during therapy. In selective situations, ristocetin is administered (25 to 50 mg./kg./24 hours) intravenously for control of susceptible organisms.

Bacitracin. Bacitracin is highly effective as a topical application or intracavity injection when the infection is caused by streptococcus, staphylococcus, or pneumococcus. Bacitracin is used for treatment of systemic infections caused by these microbes only when other drugs are contraindicated for the patient because bacitracin causes a high incidence of nephrotoxicity.

Chemotherapeutics

Sulfonamides. All the sulfonamides (Table 2-6) are weak acids that accomplish their bacteriostatic effect by interference with the biosynthesis of folic acid by bacteria. Body cells and many bacteria require preformed folic acid to meet nutritive needs because the cells are not capable of synthesis of the vitamin. Bacteria that synthesize folic acid pick up the drug substitute rather than the para-aminobenzoic acid required for folic acid synthesis. Bacterial utilization of the drug as a metabolite disrupts growth and reproduction. Body defense mechanisms are needed for removal (phagocytosis) of the microorganisms after drug inhibition of their reproduction.

Bacterial spectrum. Sulfonamides were the first anti-infective agents, and they were widely used to control infection. Long-term use of the drugs led to the development of resistant strains of bacteria. Resistant bacteria probably have become able to use the drug substitute to synthesize folic acid to meet their nutritive needs. Experience with the drugs has led to the

Table 2-6. Dosage range of anti-infective drugs: the sulfonamides

Nonproprietary name	Proprietary (trade) name	Daily adult dosage range
Phthalylsulfathiazole	Cremothalidine, Rothalid, Sulfathalidine	Oral: 50-125 mg./kg. ($\div$ 3-6)
Salicylazosulfapyridine	Azulfidine, EN-tabs	Oral: 2-12 Gm. ($\div$ 4-8)
Succinylsulfathiazole	Rolsul, Sulfasuxidine	Oral: 250 mg./kg. ($\div$ 6)
Sulfacetamide	Sulamyd, Urosulfon	Oral: 3 Gm. ($\div$ 3)
Sulfachlorpyridazine	Sonilyn	Oral: 2-4 Gm. ($\div$ 3-6)
Sulfadiazine	Coco-Diazine, Cremodiazine, Lipo-Diazine	Oral: 2-4 Gm. ($\div$ 3-6)
Sulfadiazine sodium		I.M.: 50-100 mg./kg. ($\div$ 3-4) I.V.: 50-100 mg./kg. ($\div$ 3-4)
Sulfadimethoxine	Madribon, Madriqid	Oral: 0.5-1 Gm.
Sulfaethidole	Sul-Spansion, Sul-Spantab	Oral: 1.3-3.9 Gm. ($\div$ 2)
Sulfamerazine		Oral: 2-4 Gm. ($\div$ 3-6)
Sulfameter	Sulla	Oral: 0.5-1.5 Gm.
Sulfamethizole	Microsul, Renasul, Sulfasol, Sulfstat, Sulfurine, Thiosulfil, Urosulfin, Utrasul	Oral: 2-4 Gm. ($\div$ 3-6)
Sulfamethoxazole	Gantanol	Oral: 2-3 Gm. ($\div$ 2-3)
Sulfamethoxypyridazine	Kynex, Midicel	Oral: 500 mg.
Sulfaphenazole	Sulfabid	Oral: 2 Gm. ($\div$ 2)
Sulfapyridine		Oral: 1-2 Gm. ($\div$ 4)
Sulfisomidine	Elkosin	Oral: 2-4 Gm. ($\div$ 3-6)
Sulfisoxazole	Gantrisin, Sodizole, Sosol, Unisulf	Oral: 2-4 Gm. ($\div$ 3-6)
Sulfisoxazole diolamine	Gantrisin diolamine	I.M.: 100 mg./kg. ($\div$ 3) I.V.: Same

general practice of limiting therapy to 15 days to decrease the incidence of bacterial resistance. Sulfonamides currently have a spectrum of microorganism susceptibility that includes the gram-negative meningococcus, *Haemophilus, Escherichia,* brucella, and *Enterobacter.*

Distribution. Sulfonamides are distributed in most body tissues and appear in glandular secretions (saliva, tears, sweat). They are metabolized chiefly in the liver but may be degraded by many body tissues.

Therapy with a sulfonamide is initiated with administration of a loading dose that is double the usual therapeutic dosage. The aim of therapy is to maintain blood levels of the drug at a level (12 to 15 mg./100 ml.) that will provide anti-bacterial activity. Monitoring of the blood levels is done frequently to prevent elevation above the therapeutic range.

The therapeutic effect of sulfonamides is enhanced by plasma protein binding that is characteristic of the drugs. Protein-bound drug is unavailable to tissues because the protein complex cannot cross the capillary membrane to move into tissue fluids. Loosely bound drug moves from protein-binding sites when tissue levels are lowered by metabolism or excretion of the drug. Continual replenishment of tissue levels of drug from protein-bound stores prolongs the bacteriostatic action of the sulfonamides.

Excretion. There is considerable variation in the solubility and rate of excretion of the various forms of sulfonamide. Alkalinization of the urine is planned during therapy to increase the solubility of the sulfonamide and prevent precipitation of crystals in the nephron and renal pelvis. Concurrent administration of an alkaline drug (i.e., sodium bicarbonate) maintains an alkaline urine. New combined sulfonamides are much more soluble than older forms, and less crystal precipitation occurs. Maintenance of urinary output at a level that assures solution of tubular drug (i.e., above 1200 ml.) also decreases the tendency for crystals to form.

Frequent urine examinations are done during therapy to determine whether there is crystal accumulation and renal irritation. Careful monitoring of the quantity and acidity of urine is important throughout the period during which the drugs are used.

Protein binding affects the excretion rate of the sulfonamides. Protein does not pass through the glomerular capillary of the normal nephron, and bound drug that enters the glomerular capsule remains in the circulation. Free drug or its metabolites move into the glomerular filtrate. Tubular cells are important to eventual removal of the drug from plasma. Renal tubular cells actively secrete sulfonamide into tubular urine. Tubular cells also reabsorb sulfonamides from tubular urine and return the drug to the circulating fluids. Tubular cells handle free drug, and the process of secretion and recycling returns the drug to liver or tissue sites for metabolism. Metabolized drug that returns to the nephron can pass through glomerular capillaries. The tubular recycling process delays excretion and maintains blood levels of the sulfonamide.

Differences in serum binding and rate of secretion affect the therapeutic use of the drugs. For example, 32% to 56% of an administered dose of sulfadiazine is bound to serum proteins, and 50% of the dose is excreted in the urine in 24 hours. Eighty-four percent of a dose of sulfasoxazole is bound to serum proteins, and 70% to 95% of the dose is excreted in the urine in 24 hours. Availability of approximately half an administered dose of sulfadiazine to body tissues and maintenance of the dosage level by gradual release from protein-binding sites makes it a useful drug for treatment of infections at varying tissue sites (including the brain). The slow rate of excretion (50%/24 hours) assists in maintaining therapeutic levels. In contrast, little of the administered dose of sulfasoxazole is released to body tissues (84% protein bound), but the high rate of excretion (70% to 95%/24 hours) indicates there is a constant level of drug in the renal tubule. Recycling maintains a fairly high level of the drug in tubular urine, and it is available for its therapeutic effect on urinary tract infections.

Renal tubular recycling is highest when the tubular urine is acid. Alkalinization of the urine to improve solubility of the sulfonamides slows reabsorption of the drug and increases the amount moving toward excretion.

Transport competition. Many drugs are secreted by renal tubular cells, and competition for transport or binding sites in the tubular cells may affect drug elimination. Competition may increase the blood levels of the drug requiring the same transport mechanisms for excretion (i.e., salicylates, sulfonamides, drugs with a sulfonamide component in their structure). For example, blocking of tubular secretion of oral sulfonylurea hypoglycemic drugs may cause a prolonged hypoglycemic state as the drugs accumulate.

Adverse effects. The most common use of the drugs is for short-term therapy of patients with urinary tract infections. The discomforts that patients complain about during therapy are anorexia, nausea, and vomiting. Because the problems arise when the drugs are administered orally or parenterally, direct stimulation of the chemoreceptor trigger zone of the vomiting center in the medulla is probably the source of the problem. Most patients are able to continue therapy when an antiemetic is prescribed by the physician.

The problem of greatest concern is the occurrence of blood dyscrasias (i.e., leukopenia, thrombocytopenia, erythrocytopenia) and hypoprothrombinemia. Any evidence of fever, sore throat, weakness, pallor, jaundice, or petechial bleeding is important. The drug is withheld until the problems are discussed with the physician. The probability that continued use of the drugs will precipitate bone marrow depression has led to short-term use and continued evaluation of the patient's blood values during therapy.

Allergic reactions. The incidence of reactions occurring during therapy with sulfonamides is about 5% of patients taking the drugs. Sensitization may result from topical use of sulfonamide-containing ointments or prior use of any of the drugs. Administration of the drug is discontinued by the physician if a rash appears because an irreversible and fatal syndrome (Stevens-Johnson syndrome) occasionally begins with generalized skin eruptions. High temperature, severe headache, stomatitis, conjunctivitis, rhinitis, and generalized skin rash precede the destructive cutaneous lesions of the syndrome.

Intestinal antiseptic action. Oral forms of sulfonamide are absorbed at differing rates from the gastrointestinal tract. Food or antacids decrease absorption when ingested concurrent with the drug. Phthalylsulfathiazole, salicylazosulfapyridine, and succinylsulfathiazole are used primarily for intraintestinal therapy because they are poorly absorbed from the intestinal tract. Phthalylsulfathiazole therapy results in a tenacious, stringy stool that is difficult to remove. Salicylazosulfapyridine is selectively retained in the intestinal tract, and it is metabolized in the connective tissue of the colon. When the urine is alkaline, the metabolites cause the urine to turn to an orange-yellow color. Succinylsulfathiazole produces a semifluid and gelatinous stool. Absorption of the drugs from intestinal lesions will precipitate generalized reactions comparable to those found with systemically administered drugs.

Administration. The variability in duration of action affects the frequency of administration of each of the drugs (Table 2-6). Sulfadimethoxine, sulfameter, and sulfamethoxypyridazine are administered only once a day (usually after breakfast) because they continue to have antibacterial activity for at least 24 hours. The remainder of the sulfonamides maintain consistent blood levels when administered regularly at the prescribed intervals throughout the 24-hour period.

Kidney-specific drugs

Nalidixic acid (NegGram) is administered orally (2 to 4 Gm./24 hours, divided into 4 doses) for its activity as a urinary bactericidal agent. Because 80% of the drug is excreted in the urine in 24 hours, it is effective in eradicating gram-negative urinary tract bacteria. Although nausea and vomiting are the most common problems, adverse effects are varied: dizziness, diplopia, weakness, headache, drowsiness, and pruritus. Glucuronide conjugation in the kidney may cause a false-positive reaction for glycosuria when Benedict's qualitative reagent or Clinitest is used for testing, but test tapes are not affected by the metabolites.

Nitrofurantoin (Cyantin, Furachel, Furadantin, Furalan, Macrodantin, N-Toin, Trantoin) is administered orally (5 to 7 mg./kg./24 hours, divided into 4 doses) for eradication of gram-negative urinary tract bacteria. Nausea and vomiting are the chief adverse effects, but gastritis and skin rashes occur frequently in children. Nitrofurantoin sodium is administered parenterally. The drug is incompatible with many intravenous solutions. Some of the drug is excreted in the feces, but 30% to 50% of a single dose is excreted in the urine in 12 hours. Metabolites of the drug may tint the urine brown. Alkaline urine increases renal clearance, but maximum antibacterial effect occurs in an acid tubular urine. The drug acts as a diffusible acid with increased tubular back-diffusion (tubular cycling) when the tubular urine is acid. The process maintains a higher concentration in the nephron for antibacterial action.

Methenamine is used for treatment of pseudomonas, *Enterobacter,* and proteus strains causing infections in the urinary tract. Methenamine (Uritone, Urotropin), methenamine hippurate (Hiprex), methenamine mandelate (Mandacon, Mandalay, Mandelamine, Renelate), and methenamine sulfosalicylate (Hexalet) exert antibacterial activity on the tissues by liberation of ammonia and formaldehyde. Effectiveness of the drugs is dependent on an acid urine (pH below 5.5) for maximal effect on the urea-splitting organisms. Urine acidity also reduces the incidence of bladder irritation. The usual dosage of each of the drugs is 4 Gm./24 hours, divided into 4 doses taken with an acidifying agent (ascorbic acid tablets or fruit juices). Adverse reactions are nausea, vomiting, pruritus, and skin rash. During therapy it is important to monitor the quantity and pH of urine and to obtain cultures periodically to ascertain the effectiveness of the drug.

Ethoxazene hydrochloride (Serenium) and phenazopyridine hydrochloride (Pyridium) are occasionally used for their soothing effect on irritated urinary tract tissues. They may be employed in conjunction with anti-infective agents, but the action of these drugs is limited to a local anesthetic effect on the tissues. The patient should be told to expect the startling orange-red color of the urine. The color change results from the azo dye origin of the drug.

Mycobacterium-specific drugs

Mycobacterium leprae. The low incidence of leprosy (Hansen's disease) in the world seems to contrast sharply with the number of people having the disease in biblical times. Modern drug therapy makes it possible for many of the 15 million lepers in the world to survive and to return to their homes.

Mycobacterial invasion. Prolonged and intimate contact with an individual discharging the bacillus in mucus or from surface lesions allows pathogens to enter skin or mucous membranes and cause the disease. Children are particularly susceptible, and the contact between a mother with leprosy and her child would provide the prolonged exposure required for the bacillus to gain a foothold and cause leprosy.

Invasion of the body by *Mycobacterium leprae* causes a physiologic response comparable to the body defense mechanisms occurring with other bacterial invasions. The thick lipoprotein cell wall of the bacterium resists phagocytosis by macrophage lipases, and it continues to survive within the cytoplasm of the mononuclear cell as it moves from the invasion site. Monocytes become distended with the mycobacteria that remain in their cytoplasm in neatly arranged packets shaped like cigars. Survival of the lepra during the vulnerable stages of growth and reproduction seems to be enhanced by a protective and nutritive substance natural to the cluster of bacilli. *Mycobacterium leprae* organisms spread throughout the body and may cause local lesions at varying tissue sites.

Biblical descriptions of open lesions and disfigurement by loss of terminal digits or other body parts are illustrations of the two types of leprosy: lepromatous, or nodular, and tuberculoid, or anesthetic, leprosy. *Lepromatous-type leprosy* characteristically includes ulcerated lesions and development of large nodules, or granulomas, that contain histocytes heavily laden with the mycobacterium. The tumorlike overgrowths appear on the skin and mucous membranes, and progressive enlargement gradually interferes with nerve tracts. Invasion of large nerves causes anesthesia of tissues along the related skin areas, atrophy of skin and muscle, breakdown of bone matrix, and ulceration of tissues. Spontaneous painless am-

Table 2-7. Dosage range of mycobacterium-specific agents

Nonproprietary name	Proprietary (trade) name	Daily adult dosage range
Mycobacterium leprae control: the sulfones		
Acetosulfone sodium	Promacetin	Oral: 0.5-4 Gm.
Dapsone	Avlosulfon	Oral: 50-100 mg.
Sulfoxone sodium	Diasone	Oral: 330-990 mg.
Thiazolsulfone	Promizole	Oral: 1-4 Gm.
Mycobacterium tuberculosis control		
Aminosalicylate, calcium	Pasara, Pasca	Oral: 12 Gm. (÷4)
Aminosalicylate, phenyl	Pheny-PAS-Tebamin	Oral: 12 Gm. (÷3)
Aminosalicylate, potassium	Neopasalate-K, Paskalium, Paskate, Potaba	Oral: 12-15 Gm. (÷3)
Aminosalicylate, sodium	Pamisyl, Pasara, Pasmed, Pasna	Oral: 12-15 Gm. (÷3)
Aminosalicylic acid	Para-Pas, Parasal, Pasem, Rezipas	Oral: 6-15 Gm. (÷3)
Benzoylpas, calcium	Benzapas	Oral: 10-15 Gm. (÷3)
Capreomycin sulfate	Capastat, Capromycin	I.M.: 1 Gm.
Cycloserine	Seromycin, Oxamycin	Oral: 0.5-1 Gm. (÷2-4)
Ethambutol hydrochloride	Myambutol	Oral: 15-25 mg./kg.
Ethionamide	Trecator	Oral: 0.5-1 Gm. (÷4)
Isoniazid	Armazid, Cotinazin, Dinacrin, Ditubin, INH, Isolyn, Niadrin, Niconyl, Nicozide, Nydrazid, Pyricidin, Rimifon, Tisin, Tyvid	Oral: 3-5 mg./kg. (÷2) I.M.: Same
Pyrazinoic acid amide	Aldinamide, Pyrazinamide, Tebrazid	Oral: 25-40 mg./kg. (÷3-4)
Rifampin	Rifadin, Rifaldizine, Rifampicin, Rifamycin AMP, Rimactane	Oral: 600 mg.
Viomycin sulfate	Vinactane, Viocin	I.M.: 2 Gm.

putation of terminal digits is predictable after the destruction of bone and tissues. *Tuberculoid-type leprosy* characteristically involves peripheral nerves, and the skin lesions are macular areas that are anesthetic within their margins. Tuberculoid-type leprosy follows a pattern of prolonged remission with periodic exacerbation of lesions.

Sulfone therapy. Dapsone is considered the parent sulfone, or prototype, of the sulfonamide derivatives used for control of *Mycobacterium leprae* (Table 2-7). Each of the drugs is employed in treatment of lepromatous, tuberculoid, or mixed types of leprosy. The drugs are thought to act in a manner comparable to that of the sulfonamides which provide a substitute nucleotide used by the bacteria in the synthesis of folic acid. Sulfone substitution for paraaminobenzoic acid prevents the building of folic acid necessary to mycobacterium nutrition.

All of the sulfones are administered orally once a day. After absorption from the upper small intestine, the drugs enter all tissues, and they are excreted in urine and glandular secretions. Elimination from the body is slow, and cumulative amounts of the drug add to the therapeutic effect.

Response of lesions to therapy may occur over several months. Mucosal lesions improve in three to six months. There is a gradual lessening of epistaxis, nasal obstruction, dyspnea, and hoarseness as mucosal ulceration and swelling subside. Skin lesions are somewhat slower to respond, but the heavy clusters of reticuloendothelial cells with their collections of bacteria gradually recede. The extensive lesions of skin and mucous membrane occurring with lepromatous leprosy may require from one to three years for clearance of bacilli accumulations and regression of lesions. Scarring, contractures, and deformity may be residual problems after healing.

Inflammation of nerve trunks typical of tuberculoid-type leprosy is slow to subside, and nerve tenderness may not decrease for six to nine months after initiation of therapy. Extensive anesthesia and paralysis resulting from nerve destruction are not reversed, but the anesthetic areas of skin lesions respond to sulfone therapy.

Macular lesions of tuberculoid-type leprosy may be bacteriologically negative in one and one-half to three years, but the ulcerative lesions of lepromatous-type leprosy may not be negative for three to five years after initiation of therapy.

Hemolytic anemia occurs in most patients during the initial period of sulfone therapy. Nutritional status is thought to be a contributing factor, but the anemic state usually stabilizes after the first few weeks of therapy. Patients with a fall in hemoglobin to 10 grams/100 ml. often are placed on reduced dosage of the sulfone drug until their hemologic status is improved by natural body processes and supportive therapy with combined iron and vitamin preparations.

Mild gastrointestinal disturbances occur in many patients. The chief concern is that the problems will adversely affect the eating patterns of the patient who needs body defenses to act with drugs in elimination of the bacilli.

An allergic reaction comparable to that occurring in other chronic diseases with pathogen residence in the body occurs in leprosy. The allergy is a response to the invading mycobacterium and is described as a lepra reaction. Disintegrating mycobacteria provide the allergen stimulus for antibody response. During sulfone therapy of lepromatous-type leprosy the allergic response causes diverse problems that are comparable to those occurring with serum sickness (fever, malaise, joint swelling and pain, hepatosplenomegaly), and there may be concurrent exacerbation of the existing leprous lesions. When the reaction occurs in the patient with tuberculoid-type leprosy, there is a reddening of existing skin lesions, new skin lesions appear, and neuritis increases. Lepra reaction occurring with tuberculoid-type leprosy is of shorter duration but greater severity than that with lepromatous type leprosy. Drug therapy is often discontinued until the allergic reaction subsides, and subsequent slowing of bacillus disintegration has a positive effect on the lepra reaction. Sulfone therapy may be resumed at low-dosage levels as the patient's condition improves, and the dosage is gradually increased to previous therapeutic levels.

Leprosy is considered arrested after lesions

heal, and drug therapy may continue for a long period of time. The drug regimen may include periodic "vacations" from drug therapy, and the plan may be one of the reasons that the drugs have a high safety record during the long periods of therapy.

Mycobacterium tuberculosis. Resistance of mycobacterium to phagocytosis results in sequestration of macrophage-filled bacteria in invaded tissues. Body defense mechanisms and the number of pathogens determine whether the organisms are effectively isolated or distributed widely in tissues, in which case reproduction and destruction of tissues causes tuberculosis.

The chief transmission route for the mycobacterium is droplets dispersed into the air by the cough or sneeze of an infected individual. Inhalation of the droplets or dust particles harboring surviving bacilli allows the bacillus to move toward pulmonary alveolar sites.

Primary lesions. Primary invasion by the mycobacterium precipitates a response by body defense mechanisms comparable to that occurring when other bacteria invade tissues. The thick lipoprotein wall of the mycobacterium resists destruction by macrophage lipases, and some bacteria survive in the macrophage cytoplasm. Mycobacterium-laden macrophages aggregate and are surrounded by fibrous tissue in nodules, or tubercles, that isolate the infecting organism. The center of the tubercle may become a dry, cheeselike substance through a process known as caseation. Toxic substances liberated by contained bacteria cause necrosis and liquification of cells in the tubercle. Host defenses may be sufficient to contain the pathogens, and the tubercle gradually is infiltrated with calcium phosphate. Calcified areas appear on chest x-ray films when invading organisms are confined after primary exposure. Bacilli in primary lesions may remain quiescent for years.

Secondary infection. Endogenous foci may liberate mycobacterium to cause disease when host resistance is lowered, or exogenous invasion of large numbers of pathogens may precipitate tuberculosis. About 3% of the adults with tuberculosis have primary exposure-induced disease, but initial, or primary, exposure is the chief factor in tuberculosis of children. Most adults diagnosed as having tuberculosis are thought to be infected from endogenous foci. Pulmonary tissues are the most common sites of tubercles, or cavities, but acid-fast bacilli may travel or be carried by macrophages to tissues distant from the oral portal of entry or pulmonary tubercles.

Tuberculosis prophylaxis. Isoniazid (Table 2-7) has become the most important drug for prophylaxis of individuals after exposure to tuberculosis. Isoniazid is also used for treatment of persons with positive tuberculin test reactions who have neither x-ray nor clinical evidence of tuberculosis. Isoniazid therapy may be continued for up to a year in either patient population.

Isoniazid is thought to provide protection by interfering with synthesis of the lipoprotein cell wall of the mycobacterium. Isoniazid has no effect on the natural synthesis of vitamins in bacteria, but it has an effect on the host central nervous system attributed to interference with pyridoxine levels in the body. The drug competes with pyridoxal phosphate for the enzyme (apotryptophanase) necessary for synthesis of the vitamin. Administration of pyridoxine (vitamin B_6) concurrent with isoniazid decreases the incidence of central nervous system adverse effects (i.e., hyperreflexia, paresthesias of the extremities, vertigo).

Isoniazid may cause false-positive reactions for glycosuria with cupric sulfate reagent testing methods. Benedict's qualitative reagent is slightly more sensitive than Clinitest to interference of isoniazid metabolites so that false-positive reactions occur more frequently with Benedict's solution.

Widespread distribution of isoniazid to patrons regularly eating at a cafeteria where several employees were diagnosed as having tuberculosis resulted in a high incidence of viral hepatitis–like syndrome in many of the population. A retrospective study showed a direct relationship between hepatotoxicity and alcoholism in the individuals taking isoniazid. The incident demonstrates the desirability of history taking and physical examination to discover chronic health problems before initiation of therapy. Follow-up during therapy allows evaluation of the effectiveness of the drugs and definition of emerging problems (i.e., hepatotoxicity, depression of bone marrow, skin rash). The recent practice of prescribing only one month's supply of the drug provides an opportunity for follow-up of progress and problems when the patient returns for a prescription for additional tablets.

Like all long-term pharmacotherapeutic programs for prevention of disease, isoniazid therapy is fraught with problems of the individual's commitment to following the plan when he is in a state of good health. Telephone contact with individuals that fail to return for prescriptions helps in many instances. The positive relationships established at initial contact with health team members often is a primary factor in continuance of therapy.

Tuberculosis therapy. Bacterial resistance to tuberculostatic drugs develops fairly rapidly. Combinations of drugs seems to decrease the emergence of resistant strains and decrease the incidence of adverse effects occurring when any one of the drugs is used singly for therapy. The primary group of drugs used for therapy of tuberculosis are streptomycin sulfate, isoniazid, and varying forms of aminosalicylic acid. Combination of the drugs causes a tuberculostatic effect on susceptible mycobacteria during the time they are actively dividing.

Drug therapy for the patient with tuberculosis can be a long period of treatment with frequent changes in the drug regimen to control organisms that acquire resistance to the drugs to which they they were initially susceptible. Rest and a nutritious diet are important aspects of tuberculosis therapy, as the defense mechanisms of the host are needed for phagocytosis of the nonreproducing bacteria. It is also important that the patient follow the prescribed schedule for drug use to delay the emergence of mutant strains resistant to drugs.

Drug therapy is instituted when there is clinical evidence of tuberculosis. Extensive cavitation in pulmonary areas may require surgical intervention, but drug therapy is often planned after surgery. X-ray films, sputum cultures, and gastric washings provide evidence of the presence of disease-causing *Mycobacterium tuberculosis*. The diagnosis is often made when patients arrive at the hospital for treatment of other problems. Routine chest x-ray films on admission of patients is a primary factor in the frequent diagnosis of tuberculosis. Confirmation of the x-ray findings includes examination of sputum and gastric washings, but therapy may be instituted immediately when the patient is debilitated or acutely ill. Mycobacteria are cultured for 3 weeks before a final report of growth is available.

During the acute phase of therapy, streptomycin sulfate may be administered daily for an intensive attack on the bacteria. As discussed earlier in this chapter, streptomycin sulfate increases the permeability of the cell membrane and causes misreading of the genetic construction code by the mycobacterium. The drug is the prototype of the group of antibiotics obtained from *Streptomyces,* and other derivatives of the fungus (capreomycin sulfate, cycloserine, rifampin, viomycin sulfate) are employed when streptomycin sulfate is contraindicated for the patient. The advantage of oral administration is offered by cycloserine and rifampin (Table 2-7). Bacterial resistance, neurotoxicity and nephrotoxicity are lessened by concurrent use of isoniazid and aminosalicylic acid when one of the *Streptomyces* antibiotics is employed. After the intensive period of therapy, the antibiotics may be administered two or three times a week, and the spacing of dosage decreases the incidence of neurotoxicity. Like streptomycin sulfate, each of the antibiotics employed for therapy of tuberculosis has a spectrum of effect that includes other important pathogens, but their chief use is for *Mycobacterium tuberculosis* control.

Concurrent administration of aminosalicylates with other tuberculostatic drugs is known to increase the effectiveness of the therapeutic plan, but the mode of action is not completely clear. Generic forms of the aminosalicylates (including benzoylpas) are listed on Table 2-7. The drugs are thought to interfere with bacterial synthesis of folic acid by providing a substitute for para-aminobenzoic acid during folic acid synthesis.

Gastric irritation is a common problem during therapy with aminosalicylates, but the problem may be decreased by administering the drug with meals or with an antacid. Metabolites of the drug cause a false-positive reaction for glycosuria when Benedict's qualitative reagent is employed for urine testing.

When rifampin is used with aminosalicylic acid, administration of the two agents is separated by 8 to 12 hours because rifampin absorption is decreased when the drugs are given at close intervals. The patient taking rifampin should be told that the drug may cause urine, feces, and sweat to have an orange-red hue.

Ethambutol hydrochloride, ethionamide, and pyrazinoic acid amide are second-line drugs used for treatment of patients with tuberculosis only when the primary group of drugs are ineffective in control. Each of the drugs is used as part of a combination of drugs because resistant strains develop in a manner comparable to that of the primary drugs. The drugs bind with rapidly growing mycobacterium to inhibit cell metabolism and prevent multiplication. Visual disturbances with field defects and temporary loss of vision have occurred during therapy with ethambutol hydrochloride.

Improvement in the patient's status may require a protracted period of drug therapy. X-ray films and sputum may show evidence of mycobacterium control within one month, but cavitation may require eight months before regression is evident on x-ray films. Reevaluation of progress is planned after recovery, but the patient must be aware that maintenance of his health status is important to prevention of reoccurrence of active tuberculosis.

Patient care

Concurrent with local responses to invading pathogens, there is a generalized increase in metabolic activity as the body attempts to resist the invasion. While plans are being formulated for treatment of the specific pathogen or infection site, measures should be planned to minimize the generalized effect of increased metabolic work.

Nursing guidelines. Efforts are directed at conserving energy and providing nutrients and fluids in amounts necessary to meet the increased demands of the body. A natural tendency to sleep when the temperature is elevated protects most people, but the stoic individual must be helped to understand the relationship of rest to body work.

Temperature elevation occurring with most infections is a positive physiologic mechanism that enhances phagocytosis and antibody formation. While the temperature is increased, there is a concurrent increase in cardiac and respiratory rate that assists in heat dissipation. The cardiac rate may increase 8 beats a minute with each 1.8° F. temperature increase.

Accelerated metabolic activity increases caloric costs, but the body can use its glycogen stores to meet nutritive needs for short periods of time. When the internal temperature rises, dilation of surface capillaries allows rapid heat dissipation. The quantity of water lost in the process increases the amount of fluid intake needed to maintain fluid balance. Replacement needs are predicted on the basis of normal obligatory losses (Fig. 2-2), plus the estimated

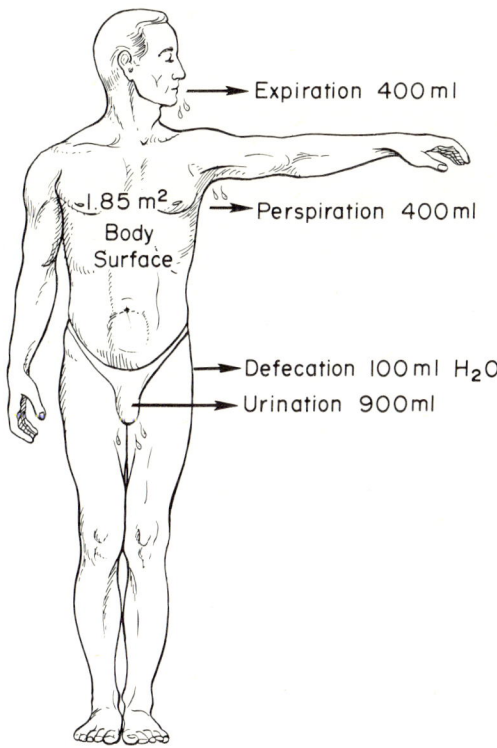

Fig. 2-2. Obligatory water output of an adult with a normal metabolic rate is approximately 1800 ml. each day. Water is the vehicle for dissipation of heat and excretion of wastes.

loss by diaphoresis (perspiration). Careful assessment of fluid balance is necessary to protect tissue hydration. Nonmeasurable or insensible losses by respiration (400 ml.) and perspiration (400 ml.) at normal metabolic rates provide guidelines for estimation of losses when an elevated metabolic rate increases respiratory rate and perspiration. Because 80% of the body's heat is dissipated through the skin surface, there will be an appreciable increase in water losses when internal temperature rises. Estimated losses by expiration and perspiration can be added to the minimal water output required to dilute metabolic waste products for urinary excretion (900 ml.). The sum of the calculations provides a guide for replacement needs of the patient with an elevated metabolic rate. The quantity and specific gravity of urine provide validating information about the adequacy of hydration and replacement needs. Excess fluid intake allows rapid renal excretion of the anti-infective drug and can decrease the effectiveness of drug therapy.

Whenever patients are responsible for self-administration of an anti-infective agent, they should understand the unique use of the drug for the particular infection. The foregoing statement is based on observations of people sharing their drugs with others who seem to have a similar problem. The predictable effect of the drug and the necessity for continued use beyond the time when there are overt signs of infection should be explained to the patient. The patient must understand the necessity for employing the drug during the entire prescribed period to assure eradication of the offending pathogen.

Assessment of drug effect. Decrease in bacterial growth will be reflected in a decrease in metabolic activity. The body temperature will gradually drop until it returns to near-normal levels. The decreased need for nutrients and oxygen will decrease cardiac and respiratory rate. Perhaps most importantly, the patient will begin to feel better. Although each of the preceding factors is important, cautious optimism and careful guidance of activity are necessary until the body replenishes reserves and equilibrium is established.

The specific attack site of the organism gradually becomes less inflamed, swollen, and painful. For example, the individual with a streptococcus infection of the oropharynx may find it possible to swallow small amounts of liquid without the excruciating pain originally present. He must understand the rationale for the 10-day therapy program required to control his streptococcal infection. With the exception of infections caused by beta-hemolytic streptococci, antibacterial therapy is continued for 48 to 72 hours after the temperature returns to normal levels and evidence of improvement is established.

Tissue or exudate cultures are obtained before initiating therapy with an anti-infective agent. Repeat cultures and bacterial susceptibility tests may be used by the physician to determine whether the bacterial invasion is being inhibited by the drug. The leukocyte count provides a guide to the status of the generalized response to the invasion. Improvement is indicated by return of leukocyte counts to the normal range (5000 to 10,000/mm.^{3}). When the patient's condition improves, revision in the administration route or dosage may be planned to protect against emergence of adverse reactions to the drug.

Assessment of drug adverse effect. The potential for yeast and fungal overgrowth during anti-infective drug therapy must be considered in planning observations throughout the pharmacotherapeutic program. The diversity of sites that can be involved makes it necessary to investigate carefully the patient's complaint of irritation or change in function (i.e., a female may complain of persistent perineal itching and vaginal discharge). Although growth characteristics often make identification relatively simple, cultures are taken prior to institution of therapy for removal of the particular organism.

Changes in physiologic function or emerging problems during therapy require prompt exploration. Alternate pathogens may gain supremacy because they are resistant to the effects of the anti-infective drug. The new organism may be an opportunist taking advantage of the decreased resistance of children and debilitated or elderly patients immediately after recovery from a major bacterial invasion. When new problems arise (i.e., increased thick, tenacious mucus, diarrhea), immediate consultation with the physician should be planned. Cultures (i.e., tracheal aspirate, stool) are used to determine whether new pathogens exist. Early therapy is important for the patient who has recently recovered from an infectious process.

Pruritus, redness, or skin rash may indicate hypersensitivity, or allergy, to the anti-infective agent. Progression of the problem may be rapid, and administration of the drug should be postponed until the physician has been consulted. Description of the areas involved, the intensity of color, and the size and height of individual elevations or plateaus on the skin are important content of the report.

Prevention of hypersensitivity, or allergic, reactions offers more protection to the patient than therapy after a problem emerges. The physician plans specific inquiry during his interview with the patient, but "minor" incidences may not be discussed by the patient during the stressful time of the diagnostic interview. Any statement of past difficulty with drugs (or other allergic reactions) should be noted and shared with nursing and medical team members. Particular allergies are printed on large labels and attached prominently on the patient's record to guard against the inadvertent administration of drugs that are known to precipitate an allergic response in the patient. The establishment of automatic stop and renewal directives in hospitals is evidence of general concern with unnecessarily long use of the highly potent and allergy-producing anti-infective drugs. Use of a prescribed anti-infective drug is limited to a definite period (i.e., 72 hours), and continued drug use requires a new prescription from the physician.

REFERENCES

Adkinson, N. F., Jr., Thompson, W. L., Maddrey, W. C., and Lichtenstein, L. M.: Routine use of penicillin skin testing on an inpatient service, The New England Journal of Medicine 285:22, 1971.

Atkins, Elisha, and Bodel, Phyllis: Fever, The New England Journal of Medicine 286:27, 1972.

Bierman, C. Warren, Pierson, William E., Zeitz, Stanley J., Hoffman, Leonard S., and Van Arsdel, Paul P., Jr.: Reactions associated with ampicillin therapy, The Journal of the American Medical Association 220:1098, 1972.

Cherry, James D., and Barta, R. A., Jr.: Some principles of pediatric, parenteral, penicillin therapy, Medical Times 95:129, 1967.

Derrington, A. W.: Oral penicillins in clinical practice, Clinical Medicine 74:17, 1967.

Downs, Ann Wright, and Cleland, Virginia S.: Bacteriuria and urinary tract infection in infancy and childhood. A review, Nursing Research 20:131, 1971.

Fair, William F.: The effect of cephaloridine on normal renal function, Journal of Urology 107:2, 1972.

Fekety, F. Robert, Jr.: Gastrointestinal complications of antibiotic therapy, The Journal of the American Medical Association 203:210, 1968.

Fox, C. Fred: The structure of cell membranes, Scientific American 226:30, Feb., 1972.

Gorini, Luigi: Antibiotics and the genetic code, Scientific American 214:102, April, 1966.

Grollman, Arthur: How drugs work: the antibiotics, Resident-Intern Consultant 1:20, Nov., 1972.

Idsøe, O., Guthe, T., Willcox, R. R., and DeWeck, A. L.: Nature and extent of penicillin side reactions, with particular reference to fatalities from anaphylactic shock, Bulletin of the World Health Organization 38:159, 1968.

Kunin, Calvin M.: Antibiotic usage in patients with renal impairment, Hospital Practice 7:141, 1972.

Olon, Lawrence P., and Holvey, David N.: Evaluation of tetracyline phosphate complex, demethylchlortetracycline hydrochloride and methacycline hydrochloride, Clinical Medicine 75:33, 1968.

Orten, James M., and Neuhaus, Otto W.: Biochemistry, ed. 8, St. Louis, 1970, The C.V. Mosby Co.

Pankey, George A.: Unusual microbial toxic reactions, Medical Clinics of North America 51:925, 1967.

Pryles, C. V.: Antimicrobial therapy in staphylococcal disease of children, Pediatric Clinics of North America 15:167, 1968.

Purcell, Robert H., and Chanock, Robert M.: Role of mycoplasmas in human respiratory disease, Medical Clinics of North America 51:791, 1967.

Reilly, Mary Jo, editor. American hospital formulary services, vol. 1, sect. 8:00, Washington, D. C., 1973, American Society of Hospital Pharmacists.

Ruddy, Shaun, Gigli, Irma, and Austen, K. Frank: The complement system of man, The New England Journal of Medicine 287:489; 492; 545; 642, 1972.

Sharon, Nathan.: The bacterial cell wall, Scientific American 220:92, May, 1969.

Smith, Alice L.: Microbiology and pathology, ed. 10, St. Louis, 1972, The C. V. Mosby Co.

Smith, Ian Maclean: Death from staphylococci, Scientific American 218:84, Feb., 1968.

Steiner, Morris: Newer and second-line drugs in the treatment of drug-resistant tuberculosis in children, Medical Clinics of North America 51:1153, 1967.

Watanabe, Tsutomu: Infectious drug resistance, Scientific American 217:19, Dec., 1967.

3

Fungus and parasite invasion

Fungus invasion
    Fungus identification
    Pharmacodynamics
    Patient care
Amebiasis
    Intestinal amebiasis
    Extraintestinal amebiasis
    Pharmacodynamics
    Patient care
Malaria
    Plasmodia invasion
    Benign tertian malaria
    Pernicious malignant malaria
    Pharmacodynamics
    Patient care
Helminth infestation
    Intestinal helminthiasis
    Extraintestinal helminthiasis
    Pharmacodynamics
    Patient care

FUNGUS INVASION

Fungus can cause superficial but persistent infection (i.e., dermatomycosis), or widely disseminated mycotic infection may affect many organ systems. The ability of the fungi to survive and multiply in an acidic or glucose-rich environment and to form granulomas affects their assessability and durability during drug therapy. For example, eradication of bone and meningeal fungus may take one to two years of sustained therapy for *Coccidioides.*

Fungus identification

The characteristic appearance and location of fungus growth on surface tissues (i.e., tinea capitis, tinea corporis, tinea pedis) facilitates identification of dermatomycoses. Scrapings of hair or skin can be cultured or examined under a microscope to verify the presence of fungus and to identify it.

Preliminary identification of the causal organism when systemic mycotic invasion is suspected may be accomplished by dermal reaction tests, using dilutions of strains of the organism indicated by the symptom complex presented by the patient. Positive tests indicate exposure, and definition of causation is incomplete until the fungus is grown on culture media. Four weeks are required before final reports of fungus growth are available. The specific dermal reaction tests for identification of pathogen exposure are presented in Chapter 4. Extracellular fluids or tissues are cultured to identify the fungus prior to initiation of therapy.

Pharmacodynamics

Many drug combinations are in common use for superficial fungal infections, and it is necessary to know the action of each ingredient to understand the predictable effect on the patient. The patient's understanding of the therapeutic plan may have a profound effect on eradication of the organism. For example, the patient who is relieved of swelling and itching by the use of a cortisone preparation may refuse to use the antifungal agent because he obtains greater relief from the drug that is minimizing the tissue response to the fungus. Explanation of the long-term plan for removal of the causative organism may increase his commitment to follow the prescribed plan of therapy.

Local fungus eradication. Griseofulvin and nystatin are available as topical and vaginal antifungal drug forms for superficial or assessable infections. Concurrent use of the systemic drugs may be planned to provide an intense attack on the fungi. For example, griseofulvin may be applied topically to the infection site while oral tablets are being taken to raise the capillary level of drug in blood nourishing the invasion site. The plan allows incorporation of griseofulvin into existing and newly formed keratinized tissue and destruction of the fungus.

Griseofulvin and similar drugs have changed the tiresome and discouraging course of treatment necessary for surface attack on fungus invading keratinized tissue (skin, nails, hair). Only 2 weeks of intensive topical and systemic treatment may be required to eradicate tinea corporis from keratinized tissue.

Griseofulvin acts as a structural analog of purine. During formation of epithelial cells, the analog is utilized for synthesis of nucleic acid in new cells. Griseofulvin-containing keratin appears at the base of the stratum corneum in 48 to 72 hours. Cellular division carries the antifungal drug as a keratin component, and newly formed tissue is resistant to invasion of fungi. Concurrent topical application of griseofulvin inhibits reproduction of fungus in superficial tissue layers. Surface layers of fungus-containing tissue are gradually shed and new keratinized tissue is fungus resistant.

Drug effect is evident when new, normal tissue appears at the surface. Infected tissue (with drug-inactivated fungi) may be present in surface layers of nondesquamated tissue. For eradication of the organism, the treatment must be continued beyond evidence of improvement. The length of the therapeutic period depends on the time necessary for keratinization of new tissue and desquamation of old tissue. The slower-growing toenails may require 6 months or longer for growth of new nail and removal of infected portions of the toenail.

Absorption of either oral form of lipid-soluble griseofulvin (Table 3-1) is enhanced when the drug is ingested with a meal high in fat content. Use of griseofulvin is relatively problem free, although patients may have some minor nonspecific complaints during therapy. The micronized form of griseofulvin produces higher serum and tissue levels of the drug, but the pharmacodynamic effect of both forms is comparable.

Both nystatin and griseofulvin are employed to suppress the fungi commonly appearing as overgrowth during anti-infective drug therapy. The saprophytes (actinomyces, candidae, aspergilli) found in the oral cavity and gastrointestinal tract are susceptible to the effects of both drugs.

Nystatin, in addition to oral tablets (Table 3-1), is available in liquid form for local treatment of *Candida albicans* in the oral cavity. The physician may prescribe use of the liquid as an agitated mouthwash or gargle. Swallowing or expectoration of the liquid will depend on the distribution of the fungal growth.

Nystatin is commonly employed for treatment of intestinal or topical *Candida* invasion. The drug is incorporated into the cell wall of the pathogen. Nystatin binds tenaciously to the cell wall sterols and causes a detergent-like effect that increases the permeability of the membrane. Destruction of fungi occurs as intracellular components leak through the permeable wall.

Systemic fungus eradication. Amphotericin B (Table 3-1) is used principally for disseminated fungal infections. Many of the less common deep mycoses (blastomycosis, coccidioidomycosis, cryptococcosis, histoplasmosis, sporotrichosis) are susceptible to destruction by the

Table 3-1. Dosage range of antifungal drugs

Nonproprietary name	Proprietary (trade) name	Daily adult dosage range
Amphotericin B	Fungizone	I.V.: 0.25-1.5 mg./kg.
Flucytosine	Ancobon	Oral: 50-150 mg./kg.
Griseofulvin	Fulvicin, Grifulvin	Oral: 0.5-2 Gm.
Griseofulvin, micronized	Grifulvin V, Grisactin	Oral: 0.25-1 Gm.
Nystatin	Mycostatin	Oral: 1.5 million-3 million U. (÷3)

drug. Amphotericin B is frequently employed when fungal growth invades vital organs.

Amphotericin B acts in a manner comparable to that of nystatin in accomplishing a fungicidal effect. Concurrent with its detergent-like effect on cell wall sterols of fungi, amphotericin B may disrupt the membrane of normal body cells, which also contain sterols. Affected cells gradually lose intracellular content. Paresthesias and muscle weakness are related to decreased cellular glycolysis and loss of potassium and magnesium ions from body cells. Potassium-containing foods or potassium supplements may replace the essential cellular component during the period of amphotericin B therapy.

Parenteral administration delivers the drug to target tissues for control of fungus invasion. Therapy is started with low dosage that is increased in a stepwise progression to the maximal level planned for therapy of the individual patient. Almost half the patients have drug-induced chills and hyperpyrexia with body temperatures up to 105° F. during therapy. Concurrent use of antipyretic drugs and an automatic hypothermal blanket are planned to control the hyperpyrexia and to allow continuance of therapy.

Nephrotoxic effects of amphotericin B often limit the course of therapy. More than three fourths of the patients receiving the drug have a gradually progressing decrease in renal function, with increasing retention of nitrogenous wastes. Renal tubular function is compromised by the direct toxic effect of amphotericin B on the tubules and concurrent constriction of renal blood vessels induced by the drug. The blood urea nitrogen (BUN) levels are analyzed daily throughout the course of therapy, and elevation of the levels above 40 mg./100 ml. may necessitate discontinuance of the drug. Cessation of therapy allows gradual return of normal renal function, and therapy may be reinstituted at a later time.

Nausea and anorexia occurring during initiation of therapy are generally controlled by concurrent use of antiemetics, and the problems tend to decrease as therapy continues. Attempts are made to minimize the number of disturbing problems during therapy so that drug administration may continue for the long period (6 weeks to 4 months) necessary to eradicate the pathogen.

Intravenous administration of amphotericin B requires a period of 6 hours of infusion to accomplish the prolonged serum levels necessary to annihilation of organ fungi. Because the drug is light sensitive in solution, the intravenous bottle and tubing are covered (i.e., with a paper bag) during the long daily infusion period. Alternate-day administration may be planned when the maximum dosage level is reached. The drug has a slow urinary excretion rate that makes it possible to maintain consistent drug levels in tissues for protracted periods once the therapeutic range is reached.

Flushing of the skin and generalized pain are adverse effects that add to the discomfort of the patient receiving the drug. Allergic reactions may occur at any time during the long period of therapy, but the incidence is highest early in the course of drug therapy. Occurrence of anaphylaxis, thrombocytopenia, or convulsions necessitates discontinuance of amphotericin B administration.

Flucytosine is an oral antifungal drug used for control of cryptococcus and *Candida albicans*. Flucytosine does not enter human cells, but in fungi the drug interferes with deoxyribonucleic acid (DNA) synthesis by disrupting pyrimidine production. During reproduction of new fungus cells the analog is picked up by the cells as they assemble nucleotides, and the drug substitute disrupts synthesis of proteins during cell construction. The antimetabolite action of flucytosine is similar to that of antineoplastic drugs which trick the cell into picking up a drug analog rather than the nucleotide needed for reproduction.

Flucytosine produces less intense adverse effects than does amphotericin B, but the former does cause skin rash and bone marrow depression (leukopenia, erythrocytopenia, thrombocytopenia). Ninety percent of the drug is excreted in the urine, and therefore monitoring of urinary output is planned to assure that the quantity of urine is sufficient to allow drug elimination.

Pyrimidines are essential to construction of cells, and inhibition of cellular development by analog substitution may affect normal body cells with high rates of mitotic activity (i.e., reticuloendothelial, intestinal, gonadal, epidermal tissues). Patient care during periods of therapy with antimetabolites is presented in detail in Chapter 26.

Patient care

The long periods necessary for eradication of systemic fungal infections and the discouraging tendency to periodic relapses make the therapeutic program a frustrating and discouraging process for the patient. Monitoring of progress and problems during therapy with the potent drugs used for treatment of systemic mycotic infection necessitates long periods of hospitalization. Discomfort caused by adverse effects and concern that the infection will progress while therapy is suspended to reestablish physiologic equilibrium are anxiety-producing aspects of the therapeutic program for the patient with systemic mycotic infection.

Many individuals with superficial fungal infection are capable of self-care. Instructions, clearly stated, and definition of specific measures to be taken during drug use should improve readiness to participate in removal of the causative fungus and prevention of its spread. For example, the patient with tinea pedis (athlete's foot) benefits by clarification of specific hygienic measures required to prevent spread of the localized fungus infection to adjacent parts of the body and to other individuals. Discussion of the contribution that sandals or comparable footwear make toward maintaining a dry, cool environment that is unfavorable to fungus growth and the necessity of discarding or laundering all materials placed in contact with infected tissues provides some of the guidelines the patient can use in managing his therapeutic plan.

AMEBIASIS

The parasites causing disease in man by invasion and erosion of the intestinal wall are *Entamoeba histolytica* (ameba), *Trichomonas hominis* (flagellate), and *Balantidium coli* (ciliate). Infestation by the ciliate is uncommon, but when present, it can extensively destroy the intestinal mucosa. Bleeding and infection of ulcerated craters may cause death.

The least destructive parasite is the flagellate. It normally maintains a saprozoic relationship in the large intestine, but occasionally it is indicted as a causative factor in bleeding of the mucosa and diarrhea. A flagellate relative, *T. vaginalis,* causes a persistent irritation, with a white frothy vaginal discharge. This flagellate eluded attempts at control until the use of amebicides for a systemic approach to trichomonad eradication was initiated. The drugs are taken by both the male and female sexual partners, and conscientious users have had remarkable relief from the troublesome *Trichomonas.* Furazolidone (Furoxone, Tricofuron) taken orally (400 mg./24 hours, divided into 4 doses) or metronidazole (Flagyl) taken orally (500 to 750 mg./24 hours, divided into 2 or 3 doses) show promise of eradicating the flagellate as a cause of vaginal infections.

Amebiasis is the term used to describe infections caused by *E. histolytica.* Like its relative *E. coli,* it sometimes is a harmless bacterial feeder. *E. histolytica* may change characteristics and destroy the lining of the intestinal tract to feed on red blood cells. It is estimated that up to 10% of the American population have amebiasis. Infection occurs after ingestion of cysts with food or other products. The capsule of the cyst is resistant to destruction by gastric acids, but the vegetative form is destroyed by human stomach acids.

Intestinal amebiasis

Cysts pass to the intestine where the digestive juices disintegrate the capsule and release the vegetative ameba. Liberated amebae digest a small cavity in the intestinal mucosal wall where they reproduce to form colonies of tiny *trophozoites.* Utilization of wall proteins for nutrients produces a large crater that extends into the submucosa. The crater looks like a flask, with the opening on the intestinal lumen. Periodic formation and liberation of quadrinucleate cysts into the feces provides a source of infection for other individuals. The diagnosis of amebiasis can be made by the appearance of cysts in the stool.

Healthy individuals may have adequate reparative function to heal, or close, ulcerated areas or craters almost as fast they are formed.

Many individuals are cyst-carriers without overt evidence of disease, and they provide the reservoir and source for spread of the cysts to others.

The most common type of amebiasis is a chronic, or latent, state that includes periodic emergence of symptoms. Patients may have vague intestinal disturbances, weight loss, and generalized muscular aching.

Lowered host resistance allows rapid proliferation of the ameba and the appearance of amebic dysentery as the colon becomes irritated by the invading pathogens. During the acute episode of violent dysentery, the stool contains blood and mucus in large quantity. Propagation of amebae may deepen intestinal wall craters enough to cause perforation during the continual propulsive movements associated with acute dysentery.

Extraintestinal amebiasis

The passage of trophozoites through the intestinal wall into the portal venous circulation to the liver may cause cavitation and abscess formation in hepatic lobes. The presence of amebae in the intestinal craters creates problems of assessability for drug therapy, but the problem is compounded when trophozoites move to hepatic, pulmonary, or brain tissues. Multiplication of trophozoites and ingestion of tissue for their nutritional needs evacuate cavities in the tissues and gradually disrupt organ function. For example, multiple craters in hepatic tissue gradually cause disruption of liver function and blood circulation through its vital metabolic tissue. Hepatitis-like symptoms are early manifestations of amebic invasion of the liver. Trophozoite activity may cause progressive destruction and abscess formation in any of the tissues invaded. Pharmacotherapy is the most desirable approach to treatment of organ abscesses because surgical incision liberates the contained amebae and other amebae traveling to the cavity from adjacent tissue sites.

Pharmacodynamics

Extraintestinal amebicides. Emetine hydrochloride (Table 3-2) is the primary drug used for control of extraintestinal amebiasis. The drug causes degeneration of the nucleus and reticulation of the ameba cytoplasm. A 10-day course of therapy is usually planned to provide an amebicidal effect on organ parasites. The 10-day course of therapy also minimizes the incidence of adverse effects, and additional protection is provided by a week-long rest period from drug therapy before a second course is started.

Emetine hydrochloride may be effective in limiting the number of amebae in an acute attack of dysentery, but it does not eliminate intestinal cysts. After the acute episode is controlled, administration of a cyst-destroying drug is necessary for eradication of cysts from sequestered sites in the intestinal lumen.

Emetine hydrochloride is slowly absorbed and slowly excreted, and the drug has been found in patients' urine 40 to 60 days after therapy has been terminated. High concentrations of the drug are found in the liver, and hepatic tissue levels account for the effectiveness of the drug in control of amebiasis in the frequently invaded liver tissue.

Emetine bismuth iodide is administered orally, and the emetine is released by the activity

Table 3-2. Dosage range of antiparasitic drugs: amebicides

Nonproprietary name	Proprietary (trade) name	Daily adult dosage range
Chiniofon	Quinoxyl	Oral: 0.75 Gm.
Diiodohydroxyquin	Diodoquin, Ioquin, Moebiquin, Yodoxin	Oral: 0.65-2 Gm. (÷1-3)
Diloxanide	Entamide	Oral: 12 mg./kg.
Diloxanide furoate	Furamide	Oral: 1.5 Gm. (÷3)
Emetine bismuth iodide		Oral: 200 mg.
Emetine hydrochloride	Glarubin	I.M.: 60 mg.
Glaucarubin	Amoebicon, Broxolin, Milibis	Oral: 3 mg./kg.
Glycobiarsol	Entero-Vioform, Vioform	Oral: 1.5 Gm. (÷3)
Iodochlorhydroxyquin		Oral: 0.75-1.5 Gm. (÷3)

of intestinal enzymes as the drug enters the intestine. The drug acts in a manner comparable to that of emetine hydrochloride to produce an amebicidal effect at intestinal and extraintestinal sites.

The cumulative tendency of emetine hydrochloride and emetine bismuth iodide increases the incidence of adverse effects on major organ function during therapy. Gastrointestinal disturbances and dizziness are common during use of the drugs. Nausea and vomiting with associated dizziness result from drug stimulation of the chemoreceptor trigger zone in the medulla and the problems occur with oral or parenteral administration of the drugs.

The incidence of adverse effects during therapy decreases appreciably when the patient is confined to bed during the period of drug administration and for several days after the course of therapy. Monitoring of cardiac status by regularly scheduled electrocardiographic tracings, and apical pulse and blood pressure monitoring are a planned component of the pharmacotherapeutic plan. Careful monitoring is planned to allow early definition of drug effect on myocardial tissue. Emetine has a direct irritating effect on cardiac tissue and may cause an increase in the heart rate, with concurrent slight decrease in systolic blood pressure. Electrocardiographic evidence of progressive cardiac failure (inversion of the T waves, prolongation of the Q-T and P-R intervals) follows the emergence of tachycardia, and therefore the drug is usually discontinued when tachycardia occurs.

Bed rest also benefits patients having generalized skeletal muscle weakness and activity-related dyspnea as adverse effects of the drugs. The gluteal site of injection of emetine hydrochloride often shows evidence of regional myositis, and the patient may complain of aching, tenderness, and stiffness of muscles adjacent to the injection site.

Intestinal amebicides. Control of parasites in the intestinal lumen can be accomplished by most of the amebicides (Table 3-2). Glycobiarsol is an arsenical that has a direct amebicidal effect. The low absorption rate from the intestinal tract makes it an effective agent with few adverse effects. The drug is eliminated in the feces, and the patient should be informed that the drug may cause his stools to be colored black. Because of its bismuth component, glycobiarsol tends to reduce peristalsis. Slowing of bowel activity for the patient with dysentery can be a positive rather than a negative effect.

Iodine-containing drugs—chiniofon, diiodohydroxyquin, and iodochlorhydroxyquin—are absorbed in very small amounts from the gastrointestinal tract. Therapy usually is continued for 3 weeks, and the course of treatment eradicates the parasites in 80% of the patients. The high iodine content of the drugs (i.e., diiodohydroxyquin contains 64% iodine) has an amebicidal effect, and the lethal effect on trophozoites decreases the production of cysts. Iodine content of the drugs causes gastrointestinal disturbances and anal itching. When the drugs are distributed to large populations for prophylactic treatment to eliminate cyst-spreading from asymptomatic carriers, many individuals complain of diarrhea while taking the drug.

Antibiotics have been employed for eradication of intestinal amebae, but the adverse effects occuring with prolonged use outweigh the advantages. The purpose of antibiotic therapy is to deprive the ameba of nutritional sources by elimination of intestinal bacteria. Antibiotics are sometimes used as part of the therapeutic plan for treatment of acute amebiasis to decrease infection at ulcerated sites on the intestinal wall.

Diloxanide, diloxanide furoate, and glaucarubin (a plant derivative) are effective and relatively problem-free drugs employed for control of intestinal amebiasis. Continual search for synthetic drugs to eliminate amebiasis as a world health problem has led to clinical trials with many compounds. Simplicity of administration, low adverse effect incidence, and low cost are important factors when the drugs are distributed widely to eliminate human reservoirs of the parasite.

Patient care

The acutely ill patient is usually receptive to the need for removal of the cause of his problem. During an acute or prolonged episode of dysentery, dehydration, emaciation, and anemia are major problems. Plans are made to meet the urgent need for electrolyte, water, and blood replacement, and strenuous attempts to eradicate the ameba may await improvement in the patient's condition.

Asymptomatic individuals who are asked to take a drug regularly for a "nonexistent" problem need help to see relevance in the plan. Only through elimination of cyst-carriers and concurrent improvement in sanitation can the extensive problem of amebic dysentery be controlled.

Amebiasis is considered completely controlled when stools are cyst free. Repeated stool examinations are necessary to assure eradication of amebae from the individual. Cyst-free stools at the end of a two-year period after termination of therapy indicates cure of the ameba invasion.

MALARIA

An increasing number of people are exposed to the hazard of contacting malaria during world travel. In countries where the disease is endemic, acquisition of the plasmodia from the bite of an infected female *Anopheles* mosquito initiates the cyclic emergence of symptoms common to the disease.

Plasmodia invasion

Initially the half million or more plasmodia injected by the mosquito travel to body tissues (i.e., the liver) where they develop to large solid parasites (trophozoites). Within the trophozoite, the nucleus divides until there are several nucleated structures (schizonts) within the walls. After 6 to 9 days, rupture of the trophozoite allows the nucleated cells to move into the bloodstream. Released schizonts are called *merozoites*. Each merozoite invades a red blood cell to repeat the trophozoite-schizont-merozoite sequence. Rupture of the red blood cell wall releases merozoites into the bloodstream, and merozoites enter intact red blood cells to repeat the cycle. Within 2 weeks there is an adequate parasitic invasion to cause clinical evidence of malaria. Synchronized release of innumerable merozoites and red blood cell debris into the bloodstream has an effect on the infected individual. The foreign proteins precipitate an antigenic response (chills, sweating, fever) that occurs in cycles representing multiples of 24 hours. The timing of symptoms in the individual correlates with the biologic clock of the particular malarial plasmodia resident in his body. Intervention of drugs or natural cellular semi-immunity may break the merozoite cycling.

The life cycle of plasmodia affects the course of the disease, plans for prevention and treatment, and transmission of malaria. Merozoites are produced by asexual division, but periodically they form male or female gametocytes that may be withdrawn from host blood by the next mosquito biting the infected individual.

Natural immunity to malaria is uncommon. The sickle cell shape of erythrocytes seen in blacks is an evolutionary adaptive characteristic protecting against development of trophozoites in the red blood cell. In the tropics it lengthens life-expectancy of the inhabitants, but inheritance of the trait causes unnecessary fragility of the erythrocytes for individuals in temperate climates.

The frequently encountered strains of plasmodia causing malaria, *Plasmodium falciparum* and *P. vivax,* each have characteristics that affect prophylaxis and therapy. *P. falciparum* maintains life activity in the human host by erythrocyte cycling. *P. vivax,* in addition to the cyclic activity in erythrocytes, forms schizonts in body tissues. Schizonts release merozoites from exoerythrocyte sites into the bloodstream after the red blood cell cycling has ceased, and a relapse may occur. *Benign tertian malaria* and *pernicious malignant malaria* are terms describing the clinical course of the disease. Identification of the plasmodium invading the individual is accomplished by examination of peripheral blood samples. Blood for examination is drawn prior to administration of antimalarial drugs because they cause merozoites to leave peripheral blood.

Benign tertian malaria

Most of the 3000 cases of malaria reported in the United States during 1972 were caused by *P. vivax,* the primary cause of benign tertian malaria. Infection with *P. vivax* results in a mild form of malaria, with recurrent exacerbations of malarial symptoms for at least two years after primary infection in untreated individuals. Though *P. vivax* is the prevalent cause of benign tertian malaria, in limited areas of the world, *P. malariae* or *P. ovale* cause a comparable clinical disease.

The characteristic triad of symptoms (chills, fever, headache) may be accompanied by muscle aching and gastrointestinal disturbances. Chills preceding body temperature elevation may be violent, shaking paroxysms, and subsequent temperature elevation may be as high as 106° F. Cyclic occurrence of chills and fever follows the biologic clock of *P. vivax* that releases metabolic by-products of merozoite activity and toxic breakdown products of erythrocytes at 48-hour intervals. Chills may last for an hour, and subsequent temperature elevation may subside in 2 to 4 hours. The episode terminates with profuse diaphoresis, and heat dissipation returns the body temperature to normal levels. Exoerythrocyte schizonts release merozoites to propagate the cyclic erythrocyte stage of the malarial symptoms.

Pernicious malignant malaria

P. falciparum causes pernicious malignant malaria. Invasion by the plasmodium causes an acute hemolytic state that releases erythrocyte debris, with subsequent embolization of small blood vessels. Erythrocyte destruction causes anemia, and the patient's clinical status may proceed to a terminal shock state within a few hours.

Incomplete degradation of hemoglobin by merozoites releases granules of pigment into the circulation. The malarial pigment stimulates reticuloendothelial phagocytes to ingest and store the products in the liver, spleen, and bone marrow. Release of malarial pigment and hemoglobin may cause jaundice, hemoglobinemia, or hemoglobinuria. The presence of hemoglobin turns the urine a reddish black color, and the entity that terminates in acute renal failure is called blackwater fever.

Increased viscosity of the blood and adhesiveness of parasitic cells causes obstruction of small vessels in major organs, and obstruction of cerebral vessels (cerebral malaria) may be fatal. Prompt parenteral administration of antimalarial drugs with concurrent measures directed at decreasing clot formation (i.e., heparinization) and improving blood flow through the cerebral microcirculation by administration of low molecular weight dextran may abort the destructive effects of the plasmodial invasion.

Disruptive effects on all major organs require immediate attention during intensive antimalarial drug therapy. Dialysis may provide an alternate route for removal of metabolic wastes during acute renal failure, or osmotic diuretics may reinstitute urine output.

Initial peripheral blood parasite counts may exceed 50,000/mm.^{3}, and the blood counts are repeated twice daily to ascertain the effectiveness of antimalarial drugs in control of the plasmodia. Prompt treatment inhibits schizogony in the erythrocytes and gradually clears the plasmodia from the bloodstream.

P. falciparum has a less clearly defined chill-fever state than does *P. vivax* because there is a continual release of parasite metabolic end products and breakdown products of red blood cells. Paroxysms may be irregular, and the patient may have a continual state of hyperpyrexia, with some modification of peaks but fewer sudden spikes than occur in benign tertian malaria.

Pharmacodynamics

Therapy terminology. Understanding of the common terminology used in malaria control aids in defining the purpose and action site of drugs employed for prophylaxis or therapy. *Causal prophylaxis* describes agents used to intercede at primary tissue sites to eradicate the plasmodium before it can begin reproduction cycles. *Radical cure* is the term employed to describe agents used to destroy tissue parasites (i.e., *P. vivax*). *Suppressive prophylaxis* and *suppressive cure* describe interruption of the blood cycle phase. Drugs employed for suppressive cure over a prolonged period of time progressively eradicate tissue parasites. *Clinical cure* describes the relief of symptoms of a patient with an acute exacerbation of malaria.

Control of the erythrocytic cycling constitutes clinical cure, suppressive prophylaxis, and suppressive cure of *P. falciparum* and *P. vivax*. Additional therapy is necessary to produce a radical cure of *P. vivax* by destruction of the exoerythrocytic sites of schizonts that periodically release merozoites into the bloodstream.

Radical cure. Primaquine phosphate (Table 3-3) is the primary drug used for radical cure of *P. vivax*. Control of tissue sources of the plasmodium usually requires 14 days of therapy after infection, and therapy is continued for a period of 8 weeks after travel to endemic areas to prevent resurgence of malaria caused by tissue sources of *P. vivax*. The drug is taken orally with meals or an antacid to decrease gastric irritation.

Suppressive cure. A dual attack on the erythrocytic and exoerythrocytic phase of benign tertian malaria caused by *P. vivax* is generally planned for residents or travelers to areas where the parasite is endemic. Primaquine phosphate may be used with chloroquine phosphate or hydroxychloroquine sulfate to provide radical cure and suppressive cure of *P. vivax*. Consistent daily use of primaquine phosphate and weekly use of chloroquine phosphate eradicates both red blood cell and tissue reservoir parasites. Chloroquine phosphate inhibits oxygen uptake and interferes with nucleic acid synthesis in the plasmodium. It also modifies the gametocytes of *P. vivax* in a manner that prevents completion of the cycle for development when the mosquito ingests infected human blood. Primaquine phosphate has a lethal effect on all gametocytes within 3 days after therapy is started.

Clinical cure. Clinical cure of acute exacerbations of either *P. vivax* or *P. falciparum* may involve the use of chloroquine hydrochloride or amodiaquine hydrochloride (Table 3-3). The drugs are rapid-acting schizonticides, and the peripheral blood may become negative for plasmodium content within 48 to 72 hours after initiation of therapy. The patient may become afebrile within 24 to 48 hours. Continuation of therapy beyond the acute illness period can produce suppressive cure of *P. falciparum*.

Suppressive prophylaxis. The slow onset of action of chloroguanide hydrochloride and pyrimethamine negates their usefulness in acute attacks of malaria, but they are employed for suppressive prophylaxis. The drugs act as folic acid antagonists, and their effectiveness occurs as plasmodium are deprived of high levels of the material essential to nucleic acid synthesis. Therapy with either of the agents is continued for 4 weeks beyond the time of last exposure to assure eradication of the erythrocyte phase of malaria. Gametocyte development in the mosquito breeder of *P. falciparum* and *P. vivax* gametocytes is inhibited by the sterilizing effect of the drugs.

Plasmodium resistance. The low incidence of adverse effects of drugs at levels necessary for control of plasmodia makes regular use of the drugs possible. Continuance of the prescribed plan for drug use is necessary to prevent emergence of drug-resistant strains of plasmodia. Therapy is based on the particular plasmodium species and known resistant strains in endemic areas of the world. Prophylaxis begins prior to

Table 3-3. Dosage range of antiparasitic drugs: antimalarials

Nonproprietary name	Proprietary (trade) name	Daily adult dosage range
Amodiaquine hydrochloride	Camoquin	Oral: 400-600 mg.
Chloroguanide hydrochloride	Paludrine, Proguanil	Oral: 100-600 mg.
Chloroquine hydrochloride	Aralen	I.M.: 0.2-1 Gm. (÷2-3)
Chloroquine phosphate	Aralen, Roquine	Oral: Gm. 0.5-1.5 Gm. (÷1-2)
Hydroxychloroquine sulfate	Plaquenil	Oral: 0.2-1.2 Gm. (÷1-2)
Primaquine phosphate		Oral: 26.3-52.6 mg.
Pyrimethamine	Daraprim	Oral: 25-200 mg.
Quinacrine hydrochloride	Atabrine	Oral: 500 mg.
Quinine dihydrochloride		I.M.: 1.8-3 Gm. (÷3) I.V.: 300-600 mg.
Quinine sulfate		Oral: 0.3-3 Gm. (÷3)
Trimethoprim	Syraprim	Oral: 0.5 Gm.

entering the endemic country and continues during the period of residence and up to 10 weeks after leaving the area. Termination of therapy will depend on the plasmodium species exposure.

P. vivax has not acquired resistance to drugs used for control, but *P. falciparum* strains that are resistant to chloroquine and other synthetic drugs employed for control of the parasite are fairly common. Emergence of resistant strains makes prophylaxis and therapy difficult. Resistant strains of *P. falciparum* in Vietnam have widened the search for additional drugs for prophylactic use. Dapsone, an agent used for control of *Mycobacterium leprae*, was employed for a short time, but the incidence of drug-related agranulocytosis terminated use of the drug. Trimethoprim (Table 3-3) is a dihydrofolate reductase inhibitor being used for control of *P. falciparum* strains that are resistant to other antimalarial drugs.

Reserve plasmodicidals. Combinations of drugs have been employed to increase the effectiveness of malaria control, and quinine is one of the drugs used when plasmodium strains show resistance to chloroquine therapy. In tropical areas of South America, natives use the readily available bark of the cinchona tree to prepare quinine alkaloids for treatment of exacerbations of *P. vivax* malaria. Though the alkaloid acts as a schizonticidal and gametocidal agent, exoerythrocytic sources of the plasmodium and continued exposure to the infected mosquito cause a high recurrence rate of malaria.

The low cost of quinine sulfate and quinine dihydrochloride makes the drugs useful for control of malaria in underdeveloped endemic countries. Alkaloids derived from the bark of the cinchona tree, including quinacrine hydrochloride, cause a fairly high incidence of adverse effects when they are employed for prolonged periods of time. The potential for damage to the auditory and vestibular branches of the eighth cranial nerve and an irritating effect on cardiac tissue cause hearing loss, vertigo, and tachycardia. The hazards inherent in wide distribution of the drugs for malaria control without supervision for detection of emerging health problems has led to the use of safer synthetic substitutes for widespread malaria control.

Quinacrine hydrochloride has a high affinity for the nucleoproteins of liver and muscle, and this characteristic provides high tissue levels of the drug for parasite control. The drug was a primary antimalarial agent during World War II, but it has been replaced by new synthetic drugs. It remains as one of the reserve antimalarial agents that are employed when resistant strains of plasmodium do not respond to other drugs.

Tissue distribution. The drugs used for malaria control are widely distributed in body tissues, with concentrations in the erythrocytes and liver at least thirty times that of serum levels. High tissue levels expand their usefulness to the control of organ ameba infestations. Antimalarial drugs are excreted slowly by the kidneys. Metabolism occurs in the liver, and small quantities of the drugs appear in the feces.

Patient care

Individuals who are not ill have a difficult time remembering to take steps to preserve their wellness. The individual who is receiving drugs to prevent malaria will remember to take the drugs daily and weekly if a definite schedule is established. The young adult probably will take daily medication regularly if a schedule is planned for him to take the drug with his evening meal. Many young people skip breakfast and grab lunch, but they eat one meal each day. The weekly dosage of the drug prescribed should be ritualistically planned to be taken on a particular day of the week.

An exacerbation of malaria exhausts the patient. Measures appropriate to any patient with sharp body temperature extremes (i.e., alternating chills as the temperature rises and profuse diaphoresis as the temperature falls) will ease the discomfort of the patient. Until drugs control plasmodium activity, the episodes occur with a regularity that is devastating to the patient. Synchronization with the biologic timing of the plasmodium assures that the self-limiting episodes will occur in the early afternoon of the cyclic day (i.e., every 3 days with the tertian cycle of *Plasmodium vivax*), and relief will be complete by late evening.

Widespread distribution of the drug for prophylactic use by residents in endemic areas is one of the programs of the World Health Organization (W.H.O.). Appearance of malarial symptoms in an individual residing in, or leaving, an endemic area is evidence of invasion by a plasmodium strain resistant to the drugs, and the drug regimen will need revision to control the disease.

Many of the drugs precipitate mild gastrointestinal disturbances that can be relieved by taking the drugs with food or antacids. The drugs are readily absorbed from the small intestine so that food will not delay absorption.

Skin dryness, pruritus, and photosensitivity (i.e., exaggerated sunburn) have been reported during drug use. Quinacrine hydrochloride is an acridine dye, and the skin may become temporarily discolored during drug therapy.

The drugs are toxic agents when taken in excessive dosage, and children are particularly sensitive to the drugs. The patient should be reminded to keep the drugs out of the reach of children. Dosage prescribed for malaria control causes some adverse effects, but the incidence of problems is more frequent when the drugs are employed at high dosage levels for their anti-inflammatory effect (i.e., rheumatoid arthritis therapy).

The antimalarial drugs have similar chemical structures, and with high dosage or prolonged use the adverse effects of one form will be similar to those of another plasmodicide. The drugs accumulate in the pigmented tissues of the eye, and there have been reports of decreased corneal sensitivity with high dosage. Peripheral retinal pigmentation and blind gaps in the visual field (scotomata) have occurred. Eighth cranial nerve damage has also been reported. During therapy any visual changes, tinnitus, vertigo, peripheral muscle weakness, or paresthesias should be brought to the attention of the physician. Specific exploration for emerging problems is planned for the patient receiving high dosage of any of the drugs.

HELMINTH INFESTATION

Helminthiasis is the term used to describe infestation with worms. The human intestinal tract has sufficient nutrients available to support the life of many parasites, and worms take advantage of the availability once their presence is established. The chief problem arising from harboring the parasites is the drain on resources when the invaders burrow into or attach to the intestinal wall.

Intestinal helminthiasis

Hookworms, *(Necator americanus* and *Ancylostoma duodenale)* enter through the skin and travel through the circulatory system to the lungs and intestinal tract. They bite into the intestinal mucosa to obtain blood from the capillaries. The continual drain on the host to meet the parasite's need for blood leads to anemia. The request that shoes be worn in shopping areas is an attempt to set up barriers to hookworm transmission.

Tapeworms *(Diphyllobothrium latum [Taenia lata],* fish tapeworm; *Hymenolepis nana [Taenia diminuta],* dwarf tapeworm; *Taenia saginata,* beef tapeworm; *Taenia solium,* pork tapeworm) attach to the intestinal wall by suckers or hooks on their head (scolex) and simply take advantage of the food available in the intestinal lumen. The intrusion site in the intestinal wall may become inflamed or infected, but the worms make no demands of their host.

Larvae of tapeworms (i.e., *T. solium)* may find a route to extraintestinal tissue sites when vomiting allows an egg-filled segment to rise to the duodenum. Intestinal enzymes digest the outer covering, and the free larvae (cysticerci) gain access to the circulation and tissues. Cysticercosis may involve any major organ. Disruption of organ function and blockage of blood supply results as larvae invasion progresses.

The most frequently encountered intestinal worm infestations are the small pinworms *(Enterobius vermicularis).* The parasites maintain residence in the host and cause only minor anal irritation. The passage of food, gum, and candy from one child to another transmits the ova readily, and many children carry pinworms in their intestines. Children seeking relief of abdominal pain often are found not to have appendicitis as expected, but pinworms. A rise in the child's blood eosinophil level indicates the body's response to foreign protein invasion.

Stool examination that reveals eggs or pinworms validates the suspicion that abdominal pain and eosinophil response are caused by pinworm invasion. In many children the parasites maintain residence in the host and cause few problems. Anal irritation is intense during the egg deposition periods of the pinworms. Scratching may spread the infestation to the vagina in females. Intestinal autoinfestation occurs as eggs are ingested during hand-mouth activities of the child. Ingested eggs produce sexually mature worms ready to deposit eggs at the anus within 35 days.

Extraintestinal helminthiasis

Liver flukes *(Clonorchis sinensis)* propagate in the intestine and biliary tract. They attach to the lumen of the tract, and they feed on the cells through their suction attachment. The effect on the host is less disruptive than that of the blood-sucking hookworm, but an increase in their number can damage the structures at attachment sites.

Extraintestinal worm infestations are resistant to eradication as larvae persist in sequestered sites in tissues. The blood flukes (i.e., *Schistosoma haematobium, S. mansoni*) and the lung flukes (i.e., *Paragonimus westermani, P. kellicotti*) require prolonged therapy to eradicate helminth larvae from tissue sites. Encysted larvae infestations from infected pork allow the *Trichinella spiralis* to invade muscle tissue in the host.

Pharmacodynamics

Eradication of any of the worms requires identification of the offending parasite. The adult forms, eggs, or larvae are present in the feces, and careful timing of collection of specimens should reveal the species. For example, a cellophane tape strip placed against the anus of a child during the night will pick up pinworms out for a nighttime excursion. Microscopic examination will reveal eggs, but worms can be seen by the naked eye.

The drugs used for control of the parasites have some specificity for particular parasites. Aspidium oleoresin (Table 3-4) is only employed for tapeworm control. Fats are withheld for 24 to 48 hours prior to administration of the drug because fats increase its absoption from the intestinal tract. A strong cathartic is given on the day prior to therapy to empty bowel contents and assure worm-drug contact. The necessity for removal of all segments of the tapeworm, including the scolex, requires that a strong cathartic be given subsequent to administration of the drug. Shortly after the post-drug cathartic, a cleansing enema is given. All stools are examined for tapeworm segments. Patients complain of nausea, abdominal pain, headache, and dizziness after the treatment.

Drugs used for tapeworm eradication vary in their mode of action on the parasite. Aspidium oleoresin paralyzes the muscle of the tapeworm, and segments of the helminth are found by straining or visually examining the stool. Dichlorophen causes the scolex to detach from the wall of the intestine, and the drug disintegrates the worm segments almost completely. Unrecognizable segments are eliminated in the feces, and the stool is a grayish white mass of tapeworm products.

Table 3-4. Dosage range of anti-parasitic drugs: antihelmintics

Nonproprietary name	Proprietary (trade) name	Daily adult dosage range
Aspidium oleoresin		Oral: 4-5 Gm. ($\div 2$)
Bephenium hydroxy-naphthoate	Alcopara	Oral: 5 Gm. ($\div 2$)
Dichlorophen	Anthiphen	Oral: 6-9 Gm. ($\div 3$)
Hexylresorcinol	Caprokol, Crystoids	Oral: 1Gm./ single dose
Methylrosaniline chloride		Oral: 180 mg. ($\div 3$)
Piperazine citrate	Antepar, Multifuge, Oxucide, Parazine, Pipizan	Oral: 2-3 Gm.
Pyrantel pamoate	Antiminth	Oral: 11 mg./kg.
Pyrvinium pamoate	Povan	Oral: 5 mg./kg.
Stibophen	Fuadin	I.M.: 1.5-12 ml.
Thiabendazole	Mintezol	Oral: 22-44 mg./kg. ($\div 1$-2)

No prior preparation or fasting is required when dichlorophen (Table 3-4) is administered, and the laxative effect of the drug is sufficient to assure removal of the tapeworm debris. Patients have abdominal cramps or colicky pain for the 4- to 6-hour period that the drug is active in the intestine.

The most versatile drug for removal of helminths is hexylresorcinol (Table 3-4). It paralyzes intestinal worms, and the inactive parasites are excreted in the feces. Hexylresorcinol is effective in removing hookworms, roundworms, pinworms, whipworms, threadworms, tapeworms, and intestinal flukes. Use of the drug is almost problem free. The gelatinous capsules are given early in the morning, and food then is withheld for 4 hours. A cathartic is given to remove the inactivated helminths from the intestinal tract.

Bephenium hydroxynaphthoate (Table 3-4) inactivates hookworms and roundworms. It blocks neuromuscular transmission and glucose transport and anaerobic glycolysis in the helminths. The bitter taste of the drug is disguised by administration of a small quantity of a strong sugar solution, milk, chocolate milk, orange juice, or carbonated beverage. Patients are asked to fast during the night and to wait two hours before eating after drug administration.

Piperazine citrate (Table 3-4) inhibits the respiratory enzymes and anaerobic metabolic reactions to inactivate pinworms. The drug is a cyanine dye, and the stool is colored bright red after administration. Elimination of helminths is accomplished with administration of a single dose unless reinfection occurs.

Methylrosaniline chloride (Table 3-4) is most frequently used for elimination of pinworms, although it is effective in control of threadworms and liver flukes in some patients. Enteric-coated tablets prevent irritation of the gastric mucosa during the 8- to 10-day course of therapy. Intestinal parasites are paralyzed by the action of the drug on their neuromuscular junctional mechanisms.

Thiabendazole (Table 3-4) is versatile as an antihelminthic agent. Interference with metabolic pathways in the worm makes it useful in elimination of hookworms, roundworms, pinworms, whipworms, and threadworms from the human host. It kills some of the larvae resulting from invasion of *Trichinella spiralis*. Thiabendazole is readily absorbed from the intestinal tract after oral administration, and peak blood levels are attained in 1 to 3 hours. The chief route of excretion is the urine, and 87% of the drug is eliminated at the end of 48 hours. About one third of the patients complain of headache, weakness, and dizziness while taking the drug.

Pyrantel pamoate (Table 3-4) aids in the elimination of roundworms, hookworms, and pinworms by blocking the neuromuscular transmission of the helminths. Paralysis of the worms removes them from the body after a single dose of the drug. The oral suspension is administered with milk or fruit juice. Nausea, vomiting, abdominal cramps, headache, and dizziness are the most common complaints of patients after administration of the drug. Absorbed drug is metabolized by the liver, but most of the drug (50%) is eliminated in the feces at the end of 48 hours after ingestion.

Stibophen (Table 3-4) is the only antihelmintic used in the United States for eradication of schistosomas. An alternate-day schedule is usually planned for the 20 intramuscular injections required for removal of the blood flukes. Stibophen is an irritating drug, and patients complain of nausea, vomiting, diarrhea, and joint and muscle pain during therapy. At the time of injection there is a drop in cardiac rate of 10 beats per minute. Concurrent electrocardiographic recording may show inversion of the T wave and prolongation of the Q-T interval. Cardiac, hepatic, and renal function are monitored throughout therapy to assure early definition of emerging problems.

Patient care

Careful attention to prescribed dosage and evacuation procedures is necessary to assure removal of the parasites and to prevent spread of eggs, larvae, or inactivated parasites. Experience with the individual drugs affects the physician's selection of a particular drug for removal of an organism known to be susceptible to several agents. As newer and less irritating agents are introduced, older drugs fall into disuse. Identification of the specific helminth invader is basic to planning the therapeutic program for eradication of the parasite.

Examination of the excreta after therapy aids in identification of drug effect. All fecal material is strained and examined closely for worms or worm segments. Magnification of material that is suspect but not clearly identifiable aids in discrimination between worms or their segments and residue of foods (fruit and vegetable fibers).

Prevention of transmission of parasites from one individual to another is an important part of health teaching. For example, the mother of a child with pinworms should understand the need for meticulous attention to hand-washing (including use of an orangewood stick for cleaning under the fingernails). It is important to stress the need for washing raw fruits and vegetables to avoid ingestion of parasites from food handlers who have parasitic infections. Eradication of pinworms from one member of the family is seldom effective in controlling transmission. Each of the family members should be examined for the presence of worms so that therapy can be planned if they are present. Hygienic measures are important adjuncts to transmission control of intestinal parasites that eject progeny into the feces.

REFERENCES

Bernhardt, Harvey E., Orlando, Joseph C., Benfield, John R., Hirose, Frank M., and Foos, Robert Y.: Disseminated candidiasis in surgical patients, Surgery, Gynecology and Obstetrics **34:**819, 1972.

Criuckshank, Robert: The influence of age and nutrition on the incidence and control of enteric infections, Medical Clinics of North America **51:**643, 1967.

Curry, Cynthia Rapp, and Quie, Paul G.: Fungal septicemia in patients receiving parenteral hyperalimentation, The New England Journal of Medicine **285:**1221, 1971.

Deller, John J., Jr.: Malaria—again a diagnostic consideration, American Family Physician **5:**68, Feb., 1972.

Febles, Francisco, Jr.: Schistosomiasis, a world health problem, American Journal of Nursing **64:**118, 1964.

Hardy, Albert V.: Current problems in enteric infections, Medical Clinics of North America **51:**609, 1967.

Hawking, Frank: The clock of the malaria parasite, Scientific American **222:**123, June, 1970.

Herban, Nancy L.: Nursing care of patients with tropical diseases, Nursing Clinics of North America **5:**157, 1970.

Marples, Mary J.: Life on the human skin, Scientific American **220:**108, Jan., 1969.

Most, Harry: Treatment of common parasitic infections of man encountered in the United States, The New England Journal of Medicine **287:**495, 698, 1972.

Reilly, Mary Jo, editor: American hospital formulary service, vol. 1, sect. 8:00, Washington, D. C., 1973, American Society of Hospital Pharmacists.

Robinson, Harry M.: Effective antifungal drugs and indications for their use, Medical Clinics of North America **51:**1181, 1967.

Smith, Alice Lorraine: Microbiology and pathology, ed. 10, St. Louis, 1972, The C. V. Mosby Co.

Werner, S. Benson, Pappagianis, Demosthenes, Heindl, Irena, and Mickel, Arthur: Epidemic of coccidioidomycosis among archeology students, The New England Journal of Medicine **286:**507, 1972.

4
Immune and allergic responses

Immune responses
    Humoral immunity
    Tissue immunity
    Sensitivity tests
Allergic reactions
    Atopic sensitization
    Acquired sensitivity: drug allergy
Histamine inhibition
    Pharmacodynamics
    Patient care
Immunity building
    Viral invasion
Immunization
    Passive immunity
    Active immunity
Inflammatory response suppression
    Pharmacodynamics
    Patient care

IMMUNE RESPONSES

Natural, or species, immunity and antibodies from maternal blood protect the newborn infant from many diseases during the first few months of life. Beyond the neonatal period long-term protection against organisms pathogenic to humans is dependent on acquisition of antibodies to the antigens that invade body tissues. Immunity can be acquired by having the disease, by introduction of live or weakened (attenuated) microorganisms that produce subclinical disease, or by injection of immune bodies from humans or animals.

Normal physiologic processes provide primary defenses against pathogen invasion. The initial antigen exposure response includes ingestion and phagocytosis of the invading pathogen by leukocytes and macrophages. After breakdown of the antigenic substance, lymphocytes return the products to reticuloendothelial tissues where antigen matching at antibody-producing cells begins the process of immunity building.

Reticuloendothelial tissues have an almost limitless ability to produce immunologically competent cells to protect against a wide variety of antigens. The flexible structure of the complex heterogenous polypeptide chains of antibodies assures that an antibody can be found to "fit" the antigen. Antigenic materials arriving at the antibody-producing plasma cells of the reticuloendothelial system find cells capable of producing antibodies that fit the antigen structure. The process is somewhat like construction of a jigsaw puzzle, and the antigen eventually rests at the cell with an antibody pattern that conforms to its shape. Production of selective antibodies is instituted once the pattern is established, and immunologically competent cells become available to defend against subsequent invasion by the same antigen.

Humoral immunity

Movement of the antibodies into the serum provides humoral immunity that lasts while the antibodies remain in the body. Survival time of antibodies varies from three months to five years or longer. Between 1% and 2% of the total circulating proteins are antibody-containing gamma globulins capable of reacting chemically with specific antigens.

Virus, bacteria, bacterial toxins, or polysaccharides provide the antigen stimulus to protective immunity building. After antibody formation, provocation by the antigen is followed by rapid movement of antibodies to the invasion site. Antibodies act in varying ways to neutralize or facilitate destruction of invading pathogens. Antibodies may form electrostatic bonds to inactive and precipitate antigens, or they may cover the surface of the pathogen to facilitate phagocytosis. Antibodies have binding sites for complement within their polypeptide chains, and binding of complement components (enzymes) after antigen-antibody union causes lysis of the pathogen membrane. In some instances, antibody-complement covering of the antigen may facilitate phagocytosis in a process called *opsonization*. Complement combines with the membrane of the phagocyte, and the pathogen is eased into the phagocytic cytoplasm. The process markedly accelerates the rate of pathogen destruction.

Tissue immunity

Defense mechanisms at the cellular level are known to confine invading virus, fungus, and some bacteria, but the mechanism for control is not completely understood. Although the antigenic substances stimulate neutrophil and macrophage activity, antibodies are not present in tissues subsequent to the invasion. It is probable that small lymphocytes responding to antigen invasion reproduce and retain the immunologic memory pattern for prompt response to subsequent invasion by the same antigenic substance. Pathogens or tissue identified as *foreign* precipitate the immune response and previously formed or committed lymphocytes respond to phagocytize the material. The cell-mediated immune process is currently under intense investigation because the immunity phenomenon is basic to rejection of tissue and organs transplanted in humans.

Antibodies recently have been isolated from the glands of the mucosa in tissues contiguous with the external environment. Tissue antibody levels provide barriers to some of the virulent viruses and bacteria that enter body orifices. The immunoglobulins are produced in tissues adjacent to their site of accumulation in mucosa rather than in the plasma cells of the reticuloendothelial system. Tissue immunity for specific antigens differs from that of serum readiness to respond to the same antigen, and there is a difference between the tissue immune bodies and serum antibodies in the same individual.

Sensitivity tests

Immunologically competent cells are available to respond to a provocative dose of the antigen that originally instituted antibody formation within one or more weeks after initial exposure. The immune status of the individual can be determined by dermal sensitivity tests, and immunization or therapy can be planned on the basis of test reactions. Biologic agents are available for detection of exposure-induced sensitivity to preparations of specific bacteria, bacterial toxins, fungi, worms, or viruses (Table 4-1).

Diluted preparations of the biologic agent (0.1 ml.) are injected intradermally on the flexor surface of the forearm, or a multiple-tine injector may be used to introduce the material into the surface of the upper arm. Local reaction at the injection site is compared with a control when one is used. A positive reaction is considered only as an indicator of exposure. The specific components of sensitivity tests have been extrapolated from the literature and appear in Table 4-1. In essence, the positive reaction is a localized antigen-induced antibody response.

Evaluation of the clinical status of the patient and culture of the causative organism are needed to verify recent disease-producing exposure because the tests indicate only that immune bodies have been formed. Tests are particularly useful to the physician in defining the presence of antibodies for the less common fungi (i.e., *Blastomyces dermatitidis, Coccidioides immitis, Histoplasma capsulatum*).

Sensitivity tests are most frequently used to determine the individual's immunity to diphtheria, mumps, or tuberculosis, and test results provide information required for planning therapy or immunization. For example, the postadolescent male may be tested with mumps skin test antigen to ascertain whether he has immunologically competent cells to protect him against the disease after he has been exposed to the virus. The unprotected male is usually

Table 4-1. Biological agents used to detect the presence of exposure-induced sensitivity

Dermal reaction tests	Antigen source	Disease exposure tested	Positive reaction after test		
			Time	Size	Appearance
Blastomycin	*Blastomyces dermatitidis*	Cutaneous or pulmonary North American blastomycosis	24-48 hr. (up to 4 days)	5 mm.+	Induration
Brucella protein nucleate	*Brucella abortus B. suis,* or *B. melitensis*	Undulant fever, or brucellosis	24-48 hr.	2-10 cm.	Erythema, edema, induration
Coccidioidin	*Coccidioides immitis* (10 strains)	Coccidioidomycosis	24-48 hr.	5 mm.+	Induration
Diphtheria toxin Diagnostic Diphtheria toxin Inactivated diagnostic (control)	*Corynebacterium diphtheriae*	Diphtheria	48-72 hr.	1-2 cm.	Redness and infiltration
Histoplasmin	*Histoplasma capsulatum*	Histoplasmosis	24-48 hr. (up to 3 days)	5 mm.+	Induration
Lymphogranuloma venereum antigen (with control)	*Lymphogranuloma venereum*	Lymphogranuloma	48-72 hr.	6 mm.+	Erythematous nodule with lighter halo
Mumps skin test antigen	Jeryl Lynn B strain of mumps virus	Mumps (epidemic parotitis)	24-36 hr.	15 mm.+	Erythema
Trichinella extract (with control)	*Trichinella spiralis*	Trichinosis	15-20 min. (up to 24 hr.)	3 mm.+	Wheal
Tuberculin Old Purified protein derivative	*Mycobacterium tuberculosis*	Tuberculosis	48-72 hr.	5-10 mm.+ 5 mm.+	Inflammation and induration Induration

inoculated against mumps after exposure to protect against bilateral orchitis and consequent sterility that is a complication of mumps.

Diagnostic diptheria toxin (Schick test toxin) is a comparative test. A control substance is injected on the alternate arm at the same time that the toxin is injected. In addition to an indication of immunologic status, the individual who reacts intensely at the control site is considered to have a sensitivity to the test materials and can be expected to have a severe reaction if toxoid is administered.

Tuberculin purified protein derivative (PPD) is available as *first test strength, intermediate test strength,* and *second test strength,* and it is used more frequently than old tuberculin because of the greater specificity attained by increasing the strength of the provocative dosage. Positive reactions are followed by x-ray examination, sputum cultures, or gastric washings to define the status of the tuberculosis invasion. Prophylactic drug therapy may be planned for the individual with a positive reaction.

ALLERGIC REACTIONS

An allergic reaction is an abnormal manifestation of the immune response, and the precipitating factor is called an allergen. An allergic reaction may be precipitated by drugs, chemicals, incompatible blood, or protein substances. Small particles, or *haptens* (i.e., chemicals, pollens, drugs), may combine with proteins, and the complex is capable of inducing an allergic response. Manifestations of the allergic response occur when allergen-antibody reactions at tissue sites cause the release of physiologically active intermediates (i.e., histamine, bradykinin) into tissues.

Atopic sensitization

Approximately 10% of the population have inherited genetic traits that cause sensitization of body tissues to varying allergens. Atopic sensitivity is a generalized body process, but there is usually a shock organ in which allergen exposure is high (i.e., nasal mucosa). Weak sensitizing antibodies (reagins) accumulate at the shock organ tissues, and each invasion elicits an allergic response. Unlike the normal immune response, a spontaneous reaction may occur without prior exposure to the allergen, and there are no circulating antibodies. *Cell-fixed antibodies* cause varying sensitivities during the life-span of the individual; that is, the child may show sensitivity to foods that is manifest as eczema or hives, but in adolescence his sensitivity may be allergic rhinitis when exposed to dust. Angioedema, bronchial asthma, eczema, gastrointestinal disturbances, and hay fever are common manifestations of atopic allergy.

Reaction of allergens with the cell-fixed antibodies causes release of histamine and other mediators that in turn cause tissue reactions, that is, hives occurring after ingestion of strawberries, gastrointestinal disturbances after ingestion of shellfish, rhinitis after exposure to pollens. Although each provocation by the allergen precipitates a response, *desensitization* is possible by long-term administration of dilutions of the allergenic substance. Periodic administration of dilutions of the allergen gradually increases the production of normal antibodies in the atopic individual. The ratio of reagins to normal antibodies changes, and complete antibodies that have a stronger affinity for the allergenic substance become available to act as *blocking antibodies.* The incidence of reagin-induced allergic responses gradually decreases as blocking antibodies inhibit reagin activity.

Desensitization is a long process that may require five or more years before allergen exposure ceases to produce an allergic response. Administration of drugs with a high allergic potential (i.e., antibiotics, hormones, horse serum) causes a high incidence of allergic responses in the individual with a history of atopic allergy.

Acquired sensitivity: drug allergy

The terms antigen and allergen describe substances that are capable of instituting the formation of antibodies. Allergen is a more specific term for the substances that institute a pathologic antibody response when exposure to an allergen occurs. Although drugs are the chief cause of allergic reactions in the nonatopic individual, comparable reactions occur when other allergens (i.e., toxins from Hymenoptera sting) precipitate antibody responses. The chief problems during allergic reactions occur as a consequence of histamine release from granules of mast cells at the site of allergen-antibody interaction.

Histaminic effect. Mast cells store concentrated histidine as granules within their cytoplasm. Peptides, polysaccharides, and antigen-antibody or allergen-antibody reactions may cause release of histamine, produced by decarboxylation of the histidine of mast cell granules. Histamine attachment to capillary and arteriole walls causes dilation, and histaminic effect on the venules is constriction. Changes in local hemodynamic relationships result as venules resist flow of blood from the capillary bed, and pressure builds in the capillary. Increased pressure and permeability of the capillary membrane allow fluid transudation into the tissue spaces. Concurrent release of bradykinin from mast cell granules is thought to intensify the irritation of nerve endings caused by histamine. The itching, pain, and irritation of allergic responses may be attributed to the presence of histamine and bradykinin at the site.

Copious quantities of histamine released at mucous membrane sites during an allergic response induce swelling, and laryngeal edema may occur when respiratory tract tissues are involved. The amine also has a direct constricting effect on bronchial tubules, which may adversely affect gas exchange. Although little is known about the normal physiologic roles of histamine, it is known to stimulate smooth muscle of the gastrointestinal tract, increase production of secretions from exocrine glands (gastric, duodenal, pancreatic, salivary, bronchial, and lacrimal glands), and dilate cerebral blood vessels. Allergic reactions cause physiologic problems ranging from uncomfortable local rash or fever to a life-threatening anaphylactic reaction due to release of histamine at widely distributed tissue sites.

Anaphylaxis. Parenterally administered substances allergenic for the individual may precipitate a widespread reaction as the allergen is disseminated to body tissues. Anaphylaxis occurs immediately after the allergen is introduced, and the reaction indicates prior exposure-induced production of antibodies that surge forth in response to the allergen presence. Allergen-antibody interaction at tissue sites causes release of histamine from mast cells, and the transudation of fluid into tissues depletes the circulating plasma. Loss of the plasma component increases the viscosity of blood and depletes the volume. Concurrent with the anaphylactic shock state, bronchial constriction and laryngeal edema occlude respiratory passages, and respiratory failure ensues. The devastating sequence of events progresses to a fatal outcome within minutes unless resuscitative measures are implemented immediately.

Maintenance of a patent airway and reinstitution of hemodynamics require prompt attention. Epinephrine hydrochloride (Adrenalin) is administered subcutaneously at intervals of 3 to 5 minutes until the patient's status improves. Epinephrine hydrochloride stimulates the myocardium and causes bronchodilation. It has a direct antagonistic effect on the histamine-induced bronchial constriction.

The potential for continued anaphylactic effect exists until the allergenic substance is metabolized or excreted. Monitoring of the patient continues until vital parameters are stable at normal levels and the predictable action time of the allergen has been exceeded.

Patients experiencing an anaphylactic reaction to a drug should be advised that subsequent use of the drug or one with similar chemical structure may precipitate an allergic response. *Medic-Alert* bracelets or other identification should be worn or carried by patients with drug allergy.

Urticaria. Generalized skin eruptions that look like giant hives or extensive plateaus in patches over the skin surface may occur when a drug is administered to a patient sensitized by its prior use. The reddish areas have white centers, and the patient complains of itching so intense that it cannot be ignored. Prompt appearance of the skin lesions indicates that antibodies produced during previous therapy with the drug or a comparable one are interacting with allergen at superficial tissue sites. Histamine release at the interaction site causes fluid accumulation in sequestered wheals.

The patient's discomfort is a primary concern when the surface lesions occur, and the physician may prescribe an antipruritic topical lotion and an antihistaminic drug to prevent progression of histamine action. Protection of the skin from injury is also a concern, and the patient is reminded to use lotion on lesions in preference to scratching. Tissue trauma allows entrance of microbes and prolongs the treatment period for the patient.

Angioedema. Histamine release consequent to allergen-antibody interaction may cause fluid accumulation in oral and respiratory tract tissues and the soft tissues in the periorbital area. Prolongation of the expiratory phase of respiration with faint wheezing demonstrates the gradual narrowing of the respiratory passages as edema progresses. Prompt discontinuance of drug administration and injection of an antihistaminic drug usually provide relief of the problems. Angioedema may accompany an urticarial reaction, or it may occur as an independent entity.

Serum sickness. A delayed response to allergen administration occurring 7 days or more after the first use of the allergenic drug is known as serum sickness. Initially the term was used to describe the entity occurring when horse serum was employed for immunization, but the symptom complex occurs when other protein substances or drugs are used for therapy. The time lag between drug administration and the allergic response is the period when antibody production is occurring. When antibodies to the allergen are produced, the generalized symptoms occur. Although the problems are somewhat comparable to those occurring with anaphylaxis, the production of antibodies is gradual, and symptoms emerge gradually. The low level (titer) of antibodies in the serum may cause intermittent periods of dyspnea and hypotension as histamine-induced tissue responses move fluid into peripheral tissues. Serum sickness may also include generalized edema, joint pain, rash, and swollen lymph glands. Discontinuance of drug administration decreases the allergen stimulus, but the reaction continues as long as the drug remains in the body to interact with antibodies. Antihistamine may be prescribed to slow the progression of symptoms. The patient's discomfort provides guides for palliative measures while the response continues.

Arthus reaction. Injection of an allergenic substance into local tissues of a patient with large quantities of bivalent antibodies may produce destruction of this local tissue, and the process is called an Arthus reaction. The allergen-antibody reaction at the tissue site causes spasticity, occlusion, and degeneration of local blood vessels. Disruption of the blood supply results in tissue necrosis, and the tissues gradually slough in a wide area around the injection site.

Delayed-reaction allergies. Antibodies that remain in the cell cytoplasm are capable of producing an allergic response to local irritation. For example, the irritating properties of some drugs (i.e., chlorpromazine) cause *contact dermatitis* on the hands of nurses who spill small amounts of it on their tissues during preparation of solutions of the drug. Contact dermatitis occurs 2 to 3 days after exposure to the allergen because cellular antibodies respond slowly to the irritant. Although prompt handwashing may decrease the exposure by removal of the irritant, rubber gloves provide maximum protection against the chemical-induced contact dermatitis.

A comparable skin reaction may occur when drugs are applied to the skin for treatment of surface lesions. Topical applications of drugs may also institute formation of antibodies, and their presence in the serum may cause an allergic response when the same drug is used for systemic therapy.

Rash and fever are delayed-reaction allergies occurring during therapy with drugs. Continuance of drug use is dependent on the extent of the reaction and the priority need for the particular drug. In allergic reactions, eosinophil levels in the serum are elevated, although the precise role of the leukocytes is not clearly understood.

HISTAMINE INHIBITION
Pharmacodynamics

Numerous drugs are identified pharmacologically as antihistamines, but many of these agents are used for problems unrelated to histamine control. The drugs included in this section have a pharmacodynamic effect in altering the vascular responses to histamine release by antigen or allergen reactions with antibodies.

Antihistamines interfere with histaminic action on small blood vessels by competing for extravascular receptors (Fig. 4-1). Histamine molecules that find a receptor site will produce dilation of arterioles, constriction of venules, and fluid transudation. To prevent histaminic effect, the antihistaminic drug must be available in quantities sufficient to bind to capillary sites prior to histamine attachment. Normal hemodynamic relationships at the tissue level are maintained when histamine is prevented from moving to receptor sites. Free histamine is readily metabolized by tissues to an inactive form.

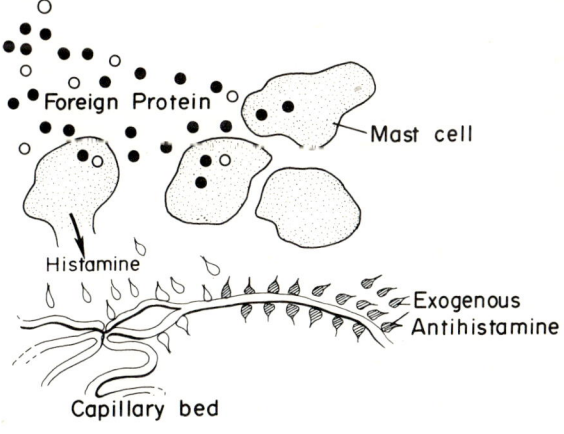

Fig. 4-1. Distention of mast cells with ingested materials (i.e., foreign protein) causes rupture of the cell membrane and release of histamine into tissues. Antihistaminic drugs interfere with histaminic effect on capillaries by competing for attachment sites on the membrane.

Table 4-2. Dosage range of drugs with antihistaminic action

Nonproprietary name	Proprietary (trade) name	Daily adult dosage range	Nonproprietary name	Proprietary (trade) name	Daily adult dosage range
Brompheniramine maleate	Dimetane	Oral: 16-24 mg. (÷3-4) I.M.: 5-40 mg. (÷4)	Diphenylpyraline hydrochloride	Cupertin, Diafen, Hispril, Sumadil	Oral: 6-8 mg. (÷3-4)
Carbinoxamine maleate	Clistin	Oral: 16-24 mg. (÷3-4)	Doxylamine succinate	Decapryn	Oral: 37.5 mg. (÷3)
Chlorcyclizine hydrochloride	Di-Paralene, Perazil	Oral: 50-200 mg. (÷1-2)	Methapyrilene hydrochloride	Cohistine, Dormin, Histadyl, Lullamin, Methoxylene, Semikon, Somnicaps, Thenylene	Oral: 200-500 mg. (÷4-5) I.M.: 10-100 mg.
Chlorothen citrate	Tagathen	Oral: 75-100 mg. (÷3-4)	Methdilazine hydrochloride	Tacaryl	Oral: 16-32 mg. (÷2-4)
Chlorpheniramine maleate	Alerin, Barachlor, Chestamine, Chlo-Amine, Chloramate, Chlor-Trimeton, Drize, Histachlor, Histadur, Histaspan, Histitrin, Histrey, Phenetron, Teldrin, Tylahist	Oral: 8-12 mg. (÷3-4) I.M.: 10 mg./single dose	Phenindamine	Thephorin	Oral: 40-100 mg. (÷4)
			Pheniramine maleate	Inhiston, Trimeton	Oral: 60-120 mg. (÷3)
			Pyrilamine maleate	Neo-Antergan	Oral: 75-150 mg. (÷3)
			Pyrrobutamine phosphate	Pyronil	Oral: 45-60 mg. (÷2-3)
			Rotoxamine tartrate	Twiston	Oral: 8-12 mg. (÷3-4)
Cyproheptadine hydrochloride	Periactin	Oral: 12-32 mg. (÷3-4)	Trimeprazine tartrate	Temaril	Oral: 10-80 mg. (÷4)
Dexbrompheniramine maleate	Disomer	Oral: 8-12 mg. (÷3-4) I.M.: 2-20 mg.	Tripelennamine citrate	Pyribenzamine	Oral: 150-200 mg. (÷3-4)
Dexchlorpheniramine maleate	Polaramine	Oral: 4-6 mg. (÷3-4)	Tripelennamine hydrochloride	Pyribenzamine, Stanzamine	Oral: 50-600 mg. I.M.: 100 mg. (÷2) I.V.: 25 mg./single dose
Dimethindene maleate	Forhistal	Oral: 1-6 mg. (÷3)			
Diphenhydramine hydrochloride	Benadryl	Oral: 100-150 mg. (÷3-4) I.M.: 10-100 mg./single dose I.V.: Same as I.M.	Triprolidine hydrochloride	Actidil	Oral: 5-7.5 mg. (÷2-3)

Antihistamines have been successfully employed to prevent anaphylactic reactions. The sequelae of cardiopulmonary arrest consequent to peripheral pooling of blood and bronchial constriction can be modified by administration of antihistamines prior to the use of allergy-producing drugs. The antihistamines attach to membrane sites before histamine is released by the interaction of allergen-antibody complexes at tissue sites. For example, antihistamines given before intravenous administration of radiopaque dyes known to have a high potential for causing allergic responses prevent anaphylactic reactions. The same protection can be afforded an individual with atopic allergy who requires therapy with an agent containing a component known to precipitate generalized allergic responses.

Antihistamines can prevent the progression of a histamine-initiated response, but the drugs do not reverse the effects occurring from histamine prior to drug use. For example, progression of an urticarial response may be halted by administration of an antihistamine, but existing areas of erythema and edema are dependent on normal physiologic mechanisms for resolution. The blockade of histaminic action in tissues also halts the irritation of nerve endings, and the itching or burning sensation subsides. For the patient with an urticarial response, the decreased rubbing and scratching of tissues lessens the danger of superimposed tissue injury and infection.

There are differences in the potency of individual antihistamines (Table 4-2), but their action in the body is similar. The incidence of effects and adverse effects among the large number of antihistiminic drugs is comparable. The wide distribution of the agents in all body tissues makes them effective at the varying sites affected by excess histamine release. The antihistamines are metabolized in the liver, lungs, and kidneys before excretion into the urine.

Some effect is seen 15 to 30 minutes after oral administration. The variation in duration of effective levels is reflected in the differing time periods for administration of the drugs (Table 4-2).

Individual factors influence responses to the drugs and the incidence of adverse effects. Each of the antihistamines has some antiemetic, anticholinergic, and central nervous system depressant effect. The sedative effect of an antihistamine is a primary consideration in selection of a particular drug for the patient.

Drowsiness and dizziness are manifestations of central nervous system depression seen in the first days of therapy, but most patients develop tolerance to the effects in 2 to 3 days. Carbinoxamine maleate, rotoxamine tartrate, and diphenhydramine hydrochloride cause drowsiness or dizziness in 50% of the patients taking them. In contrast to the central nervous system depression, children and some older patients sometimes have episodes of excitation or irritability, which indicate central nervous system stimulation. After administration, headache and hypotension occur in some patients. Topical application may cause sensitization, and use of the drugs for a patient with atopic allergy may precipiatate an allergic response.

Many of the drugs are available in an extended-release form that decreases the amount of drug free in the tissues during any period of time. These preparations decrease the incidence of drowsiness, dryness of the mouth, and gastrointestinal disturbances (nausea, vomiting, anorexia, diarrhea, constipation) common during use of antihistamines.

Patient care

The supportive measures necessary to decrease the disruptive effects of the physiologic problem will depend on the site of the histaminic tissue response. For example, local application of cooling lotions or bathing may decrease the skin irritation occurring with an urticarial reaction but dietary modification will be necessary when the response affects the gastrointestinal tract. Plans for nursing measures to relieve the basic problem are continued throughout drug therapy. Antihistaminic drugs halt the histaminic effect, but they do not affect tissue damage caused by the allergen or by the patient during the intense reaction period. For example, the patient with urticaria may have scratches or other lesions on the skin that require meticulous cleaning and measures to promote healing.

The patient who is responsible for self-medication must understand the rationale for maintaining the prescribed schedule for use of the drug and continuance of therapy beyond the time of response cessation. Suggesting that the drug be taken with milk or a snack may decrease the incidence of gastric irritation.

Not all patients will take advantage of the period of drowsiness to rest and relax. The patient must understand the hazards of driving a motor vehicle or doing hazardous work when slight drowsiness may affect alertness and reaction time. The patient should also know that alcohol will potentiate the central nervous system depressive effect of the drug.

66 Drugs used to control infection and inflammation

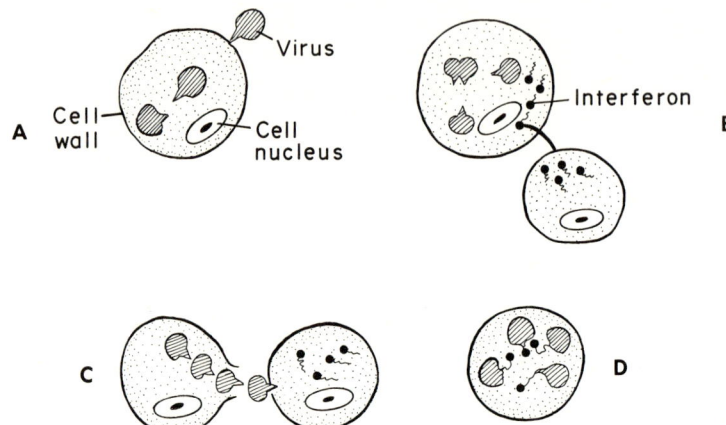

Fig. 4-2. Viral resistance is provided by interferons produced in the invaded cell. **A,** Viruses penetrate the membrane and enter the cell. **B,** Viruses utilize the cellular contents to obtain nutrients for multiplication. The invaded cell produces interferons that move out into adjacent cells. **C,** Virus activity depletes cell stores, and viruses move out toward another nutrient source. **D,** Viruses entering the cell are inactivated by interferons.

The drugs have a fairly high therapeutic index, but accidental overdosage has caused central nervous system excitation leading to convulsions and death in children. The patient should be encouraged to place the drug out of the reach of children.

IMMUNITY BUILDING
Viral invasion

Agents have been developed for immunity building against the invasion of some viruses, but the common cold still exists. The self-limiting nature of the problem makes it one that perhaps can wait solution. Latent viruses have been indicted as a cause of crippling chronic disease, and measures for eradication of causative viruses are sought as part of the disease control program.

The characteristics of viruses make eradication of the organism difficult. After entrance into the body, the virus enters normal cells and becomes an integral part of the cellular residence. Viruses use cellular ribosomes in the manufacture of deoxyribonucleic acid (DNA) and ribonucleic acid (RNA) necessary to production of additional viral cells. During the time of intracellular viral growth, the cells produce a substance known as interferon (Fig. 4-2). The interferon moves out of the virus-infected cell and enters another normal cell in the area. The interferon stimulates production of a protective protein in the new cell. When the original host cell becomes distended with viral progeny, the membrane ruptures, and liberated viruses enter adjacent cells. Interferon-containing cells block viral activity, and the virus cannot survive. Nature has provided a source of protection against viral invasion, but the amount of interferon is insufficient to abort a massive invasion. Building blocks for interferons (polynucleotides) are currently being manufactured for antiviral therapy. Antibodies formed in response to the virus invasion must inhibit the action of viruses during subsequent invasion as soon as they enter the body because the organisms quickly move to protected areas in cells where antibodies cannot reach them.

Host survival of most viral invasions is probable, but problems exist when the viruses remain in the cells and form latent *genomes.* As genomes viral hereditary materials can be carried by body cells for long periods, with genetic components for virus formation as an integral part of the descendent cells. Precipitating factors in the host environment are thought to stimulate resurgence of the virus form and symptoms of disease. For example, the virus invasions during the influenza epidemic after World War I affected many people. Epidemio-

Immune and allergic responses   67

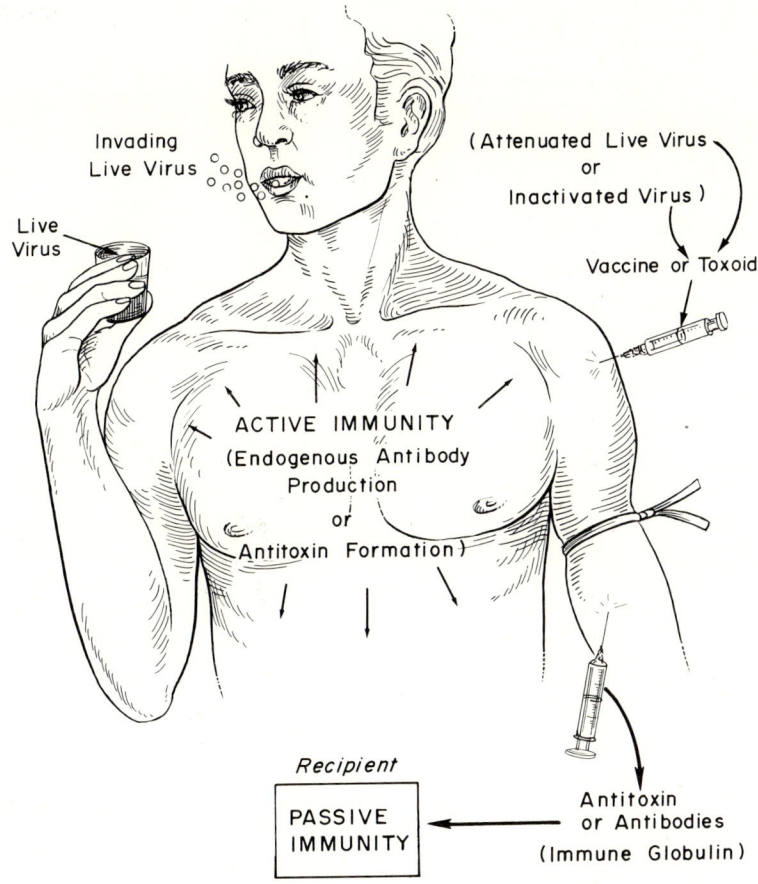

Fig. 4-3. Relationship between active and passive immunity in man (schematic).

logic studies indicate a clear relationship between individuals with influenza (or subclinical influenza) and individuals who currently have Parkinson's disease. The virus-genome-virus sequence seems to explain the origin of a debilitating disease thirty or forty years after the initial viral invasion.

Amantadine hydrochloride (Symmetrel) is the only oral antiviral drug in common use. The drug is given (200 mg./24 hours, divided into 2 doses) as a prophylactic agent when exposure to virus cannot be prevented and the effects of disease would be detrimental to the patient. The drug acts by preventing entrance of the virus into the host cells so that the drug must be in the tissues prior to invasion of the virus. Adverse effects of the drug are manifestations of central nervous system depression or stimulation (i.e., drowsiness, insomnia).

The search for antiviral agents continues. Extensive double-blind studies are being conducted to ascertain the effectiveness of idoxuridine in control of *herpes simplex encephalitis.* The objectives are to control the residual functional problems of patients surviving the disease entity and to decrease mortality from the viral invasion.

IMMUNIZATION

Antibody formation is dependent on exposure to the pathogen, and the individual is deficient in specific antibodies on initial antigen exposure. One week to several months are required to provide protection after exposure by antibodies formed in response to antigen invasion. Infants are protected for the first few months of life by residual maternal antibodies that cross the placenta, but subsequent antibody production is dependent on periodic challenges by antigens. Protective immunization is planned to correlate with the development of the physiologic mechanisms for antibody formation near the termination of the infant's first year of life.

Active immunity can be obtained by inadvertent exposure to pathogens that leads to clinical or subclinical disease or by planned introduction of vaccine or toxoid that stimulates endogenous antibody production or antitoxin formation (Fig. 4-3). Prompt but short-lived antibody protection can be attained by antitoxin or antibodies received from injections of serum from protected humans or animals.

Passive immunity

Protection after exposure to pathogens or toxins can be provided by serum-containing antibodies that immediately begin to neutralize antigens and prevent serious consequences of the invasion. Antibody protection is provided by administration of antibody-laden serum from an animal (usually a horse) or from humans known to have immunologically competent cells. A list of serum products follows.

Antitoxins*
  Antilymphocyte serum
  Antirabies serum
  Antivenin, spider bite†
  Crotaline antivenin, polyvalent‡
  Diphtheria antitoxin
  Gas gangrene antitoxin, pentavalent§
  Tetanus antitoxin§
Antibodies‖
  Immune serum globulin (human)¶
  Pertussis immune human serum
  Pertussis immune human serum, concentrated
  Rh_o (D) immune globulin (human)
  Tetanus immune globulin (human)
  Vaccinia immune globulin (human)

Animal serum globulins. Hyperimmunity of animals is accomplished by regularly injecting preparations of virus or toxin-producing bacteria that progressively raise the antibody titer as the strength of the challenging substance is increased. Preparations of animal serum provide passive immunity to the individual inoculated after exposure. For example, antivenom may be used to protect the individual bitten by a snake or spider. The bite of a spider, snake, or rabid animal is an unpredictable event without precedent for the individual, and antibodies are not available in the victim's serum. Venom injected by the bite of a snake or spider travels from the injection site into body tissues and may cause acute illness. Administration of antibody-containing serum parenterally and infiltration of the serum around the entry site provides antibodies for neutralization of the venom. Immobilization of the affected area is planned concurrently to decrease venous flow and retard venom absorption from the entry site.

Contaminated or puncture wounds provide protection and enhance the propagation of anaerobic organisms. When wounds occur in previously unchallenged individuals, bacillus growth and liberation of tissue-destroying toxins can be prevented by administration of gas gangrene and tetanus antitoxin. Concurrent debridement and cleansing of the wound are necessary to enhance wound healing and inhibit the growth of anaerobic organisms.

Planned immunization of children with diphtheria toxoid limits the need for protective sera, but exposure of an unprotected individual to diphtheria bacillus necessitates the use of diphtheria antitoxin. The serum is usually administered intravenously, but it may be given intramuscularly to ambulatory contacts of the infected individual.

Use of horse serum carries with it the hazard of sensitivity reactions because horse serum contains a large number of foreign proteins. Prior to use, sensitivity tests are performed. A

---

*Antibodies prepared from horse or bovine serum
†Black widow spider venom used to stimulate antivenin production.
‡Eastern and western diamondback, Central and South American rattlesnake, and Fer-de-lance venom used to stimulate antivenin production.
§Available as a combined solution for single injection.
‖Products contain the globulin portion of serum from immunized humans
¶Extensive geographic collection of placental extracts provides antibodies against hepatitis, rubella, rubeola, and poliomyelitis viruses.

minute amount of the serum is diluted with sodium chloride solution (1:10) and injected into the intradermal tissue or into the conjunctival sac. Redness or swelling in the area of the serum test site is indicative of sensitivity to horse serum. Individuals with atopic allergies usually show sensitivity to horse serum.

Use of the serum in the presence of a positive reaction requires dilution and administration of small amounts (0.5 ml.) of serum at 30-minute intervals. If no reaction follows the first few injections, the remainder may be given by intramuscular injection. Epinephrine hydrochloride solution (1:1000), a rubber airway, and oxygen should be available for use if an anaphylactic response should occur. Distribution of the injected serum may be delayed by application of a tourniquet when the serum is injected into an extremity. Serum sickness, discussed earlier in the chapter, may occur 7 to 10 days after the introduction of horse serum. Bovine serum is available as a well-tolerated substitute serum for individuals with intolerance to horse serum.

Human serum globulins. Immune globulins from human serum are also employed to provide antibody protection. Pooled gamma globulin products obtained from previously challenged human sources provide globulin concentrations up to twenty-five times that of normal human plasma. Intramuscular injection of globulins causes a large, reddened, tender nodule at the injection site that remains up to 4 days. A slight rise in body temperature may occur after administration. Immune globulins supply antibodies to the individual, but the infection may be spread to contacts until the antibodies and normal defense mechanisms complete attenuation or eradication of the invading virus.

Passive immunity may be provided to protect the individual against his own internally produced antibodies. Both antilymphocyte serum and Rh_o (D) immune globulin are agents used to protect against emergence of immune bodies harmful to the host in which they are produced.

Antilymphocyte serum is employed to prevent the production of lymphocytes after organ transplantation. Immune responses are the usual cause of tissue rejection. The injected antibodies attack and destroy the small lymphocytes in the tissue recipient and lessen the rejection response. After the first few injections the recipient begins to produce antibodies against the serum and its effectiveness decreases.

Rh_o (D) globulin is administered intramuscularly (within 72 hours after delivery) to suppress formation of antibodies in the Rh-negative mother after separation of an Rh-positive baby. Blood from the umbilical cord is used to determine the Rh status of the newborn infant. Administration of Rh_o (D) immune globulins prevents antibody formation naturally stimulated by the incompatible placental products at the delivery. The natural antibodies may initiate an antigenic response that prevents subsequent Rh-positive fetal development or destroys the fetal erythrocytes (erythroblastosis fetalis). The commercial products are relatively new, and they are expensive (approximately $75 a vial). Public health department biologic laboratories have begun production, and the cost of administration is about half that of commercial products.

Accidental inoculation (transinoculation) of individuals with vaccine from a recent smallpox vaccination may cause extensive lesions in the second recipient of the vaccine. Vaccinia immune globulin is distributed without charge from the National Communicable Disease Center for treatment of transinoculation-induced disease. The globulin reduces the severity and sequelae of the infection.

Intercontinental collection of immune serum globulin from human placenta provides antibodies for protection of individuals exposed to varying viruses. Initial use of the globulins was limited to children and pregnant women exposed to viral disease (i.e., hepatitis), but expansion of collection sources to include placental extraction made copious quantities of globulin available. For example, immune serum globulin (human) is available for administration as a prophylactic measure to travelers leaving the United States for countries where infectious hepatitis is endemic.

Active immunity

Challenging the individual's physiologic immune responses stimulates the production of

70 Drugs used to control infection and inflammation

Table 4-3. Agents used for active immunization against bacterial toxins, rickettsia, and viruses

Immunizing agents	Inoculation plan		Duration of immunity	Local and general reaction to inoculation
	Schedule	Frequency		
BCG vaccine, attenuated (bacillus Calmette-Guérin strain of *Mycobacterium tuberculosis*)	Preexposure (post negative dermal reaction testing)	1 injection	4 yr.+	Attenuated, primary tuberculosis lesion (8 mm.) at injection site in 1-5 wk. Lymphangitis, urticaria
Cholera vaccine, inactivated (*Vibrio cholerae*)	Preexposure	3 injections at 1 wk. intervals	3-6 mo.	Pain and swelling at injection site Malaise, fever, chills
Diphtheria toxoid*† (*Corynebacterium diphtheriae* toxin)	Age 6-8 wk. or preexposure	3 injections at 4 wk. intervals	5 yr.+	Soreness, redness at injection site lasting up to 2-3 days
Influenza vaccine Bivalent, inactivated‡ (type A_2 Japan; type A_2 Taiwan; type B_2 Massachusetts) Monovalent, inactivated‡ (type A Asian strain) Polyvalent, inactivated‡ type A PR; type A_1 Ann Arbor; type A_2 Japan; type A_2 Taiwan; type B_2 Massachusetts)	Preexposure	2 injections at 2 mo. intervals	1 yr.+	Redness, tenderness at injection site Mild fever, general malaise, backache, headache
Measles virus vaccine, live, attenuated‡§|| (Edmonston, Schwarz, or Enders strains)	Age 12 mo. or preexposure	1 injection	4 yr.+	Fever, rash Occasionally: mild cough, coryza, Koplik's spots lasting 2-5 days
Mumps virus vaccine inactivated‡	Preexposure	2 injections at 4 wk. intervals	6-12 mo.	Tenderness, erythema, and induration at injection site Fever, skin rash, general malaise
Live, attenuated‡|| (Jeryl Lynn B strain)	Age 12 mo. or preexposure	1 injection	2 yr.+	Soreness and erythema at injection site Fever
Pertussis vaccine, inactivated*† (*Bordetella pertussis*)	Age 6 mo. or preexposure	3 injections at 1 mo. intervals	1-4 yr.	Redness and soreness at injection site in first 24 hr. Occasionally: loss of appetite
Plague vaccine, inactivated (*Pasteurella pestis*)	Preexposure	2 injections at 1 wk. intervals	4-6 mo.	Swelling, erythema, induration at injection site Slight fever, malaise, headache

*Available in combined solution for single injection.
†Available as alum-precipitated, aluminum hydroxide–adsorbed, or aluminum phosphate–adsorbed preparations.
‡Product may be from chick or fowl media.
§Product may be from canine media.
\|\|Vaccine contains an antibiotic.
¶Product may be from rabbit brain media.

Table 4-3. Agents used for active immunization against bacterial toxins, rickettsia and viruses—cont'd

Immunizing agents	Inoculation plan		Duration of immunity	Local and general reaction to inoculation
	Schedule	Frequency		
Poliomyelitis vaccine				
Attenuated*‖ (type 1 Brunhilde; type 2 Lansing; type 3 Leon)	Age 6-12 wk. or preexposure	3 injections at 1 mo. intervals	4 yr.+	Mild localized reaction at injection site General malaise, low-grade fever
Live, oral, monovalent‖ (types 1, 2, 3 Sabin strains)	Age 6-24 wk. or preexposure	1 drink of each type at 6 wk. intervals	4 yr.+	
Live, oral, trivalent‖ (types 1, 2, and 3 Sabin strains)	Age 10-12 mo. or preexposure	1 drink 6 mo. after monovalent series	4 yr.+	
Rabies vaccine, inactivated‡¶	Preexposure and postexposure	2 injections at 1 mo. intervals	6 mo.	Transient stinging, tenderness, erythema, induration at injection site Regional lymphadenopathy
Rocky Mountain spotted fever vaccine, inactivated‡ (Rickettsia rickettsii)	Preexposure	3 injections at 1 wk. intervals	1 yr.	Slight soreness at injection sight
Rubella virus vaccine, live‡§‖ (Cendehill or HPV-77 strains)	Age 12 mo. or preexposure	1 injection	4 yr.+	Induration, pain at injection site Occasionally: transient arthralgia, skin rash, fever
Smallpox vaccine, attenuated‡‖ (vaccinia virus)	Age 15-18 mo. or preexposure	1 injection	3 yr.+	Pustulation, crusting at injection site Maculopapular rash, fever, lymphadenitis Accidental trans-inoculation
Tetanus toxoid*† (Clostridium tetani toxin)	Age 6-8 wk. or preexposure	3 injections at 4 wk. intervals	5 yr.+	Redness, edema at injection site for 2-3 days
Typhoid vaccine, inactivated (Salmonella typhi)	Preexposure	3 injections at 1-4 wk. intervals	1 yr.	Redness at injection site Malaise, fever, headache
Typhoid and paratyphoid vaccine, inactivated (Salmonella typhi, S. paratyphi, S. schottmülleri)	Preexposure	3 injections at 1 wk. intervals	1 yr.	Edematous swelling, pain at injection site for 48 hr. Fever, malaise, headache, nausea
Typhus vaccine, inactivated‡ (Rickettsia prowazeki)	Preexposure	2 injections at 1 wk. intervals	6 mo.	Redness at injection site Malaise, headache
Yellow fever vaccine, attenuated‡	Preexposure	1 injection	6 yr.	Fever, generalized aching 1 wk. after injection

antibodies specific to the antigen introduced. Duration of immunity is related to the virulence of the biologic agent used to stimulate the response. Live or attenuated microorganisms provide the highest level stimulus to antibody production; consequently antibodies are available in large numbers over a long period of time. Inactivated microorganisms provide less stimulus, and the duration of effectiveness is considerably shorter (Table 4-3).

Use of microorganisms (or toxoids) constitutes the intentional production of subclinical disease to stimulate production of antibodies at (or close to) a level that would result from exposure to the disease. At the end of the predictable period of protection, subsequent exposure may precipitate disease unless additional challenge is provided as a booster of the antibody level.

Diverse media are used to develop the immunizing agents; therefore it is necessary to ascertain the particular media and the patient's sensitivity to specific products (i.e., egg protein, canine dander) prior to administration. Many of the products are available in a form designed to prolong absorption (i.e., precipitated, or adsorbed). Prolongation of drug absorption delays the onset of effect, but it also increases antibody titers by slowly releasing antigen from the injection site. The additives, or *adjuvants,* are irritating to tissues, so a small air bubble is left in the syringe to be injected after the solution. The procedure prevents escape of adjuvant into the injection tract tissues. A small nodule may remain for some time after the injection. The varying potency of each vaccine affects the amount of the immunizing agent (0.5 to 1 ml.) required to provide protection, and specific information is provided on the package inserts accompanying each agent.

Poliomyelitis vaccine (Sabin strains) is the only live virus preparation for oral use. Successful suppression of poliomyelitis epidemics has grown out of the planned spread of the virus in attenuated form from the individual taking the vaccine to other nonprotected contacts. The efficacy of the virus is dependent on its reproduction in the host gastrointestinal tract. Administration of the vaccine is most effective when planned to avoid the high incidence of enteroviral infections occurring from May through October in temperate climates.

The desirability of providing immunity with methods other than injection of antigen has led to experiments with oral agents. Bacillus Calmette-Guérin (BCG) vaccine is being tested as an aerosol spray for tuberculosis immunity building in children. A plan for controlled exposure to virus in a small mobile cubicle has been implemented, and early tests of immunologically competent cells show effectiveness of the method for mass protection of school-age children.

Studies of the incidence of communicable diseases have affected trends in planned immunization programs. Smallpox vaccination was considered mandatory for children until a few years ago, and vaccination of children between 12 and 24 months of age was a routine component of child health care programs. The high incidence of vaccinia reactions caused by contamination of tissues apart from the vaccination site resulted in pustules covering the body surface and acute illness. The incidence of vaccinia reactions rose above the rate of reported cases of smallpox and routine vaccination was halted. Reexamination of the plan may be appropriate, since recent reports indicate the incidence of smallpox is rising. Only about half the children under 4 years of age are vaccinated, and the incidence of smallpox has tripled in recent years.

Immunization with rubella virus vaccine is the only plan for vaccination that is directed at a target population other than the individuals being immunized. Children are immunized to protect the mother against rubella when she is pregnant. Fifteen to 20% of the women of child-bearing age are susceptible to the disease and would have clinical or subclinical rubella if an epidemic occurred. The rubella epidemic of 1964 caused nonprotected women to deliver infants that had problems described as a rubella syndrome (deafness, blindness, congenital heart disease, mental retardation). Protection of the fetus against rubella virus exposure is accomplished by decreasing the exposure of women of child-bearing age by vaccination of children.

Table 4-3 has been prepared as a guide to defining the immunizations advisable for individuals in the community. It is offered as a base for informed health teaching in contacts with patients. For example, the individual who has received monovalent influenza vaccine will need help to understand the concept of *influenza strain shift* necessitating annual immunization for prevalent strains of influenza expected to be present in the area during the year. Preparing him for local or generalized discomforts known to occur after immunization may help him to accept them as usual and a small price to pay for disease prevention.

The immunizing agents are disease specific, and it is necessary to explore the problems relative to the diseases to fully appreciate the importance of immunization to humanity. Each of the agents represents a long search for a specific disease-suppressing immunizing agent to decrease the susceptibility of the host.

INFLAMMATORY RESPONSE SUPPRESSION

The natural role of glucocorticoids in mobilization of carbohydrates and in suppression of the inflammatory and immune response provides stabilizing and protective mechanisms against some of the disruptive effects of varying physiologic and emotional stressors. Normal physiologic responses to intense or sustained stressors result in higher plasma levels of glucocorticoids, aldosterone, and androgens caused by the release of the hormones from the adrenal cortex.

The natural stimulus for liberation of the adrenocorticoids arises in the hypothalamic *corticotropin-releasing center.* Hypothalamic release of *corticotropin-releasing factor* stimulates anterior pituitary centers to release the adrenocorticotropic hormone (ACTH) necessary to adrenal cortex stimulation (Fig. 4-4). The adrenal cortex responds to stimulation by synthesizing adrenal steroids from cholesterol and releasing hormones into the circulation.

The steroids most involved in tissue responses to trauma are the glucocorticoids; therefore the natural mechanisms for production of glucocorticoid is the focus of this section. The chief glucocorticoid is *cortisol* (95%),

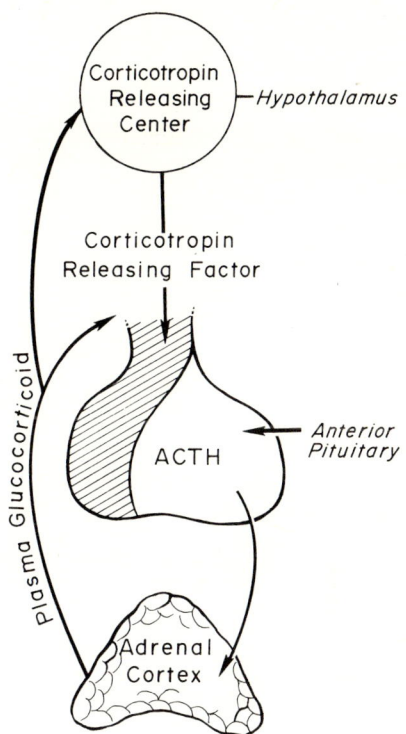

Fig. 4-4. Hypothalamic-pituitary-adrenal hormonal interaction maintains physiologic plasma glucocorticoid levels.

although *corticosterone* and *cortisone* are also present in adrenocortical secretions.

The hypothalamic-pituitary-adrenal hormonal interaction is a negative feedback mechanism that maintains physiologic levels of glucocorticoids in the plasma. The inverse relationship between glucocorticoid levels and ACTH increases ACTH release when plasma glucocorticoid levels are low. Physiologically normal levels of plasma glucocorticoid decreases the release of ACTH. Stressors increase glucocorticoid availability by stimulating the hypothalamic-pituitary release of ACTH. Stressor stimulation overrides the negative feedback mechanism, and glucocorticoids are released at higher levels than those reached in nonstress periods.

Glucocorticoids are involved in carbohydrate, protein, and fat metabolism. Stress-induced elevation of cortisol levels stimulates hepatic glyconeogenesis and protein synthesis and inhibits peripheral tissue protein synthesis. Pro-

74 Drugs used to control infection and inflammation

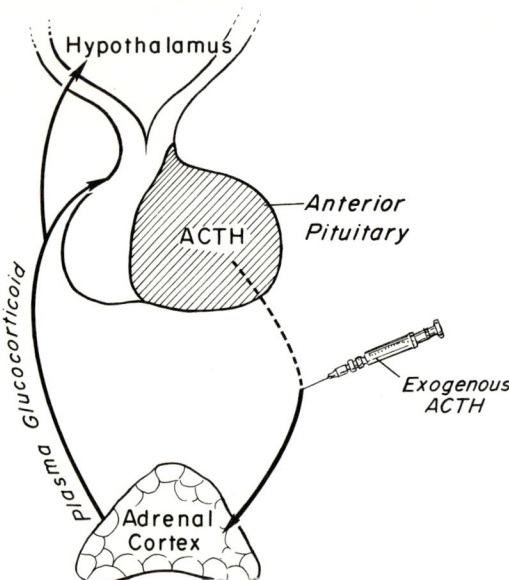

Fig. 4-5. Exogenous ACTH provides the stimulus for adrenocorticoid release, including glucocorticoid. Elevated plasma glucocorticoid levels inhibit subsequent release of endogenous ACTH.

vision of carbohydrates and maintenance of protein production in the liver are a physiologic adaptive mechanism to sustain the individual during periods of stress.

Pharmacodynamics

Pituitary hormone administration. Replacement of the pituitary hormone by exogenous administration is necessary when pituitary function is decreased or when the gland has been removed. In the presence of normal adrenal glands, ACTH may be administered to stimulate glucocorticoid production for control of acute inflammatory responses. When high plasma levels of glucocorticoids are needed, it is more usual for the glucocorticoids rather than ACTH to be administered.

Administration of ACTH stimulates production and release of glucocorticoid hormone, and increased plasma glucocorticoid levels decrease the production of endogenous ACTH during therapy (Fig. 4-5). ACTH administration stimulates production of all adrenocorticoid hormones; therefore use of ACTH is accompanied by elevated plasma levels of the chief adrenocorticoids: aldosterone, cortisol, and androgen.

Administration. ACTH, or corticotropin (Acthar), must be administered parenterally for systemic effect because the digestive juices destroy the polypeptide compound. Aqueous ACTH is administered intravenously over a period of 8 hours to maintain a 24-hour period of pharmacodynamic activity. When administered intravenously, the drug is rapidly destroyed, but slow infusion provides the adrenocortical stimulation necessary to sustained plasma levels of the adrenal hormones. Intramuscularly administered aqueous ACTH is rapidly utilized in the body, and maintenance of therapeutic levels requires a plan for administration of the drug (3 to 25 units) at regular 6-hour intervals.

ACTH is available in repository and zinc hydroxide formulations that may be given once daily for pharmacodynamic activity that persists for 18 to 24 hours. The addition of gelatin to ACTH also prolongs the effect of repository corticotropin (ACTH gel, Corticotropin-gel, Depo-ACTH, Cortrophin gel, H.P. Acthar gel).

Discontinuance of drug therapy includes a plan for gradual decrease in dosage to allow time for normal adrenal responses to endogenous ACTH to be firmly established. Rapid withdrawal after high dosage may precipitate problems related to adrenocortical hypofunction during the first 2 to 5 days after stopping administration of the ACTH.

Adverse effects. The direct relationship between ACTH administration and glucocorticoid release makes it possible to view some of the effects and adverse effects of ACTH within the framework of glucocorticoid administration. Increased levels of mineralocorticoid (aldosterone) may cause sodium ion retention and potassium ion losses during therapy with ACTH. Limiting sodium ion intake and providing potassium ion supplements may maintain balance and prevent edema. Specific effects and problems during administration of mineralocorticoids will be presented in Chapter 6. Excess androgen release results in signs of masculinization and hirsutism. Therapeutic effects of androgens will be presented in Chapter 27.

Glucocorticoid administration. Exogenous glucocorticoids are most frequently used to

Immune and allergic responses 75

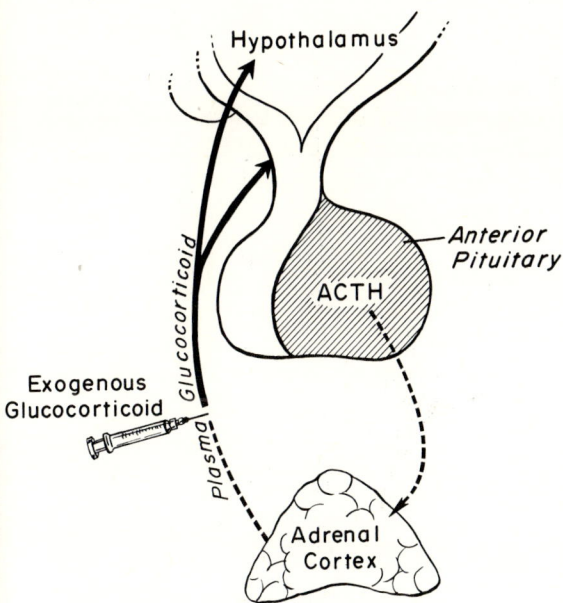

Fig. 4-6. Exogenous glucocorticoid raises the plasma level and decreases ACTH release from the pituitary gland. In the absence of ACTH stimulation the adrenal gland ceases to provide endogenous glucocorticoid, and dependence on exogenous glucocorticoid is established.

produce high plasma levels of the hormone required for suppression of inflammatory and immune responses in acute situations, although they are used for chronic illnesses in selected situations when other control measures are ineffective. For example, glucocorticoids may be administered to control inflammatory responses when physiologic defense mechanisms mobilized in response to tissue trauma (i.e., surgery, immune responses, or injury) impinge on vital organ function and disrupt physiologic processes. Glucocorticoids are also employed when tissue response to the individual's own body proteins (autoimmunity) causes an inflammatory response in collagen fibers of the skin, bone, ligaments, and cartilage that progressively cripples or limits the function of the individual.

Glucocorticoids suppress the inflammatory response by interfering with the chief physiologic factors that promote and maintain the sequestration of fluid and irritants. Glucocorticoids decrease the transudation of fluid from capillaries and infiltration of leukocytes at tissue sites. The hormone also stabilizes lysosome membranes, thereby decreasing spill of tissue enzymes that propagate the inflammatory process.

Glucocorticoids cause an initial brief output of antibodies, but the hormone decreases immune responses by inhibiting antibody production. Suppression of immune bodies is therapeutic in autoimmunity or in control of immune responses during tissue transplantation.

Glucocorticoid administration supplies the hormone in amounts calculated to meet the individual needs of the patient. Exogenous glucocorticoid administration raises the plasma level and decreases both ACTH and endogenous glucocorticoid production (Fig. 4-6). Administration of the glucocorticoids is planned to maintain a consistent plasma level of hormone throughout the 24-hour period. Inactivity of the adrenal cortex during exogenous administration makes it necessary to follow carefully the prescribed plan for gradual discontinuance of drug administration. For example, prednisone dosage may be lessened from 30 mg./24 hours, divided into 3 doses, to 20 mg./24 hours, divided into 2 doses, for 2 days, and finally 10 mg./24 hours, divided into 2 doses, for 5 days. The gradual decrease in dosage provides time for the adrenal gland to resume activity. Long-term administration of glucocorticoids may be interrupted for short rest periods during which ACTH may be administered to stimulate natural adrenal hormone production.

Fludrocortisone acetate (Table 4-4) is a synthetic glucocorticoid that also has mineralocorticoid activity. Administration of the drug may result in greater sodium ion retention and potassium ion depletion than those occurring with other glucocorticoids. The manifestations of mineralocorticoid effect are additive to the glucocorticoid effect. Only in rare instances will other forms of the glucocorticoids cause comparable mineralocorticoid-like effects.

There are variations in the particular products used for therapy, but all the drugs increase the amount of glucocorticoid available in the body. The physician's selection of a particular drug is related to dosage and route of administration appropriate to therapy of the patient's

Table 4-4. Dosage range of glucocorticoids

Nonproprietary name	Proprietary (trade) name	Daily adult dosage range	Nonproprietary name	Proprietary (trade) name	Daily adult dosage range
Betamethasone	Celestone	Oral: 0.6-8.4 mg.	Methylprednisolone acetate	Depo-Medrol	I.M.: 3-300 mg. (÷4)
Betamethasone sodium phosphate and acetate	Celestone Soluspan	I.M. 1.5-12 mg./wk (÷2)	Methylprednisolone sodium succinate	Solu-Medrol	I.M.: 10-160 mg. (÷4) I.V.: Same
Cortisone acetate	Cortivite, Cortogen, Cortone	Oral: 12.5-400 mg. (÷4) I.M.: 100-300 mg. (÷3)	Paramethasone acetate	Haldrone	Oral: 1.5-12 mg. (÷3-4)
Dexamethasone	Decadron, Deronil, Dexameth, Gammacorten, Hexadrol	Oral: 0.5-10 mg.	Prednisolone	Co-Hydeltra, Delta-Cortef, Hydeltra, Meticortelone, Paracortol, Prednis, Sterane, Sterolone	Oral: 5-50 mg. (÷4)
Dexamethasone sodium phosphate	Decadron phosphate	I.M.: 2-80 mg. (÷3-4) I.V.: Same	Prednisolone acetate	Sterane	I.M.: 5-50 mg. (÷4)
Fludrocortisone acetate	Alflorone, F-Cortef, Florinef	Oral: 0.1-2 mg.	Prednisolone butylacetate	Hydeltra T.B.A.	I.M.: 5-50 mg. (÷4)
Fluprednisolone	Alphadrol	Oral: 0.075-22.5 mg. (÷4)	Prednisolone sodium hemisuccinate	Meticortelone soluble	I.V.: 100-200 mg. (÷2-4)
Hydrocortisone	Cort-Dome, Cortef, Cortifan, Cortisol, Cortril, Hydrocortone	Oral: 10-350 mg. (÷4)	Prednisolone sodium phosphate	Hydeltrasol	I.M.: 10-100 mg. I.V.: Same
Hydrocortisone sodium succinate	Solu-Cortef	I.M.: 50 mg./kg. I.V.: Same	Prednisone	Deltasone, Deltra, Meticorten, Paracort	Oral: 5-75 mg. (÷4)
Meprednisone	Betapar	Oral: 2-64 mg. (÷3-4)	Triamcinolone	Aristocort, Kenacort	Oral: 4-100 mg. (÷3-4)
Methylprednisolone	Medrol, Wyacort	Oral: 3-300 mg. (÷4)	Triamcinolone acetonide	Kenalog	I.M.: 40-80 mg. weekly
			Triamcinolone diacetate		I.M.: 40-80 mg. weekly

problem. The drugs are administered by all body routes including intra-articular, intrasynovial, and topical areas.

Glucocorticoids have an effect on almost every organ in the body, and it can be predicted that drugs with wide-spectrum therapeutic effect will also have many adverse effects. Many of the problems during drug use are extensions of the planned pharmacodynamic action. The patient must understand and participate in plans for maximizing the effect of therapy and preventing extension of problems arising concurrent with drug use.

Patient care

Use of the glucocorticoids is often instituted in situations in which the patient is in acute distress with a generalized allergic or inflammatory process (i.e., bronchial asthma, arthritis). During the acute phase the patient's attention is directed at each indication of suppression of the life-threatening or painful entity. Administration of glucocorticoids shows some target tissue effect within 24 to 48 hours of initiation of therapy. Glucocorticoids prevent the damaging effects of the inflammatory response, but they do not treat the basic dis-

Immune and allergic responses 77

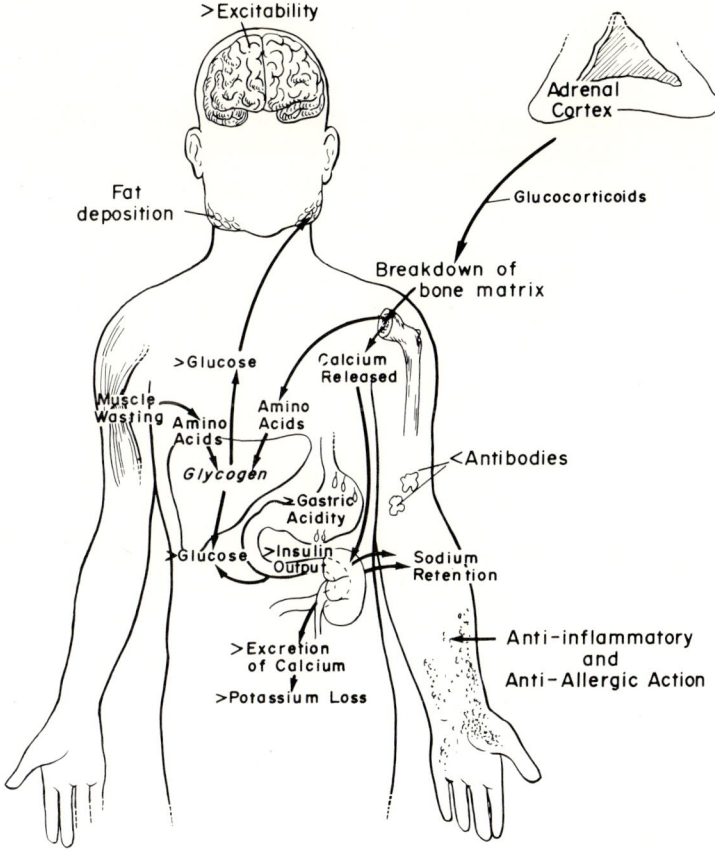

Fig. 4-7. Principle biochemical actions of glucocorticoids are protein breakdown, glyconeogenesis, and lipogenesis. The pharmacotherapeutic effect on traumatized tissue is often the basis for administration of the drugs. Gastric acidity and cation imbalances present problems during therapy.

ease or condition that initiates the response.

Assessment of drug effect. Modification of the inflammatory response may mean increased mobility for the patient, but he should be encouraged to modify activity to prevent damage to areas with residual inflammation. Speed of return to previous activity levels will depend on the status of the patient. During the period of reduced activity, plans directed at maintenance of tissue integrity are an important aspect of care.

Concurrent with inflammatory or immune response suppression, some of the positive effects regularly seen during therapy with glucocorticoids are a feeling of well-being and improvement in appetite with consequent weight gain. To enhance drug effect and decrease protein depletion, the patient on long-term therapy should be encouraged to maintain a liberal protein intake. Anabolic agents sometimes are used to improve amino acid synthesis and counteract the catabolic effects of glucocorticoids on muscle tissue. Rapid protein catabolism increases serum and urinary urea levels, and monitoring of blood urea nitrogen levels (BUN) and quantity of urinary output provide an indication of effective elimination of the metabolic waste.

Assessment of adverse effects. Some of the effects occurring during drug administration are gastrointestinal bleeding, changes in the musculoskeletal structures (osteoporosis, muscle wasting, weakness), and increased lability of glucose balance in patients with diabetes. Consideration of the diverse problems presented during use of glucocorticoids for control of an extensive inflammatory response will help to identify and clarify some of the interrelated problems occurring during therapy (Fig. 4-7).

Glucocorticoids increase gastric acidity, and the acid content is irritating to the gastric mucosa. Long-term administration of glucocorticoids causes a high incidence of ulceration. Administration of the drugs with milk or a snack may decrease gastric irritation, and the physician usually prescribes an antacid to neutralize gastric contents between meals. Antacids are often administered on an alternating schedule with milk or cream to provide maximum protection of the mucosal lining. Testing of all stools and vomitus for microscopic amounts of blood is a routine established during glucocorticoid therapy to assure early definition of gastrointestinal bleeding.

Glucocorticoids accomplish glyconeogenesis, which increases available nutrients and supplies glucose for tissue needs. Breakdown of bone matrix and muscle protein weakens the musculoskeletal structure. The catabolic process also mobilizes calcium and potassium ions, and urinary elimination of the vital electrolytes increases. Long-term use of the glucocorticoids increases the fragility of bones and decreases muscle strength. Throughout long-term therapy, dosage levels are maintained at the lowest level that will control the patient's problems because the musculoskeletal effects of the glucocorticoids have an adverse effect on the functional capacity of the patient. The patient must be alert for changes that affect his ability to function, and he should be helped to modify activity and correct hazardous situations within his home (i.e., loose scatter rugs, highly waxed floors) that could lead to accidents.

Glyconeogenesis increases the availability of carbon, hydrogen, and oxygen components for fat synthesis, and lipids are deposited in the mandibular area during prolonged therapy. The effect initially appears to be a soft and pleasant change in facial contour, but as deposition increases, the classic moon face appearance is evident. Fat deposition also occurs in supraclavicular and abdominal tissues, but facial deposits are more easily identified.

Elevation of circulating glucose levels increases the need for insulin for utilization of the carbohydrate. The increased demand for insulin places a burden on the productivity of the pancreas, which may cause a drug-related diabetic state. Patients with diabetes mellitus are prone to sharp and sudden changes in hypoglycemic and hyperglycemic states, which make control difficult when glucocorticoids are prescribed. Routine tests of blood sugar levels and regularly scheduled tests for sugar and acetone content of the urine are planned for all patients receiving glucocorticoids.

Suppression of the inflammatory and immune responses is a planned effect of glucocorticoid therapy, but the patient is gradually deprived of the normal physiologic defense mechanisms that control invasion of pathogens. Protection from exposure to infection is a necessary component of the patient's care. Prophylactic use of anti-infective drugs may be prescribed by the physician. Specific assessment of changes in the patient's status include observation of changes in respiratory tract secretions and the healing status of wounds and lesions. Cultures of exudate that are obtained promptly after evidence of change may allow initiation of anti-infective drug therapy before the pathogen obtains a foothold in a patient with decreased defenses.

Central nervous system stimulation may be a positive effect if it is confined to mood elevation, but patients may have changes ranging from euphoria to psychosis. Base-line personality traits are important in definition of changes. The patient's family may be the best source for information about pretreatment personality in the acutely ill patient. Patients frequently complain of an inability to sleep because their "minds are racing."

The glucocorticoids may be employed as a vital part of hormone replacement therapy for the adrenalectomized individual. Total dependence on exogenous glucocorticoids necessitates conscientious use of the drug. Evidence of insufficient plasma levels of the hormone would be comparable to those seen in the patient during sudden withdrawal of glucocorticoids (i.e., weakness, abdominal pain, circulatory collapse, nausea, vomiting).

The dramatic changes resulting from use of

glucocorticoids often overshadow the problems occurring during therapy. Maintaining balance between therapy and emergence of adverse effects is important to continued use of drugs that may be the patient's lifeline.

REFERENCES

Ascari, W. Q., Allen, A. E., Baker, W. J., and Pollack, W.: Rh$_o$ (D) Immune globulin (human): evaluation in women at risk of Rh immunization, Journal of the American Medical Association **205**:71, 1968.

Calafiore, Dorothy C.: Eradication of measles in the United States, American Journal of Nursing **67**:1871, 1967.

Clarke, C. A.: Prevention of "Rhesus" babies, Scientific American **219**:46, Nov., 1968.

Cooper, Louis Z.: German measles, Scientific American **215**:30, July, 1966.

Craven, Ruth Falk: Anaphylactic shock, American Journal of Nursing **72**:718, 1972.

Dean, Geoffrey: The multiple sclerosis problem, Scientific American **223**:40, July, 1970.

Edelman, Gerald M.: The structure and function of antibodies, Scientific American **223**:34, Aug., 1970.

Ehrenkranz, N. Joel, Ventura, Arnoldo K., Cuadrando, Raul R., Pons, William L., and Porter, John E.: Pandemic dengue in Caribbean countries and the southern United States, The New England Journal of Medicine **285**:1460, 1971.

Francis, Thomas, Jr.: Epidemic influenza: immunization and control, Medical Clinics of North America **51**:781, 1967.

Frazier, Claude A.: Diagnosis and treatment of insect bites, Clinical Symposia **20**:75, 1968.

Goodman, Louis S., and Gilman, Alfred, editors: The pharmacological basis of therapeutics, ed. 4, New York, 1970, The Macmillan Co.

Grant, Michael E., and Prockop, Darwin J.: Biosynthesis of collagen, The New England Journal of Medicine **286**:291, 1972.

Grossberg, Sidney E.: The interferons and their inducers, The New England Journal of Medicine **287**:13, 79, 1972.

Guillemin, Roger, and Burgus, Roger: The hormones of the hypothalamus, Scientific American **227**:24, Nov., 1972.

Hilleman, Maurice R., and Tytell, Alfred A.: The induction of interferon, Scientific American **225**:26, July, 1971.

Hirschhorn, Norbert, and Greenough, William B., III: Cholera, Scientific American **225**:15, Aug., 1971.

Holden, Melvin, Dubin, Michael R., and Diamond, Paul H.: Negative intermediate-strength tuberculin sensitivity in active tuberculosis, The New England Journal of Medicine **285**:1506, 1971.

Horstmann, Dorothy M.: Lagging immunity in our children, The New England Journal of Medicine **285**:1432, 1971.

Janeway, Charles A.: Progress in immunology, Journal of Pediatrics **72**:886, 1968.

Johnson, Richard T.: Effects of viral infection on the developing nervous system, The New England Journal of Medicine **287**:599, 1972.

Kilbourne, Edwin D.: Influenza: the vaccines. In Hospital practice symposium on influenza, New York, 1971, HP Publishing Co., Inc.

Lister, Joann: Nursing intervention in anaphylactic shock, American Journal of Nursing **72**:720, 1972.

Luria, Salvador E.: The recognition of DNA in bacteria, Scientific American **222**:88, Jan., 1970.

McCombs, Robert P.: Diseases due to immunologic reactions in the lungs, The New England Journal of Medicine **286**:1186, 1245, 1972.

Meade, Gordon M.: Contemporary tuberculin testing, American Family Physician **5**:68, May, 1972.

Mountcastle, Vernon B., editor: Medical physiology, ed. 13, vol. 1, St. Louis, 1974, The C. V. Mosby Co.

Morrison, Shirley T., and Arnold, Carolyn R.: Patients with common communicable diseases: preventive measures, treatment, and rehabilitation, Nursing Clinics of North America **5**:143, 1970.

Orten, James M., and Neuhaus, Otto W.: Biochemistry, ed. 8, St. Louis, 1970, The C. V. Mosby Co.

Peters, William P., Holland, James F., Senn, Hansjoerg, Rhomberg, Walter, and Banerjee, Tarit: Corticosteroid administration and localized leukocyte mobilization, The New England Journal of Medicine **286**:342, 1972.

Puschak, Russell, Young, Muriel, McKee, Thomas V., and Plotkin, Stanley A.: Intranasal vaccination with RA 27-3 attenuated rubella virus, Journal of Pediatrics **79**:55, 1971.

Reilly, Mary Jo, editor: American hospital formulary service, vol. 1, sect. 4:00; vol. 2, sect. 68:00, 80:00, Washington, D.C., 1973, American Society of Hospital Pharmacists.

Remington, Jack S.: The compromised host, Hospital Practice **7**:59, April, 1972.

Rose, Harry M.: Influenza: the agent. In Hospital practice symposium on influenza, New York, 1971, HP Publishing Co., Inc.

Rosenthal, Sol Roy: BCG vaccine, American Family Physician **5**:98, Feb., 1972.

Ross, Russell: Wound healing, Scientific American **220**:40, June, 1969.

Russell, Findlay E.: Injuries by venomous animals, American Journal of Nursing **66**:1322, 1966.

Sherman, William B.: Atopic hypersensitivity, Medical Clinics of North America **49**:1597, 1965.

Smith, Alice Lorraine: Microbiology and pathology, ed. 10, St. Louis, 1972, The C. V. Mosby Co.

Speirs, Robert S.: How cells attack antigens, Scientific American **210**:58, Feb., 1964.

Tomasi, Thomas B., Jr.: Secretory immunoglobulins, The New England Journal of Medicine **287**:500, 1972.

Vaheri, Antti, Vesikari, Timo, Oker-Blom, Nils, Seppala, Markku, Parkman, Paul D., Veronelli, Jorge, and Robbins, Frederick C.: Isolation of rubella-vaccine virus from human products of conception, The New England Journal of Medicine **286**:1071, 1972.

Van Heyningen, W. E.: Tetanus, Scientific American **218**:69, 1968.

Wyll, Shelby A.: The current status of measles (rubeola) in the United States, Journal of the Kentucky Medical Association **70**:99, Feb., 1972.

UNIT TWO
DRUGS USED TO CONTROL EXCRETION OF FLUID, METABOLIC WASTES, AND TOXICANTS

5 Pulmonary ventilation

6 Fluid balance

7 Tissue toxicants and debris

8 Enteric elimination

9 Emesis

10 Gastric acidity and intestinal motility

5

Pulmonary ventilation

Arterial blood gases
Acid-base shift
Medullary chemoreceptors
Arterial chemoreceptors
Pressure differentials
Secretion mobilization
Drug therapy
Bronchial constriction
    Pharmacodynamics
    Patient care
Respiratory depression
    Pharmacodynamics
Retained secretions
    Pharmacodynamics
    Patient care

Periodic inspiration and expiration cycles and patent air passages are primary factors in maintenance of gas exchange. Diffusion of gases across the alveolar capillary membrane perfuses the blood with oxygen necessary for body needs and removes the carbon dioxide produced during physiologic work (Fig. 5-1).

Normal ventilation-perfusion ratios at the alveolar capillary membrane occur as a consequence of complex neural and chemical stimuli that influence the *volume, pressure,* and *time factors* involved in gas exchange. Interaction between varying compensatory mechanisms provides the adjustments required by changing metabolic activity, and the same mechanisms may maintain gas exchange when external or internal factors disrupt pulmonary ventilation.

Arterial blood gases

Monitoring of the arterial blood gas content allows identification of the effectiveness of ventilation-perfusion ratios in maintaining gas exchange. Disruption of the volume, pressure, or time factors at either side of the alveolar capillary surface causes a shift in the partial pressures of arterial blood gases. For example, shallow respirations or continued partial airway obstruction by thick, tenacious secretions changes ventilation factors and causes lowered arterial blood oxygen content and elevated arterial blood carbon dioxide content.

Acid-base shift

Increased carbon dioxide content of the blood (hypercapnia) increases the formation of carbonic acid in circulating fluids. Retention of carbon dioxide changes the bicarbonate:carbonic acid ratio from the 20:1 value of physiologic equilibrium. When the level of carbonic acid increases (i.e., with respiratory depression) acidosis has an adverse effect on normal physiologic processes. Renal compensatory mechanisms are capable of removing excess hydrogen ions to correct the acidotic state, but the process is very slow.

Medullary chemoreceptors

Chemoreceptors in the respiratory centers of the upper ventral surface of the medulla are stimulated by the increased hydrogen ion content of the carbonic acid (H_2CO_3), and efferent neural impulses to pulmonary tissues increase the rate and depth of respiratory excursions. The high concentration of carbonic acid in spinal fluid bathing the medulla is the source of the medullary center stimulus. Increase in the volume and in the time of respirations instituted by the compensatory mechanisms increases the carbon dioxide expiration rate

84 Drugs used to control excretion of fluid, metabolic wastes, and toxicants

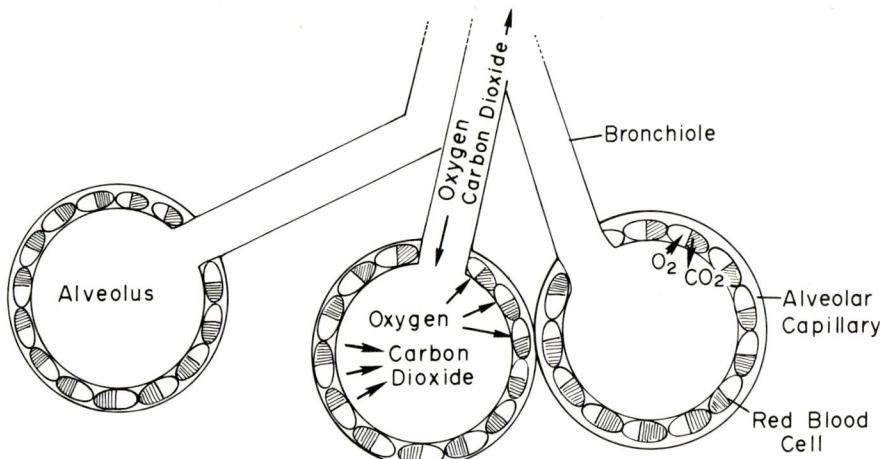

Fig. 5-1. Red blood cells enter the alveolar capillary bed with carbon dioxide (CO_2) attached to hemoglobin. Pressure differentials cause CO_2 diffusion into alveolar spaces, and oxygen (O_2) replaces it on the hemoglobin attachment site.

($H_2CO_3 \longrightarrow H_2O + CO_2$), and the resulting decrease in carbonic acid returns the pH of blood toward the normal alkaline value (pH 7.4).

The response of medullary chemoreceptors to hydrogen ion stimuli improves exchange of both carbon dioxide and oxygen at the alveolar capillary membrane. Although excess carbon dioxide institutes the sequence of events leading to respiratory changes, improved oxygen exchange is a natural consequence of the increased rate and depth of respiration.

Arterial chemoreceptors

Chemoreceptors in the carotid artery and aorta respond to hypoxia or hypercapnia. Chemoreceptor-initiated neural impulses are routed through the medullary inspiratory centers to the lungs. The stimuli increase the rate and volume of respirations. The carotid and aortic bodies are thought to be secondary mechanisms that become active when chronic levels of hypercapnia decrease the sensitivity of the medullary centers to carbonic acid. Patients with chronic obstructive lung disease may become dependent on the response of the arterial centers to hypoxia for respiratory control because medullary centers become desensitized to the chronically elevated levels of carbon dioxide.

Pressure differentials

Constriction or partial obstruction of the bronchi initially causes an increase in the respiratory rate (hyperpnea). Hypercapnia stimulates vasomotor centers in the medulla and pons, and tachycardia ensues. Changed respiratory and cardiac time factors increase the alveolar ventilation rate and the circulation of blood in pulmonary capillaries. Pressure differentials naturally causing diffusion of gases across the alveolar capillary membrane can be maintained by the changed time factors.

Carbon dioxide pressures. The increased rate of expiration removes retained carbon dioxide from the alveoli, and the lower alveolar concentration speeds the movement of carbon dioxide from venous blood into the alveoli. The process gradually returns the partial pressure of carbon dioxide in the alveoli to the normal level (40 mm. Hg), which maintains the pressure differential required for movement of capillary carbon dioxide at 46 mm. Hg partial pressure toward the lower carbon dioxide concentration of the alveolar space.

Oxygen pressures. Diffusion of oxygen across the alveolar capillary membrane is also increased when the rate of respiration and circulation is accelerated. Inspiration provides sufficient oxygen to perfuse the increased quantity of blood circulating through the capillary bed. The differential between partial pressure of oxygen in the alveoli (100 mm. Hg) and that of capillary blood (40 mm. Hg) is basic to the diffusion of oxygen. Arterial blood leaving the capillary bed has an oxygen content of at least 100 mm. Hg.

Secretion mobilization

Activity tolerance is adversely affected by decreased gas exchange. For example, the individual with large amounts of tenacious bronchial secretions (i.e., respiratory tract infection) will breathe heavily with minimal activity. He may stop to rest and catch his breath while dressing. Taking his pulse at this time would reveal an increased cardiac rate. The increased rate and depth of respirations move secretions to the cough-sensitive areas of the main bronchus, and coughing clears the respiratory tree of excess mucus, after which the individual may continue with the planned activity.

Drug therapy

Drugs used to control ventilation have a positive effect in maintaining normal gas exchange at the alveolar level. By varying modes of action, the drugs dilate bronchial structures, increase the rate and depth of respirations, control cough, or liquefy secretions.

BRONCHIAL CONSTRICTION

Bronchial constriction is a recurrent problem of individuals with atopic traits causing allergic responses in tissues of the respiratory tract. Constriction of the bronchi or bronchioles decreases the movement of carbon dioxide and oxygen during respiration. Gases trapped in pulmonary lobes distal to the areas of constriction distend the alveoli, and alveolar architectural changes may result from prolonged distention.

For the patient the struggle to breathe with acute bronchial constriction is an intolerable physical burden. The accessory muscles are used to support efforts to breathe. Acute respiratory distress in children moves rapidly from initial restlessness, apprehension, and increased respiratory and cardiac rate to overt evidence of the struggle to breathe. Sternal retractions and nasal flaring are overt signs of increased respiratory work. Cyanosis appears as oxygen deprivation continues, and respiratory failure would be a natural outcome if the distressing situation were allowed to progress. The feeling of suffocation causes a high anxiety level, and administration of prompt-acting bronchodilating drugs provides relief of the intolerable situation.

Pharmacodynamics

Bronchodilators. In acute emergency situations, epinephrine hydrochloride is used for its prompt bronchodilating action. The potent bronchodilator is needed for reversal of the diffuse constriction that may completely occlude the air passages in anaphylactic reactions. Theophyllines provide comparable relief in the patient with bronchial asthma who has constriction of the upper air passages, but the onset of effect is slower than that of epinephrine hydrochloride.

Theophyllines. In addition to the drugs readily identified by the nonproprietary name, aminophylline, dyphylline, and oxtriphylline are theophyllines (Table 5-1). The drugs are effective bronchodilators when used by adults, but some of the theophyllines are ineffective when administered to children.

The theophyllines relax the smooth muscle of the bronchus, and respiratory volume may show a 24% increase after administration. Theophyllines differ in specific responses obtained by patients but have comparable pharmacodynamic effects. In addition to the effect on dilation of bronchi, the theophyllines have a direct stimulatory effect on the myocardium, which may lead to a 26% increase in cardiac output. Improvement in circulation coupled with a direct action on renal tubules results in a diuretic action. At the renal tubule the drugs increase the excretion rate of sodium and chloride ions, with concurrent elimination of water required as a diluent in tubular urine.

Aminophylline is the drug most frequently used for treatment of acute bronchial constriction, and intravenous administration provides dramatic relief. Oral or rectal forms of the drug may be administered after the acute asthmatic attack to provide prolonged relief of bronchial constriction. Theophylline formulations used as retention enemas or rectal suppositories provide therapeutic blood levels of the drug in 30 to 60 minutes after administration. Pocket-size nebulizers provide a handy supply of nebulized drug. The patient should have clear instructions about spaced use of the nebulized drug since topical bronchial irritation by the drug can cause bronchospasm.

ADVERSE EFFECTS. Intravenous administration relieves bronchospasm almost immediately, but adverse effects appear regularly if the drugs are administered rapidly. The chief adverse effects result from action of the theophyllines on smooth muscle of peripheral vessels, which leads to dilation. Hypotension and flushing are overt signs of the vasodilating action. Cerebral vascular resistance caused by the theophyllines results in decreased oxygenation during rapid intravenous administration, and the patient may complain of headache and dizziness. The stimulatory effect of the drug on the heart may cause palpitation and precordial pain. Effective intravenous use of the theophyllines for treatment of acute bronchial constriction requires that a 4- to 5-minute period be used as a guide for slow administration. Intramuscular injection is the least desirable route for administration of the theophyllines because local pain occurs at the injection site and pain persists for several hours after administration.

The gastric irritation of the drugs may be lessened by administration of the oral forms with or after meals. Use of enteric-coated forms or concurrent use of antacids is generally part of the prescribed therapeutic plan. The oral drugs tend to be cumulative; therefore the patient should follow the prescribed spacing of dosage carefully.

Adrenergic drugs. Bronchial constriction is seldom an entity occurring alone. Concurrent tissue edema and accumulation of thick tenacious secretions add to the problem of bronchial constriction that obstructs respiratory passages. Epinephrine hydrochloride is the drug most frequently used when the life-threatening anaphylactic reaction causes constriction and edema that block the bronchial passages.

In less acute situations less potent adrenergic drugs are employed for their local effect in relaxing the musculature and decreasing both glandular and tissue fluid in the bronchus. Methoxyphenamine hydrochloride, phenylpropanolamine hydrochloride, and pseudoephedrine hydrochloride (Table 5-1) are administered orally to maintain the patency of the

Table 5-1. Dosage range of drugs used for bronchodilator effect

Nonproprietary name	Proprietary (trade) name	Daily adult dosage range
Aminophylline*		Oral: 300-800 mg. (÷3-4) I.M.: 250-500 mg./single dose I.V.: Same as I.M.
Dyphylline*	Dilor, Iphyllin, Neothylline	Oral: 0.6-2.4 Gm. (÷3) I.M.: 500 mg./single dose
Methoxyphenamine hydrochloride	Orthoxine	Oral: 300-800 mg. (÷6-8)
Oxtriphylline*	Choledyl	Oral: 0.8-1.6 Gm. (÷4)
Phenylpropanolamine hydrochloride	Propadrine	Oral: 150-200 mg. (÷3-4)
Pseudoephedrine hydrochloride	Sudafed	Oral: 180-240 mg. (÷3-4)
Theophylline*	Aqualin, Elixophyllin, Optiphyllin	Oral: 0.2-1 Gm. (÷3)
Theophylline calcium salicylate*	Phyllicin	Oral: 0.2-1.5 Gm. (÷2-4)
Theophylline ethanolamine*	Monotheamin	Oral: 400-800 mg. (÷2)
Theophylline sodium acetate*	Theocin	Oral: 0.8-1 Gm. (÷3-4)
Theophylline sodium glycinate*	Dorsaphyllin, Glynazan, Pemophyllin, Synophylate, Theoglycinate	Oral: 1.2-6 Gm. (÷4-6) I.V.: 1.2-3.2 Gm. (÷3-4)

*Theophyllines.

respiratory tract structures when bronchitis and related problems occur.

There are many other sympathomimetic, or adrenergic, drugs that are used as components of inhalers for the patient with chronic episodic bronchoconstriction (i.e., bronchial asthma). Preparations may contain phenylephrine, ephedrine, or epinephrine. Local contact of the drugs with the bronchial membranes causes vasoconstriction, with a subsequent decrease in congestion or edema of the tissues. Prolonged use of any of the preparations may cause trauma to the delicate mucosal tissues, with emergence of injury-induced edema (congestive rebound).

Oral use of the adrenergic drugs may cause adverse effects due to adrenergic action on noninvolved tissues, but the incidence is relatively low. The only problematic effect is a transient elevation in the pulse and systolic blood pressure, and the patient may complain of dryness of oral tissues.

Isoproterenol hydrochloride (Isuprel hydrochloride) has a bronchodilation effect comparable to that of aminophylline in intensity. Isoproterenol hydrochloride is a potent adrenergic drug, and concurrent effects on the cardiovascular system are usually seen when the drug is used for its bronchodilator effect. Its action on cardiac beta receptors may cause tachycardia, and action at the beta receptors of peripheral blood vessels may cause vasodilation with consequent hypotension. Tachycardia and hypotension may occur when the drug is employed by any route (including inhalation), and the problems may cause the patient to discontinue use of the drug. The disturbing dizziness occurring as a consequence of hypotension may be lessened by modification of activity immediately after use of the drug.

Patient care

Many measures are used concurrently with drug administration to facilitate the breathing of the patient who seems to be struggling for each breath during an acute attack. An upright sitting position while receiving oxygen or using a respirator may decrease the work of breathing and allow maximum expansion of the thoracic cage. After an attack the patient is exhausted, but the fear of recurrence makes relaxation difficult. The physician may prescribe drugs to sedate the patient and decrease his anxiety.

The child with recurrent laryngotracheobronchitis (croup) has an interim period during which slight environmental changes (temperature, smoke, humidity) may precipitate a cough that sounds like a barking dog. Frequent demonstration of the cough may be used as a mischievous prank or as an attention-getting mechanism. Cough-induced drying and irritation of bronchial mucosa makes it necessary to assist the mother in finding ways to decrease cough stimuli. Her ongoing plan must also include provision of adequate fluids, prevention of exposure to individuals with infections, and maintenance of the physiologic resistance status of the child. Adding moisture to the environment during sleep hours with a cold air humidifier or placing open water containers on or near artificial heat sources (i.e., a pan of water on a steam radiator) decreases the detrimental effects of artificial heat on sensitive mucous membranes.

Prevention of exposure to respiratory tract infections and avoidance of other precipitating factors, that is, sudden environmental temperature extremes, emotion-laden situations, may decrease episodes of respiratory tract obstruction for the patient with a chronic respiratory tract problem.

RESPIRATORY DEPRESSION

Cessation of breathing (apnea) is incompatible with life. The urgency for reinstituting breathing makes stimulants a necessary part of the armamentarium of drugs and resuscitative devices available for treatment of acute respiratory depression (that is, drug intoxication, or overdose, respiratory depression after an anesthetic, pulmonary arrest). In most situations the drugs are used in conjunction with other pulmonary resuscitative measures. Many individuals will be intubated (Fig. 5-2) to provide a route for administering oxygen during the apneic period. Connection of the endotracheal tube to a respirator makes it possible to manually or automatically regulate the respiratory cycle. Intubation also facilitates removal of secretions by periodic deep endotracheal suctioning.

88 Drugs used to control excretion of fluid, metabolic wastes, and toxicants

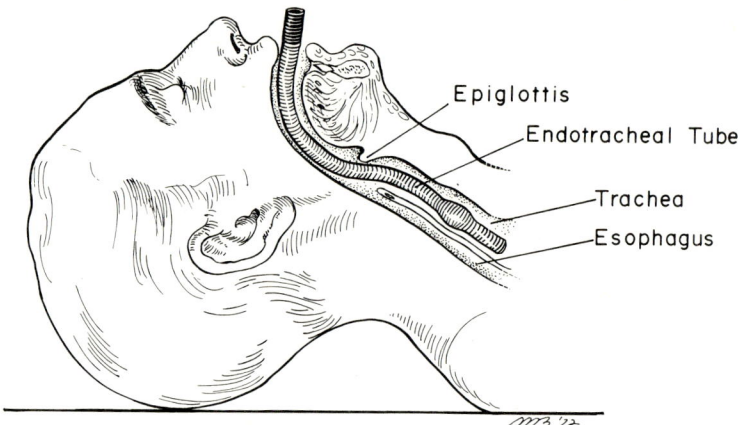

Fig. 5-2. Endotracheal tube in place.

Pharmacodynamics

Respiratory stimulants. Aromatic spirits of ammonia is probably the simplest form of respiratory stimulant. It acts to increase the depth of respiration by reflex stimulation of the medullary centers. The drug acts as a peripheral irritant to sensory nerve receptors in the pharynx, esophagus, and stomach. Afferent messages reaching the control centers accelerate the rate and depth of breathing. Inhalation of the pungent vapor or sipping a small amount of the drug diluted in 2 to 4 ml. of water will cause sufficient irritation to stimulate respirations.

Caffeine and sodium benzoate (Table 5-2) acts to stimulate physiologic responses and increase the volume and rate of respirations. The stimulatory effect on central nervous system, cardiac, and respiratory centers after intramuscular administration generally improves the vital processes of the patient.

Doxapram hydrochloride, ethamivan, and nikethamide (Table 5-2) are used intravenously to reinstitute respiration when medullary control center depression occurs. Oral forms of respiratory stimulants or central nervous system stimulants may be employed to improve moderately depressed respiratory cycles.

The drugs act to increase the rate and tidal exchange by a direct action on the medullary respiratory centers; the drugs also have a minor effect on the carotid and aortic chemoreceptors that supports medullary center stimulation of

Table 5-2. Dosage range of drugs used as respiratory stimulants

Nonproprietary name	Proprietary (trade) name	Adult dosage range
Caffeine and sodium benzoate		I.M.: 0.5-1 Gm.
Doxapram hydrochloride	Dopram	I.V.: 0.5-4 mg./kg.
Ethamivan	Emivan	Oral: 20-60 mg. I.V.: 1-2 mg./kg.
Nikethamide	Coramine, Nikethyl	I.V.: 0.25-1.25 Gm.

respiration. There is a concurrent drug-related increase in many of the parasympathetic nervous system–related body responses. For example, there is increased motility of the gastrointestinal tract and increased production of gastric and salivary gland secretions. Increased motility of the urinary bladder makes it necessary to insert a catheter in the bladder of the comatose patient.

Intravenous injection of the drugs initiates a response within a minute after administration. The patient with respiratory depression is observed carefully, and arterial blood gases, blood pressure, heart rate, and deep tendon reflexes are monitored during the period of unconsciousness.

Responsiveness is evidenced in the patient with drug intoxication (i.e., barbiturates) by grimacing or twitching and return of the corneal and pupillary reflexes. Additional dosage may be planned to maintain the foregoing reactions until full responsiveness occurs. Intervals for administration are planned on the basis of the predictable action time of the drugs (10 to 30 minutes), and repeated dosage may be planned to correlate with the cessation of pharmacodynamic effect. The drugs may be administered periodically until cerebral and respiratory function returns.

ADVERSE EFFECTS. The centrally acting drugs may stimulate adjacent midbrain centers. Coughing, sneezing, bronchospasm, laryngospasm, or elevation of the systemic blood pressure (due to mild peripheral vasoconstriction) jeopardizes the progress of the patient during therapy with respiratory stimulants. Because adverse effects occur most frequently during intravenous drug therapy, observation of the patient is important during parenteral administration.

Hyperventilation occurring after correction of respiratory depression is as hazardous to the patient as hypoventilation. A decrease in carbonic acid occurring with hyperventilation causes constriction of the cerebral vessels and decreased blood flow to cerebral tissues.

Narcotic antagonists. Respiratory depression or respiratory arrest induced by overdose of addictive analgesics (narcotics) is treated by administration of specific narcotic antagonists. Levallorphan tartrate (Lorfan), nalophine hydrochloride (Nalline), or naloxone hydrochloride (Narcan) acts pharmacodynamically by competing with narcotics for receptor sites at the respiratory center to lower the threshold for carbon dioxide stimulus to respiration. Intravenous injection of the drugs produces almost immediate response. Narcotic antagonists may be injected into the umbilical vein of newborn infants with narcotic-induced respiratory depression. The decrease in narcotic-induced depression of medullary respiration control centers increases the rate and volume of respirations, and the carbon dioxide levels move toward the normal range. Use of the agents may lead to withdrawal symptoms in the presence of narcotic addiction.

Nalorphine hydrochloride tends to cancel the analgesic effect of narcotics by competing at varied receptor sites, in addition to respiration center sites. Levallorphan tartrate improves respiration without abolishing the analgesia level.

Nalorphine hydrochloride and levallorphan tartrate induce respiratory depression when given in the absence of narcotic-induced depression, but naloxone hydrochloride is active only in the presence of narcotic-induced respiratory depression. The differentiation becomes important when an emergency situation arises in which it is unclear whether respiratory depression is related to narcotic overdosage or other agents. The narcotic antagonists are only effective in displacement of narcotics from the respiratory centers. Naloxone hydrochloride also reverses the respiratory depression caused by the analgesic pentazocine lactate.

Depression of all phases of respiration is the most critical aspect of narcotic overdosage. Improvement of the rate and tidal exchange is an important outcome of therapy with narcotic antagonists. Respiratory distress may reoccur when circulating narcotic reaches the respiratory receptors after termination of narcotic antagonist action. Drowsiness may be the early sign that circulating drug levels are high, and a second dose of the narcotic antagonist is usually administered.

Prolonged respiratory depression requires the use of intravenous bicarbonate to correct acidosis, and plans for hydration and electrolyte replacement are established. The patient who remains unconscious will require insertion of a bladder catheter during the period of intravenous fluid replacement.

Additional measures are necessary to maintain a patent airway during the acute period of depression. When the patient is unable to cough to remove excess secretions, suction may be employed to clear the airway. Respirators for control of ventilation and other assistive devices are used according to the status of the individual patient. Each patient is observed

90 Drugs used to control excretion of fluid, metabolic wastes, and toxicants

carefully to ascertain whether respiratory status continues to accomplish effective perfusion of the circulating blood.

RETAINED SECRETIONS

Coughing is a protective mechanism intended to remove secretions of glands lining the tracheobronchial tree and the particles trapped by the cilia during inspiration. The pharynx, trachea, and bronchus are supplied with highly sensitive afferent nerve endings that are stimulated by secretions, irritation, or edema. The afferent nerves take messages via the vagus nerve to the medullary centers where an integrated series of motor impulses is stimulated to initiate the multiple physical responses involved in coughing. Forceful cough may produce secretions that can be expectorated, but many individuals swallow rather than expectorate small amounts of mucus raised with weak coughing. Either practice removes secretions from the respiratory tree and removes the mucus barrier to maximum gas exchange.

Pharmacodynamics

Cough suppressants. Coughing becomes destructive rather than protective when it is continued, spasmodic, and nonproductive. The work of coughing exhausts the individual, and mucous membranes become dry and irritated by the continued expulsive movement of air.

Suppression of cough requires careful evaluation of the etiology of the problem. In the presence of pulmonary secretions, cough is required to clear the respiratory structures. Excessive cough, though productive, tires the individual and increases metabolic work. Drugs may contain a suppressant that modifies the frequency of cough without eliminating the protective cough pattern. Many of the cough preparations available for therapy represent formulations that provide a balanced control of cough rather than complete suppression.

Narcotic suppressants. Most narcotics act as cough suppressants, and codeine is frequently used as a component of cough preparations that provide balanced cough control. Several agents are available that decrease coughing without the adverse effects of narcotics. Dextromethorphan hydrobromide, hydrocodone bitartrate, levopropoxyphene napsylate, and noscapine (Table 5-3) are derivatives of narcotics, but the preparations have been refined to limit sedative effects. These drugs act on the medullary control center to suppress cough, and their pharmacodynamic effect is evident 15 to 30 minutes after oral administration. Serum levels of the drugs last for 3 to 6 hours. The cough suppressants seldom precipitate adverse effects, although some hypersensitive individuals may complain of nausea when the formulations contain a narcotic. The drugs are frequently found in formulations containing other drugs.

Antihistaminic suppressants. Cough preparations containing antihistamines are frequently employed for control of allergy-stimulated

Table 5-3. Dosage range of drugs used to suppress nonproductive cough

Nonproprietary name	Proprietary (trade) name	Daily adult dosage range
Benzonatate*	Tessalon	Oral: 300-600 mg. (÷3) I.M.: 15 mg. (÷3) I.V.: Same as I.M.
Carbetapentane citrate*	Toclase	Oral: 45-120 mg. (÷3-4)
Chlophedianol hydrochloride†	Ulo	Oral: 75-100 mg. (÷3-4)
Dextromethorphan hydrobromide‡	Dormethan, Methorate, Romilar	Oral: 10-80 mg. (÷1-4)
Diphenhydramine hydrochloride elixir†	Benadryl elixir	Oral: 25-200 mg. (÷2-4)
Hydrocodone bitartrate‡	Codone, Dicodid	Oral: 15-40 mg. (÷3-4)
Levopropoxyphene napsylate‡	Novrad	Oral: 300-600 mg. (÷6)
Noscapine‡	Nectadon	Oral: 45-120 mg. (÷3-4)

*Local anesthetic cough suppressant.
†Antihistaminic cough suppressant.
‡Narcotic cough suppressant.

cough. Chlophedianol hydrochloride and diphenhydramine hydrochloride elixir are used for their effect at the tissue level where minimal histamine-induced edema causes irritation of the cough-sensitive nerve endings in the tracheobronchial structures. In addition to local action, the drugs produce a mild sedative effect that provides rest from the sleep-disturbing paroxysms of allergy-induced cough.

Local anesthetic suppressants. Benzonatate and carbetapentane citrate have local anesthetic properties that inhibit the cough reflex at the afferent endings of the vagus nerve and at medullary transmission sites. The drugs produce a slight numbness of the oral mucosa if the preparations are held in the mouth. Although nausea and drowsiness are reported to occur occasionally with each of the drugs, it is difficult to evaluate whether drowsiness is related to exhaustion from tiring episodes of coughing or to the action of the drug.

Expectorants and mucolytics. The hydration status of the individual is a primary factor in the production of secretions with adequate fluid content to allow expulsion by cough. The secretions raised contain particulate matter that has been entrapped by the cilia projecting from the epithelial lining of the tract. Removal of secretions has a cleansing and protective effect on the respiratory tree.

Drugs employed to facilitate removal of respiratory tract secretions (Table 5-4) are classified as expectorants or mucolytics, but both groups increase the production of thinner, less viscid secretions. Protection of bronchial tissues is a positive pharmacodynamic side effect of secretion production.

Expectorants. Expectorants are often used in mixed preparations. Hydriodic acid may damage the teeth and is therefore diluted before administration. Added protection can be provided by drinking the diluted drug with a straw.

Elixir of terpin hydrate is usually combined with codeine in a cough preparation. The high alcohol content of the elixir (42.5%) provides the expectorant action when the drug is combined with codeine for cough control.

Tripelennamine is an antihistamine that is available as an elixir. It is frequently prescribed for control of persistent nighttime cough. It may cause slight drowsiness when given to children.

Mucolytics. Each of the mucolytic drugs acts by raising the osmolality of the bronchial glandular secretions, and fluid moves to dilute the secretions. The resulting secretions are thinner, and the improved ease of removal maintains the patency of the tracheobronchial lumen. Several drugs in clinical use liquefy secretions by a direct effect on the *mucin macromolecules.* The agents (i.e., tyloxapol, sodium ethasulfate, acetylcysteine) are administered topically as aerosols.

Calcium iodide, iodinated glycerol, and potassium iodide are employed in acute situations for their mucolytic action. The drugs are irritating to the gastrointestinal tract, and skin eruptions have occurred. The chief concern is the possibility that patients will continue to use the drugs for long periods of time, although the bitter taste tends to decrease interest in taking the drugs at any time. *Iodism* occurs with prolonged use. The entity includes inflammation of most of the tissues of the respiratory tract, skin eruptions, and accumulation of fluid in the nasal passages, lungs, and eyelids. The patient

Table 5-4. Dosage range of drugs used to remove respiratory tract secretions

Nonproprietary name	Proprietary (trade) name	Daily adult dosage range (oral)
Expectorants		
Hydriodic acid, diluted		1.8-4 ml. ($\div 3$)
Terpin hydrate elixir		40-80 ml. ($\div 8$)
Tripelennamine citrate	Pyribenzamine	32-64 ml. ($\div 8$)
Mucolytics		
Calcium iodide		1.8-3.6 Gm. ($\div 6$)
Glyceryl guaiacolate	Robitussin	0.6-1.2 Gm. ($\div 6$)
Iodinated glycerol	Organidin	240 mg. ($\div 4$)
Potassium iodide	Enkide	3.6-7 Gm. ($\div 12$)

Patient care

Liquefying tenacious secretions facilitates removal by cough or suction and decreases obstruction of the respiratory passages. An adequate amount of extracellular fluid is necessary to enhance action of the drugs; therefore encouraging the patient to take fluids will maximize drug effect. The patient should be positioned to allow removal of secretions (i.e., postural drainage) after taking the medication. Throughout the period when secretions are obstructing the airway, the patient should be positioned to allow maximum ventilation. Deep-breathing exercises and side-to-side position changes move retained secretions from peripheral pulmonary sites to the cough-sensitive areas of the bronchus. When the patient can tolerate a side-lying position without elevation of the headrest, the secretions at the bases of the lungs drain toward the larger bronchial structures. The vibratory action of a back rub may provide the added impetus to upward movement of secretions that allows expulsion with cough.

Efficacy of the drugs may be seen as a change from thick, sticky, adherent secretions to mucoid secretions easily raised from the pharynx or trachea. Drug administration should be planned to avoid meal hours because the increased secretions may precipitate cough and vomiting of the foods recently ingested.

REFERENCES

Ayres, Stephen M., and Lagerson, Joanne: Pulmonary physiology at the bedside: oxygen and carbon dioxide abnormalities, Cardiovascular Nursing 9:1, Jan.-Feb., 1973.

Belling, Dorothy I.: Complications after open-heart surgery, Nursing Clinics of North America 4:123, 1969.

Betson, Carol: The nurse's role in blood gas monitoring, Cardiovascular Nursing 7:83, Nov.-Dec., 1971.

Broughton, Joseph O.: Chest physical diagnosis for nurses and respiratory therapists, Heart & Lung 1:200, 1972.

Burrows, Benjamin: Pulmonary diffusion and alveolar-capillary block, Medical Clinics of North America 51:427, 1967.

Cherniack, Reuben M.: Chronic obstructive lung disease: it's not what what you do, but how you do it, Resident-Intern Consultant 1:44, May, 1972.

Collart, Marie E., and Brenneman, Janice K.: Preventing postoperative atelectasis, American Journal of Nursing 71:1982, 1971.

Crossman, P. F., Bushnell, L. S., and Hedley-White, J.: Dead space during artificial ventilation: gas compression and mechanical dead space, Journal of Applied Physiology 28:94, 1970.

Farber, Seymour M., and Wilson, Roger H. L.: Chronic obstructive emphysema, Clinical Symposia 20:35, 1968.

Foley, Mary F.: Pulmonary function testing, American Journal of Nursing 71:1134, 1971.

Fontana, Vincent J.: Status asthmaticus, Hospital Medicine 8:84, Jan., 1972.

Griffith, Elizabeth Welk: Nursing process: a patient with respiratory difficulty, Nursing Clinics of North America 6:145, 1971.

Kauffman, Leon A.: Complications of respiratory failure, American Family Physician 5:110, April, 1972.

Keltz, Harold: The effect of respiratory muscle dysfunction on pulmonary function, American Review of Respiratory Diseases 91:934, 1965.

Kurihara, Marie: Assessment and maintenance of adequate respiration, Nursing Clinics of North America 3:65, 1968.

LaForce, R. C., and Lewis, B. M.: Diffusional transport in the human lung, Journal of Applied Physiology 28:291, 1970.

Levine, Edwin Rayner: Inhalation therapy—aerosols and intermittent positive pressure breathing, Medical Clinics of North America 51:307, 1967.

Lewis, J. W., Bentley, K. W., and Cowan, A.: Narcotic analgesics and antagonists, Annual Review of Pharmacology 11:241, 1971.

Mitchell, R. A.: Respiration, Annual Review of Physiology 32:415, 1970.

Murphy, Eleanor R.: Intensive nursing care in a respiratory unit, Nursing Clinics of North America 3:423, 1968.

Peters, Richard M., and Hedgpeth, E. M., Jr.: Acid-base balance and respiratory work, Journal of Thoracic and Cardiovascular Surgery 52:649, 1966.

Petty, Thomas L.: Respiratory failure and the heart, Heart & Lung 1:84, 1972.

Said, Sami I.: Role of pulmonary surfactant in health and disease, Medical Clinics of North America 51:391, 1967.

Schwaid, Madeline C.: The impact of emphysema, American Journal of Nursing 70:1247, 1970.

Sedlock, Stephanie Ann: Detection of chronic pulmonary disease, American Journal of Nursing 72:1407, 1972.

Senior, Robert M., and Fishman, Alfred P.: Disturbances in alveolar ventilation, Medical Clinics of North America 51:403, 1967.

Sitzman, Judith: Respiratory problems and the nurse's changing responsibilities, Cardiovascular Nursing 6:41, May-June, 1970.

Slonim, N. Balfour, and Chapin, John L.: Respiratory physiology, St. Louis, 1967, The C. V. Mosby Co.

Szidon, Jan P., Pietra, Giuseppe G., and Fishman, Alfred P.: The alveolar-capillary membrane and pulmonary edema, The New England Journal of Medicine **286**:1200, 1972.

Turner, Howard G., Jr.: The anatomy and physiology of normal respiration, Nursing Clinics of North America **3**:383, 1968.

Winter, Peter M., and Lowenstein, Edward: Acute respiratory failure, Scientific American **221**:23, Nov., 1969.

6

Fluid balance

Renal controls
    Osmotic pressures
    Hormone controls
    Thirst center response
Fluid imbalance
    Pharmacodynamics
    Patient care

Physiologic mechanisms for control of fluid also maintain levels of extracellular and intracellular solutes. Equilibrium maintenance is an exquisite interaction between hormonal, hemodynamic, and renal transport control factors that preserve physiologic fluid balance.

Renal controls

The kidneys play an important role in control of fluid and electrolyte balance. From the copious amount of fluid filtered by the glomeruli (130 ml./minute), only 1% is excreted as urine. The decrease results from reabsorption of fluid along the pathway to the renal pelvis. About 86% is reabsorbed in the proximal tubules and 13% in the distal tubules. The end result is a renal urine output of 1 ml./minute.

Movement of electrolytes across the tubular cells maintains equilibrium between electrically charged ions in the peritubular and tubular fluids. Movement of electropositive ions from the tubular fluid to the peritubular fluid causes electronegativity within the tubule lumen, and electronegative ions move toward the peritubular fluid. For example, active reabsorption of sodium ions at the tubular cells rapidly moves the cations into the peritubular fluid, and anions (primarily chloride ions) from the electronegative tubular urine rapidly move to the electropositive sodium ions. Tubule epithelial cells are especially permeable to chloride ions; therefore the anions most frequently move with sodium ions and other cations, but other anions (i.e., phosphate, bicarbonate) also cross the tubule epithelial cells.

Proximal tubule transport mechanisms. Nephrons conserve 85% of the sodium ions from the glomerular filtrate by reabsorption from the lumen of the proximal tubules. Throughout the nephron unit, sodium ions are reabsorbed by active-transport mechanisms involving the dehydration of carbonic acid in renal tubular cells. Carbonic anhydrase is the enzyme involved in the process that results in the formation of bicarbonate ions and release of hydrogen ions:

$$H_2CO_3 \; (+ \text{ carbonic anhydrase}) \rightleftharpoons HCO_3 + H^+$$

Movement of hydrogen ions into the lumen of the proximal tubule, where they combine with anions in the fluid, contributes to the acidity of tubule contents. The movement of hydrogen ions into tubular fluid occurs as an exchange mechanism that moves sodium ions into peritubular blood. Sodium ions combine with the anions bicarbonate or chloride, and the process moves most of the products of glomerular filtration into peritubular blood. Approximately 90% of the bicarbonate ions from the filtrate are returned to the peritubular blood as a result of the active-transport mechanism for sodium ions in the proximal tubule. The process also involves movement of isosmotic

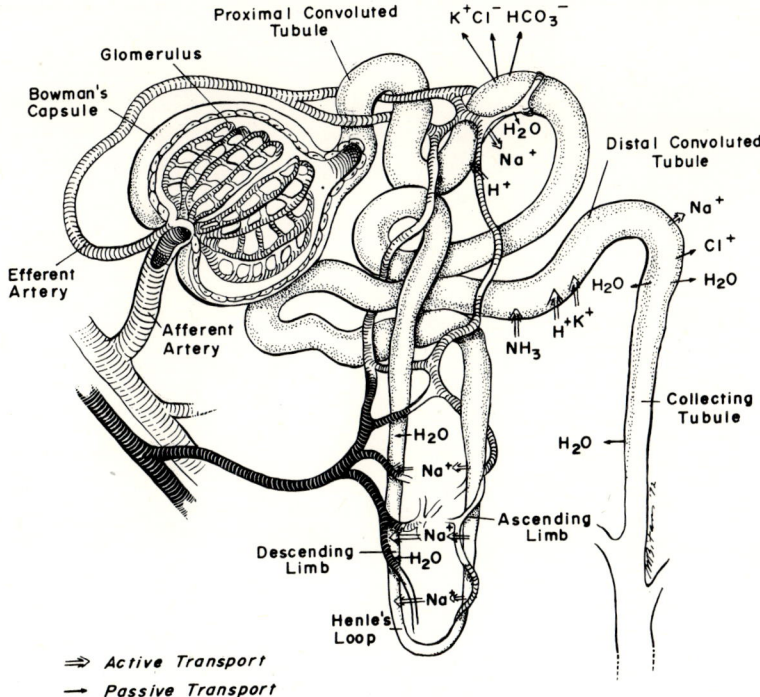

Fig. 6-1. Active and passive movement of water and electrolytes between the blood and the nephron unit affects the volume and composition of retained and excreted fluid.

amounts of water from the tubule lumen (Fig. 6-1).

The transport of potassium ions across the tubule cells increases the potassium ion content of peritubular blood. The mechanism for potassium ion transport may be active rather than passive, but components of an active exchange mechanism have not been identified.

Henle's loop transport mechanisms. The ascending limb of Henle's loop is the site of active transport of 15% of the filtered sodium ions into peritubular blood. The walls of the ascending limb are impermeable to water; therefore sodium ions move without accompanying quantities of water. Descending limb structures are highly permeable to sodium ions and water, and the proximity of the parallel limbs (Fig. 6-1) in the renal medullary tissues allows continuous active transport of sodium ions into the descending tubule. The process includes passive transport of water from peritubular blood or tissues into the descending limb. The cycling process is known as the *counter-*

current mechanism. Cycling and addition of sodium ions from the filtrate continually moving into the tubule maintain a high osmolality of tubule contents at the medullary tip of Henle's loop.

Distal tubule transport mechanisms. In the distal and collecting tubules active reabsorption of sodium ions creates a negative electric potential in the tubule lumen. The electronegativity of the tubular urine attracts potassium ions across the tubule epithelial cells. Diffusion of potassium ions at the distal aspects of the nephron is an important mechanism for control of serum potassium ion levels. Active transport of potassium ions at the distal tubule is partially influenced by the action of aldosterone.

Active transport of hydrogen ions contributes to the control of acid-base balance necessary to physiologic equilibrium. Hydrogen ions are held in tubular fluid in combination with ammonia from tubular cells. Glutaminase in the tubular cells converts glutamine to form ammonia (NH₃) and glutamic acid. Active transport of the ammonia ion into tubular urine allows combination with hydrogen and chloride ions to form ammonium chloride (NH₄Cl). In a comparable enzymatic process, oxidase converts other amino acids (i.e., asparagine) in tubule cells to ammonia ions. Either enzymatic process contributes to removal of hydrogen ions from the body and to acidification of the urine.

Collecting tubule mechanisms. Final steps in concentration of urine are completed at collecting tubule sites. Active reabsorption of sodium ions passively moves chloride ions and isosmotic amounts of water from the tubule contents before the final urine product enters the renal pelvis.

Osmotic pressures

The normal hydrostatic and colloidal osmotic pressure relationships in the hemodynamic system maintain fluid balance at capillary tissue sites. Considerable latitude exists between capillary and tissue pressures before problems emerge. The margin of safety for capillary pressure elevation or decreased osmotic pressure normally prevents transudation of fluid into tissue spaces. Lymph channels remove protein from tissue spaces to maintain functional colloidal osmotic pressures, and lymph drainage increases when excess fluid raises the pressure in interstitial spaces.

Hormone controls

Many hormones contribute to fluid accumulation or elimination concurrent with their natural physiologic action (i.e., estrogens), but *aldosterone* and *antidiuretic hormone* (ADH) are the biologic hormones specifically involved in solvent-solute maintenance (Fig. 6-2).

Aldosterone action. Volume receptors in the adrenal cortex release aldosterone in response to local stimuli or messages relayed from cerebral-hypothalamic centers by tropic hormones (i.e., adrenoglomerulotropin). Volume receptors may be stimulated by decreased volume, lowered sodium ion content, or elevated potassium ion content of fluids bathing the adrenal centers. Aldosterone controls the ratio between potassium and sodium ions in extracellular fluids.

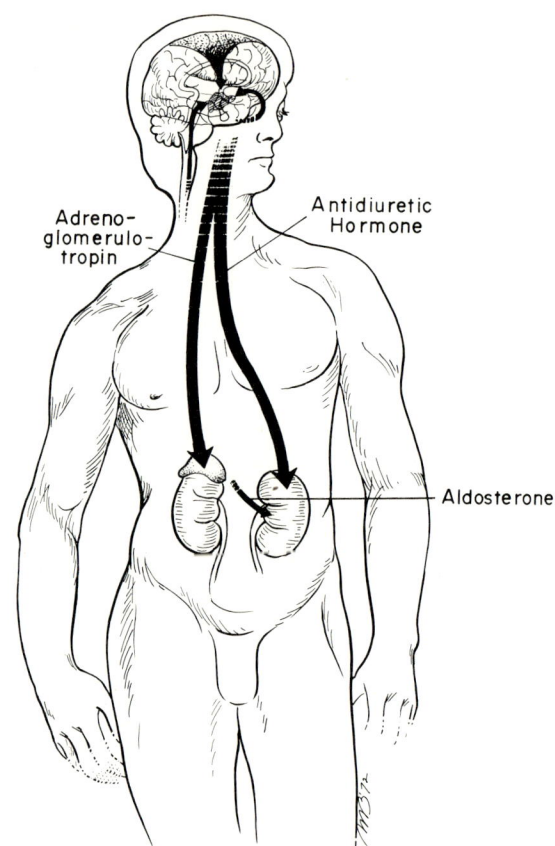

Fig. 6-2. Volume receptors, osmoreceptors, and emotional factors stimulate release of hormones that control the volume and osmolality of extracellular fluids.

Psychologic or physiologic stressors (i.e., trauma, surgery) may continually stimulate the volume receptors. A slight increase in body weight can occur secondary to accumulation of sodium and water in tissues.

Edema may occur consequent to elevated aldosterone levels produced by the hormone *renin,* which is released in *renal autoregulation* of blood pressure. Diminished blood supply in the afferent renal arterioles causes release of renin from cells in the arteriole walls. Renin action on its plasma substrate releases *angiotensin I,* which is converted in the blood to *angiotensin II.* The potent vasoconstricting action of angiotensin II is a primary factor in renal regulation of blood pressure, and it also directly stimulates secretion of aldosterone in the adrenal cortex.

Liberated aldosterone travels to effector sites in the nephron to increase reabsorption of sodium ions in the ascending limb of Henle's loop and in the distal convoluted tubule (Fig. 6-1). Active reabsorption of sodium ions is accompanied by passive movement of water. During the transfer, potassium ions are exchanged and are excreted in the urine.

Like other complex physiologic processes, regulation of the tone of renal arteries is affected by many factors. In addition to the vasoconstricting action of renin on renal arterioles, circulatory baroreceptor reflexes may cause constriction of the afferent arterioles and decrease glomerular filtration. The mechanism is one of the factors contributing to the low urine output seen in shock states.

Antidiuretic hormone action. Antidiuretic hormone is synthesized in the hypothalamus and released from posterior pituitary storage sites in response to deficits of body fluid. Hyperconcentration of the extracellular fluids bathing hypothalamic osmoreceptor tissue draws fluid from the osmoreceptors, and the internal dehydration stimulates release of ADH. The hormone travels to nephron effector sites (distal tubules) to increase reabsorption of water (Fig. 6-1). Return of extracellular fluid lowers the osmolality (specific gravity) of the serum, and ADH is no longer liberated by the osmoreceptors.

Clinical determination of serum osmolality (or osmolarity) can be evaluated by measurement of the serum sodium ion level. Sodium is the chief cation solute of the extracellular fluids; therefore the sodium ion level reflects the ratio of solute to solvent (specific gravity) of the serum. Serum osmolality above 290 or a serum sodium ion level above 140 mEq./liter stimulates ADH release.

Excess drinking of liquids, psychic factors, and some central nervous system depressants (including alcohol) may inhibit ADH secretion and increase urinary output. Increased blood volume with concurrent filling of the atria and great veins stimulates volume receptors, and consequent lowering of antidiuretic hormone increases urinary output. Each of the foregoing factors represents direct depression of the hypothalamic-thalamic centers or hemodilution as inhibitors of ADH release.

Thirst center response

Concurrent with the stimulation of hypothalamic osmoreceptor centers, thirst centers in adjacent tissue are stimulated. Thirst is one of the most primitive drives, and excitation of the centers initiates the sensation that leads the individual to increase fluid intake. A serum sodium ion level above 145 mEq./liter will cause extreme thirst, and it may be the only specific complaint of the patient with disturbed fluid balance. Osmoreceptors and thirst centers act synergistically to maintain normal osmolality of extracellular fluid.

FLUID IMBALANCE

Man's physiologic ability to manage fluid control at a highly sophisticated level is exquisite but not infallible. Any contrivance with numerous interdependent parts is subject to disruption in a component and consequent malfunction in the total system. Pathology in any one of the organs or systems of control can cause excess retention or elimination of fluid. For example, decrease in the synthesis of aldosterone by adrenal medullary volume receptors causes excess sodium ion losses from the body, with consequent dehydration. Problems may extend beyond the source of supply. For example, hepatic degradation of aldosterone is necessary to maintain physiologic levels of the hormone in the body. When liver function is impaired, excess aldosterone activity may cause sodium ion (and fluid) accumulation and loss of potassium ions.

Accumulation of interstitial fluid interferes with cellular function. The urgency for intensive fluid removal is related to the site of edema emergence. Although peripheral edema can be tolerated, there are sites where immediate removal of excess fluid is mandatory to reinstitute function in vital organs. For example, the pressure of a fluid-filled abdomen (ascites) may limit diaphragmatic movement and depress respirations. Intracranial fluid accumulation carries with it the life-threatening potential for displacement of cranial structures and medullary herniation. Pulmonary edema may compromise respirations as the patient literally drowns in alveolar fluid. In each of the foregoing situations tissue fluid must be removed promptly.

Dehydration of tissues deprives the body of the medium necessary for temperature regulation, enzymatic and bioelectrical reactions, and cushioning and lubrication of organs and joints. Treatment of the basic problem may be planned over a period of time, but extracellular solvent-solute relationships must be converted to normal levels promptly.

Pharmacodynamics

Drugs may be employed to replace, potentiate, or interrupt normal physiologic mechanisms for fluid control. Sequestration of excess fluid in tissues (edema) is the most frequent manifestation of fluid imbalance, and diuretics that act at varying sites of the nephrons are used for control of the electrolyte and water imbalance.

Antidiuretic hormone replacement. Hormone extracts of the posterior portion of the pituitary gland (Pituitrin) have a triple physiologic action (pressor, antidiuretic, oxytocic activity). Vasopressin (Pitressin) and vasopressin tannate (Pitressin tannate) are extracts of the pituitary hormone that have been purified to remove oxytocic activity. The vasopressin extracts are in essence pharmacodynamic substitutes for the natural ADH hormone, and they are administered intramuscularly to replace ADH when the patient has *diabetes insipidus* caused by compromised pituitary or hypothalamic function. In addition to intramuscular forms of vasopressin, the extract is available as a powder for nasal insufflation.

The concurrent effects of vasopressin on smooth muscle (pressor activity) necessitates observation of the patient for an increase in blood pressure and evidence of contraction of smooth muscles in the viscera (i.e., gastrointestinal tract, bladder, uterus). The effect on smooth muscles may be a planned therapeutic use of the drug.

The patient without ADH control is encouraged to drink liberally in amounts to equal his urinary output, and he eliminates copious amounts of dilute urine (low specific gravity). During the time the drug is being used, fluids are restricted, and the drug effect on water conservation causes the urine to be more concentrated (high specific gravity).

Lypressin (Diapid) is a synthetic form of ADH. The drug is only available as a nasal spray that the patient uses whenever urinary frequency or thirst increases significantly. Although the drug has little pressor activity, excessive use may precipitate vasoconstriction. The patient should be told to use the spray more frequently rather than to increase the 2-spray dosage plan. Patients are instructed to hold the head upright (vertical) to avoid inhalation of the drug during the spray procedure.

Aldosterone replacement. Physiologic aldosterone represents 95% of the natural mineralocorticoid produced by the adrenal volume receptors. The remaining mineralocorticoids, corticosterone and deoxycorticosterone, control only 5% of the biologic effect on nephron reabsorption of sodium ions and excretion of potassium ions. Synthetic forms of deoxycorticosterone are used for hormone replacement, in conjunction with other adrenal hormone substitutes, for individuals with adrenocortical insufficiency (hypoadrenal syndrome).

Deoxycorticosterones stimulate reabsorption of sodium ions from the renal tubules and decrease glandular elimination of sodium ions (i.e., salivary, sweat, gastrointestinal glands). For the patient with adrenal dysfunction, restoration of sodium and potassium ion balance as well as extracellular and intracellular fluid levels has a positive effect on hemodynamic function, nutrient utilization, and nitrogen excretion.

Deoxycorticosterone acetate (Cortate, Cortinaq, Decortin, Decosterone, Descotone, Doca, Percorten, Steraq) is administered sublingually (4 to 15 mg./24 hours divided into 2 or 3 doses). Deoxycorticosterone trimethylacetate is administered intramuscularly once a month (25 to 75 mg.). Drug pellets may be implanted in the subcutaneous tissues for 9- to 12-month periods of control.

While the patient is taking the drug, sodium chloride intake is encouraged at the highest tolerable rate (i.e., frequent snacks of saltines, salted popcorn) because increased salt intake decreases the amount of drug required. Potassium ions are readily removed by drug action on the renal tubules so that potassium ion intake is unrestricted during therapy.

Diuretics. Diuretics may provide immediate or long-term control of fluid accumulation, but they do not directly affect the etiologic factor leading to fluid sequestration. Diuretics are drugs that mobilize fluid or sodium ions from interstitial spaces, improve circulation to the kidneys, or decrease reabsorption of sodium or water from renal tubules. Drug action sites in the nephron influence electrolyte and acid-base problems occurring during diuretic drug therapy.

Aldosterone antagonists. Spironolactone (Aldactone) acts as an antagonist to aldosterone by interfering with the hormone-induced reabsorption of sodium ions at distal tubule sites. By inhibiting active-transport mechanisms in the tubule cells, sodium ions are excreted and potassium ion loss is lessened. Spironolactone is called a *potassium-sparing diuretic,* and it is often used in conjunction with other diuretics that cause potassium loss. When used with other diuretics that prevent sodium ion reabsorption at the proximal tubules, spironolactone has an additive effect on sodium ion excretion.

Long-term use of spironolactone may cause consistently low serum sodium ion concentrations that stimulate an increase in aldosterone secretion. The chief adverse effects occurring during therapy are mild headache and hyponatremia. Mild acidosis may occur as a result of the tendency of the drug to decrease ammonium excretion. Oral administration (100 to 300 mg./24 hours, divided into 1 to 3 doses,) slows the onset of initial action for up to 3 days but facilitates use of the drug for long-term therapy.

Triamterene (Dyrenium), although not an aldosterone antagonist, acts in a manner mimicking the effect of spironolactone. The principal effector site is the distal tubule, and it removes sodium ions while conserving potassium ions. The synergistic effect with other diuretics acting at the proximal segments of the renal tubule is comparable to that of spironolactone. The chief difference in pharmacodynamic action between the two drugs is the direct effect of triamterene on the nephron sites rather than through blocking aldosterone effect. Like spironolactone, it is often used in conjunction with other diuretics.

Most of the adverse effects occurring during therapy with triamterene relate to gastrointestinal irritation and may be relieved by administration of the drug with or immediately after meals. Other reported adverse effects are manifestations of tissue dehydration or hyponatremia. The daily oral dosage range of triamterene is 100 to 300 mg. given in 1 to 3 doses.

Carbonic anhydrase inhibitors. Carbonic anhydrase is an enzyme acting in many body tissues to hydrate carbon dioxide (CO_2) and dehydrate carbonic acid (H_2CO_3) in a reversible reaction necessary to maintenance of acid-base balance:

$$CO_2 + H_2O \rightleftharpoons H_2CO_3 \rightleftharpoons H^+ + HCO_3^-$$

Formation of bicarbonate (HCO_3^-) in renal tubular cells is a mechanism that contributes to maintenance of the normal base bicarbonate–carbonic acid ratio (20:1) of circulating fluids. Enzymatically induced dehydration of carbonic acid in the proximal and distal tubule cells releases hydrogen ions for exchange with sodium ions from tubular urine. Hydrogen ions liberated into tubular urine combine with phosphate ions (HPO_4^-), and the weak acids are excreted into the renal pelvis. Sodium ions combine with bicarbonate ions in the tubule cells, and the molecules return to the circulating fluids to influence the acid-base ratio (Fig. 6-3).

Carbonic anhydrase inhibitors decelerate the reversible bicarbonate reaction by interfering with enzymatic activity at each step in the reaction. The net effect is a decrease in formation of sodium bicarbonate in tubule cells and retention of sodium ions in tubular urine (Fig. 6-3). Blocking of tubule cell secretion of hydrogen ions reduces the reabsorption of sodium and bicarbonate ions. Sodium and hydrogen ion exchange is reduced throughout the nephron, but the exchange of potassium ions for sodium ions in the distal tubule may be increased (Fig. 6-1). The exchange increases potassium ion losses, and hypokalemia may occur.

Sodium ion content in the tubule lumen osmotically holds water. Passive transport of bicarbonate, chloride ions, and water is lower when active transport of sodium ions is decreased by carbonic anhydrase inhibitors. The

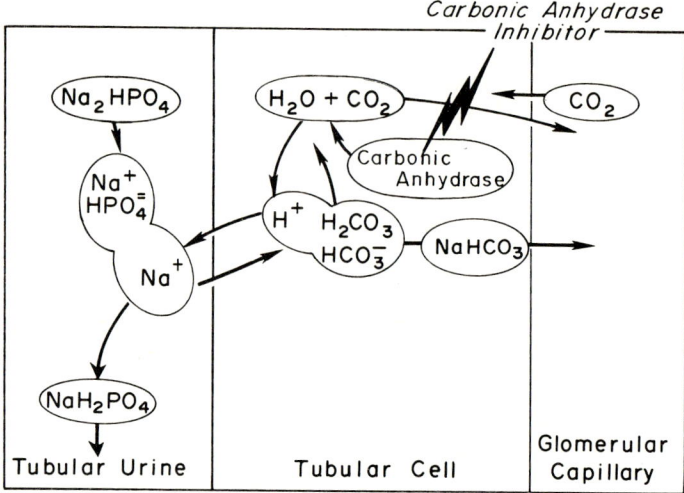

Fig. 6-3. Carbonic anhydrase inhibitors interfere with enzymatic conversion in the carbonic acid–base bicarbonate interaction necessary to formation and return of sodium bicarbonate to circulating fluids.

physiologic outcome is an increased excretion of hypotonic urine, a moderate increase in acidity of body fluids, and an increase in the alkalinity of the urine.

Carbonic anhydrase inhibitors are sulfonamide derivatives, and some of the adverse effects are similar to those of the sulfonamide group (i.e., fever, skin rash, depression of bone marrow with long-term use). Consistently high urine formation during diuretic therapy prevents the sulfonamide-related problems of crystal accumulation and stone formation in the renal pelvis. Gastrointestinal disturbances and paresthesias in the extremities occur during administration of the diuretics.

Each of the carbonic anhydrase inhibitors—acetazolamide, dichlorphenamide, ethoxzolamide, and methazolamide—is available for oral use (Table 6-1). The physician's decision to employ a particular drug is based on the potency of the agent in producing diuresis and the planned duration of therapy. Control of acidosis during long-term therapy may be accomplished by using intermittent schedules that allow periodic renal control of the base bicarbonate–carbonic acid ratio.

Sodium transport inhibitors. The group of drugs traditionally employed for control of edema caused by sodium retention are classed pharmacologically as *mercurials*. The drugs block the sulfhydryl-containing enzymes that control tubule transport systems for sodium ions in the nephron by releasing small amounts of mercurial ions in the tubule cells. The chief sites of sodium ion blocking are thought to be at the active-transport sites in proximal and distal tubules. Mercurials may inhibit transport of 20% to 30% of the sodium ions from the glomerular filtrate, and isosmotic amounts of water remain as solvent in the tu-

Table 6-1. Dosage range of diuretics: carbonic anhydrase inhibitors

Nonproprietary name	Proprietary (trade) name	Daily adult dosage range
Acetazolamide	Diamox	Oral: 5 mg./kg.
Acetazolamide sodium	Diamox sodium	I.V.: 5 mg./kg.
Dichlorphenamide	Daranide, Oratrol	Oral: 25-200 mg. ($\div$1-3)
Ethoxzolamide	Cardrase, Ethamide	Oral: 62.5-750 mg. ($\div$2-4)
Methazolamide	Neptazane	Oral: 100-300 mg. ($\div$2-3)

bular urine. Blocking of sodium ion transport effected by mercurials affects passive transport of chloride ions and water, and a large amount of tubular fluid is delivered to collecting tubule sites. Potassium and hydrogen ion exchange for sodium ions at collecting tubule sites increases the output of the electrolytes, and hypokalemic alkalosis may occur with prolonged therapy. Excessive use of mercurials may cause destruction of tubule cells.

Meralluride or mercaptomerin sodium is administered parenterally for edema control (Table 6-2). Because the drugs are irritating to tissues, the patient may complain of pain at the site of injection. Chlormerodrin may be administered orally for control of moderate fluid accumulation.

Many patients are hypersensitive to the mercurial drugs. Test doses of the drug are administered at initiation of therapy, and supervision of the patient is planned while he is taking the drug. In sensitive patients a variety of problems may arise: pruritus, skin rash, gastrointestinal disturbances (including stomatitis), vertigo, and headache.

Thiazides are the most widely used diuretics for control of edema. The drugs interfere with sodium ion transport at the ascending limb of Henle's loop, and a decrease of sodium ion transport into the descending limb is part of the countercurrent mechanism. Active transport of sodium is also impaired at distal tubule sites by a thiazide effect that inhibits carbonic anhydrase activity. As tubular fluid flows to collecting tubule sites, potassium ion exchange for sodium ions progresses at a rapid rate, and the process causes increased potassium ion excretion. Hydrogen ion exchange remains at normal levels; therefore the chief concern during therapy with the thiazides is potassium replacement to prevent hypokalemia.

Thiazides have an action onset time of 2 hours when administered orally. Some of the thiazides continue to have a diuretic effect for 24 hours or more (i.e., bendroflumethiazide, chlorthalidone, cyclothiazide, hydroflumethiazide, methyclothiazide, polythiazide, quinethazone, trichlormethiazide). Thiazides with a peak diuretic effect of 4 hours and approximately a 12-hour diuretic action are benzthia-

Table 6-2. Dosage range of diuretics: sodium transport inhibitors

Nonproprietary name	Proprietary (trade) name	Daily adult dosage range
Bendroflumethiazide*	Benuron, Naturetin	Oral: 5-20 mg.
Benzthiazide*	Aquatag, Exna	Oral: 50-200 mg. (÷2)
Chlormerodrin†	Neohydrin	Oral: 55-110 mg.
Chlorothiazide*	Diuril	Oral: 0.5-2 Gm. (÷1-2)
Chlorothiazide sodium*	Diuril sodium, Lyovac	I.V.: 0.5-2 Gm. (÷1-2)
Chlorthalidone*	Hygroton	Oral: 50-200 mg.
Cyclothiazide*	Anhydron	Oral: 1-8 mg.
Ethacrynate sodium	Edecrin sodium, Lyovac sodium Edecrin	I.V.: 0.5-1 mg./kg.
Ethacrynic acid	Edecrin	Oral: 50-400 mg. (÷2)
Flumethiazide*	Ademol	Oral: 0.5-2 Gm.
Furosemide	Lasix	Oral: 40-600 mg. (÷1-2) I.M.: 20-40 mg. (÷1-2) I.V.: Same as I.M.
Hydrochlorothiazide*	Esidrex, Hydro-Diuril, Oretic	Oral: 25-200 mg. (÷1-2)
Hydroflumethiazide*	Saluron	Oral: 50-200 mg. (÷1-2)
Meralluride†	Mercuhydrin	I.M.: 130-260 mg.
Mercaptomerin sodium†	Diucardyn, Thiomerin	I.M.: 60-250 mg.
Methyclothiazide*	Enduron	Oral: 2.5-20 mg. (÷1-2)
Polythiazide*	Renese	Oral: 1-12 mg. (÷1-3)
Quinethazone*	Hydromox	Oral: 50-200 mg. (÷1-2)
Trichlormethiazide*	Metahydrin, Naqua	Oral: 2-16 mg. (÷1-2)

*Thiazides.
†Mercurials.

zide, chlorothiazide, flumethiazide, and hydrochlorothiazide (Table 6-2). The variation in onset time, peak effect, and duration of action influence plans for administration of the drugs. Administration is planned to accomplish diuresis without disturbing the sleep patterns of the patient. Because the drugs are effective in decreasing total circulating blood volume, they are often used as part of the total therapeutic plan for patients with hypertension.

Thiazides sometimes induce symptoms of *gout* secondary to increased urate retention and hyperuricemia. Drugs that enhance the excretion of uric acid (uricosuric agents) may be prescribed for concurrent use with oral thiazides. Other adverse effects of thiazides include gastrointestinal irritation, central nervous system manifestations (dizziness, vertigo, paresthesias, headache), or dermatologic reactions (skin rash, or urticaria).

Ethacrynate sodium and furosemide, when administered intravenously, are potent diuretics that provide prompt diuresis in patients with life-threatening pulmonary edema. Oral administration of ethacrynic acid or furosemide produces diuresis in 30 to 60 minutes.

Administration of the large dosage required for rapid diuresis causes dilation of the renal arterioles, with consequent increase in glomerular filtration rate. The potent effect of the drugs is partially related to their action at proximal tubule sites where there is some inhibition of sodium chloride (and water) reabsorption. The chief action of the drugs is interference with active transport of sodium ions in the ascending limb of Henle's loop.

Potassium and hydrogen ion exchange for sodium ions in collecting tubule sites causes losses of the electrolytes. Hypokalemia and alkalosis may result from electrolyte losses when therapy with large dosage is prolonged. Potassium replacement is usually planned as part of the diuretic therapy program. Intermittent schedules for diuretic use (i.e., administration every other day) may be planned to allow maximum diuresis with minimal loss of electrolytes.

Urate excretion is accelerated during intravenous therapy with ethacrynate sodium or furosemide, but long-term oral administration may cause urate retention and hyperuricemia. Uricosuric drugs may be used as prophylaxis against emergence of gout, or the drugs may be employed to control symptoms in patients having joint involvement.

Renal blood flow increase. Theophylline calcium salicylate (Phyllicin) and theobromine calcium salicylate (Theocalcin) are both identified pharmacologically as *xanthine* drugs. As a group the xanthines have a direct stimulatory effect on the myocardium, which may increase the cardiac output up to 26%. The increased blood flow accelerates the rate of glomerular filtration and consequently the production of urine. Concurrent dilator effect of the drugs on renal afferent arterioles increases the excretion rate of sodium and chloride ions. Combination of the two factors has a positive effect in removal of excess fluid and sodium from the body, although in most instances there is only a threefold to fivefold increase in urine output.

The absence of sodium in the products extends their use to patients with sodium-restricted intake. The presence of a salicylate component limits their usefulness for patients receiving anticoagulants for long-term control of prothrombin formation. Salicylates and oral anticoagulants act at similar sites in the hepatic coagulation process, and concurrent use of the drugs interferes with control of prothrombin levels.

The drugs are administered orally: theophylline calcium salicylate, 0.25 to 1 Gm./24 hours, divided into 2 to 4 doses, and theobromine calcium salicylate, 1.5 to 3 Gm./24 hours, divided into 3 doses. Administration of the drugs at or after meals may decrease symptoms of gastrointestinal irritation (i.e., nausea, vomiting, diarrhea, abdominal cramps). The drugs are metabolized in the liver and excreted in the urine.

Osmotic diuretics. Osmotic diuretics are most useful when fluid accumulation is related to increased production of fluid, obstruction to fluid removal, or fluid transudation caused by elevated intravascular pressure. Osmotic diuretics act by increasing the osmolality of the plasma. Increased plasma solute causes osmotic movement of fluid from sequestered sites. There is a transient expansion of plasma volume that is reversed as fluid is removed by the kidneys. Increased osmolality of renal tubular fluid opposes reabsorption of water in the nephron unit, and elimination of urine increases. One concern during therapy is the possibility of generalized tissue dehydration. When osmotic diuretics are used to reverse an oliguric state, an alternate route for removal of fluid is planned (i.e., peritoneal, hemodialysis) if urine output does not result from therapy.

Glycerin, 50% (Glyrol, Ophthalgan, Osmōglyn) is the only osmotic diuretic that is administered orally (120 ml., divided into 4 doses). It is used chiefly to move accumulated fluid in ocular or cranial sites toward the circulating plasma. The oral preparation is flavored with a tart citrus base to disguise the taste, but many patients find the drug unpalatable. To decrease the incidence of vomiting after ingestion, the drug may be poured over cracked ice and served with a soda straw. Asking the patient to remain recumbent for a short time after taking the drug modifies both the emesis pattern and cerebral dehydration–related headache.

Slightly more than the usual daily dosage amount (150 ml.) of 50% glycerin supplies 375 calories, or 18% of a 2000-calorie diet. Most of the orally administered dose is incorporated into neutral fat molecules as the triglyceride, and less than 14% is excreted by the kidneys. Onset of action after oral use is 10 minutes, with peak effect in 30 to 120 minutes.

Mannitol (Osmitrol) is an osmotic agent frequently administered intravenously (50 to 200 Gm.) for relief of fluid accumulation. When employed to improve renal output, a test dose of 200 mg./kg. may be administered to ascertain whether urine output will be improved by the drug. The remainder of the drug is given if the urine output is 40 ml./hour after administration of the initial test dose. Mannitol increases the osmotic pressure of glomerular filtrate and tubular contents to a level that tenaciously holds water, and copious amounts of dilute urine are produced. Mannitol is almost entirely excreted by the kidneys. Adverse effects may be related to changes in hydration of cerebral centers (i.e., nausea, vomiting, headache, thirst).

Sterile urea (Ureaphil, Urevert) promotes diuresis by elevation of the osmotic pressure of the glomerular filtrate. Although the drug is an effective osmotic diuretic, the time lag occurring while the solution is prepared for intravenous administration lessens its usefulness in emergency situations (i.e., intracranial fluid accumulation).

Dextrose, 50%, is used intravenously in the same situations as are other osmotic diuretics. Dextrose increases fluid output by acting osmotically in tubular urine, but much of the administered dose is actively reabsorbed in the proximal tubule. Excess over renal threshold levels for dextrose allows adequate tubule content for osmotic effect, therefore intravenous dosage is high when osmotic removal of fluid via renal routes is desired. A hundred milliliters of 50% dextrose provides 200 calories, and the calorie content may influence the physician's selection of dextrose as an osmotic diuretic for removal of fluid when the patient has diabetes mellitus.

Albumin replacement. Maintenance of blood volume is the function of the total circulating protein mass (mainly albumin) that exerts the pressure holding fluid in the vasculature (oncotic pressure).

Depletion of fluid volume unaccompanied by loss of blood cells causes hemoconcentration, identified by analysis of the hematocrit level (normal: males, 42 to 50 mm./100 ml.; females, 40 to 48 mm./100 ml. blood). The rise in hematocrit levels indicates normal quantity of blood cells in a decreasing plasma volume.

When albumin levels are depressed, absence of opposition allows hydrostatic pressure to force fluid into extracellular spaces. Edema develops gradually when levels of total circulating proteins are low, and the blood volume is gradually decreased.

When protein depletion has allowed tissue fluid accumulation, albumin replacement acts osmotically to draw fluid from tissue spaces into the vasculature. Oral or parenteral intake may be withheld for 8 hours after administration to maximize the oncotic effect. Prophylactic replacement of albumin in a dehydrated patient requires that a diluent accompany the intravenous albumin administration and additional fluid intake be provided.

Replacement products vary in the amount of dilution natural to the product. Because the same proprietary, or trade, name is used for the product whether it has 5% or 25% albumin content, it is important to note carefully the *percent* designation, in addition to the generic designation of normal human serum albumin.

Differences in planned therapeutic effect influence the rate of administration. Use of albumin as a plasma expander to replace losses of blood or plasma requires that the drug be administered rapidly. A slower rate of administration (2 ml./minute) is indicated when the product is employed to reverse a hypoproteinemic state and attract tissue fluid to the vasculature.

Normal human serum albumin contains 60 mg. sodium ion/20 ml.; therefore a salt-poor form of albumin (0.07 mg./20 ml.) is used for the patient on restricted sodium ion intake. Each 20 ml. vial of normal human serum albumin administered intravenously is capable of drawing approximately 70 ml. of fluid into the vasculature in 15 minutes. The pharmacodynamic effect results in an elevation of the blood pressure level and a gradual return of the hematocrit level to the normal range.

Plasma protein fraction (human) acts in a manner comparable to albumin replacement but replaces additional proteins. The solution contains 4.4% albumin, 0.35% alpha globulin, and 0.25% beta globulin. Pharmacodynamic effect is comparable to that of albumin, and plasma protein fraction (human) maintains the blood volume increase for up to 48 hours. Biochemical similarity between plasma protein fraction and normal 5% human serum albumin makes them generally interchangeable. Patients occasionally have a rash that occurs as an allergic reaction to introduction of albumin. The rash may occur during or immediately following albumin administration.

Patient care

The location and duration of fluid accumulation will affect the functional problems and the responsibilities of the patient during therapy. In nonacute situations the patient's understanding of the therapeutic regimen is important to the outcome of the plan. Drug administration, fluid limitation, or sodium restriction can be supervised when the patient is hospitalized, but his adherence to the schedule at home is dependent on his understanding of the rationale and details of the plan. Therapy will be more effective if the regimen fits the patient's individual physiologic and living patterns.

Nursing guidelines. Data indicating the amount of accumulated fluid provides baseline information for planning nursing care and for evaluating drug effect. The site of fluid collection affects whether assessment can be indirect or direct. For example, definition of the presence or progress of excess intracranial fluid includes tabulation of clues indicating neurologic function (indirect assessment). Edema in peripheral areas can be directly assessed by observation and measurement of distended tissues (i.e., size of the ankle, calf, abdomen) and weighing the patient. Weight changes provide a guide to the effectiveness of the diuretic in removing tissue fluid (1 pound = 1 pint).

Consistency of measurements assures accurate analysis of fluid accumulation. Use of a ball-point pen to mark the upper and lower margins of the measuring tape on the extremity or abdomen assures that each subsequent measurement is at a comparable area on the body.

Regularly scheduled weighing times (i.e., before breakfast) and consistency of clothing worn by the patient decreases such interfering variables as the weight of each item of clothing or food ingested. Variations in accuracy of scales makes it helpful if the same scale is used for comparative weight analysis.

Acute situations in which fluid accumulation jeopardizes the physiologic status of the patient require fine monitoring of fluid balance. In situations in which maintenance of fluid balance necessitates titration of fluid replacement with output of fluid by all routes (i.e., urine, wound drainage, insensible losses by perspiration and respiration) it may be necessary to weigh diapers, bedding, or dressings to define the total output. In most patient situations the carefully tabulated record of intake and output by all routes provides the base for definition of fluid balance and replacement needs.

Rigid fluid restrictions (i.e., 1500 ml./24 hours) require monitoring and recording all liquids ingested. Only in extreme situations is the amount of fluid contained in foods included in the restriction, but foods that become liquids at body temperature (i.e., ice cream, Jell-O) and intravenous infusions are calculated.

Maintenance of nutrition requires that a preplanned amount of liquid accompany foods served; therefore a plan for "saving" fluids for mealtime is required, and the amount calculated is deleted from interim fluids allowed. It is important to provide for replacement of liquids the patient is unable to drink at mealtime.

Administration of medications requires concurrent fluid intake, and the amount allocated also must be planned within the 24-hour restriction schedule. Attention to humidity of the room air, application of lubricants to the lips, and spacing of small amounts of fluid intake may make the rigid restriction schedule less traumatic to the patient.

Fluid restriction schedules are most effective when the patient participates in planning and maintaining the restriction. The patient's definition of times when thirst is most acute allows planning to meet his needs and increases the potential for success of the program.

Assessment of general tissue hydration provides base lines against which to measure changes during therapy. Excessive amounts of sequestered fluid can deplete the extracellular fluid volume. In addition to evidence of tissue dehydration (dry and furrowed tongue, decreased skin turgor), hemoconcentration and depleted blood volume will be reflected in hypotension, elevated hematocrit level, or an increase in the serum sodium ion level. Depressed pressor receptor (aortic and carotid) response to decreased blood volume will be evident when the blood pressure is taken with the patient standing rather than in a supine position. Each of the assessments influences planning of nursing measures to enhance the effect of the total plan for control of fluid accumulation and excretion.

Assessment of drug effect. Diuretics are given to remove fluid, and any change in function or size of accumulation sites serves as an indicator of the progress of therapy. The final pathway of excretion is the kidney; therefore changes in the amount and concentration (specific gravity) of the urine provide important clues to diuretic drug effect. After initial administration of the drug, urine output should rise sharply above the normal level of 50 ml./hour. Unconscious patients have an indwelling catheter during diuretic therapy to assure prompt removal of the copious urine outflow. Whenever possible, the patient should be told to expect an increase in the frequency and the volume of urination after drug administration. Regularly scheduled diuretic drug use maintains a steady state of fluid elimination without sharp peaks in urine output.

The aim of therapy for patients with generalized edema is a weight loss of 1 to 2 pounds/24 hours. Many patients view the change as loss of tissue mass, and so the relationship between weight loss and fluid decrease must be explained clearly.

Assessment of drug adverse effect. Specific assessment of fluid and ion depletion is indicated throughout diuretic drug therapy. In the hospital setting frequent serum samples will be examined. Serum values provide vital evidence of change before overt problems appear. Decrease in cation levels in extracellular or intracellular fluid modifies the isotonicity and electrodynamic activity essential to membrane function.

Potassium deficit. Serum potassium ion levels reflect the amount of intracellular potassium ions (Fig. 6-1) because extracellular potassium ions are actively incorporated into the cell to maintain the cation level. When there is a deficiency in the supply of available potassium ions, sodium ions move to replace the intracellular cation deficit. The shift leads to hyperpolarization of membrane fibers, thus disrupting the polarization-depolarization sequence necessary to fiber response to stimuli. The change would be evident in lethargy of the patient. Muscle paralysis occurs with extreme hypokalemia. Potassium ion levels approaching the low normal range (normal: 3.5 to 5 mEq./liter) portend decreased muscle contraction and nerve impulse transmission.

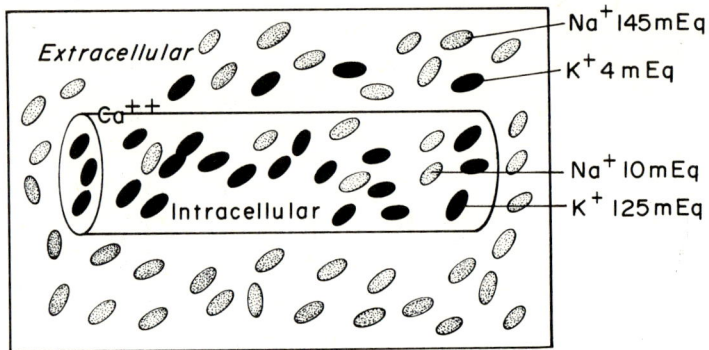

Fig. 6-4. Differences between extracellular and intracellular cations affect the bioelectrical activity of cell membrane.

Potassium replacement. Potassium ion levels may be maintained by addition of potassium-rich foods to the diet (meats, bananas, citrus fruits, melons) or by using commercial supplements. Potassium chloride is frequently employed for prophylactic or therapeutic maintenance of potassium ion levels because deficit of the cation is associated with anion decrease. Liquid forms have an unpleasant taste and should be given in citrus fruit juice. The potential for overcorrection of potassium ion deficit is minimal with oral replacement because potassium is nonselectively excreted.

Onset of hyperkalemia is possible with intravenous administration; therefore the infusion is run slowly. Potassium chloride solutions are irritating to venous tissues, and the patient will complain of a burning sensation if the infusion is run rapidly. During intravenous replacement therapy, the rate and rhythm of the apical pulse must be monitored because hyperkalemia increases myocardial irritability. When there is a change in the pulse, objective validation with an electrocardiographic recording will assist in defining the specific problem. Peaking of the T wave on the recording is early evidence of increasingly hyperkalemia.

There are several oral agents commercially available for potassium supplementation: potassium gluconate (Kaon); Randall's solution, which contains potassium acetate, potassium bicarbonate, and potassium citrate (potassium Triplex); and some effervescent forms that are palatable. Consistent use of the supplement is planned to decrease the incidence of physiologic problems arising with depletion of the intracellular cation.

Sodium deficit. Decreased serum sodium levels (normal: 135 to 145 mEq./liter) may occur during diuretic therapy when the patient restricts salt intake below the suggested level or when he is persistently diaphoretic (fever, hot environment). The basic physiologic problems, like those occurring with intracellular cation depletion, relate to decreased isotonicity and electrodynamic activity. Manifestations of deficit are comparable to those experienced by any individual after strenuous exercise in the hot sun: weakness, nausea, dryness of the mouth, drowsiness, and leg cramps. Correction of the deficit decreases the symptoms. Sodium ion depletion has a cancellation effect on diuretics dependent on inhibition of sodium transport in the nephron. The absence of sodium ions in tubular urine allows reabsorption of water to proceed, and edema may persist. Hypertonic sodium chloride with concurrent restriction of water intake may be planned to correct the imbalance and reinstitute effective diuretic therapy.

REFERENCES

Abbey, Jane C.: Nursing observations of fluid imbalance, Nursing Clinics of North America **3**:77, 1968.

Basch, R. I., and Merrill, J. P.: Effect of sodium balance on intrarenal distribution of blood flow in normal man, Journal of Applied Physiology **28**:312, 1970.

Cannon, Paul J.: Physiology of the diuretics: how they work, how to pick the best one, Resident and Staff Physician **18**:31, April, 1972.

Clark, James E., and Caedo, Rose-Elaine: Fluid and electrolyte management in renal failure, American Family Physician **5**:124, Feb., 1972.

Crosbie, Delores, Mink, Mariann, and Mullen, Elaine: Metabolic studies in a child with antidiuretic hormone syndrome, Nursing Clinics of North America **4**:155, 1969.

Downing, Shirley R.: Nursing support in early renal failure, American Journal of Nursing **69**:1212, 1969.

Evarts, Charles M.: Low molecular weight dextran, Medical Clinics of North America **51**:1285, 1967.

Hayslett, J. P., Domoto, D. T., Kashgarian, M., and Epstein, F. H.: Role of physical factors in the natriuresis induced by acetylcholine, American Journal of Physiology **218**:880, 1970.

Heath, Joleen Klocke: A conceptual basis for assessing body water status, Nursing Clinics of North America **6**:189, 1971.

Hultgren, Herbert N., and Flamm, M. D.: Pulmonary edema, Modern Concepts of Cardiovascular Disease **38**:1, 1969.

Knox, F. G.: Effects of increased proximal delivery of furosemide natriuresis, American Journal of Physiology **218**:819, 1970.

Lapides, Jack, Bourne, Richard B., and MacLean, Lloyd R.: Clinical signs of dehydration and extracellular fluid loss, Journal of the American Medical Association **191**:141, 1965.

McDonald, K. M., Rosenthal, A., Schrier, R. W., Galicich, J., and Lauler, D. P.: Effect of interruption of neural pathways on renal response to volume expansion, American Journal of Physiology **218**:510, 1970.

Merrill, John P.: Acute renal failure, Journal of the American Medical Association **211**:289, 1970.

Mountcastle, Vernon B., editor: Medical physiology, ed. 13, vol. 1, St. Louis, 1974, The C. V. Mosby Co.

Orten, James M., and Neuhaus, Otto W.: Biochemistry, ed. 8, St. Louis, 1970, The C. V. Mosby Co.

Reilly, Mary Jo, editor: American hospital formulary service, vol. 2, sect. 40:28, Washington, D. C., 1973, American Society of Hospital Pharmacists.

Ritchie, Mignon: Heart failure—the geriatric patient, Nursing Clinics of North America **3**:663, 1968.

Rothschild, Marcus A., Oratz, Murray, and Schreiber, Sidney S.: Albumin synthesis, The New England Journal of Medicine **286**:816, 1972.

Santos-Martinez, J., and Selkurt, E. E.: Renal lymph and its relationship to the countercurrent multiplier system of the kidney, American Journal of Physiology **216**:1548, 1969.

Schneider, William J., and Boyce, Barbara A.: Complications of diuretic therapy, American Journal of Nursing **68**:1903, 1968.

Schrier, R. W., and de Wardener, H. E.: Tubular reabsorption of sodium ion, The New England Journal of Medicine **285**:1231, 1971.

Smith, Barbara C.: Congestive heart failure, American Journal of Nursing **69**:278, 1969.

Swendsen, Leslee: Nursing care of the infant with congestive heart failure, Nursing Clinics of North America **4**:621, 1969.

Uttiger, Robert D.: Disorders of antidiuretic hormone secretion, Medical Clinics of North America **52**:381, 1968.

Wilkinson, Harold A., Wepsic, James G., and Austin, George: Diuretic synergy in the treatment of acute experimental cerebral edema, Journal of Neurosurgery **34**:203, 1971.

Yu, Paul N.: Lung water in congestive heart failure, Modern Concepts of Cardiovascular Disease **40**:27, June, 1971.

Zimmerman, Jack E.: Respiratory failure complicating post-traumatic acute renal failure: etiology, clinical features and management, Annals of Surgery **174**:12, 1971.

7
Tissue toxicants and debris

Environmental poisons
Heavy metal poisoning
    Poison control centers
    Pharmacodynamics
    Patient care
Retained metabolic products
    Pharmacodynamics
Tissue fluid and debris
    Pharmacodynamics

Current concern with environmental pollutants has stimulated public interest in sources of contamination from insecticides, heavy metals (i.e., lead, mercury), and radioactive materials. Positive steps are being taken to decrease exposure and eliminate sources of products hazardous to man.

Environmental poisons

The effect of insecticides on life processes has been identified. *Organophosphorus* compounds inhibit the vital enzyme *cholinesterase* in living systems, and storage of *chlorinated hydrocarbons* in body lipids adversely affects neurologic function. Humans may tolerate the effects of insecticides, but the compounds are lethal to many other living creatures.

The impact of insecticides on ecologic systems remains a concern as man seeks ways to retain balance in his environment. The universality of the problem of ecologic balance makes it seem distant to the average citizen, but there are pollutants over which the individual has greater control. For example, public concern with the neurotoxic and potentially lethal effects of mercury accumulation in body tissues has sharply decreased fish consumption. The protective action taken by individuals does not discriminate between varying levels of mercury in fish, and widespread cessation of fish eating has jeopardized the fishing industry.

HEAVY METAL POISONING

Heavy metals may enter the body by ingestion, inhalation, or absorption through the skin. Sequestration of the metals in tissues disrupts enzymatic processes because the heavy metals have an affinity for the *sulfhydryl groups* involved in many enzymatic processes.

Prophylactic and therapeutic programs for control of lead poisoning have been implemented in response to public concern with the debilitation and encephalopathy occurring in children who are exposed to the heavy metal. Recent research indicates that the teething infant who gnaws on the bars of a crib covered with lead-based paint could ingest enough lead to adversely affect reticuloendothelial tissues. Bacterial invasion of the gastrointestinal or upper respiratory tract, which frequently occurs in infants, could become lethal infections in the absence of defense mechanisms of the reticuloendothelial tissues. Widely publicized warnings about the hazards of poisoning have decreased the use of lead-based paint on children's furniture and playthings.

Planned programs for examination of children in substandard housing areas include testing for urine and tissue lead content. Children are examined for generalized effects of lead on muscle tissues (i.e., abdominal pain, weakness of the extensor muscles of the wrists). Accumulation of lead deposits causes typical gingival lead lines and signs of brain damage (i.e., behavioral problems, mental retardation). Therapeutic measures are planned for children with lead deposits in their tissues. Prevention of poisoning offers the greatest protection for children, and education of the public about hazards and measures to use for control is a planned program of many public health agencies.

Elimination of some of the generally available sources of heavy metals in the natural environment of children and decreasing sources of contamination by heavy metals in industry are positive steps toward solution of an identified problem. Accidental ingestion of drugs containing the heavy metals (i.e., iron tablets, mercurial diuretics, arsenic-containing drugs) remains one of the major health problems of children.

The tissue site invaded by the heavy metal affects the functional problems demonstrated and the therapeutic approach necessary for removal of the poison. For example, when a child swallows iron tablets, prompt use of an emetic may remove the entire amount of drug from the stomach, and the problem may be terminated. In another situation, the child in the hand-mouth phase of development may put peeling bits of sweet-tasting lead-based paint into his mouth as he stands at the windowsill each day. In the latter situation, lead ingestion may exceed the rate of excretion. Gradually the excess lead becomes deposited in tissues (including bone). Lead accumulation in central nervous system tissues disrupts function and causes acute toxic effects (i.e., convulsions, coma).

Poison control centers

Poison control centers maintain files of information about contents of drugs and the innumerable commercial products (i.e., household cleansers, aerosols, detergents) that contain substances harmful to humans. Contact with the center and identification of the particular product ingested results in rapid identification of the components of the product that are pathologic. Emergency measures to halt absorption of the poison from the gastrointestinal tract or other contaminated surface (i.e., skin, eyes) are recommended by poison control center personnel on the basis of stored data.

Contact with the center can be made by either physician or private citizen. The service allows prompt use of specific measures for the particular poison. Follow-up contact with the physician is recommended for evaluation of the effectiveness of emergency measures and control of predictable effects of absorbed portions of the poison.

Pharmacodynamics

Drugs used to remove excess amounts of heavy metals from serum or from sequestered sites in tissues act by forming chelates (from the Greek word *chele,* meaning claw). Chelating drugs remove heavy metals by mutual sharing of valence forces to form a chemical union with the metal. Chelation inactivates heavy metals when the new molecule (chelate) is formed (Fig. 7-1). Chelates are water-soluble metal complexes with little ionizing potential, and they move into the vascular bed to be eliminated in urine or feces. Chelates are less irritating to excretory routes than are the heavy

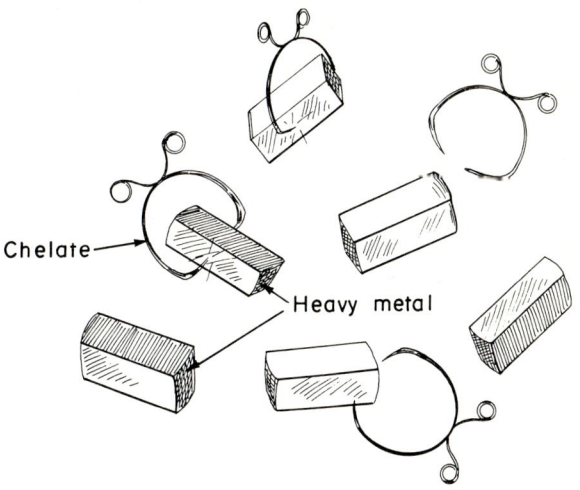

Fig. 7-1. The pincer grasp of chelates removes heavy metals from tissue storage sites. The combined chelate–heavy metal product enters the circulation and is eliminated from the body.

metals. Chelating drugs are capable of removing many different metals, but there is some specificity in clinical use of the drugs.

Calcium chelation. Disodium edetate (Table 7-1) is capable of chelating several heavy metals, and it offers an excellent example of the problems that occurred when chelates were introduced. Pharmacotherapeutic plans for removing heavy metals were fraught with the hazard of concurrent removal of calcium ions by the chelating action of disodium edetate. Recent clinical use takes advantage of the high affinity of disodium edetate for calcium ions (nonheavy metal), and the drug is employed primarily for patients with hypercalcemia. The drug is used as an emergency measure to decrease serum levels and the mobile reserves of calcium ions. The process tends to move calcium ions from deposits, or nodules, in the body to replace the serum deficit caused by chelation of circulating calcium ions, and the process increases calcium ion availability to drug action. One gram of disodium edetate can chelate 120 mg. of calcium ions.

Calcium ions are necessary from many physiologic processes (i.e., nerve conduction, muscle contraction, clotting mechanisms, vascular tone), and removal of the cation is carefully controlled to maintain the normal circulating levels of calcium ions. A replacement drug (i.e., calcium gluconate) should be readily available for use if the serum calcium ion level drops precipitously. Hypocalcemia can cause cardiopulmonary arrest or convulsions; therefore the serum levels of calcium ion are monitored during administration of disodium edetate.

As a precautionary measure the patient is placed in a recumbent or sitting position to decrease the incidence of hypotension during the time of drug administration. Patients sometimes have nausea, diarrhea, and skin rash in the facial area during therapy. Adverse effects occur most frequently with rapid intravenous administration.

Lead chelation. Calcium disodium edetate (Table 7-1) is similar to disodium edetate, but addition of the calcium component decreases the affinity for calcium ions in the chelating process. The chief clinical use of calcium disodium edetate is for removal of lead from deposits in the body, but the drug can form chelates with many other metals (cadmium, chromium, copper, iron, manganese, nickel, zinc).

Mobilization of lead is highest in the first 24 to 48 hours after administration is initiated. Intensive therapy includes continuous intravenous drip for 2 to 3 days. A rest period is planned after 3 to 5 days of therapy to allow redistribution of lead and increase its accessibility to the chelating drug. In the process of lead removal from blood and tissue depots, calcium is exchanged for the lead. Chelates are excreted in the urine 6 hours after initiation of intravenous therapy, and the peak excretion period is 24 to 48 hours.

The chief concern during therapy is the occurrence of acute necrosis of proximal convoluted tubules in the nephron. Urinary output of the patient is monitored during therapy to determine lead content and quantity of urine. Patients occasionally complain of malaise, fatigue, and numbness of the extremities. Onset of adverse effects of the drug may include specific complaints of gastrointestinal disturbances, fever, or pain in muscles and joints.

Iron chelation. Iron ingestion ranks fourth among prevalent agents causing poisoning of children in the United States. Spontaneous emesis caused by the irritating effects of the drug or by an emetic (i.e., ipecac) may produce

Table 7-1. Dosage range of chelating drugs

Nonproprietary name	Proprietary (trade) name	Daily adult dosage range
Calcium disodium edetate	Calcium Disodium Versenate	Oral: 4 Gm. (÷2) I.V.: 75 mg./kg.
Deferoxamine mesylate	Desferal	I.M.: 1-6 Gm. (÷ 6) I.V.: Same
Dimercaprol	BAL	I.M.: 15-18 mg./kg. (÷ 6)
Disodium edetate	Endrate	I.V.: 50 mg./kg
Penicillamine	Cuprimine	Oral: 1-5 Gm. (÷ 4)

enough black-colored vomitus to indicate removal of most of the iron (usually iron tablets) ingested. When there is a question whether emesis has adequately removed the heavy metal, x-ray examination of the abdomen may reveal the presence of residual iron in the gastrointestinal tract. Ingestion of 500 mg. or more of iron without adequate emesis usually is considered an indication for intravenous infusion of the iron-chelating drug. The urgency for removal is related to the toxic effect of iron on cerebral, hepatic, renal, and respiratory function.

Deferoxamine mesylate (Table 7-1) has a specific affinity for iron, and it complexes with the heavy metal to form the chelate *ferrioxamine*. Deferoxamine mesylate removes ferric iron from the loosely bound storage forms (ferritin, transferrin) and hemosiderin, but it has no effect on iron attached to hemoglobin. Renal excretion of the chelate *ferrioxamine* causes reddish coloring of the urine. Ferrioxamine is dialyzable; therefore an alternate route for elimination is available in the presence of renal failure.

Intramuscular injection is the preferred parenteral route for administration, but patients complain of pain at the injection site. All patients receiving deferoxamine mesylate are observed for onset of skin rash, blurred vision, abdominal pain, leg cramps, tachycardia, and fever. Long-term use for iron-storage disease (hemochromatosis) has precipitated allergic reactions.

Copper chelation. Penicillamine (Table 7-1) is related to penicillin, but it has no bacterial activity. It is used chiefly for chelation of copper, although it can form chelates with iron, mercury, or lead. Penicillamine is the specific drug employed for removal of the cuprous copper that causes *hepatolenticular degeneration* in the rare hereditary disease resulting from a defect in copper metabolism (Wilson's disease). Long-term use of the drug decreases the deposits of copper in liver and brain tissue that are life-threatening to youngsters with the disease. Therapy includes measures directed at maintenance of a negative copper balance, and dosage of penicillamine is titrated with urinary copper excretion. Concurrent ingestion of copper in foods and fluids is monitored carefully, and exchange resins may be used to prevent absorption of trace amounts of copper from the gastrointestinal tract.

Hypersensitivity reactions to penicillamine occur, but the adverse effects of greatest concern are leukopenia and thrombocytopenia. Blood values are followed closely during the therapeutic program. Petechial bleeding or changes in behavior should be brought to the attention of the physician promptly. Body temperature regulation is affected by the level of copper in thalamic tissues, and depletion of copper may cause hyperpyrexia. The body temperature is taken nightly to assure early identification of fever onset during therapy.

Arsenic, mercury, and gold chelation. Dimercaprol (Table 7-1) is a chelating agent used for removal of toxic levels of the heavy metals that inhibit enzyme systems (i.e., pyruvate-oxidase). The chief use of dimercaprol is for chelation of arsenic, mercury, or gold, but the drug is sometimes employed for removal of copper and in patients with encephalopathy for removal of lead. *Mercaptide* is the chelate formed, and it is excreted in urine within 6 to 24 hours after initiation of parenteral therapy with dimercaprol. Prompt removal of arsenic or mercury is required to prevent toxic effects of the metals on body tissues. Arsenic accumulation causes agranulocytosis, and mercury accumulation causes irreversible tissue damage.

Patient care

The individual with an inborn error of metabolism (i.e., Wilson's disease) requires lifelong therapy to decrease the toxic effects of retained metals. Concurrent therapy is directed at maximizing elimination of the metal while decreasing the amount entering the body from food sources.

The timing of initial therapy related to the period of heavy metal ingestion is an important factor when the toxicants enter the body. The individual accidentally or intentionally taking a drug or other contaminant requires prompt therapy to remove residual material or block its absorption from the gastrointestinal tract into the circulation.

In an emergency situation the physician (or

poison control center) will suggest measures appropriate to the agent ingested. In some instances common foods or fluids are recommended for binding of poisons in the gastrointestinal tract. For example, the tannic acid of strong tea binds some drugs and heavy metals (i.e., cobalt, copper, lead, mercury, nickel, zinc); protein content of milk or egg white binds some poisons (i.e., mercuric chloride); and pectin content of fresh apples binds electrolytes of some drugs (i.e., magnesium citrate). Many ingested chemicals are irritating to the gastrointestinal tract lining, and hemorrhage may occur when motility of the tract is increased by enemas or emetics. Removal of the material by gastric lavage may be necessary.

Removal of the toxicant from circulating fluids or tissues may be accomplished by the chelating drugs, or in some instances dialysis may be used to remove the material. Concurrent supportive therapy required by the patient will depend on the disruptive effects of the metals on physiologic function in sites where metals are sequestered.

Trace elements of many metals are important to normal physiologic processes. For example, iron is a necessary component in the oxygen-carrying function of hemoglobin. Abnormally high levels of iron interfere with normal enzymatic function and cellular equilibrium; therefore the levels must be reduced.

It is probable that new drugs capable of chelating metals will be developed in the near future. In addition to removal of excess heavy metals, chelation is a factor in maintaining physiologic processes. For example, hemoglobin and vitamin B_{12} are natural chelates found in the body. Chelation is a factor in maintaining physiologic levels of trace metals in the body and in potentiating the effectiveness of many pharmacotherapeutic agents. For example, aspirin is thought to provide an antipyretic effect by delivery of chelated copper to thalamic temperature control centers.

RETAINED METABOLIC PRODUCTS

Preparation of ingested protein materials for body use requires enzymatic conversion in the gastrointestinal tract. Various proteolytic enzymes (trypsin, chymotrypsin, peptidases) prepare the protein for absorption and assimilation to meet energy and building needs. In the process of breaking the protein into its component parts, each of the ionic materials is available for building new products or for formation of amino acids. Complexes of carbon, hydrogen, and oxygen ions can be assembled to form carbohydrates or fats. Nitrogen ions (and trace metals) are necessary for formation of amino acids. Building of carbohydrates and fats from protein frees nitrogen ions, and the ammonia product (NH_3) passes to the liver. Hepatic metabolic pathways convert ammonia to urea. After conversion, urea enters the hepatic veins and moves toward contact with the arterial circulation and excretion by the kidneys.

Excess ingestion of protein or high-protein tube feedings increases the amount of ammonia delivered to the liver. Excess tissue destruction or gastrointestinal tract hemorrhage may increase the endogenous sources of nitrogen and raise the quantity of ammonia entering the hepatic metabolic cycle. In either situation the amount of urea leaving the liver will be increased, and kidney elimination of the metabolic waste proceeds at a rapid pace.

The chief intracellular cation is potassium, and initial breakdown of protein liberates potassium chloride from the food or tissue source. Potassium chloride enters the serum by diffusing across the gastrointestinal membrane, and it is available in the serum to meet cellular needs. Excess amounts of the molecule are nonselectively excreted by the kidneys. Potassium chloride is not a metabolic waste because it can be reused by the body. Excess amounts of potassium chloride in the serum disrupts the electrophysiologic properties of nerve and muscle membranes. Elevated serum potassium ion levels occur during rapid parenteral administration of potassium chloride or excessive protein catabolism.

From the foregoing description of natural travel routes of ammonia, urea, and potassium ions, it is evident that excessive amounts will appear in the blood when tissue destruction is high or when excretion routes are obstructed. Renal shutdown closes the excretion route for urea and potassium chloride, and sluggish hepatic function slows the conversion of ammonia to urea. Diverse physiologic problems occur when either of the major organs cease their detoxification, excretion, and elimination activities; retention of ammonia, urea, or potassium ions presents complex acute physiologic problems for the patient.

When the routes for elimination of metabolic products are closed, alternate routes must be established because abnormally high blood levels of ammonia, urea, or potassium chloride are incompatible with life. Urgent need for removal of urea and potassium ions may require peritoneal dialysis or hemodialysis, but in less acute situations, drugs may be used to remove the products from the body. In the absence of functioning kidneys, dialysis is required to lower elevated blood urea levels.

Pharmacodynamics

Potassium ion removal. Potassium has a narrow range of normal limits in the serum (3.5 to 5.0 mEq./liter), and elevation above the higher limit rapidly causes irritability of cell membranes. Early changes occur in the cardiac rate and rhythm, and the patient is monitored continually when potassium levels are high. Electrocardiographic recordings show changes indicating increasing cardiac irritability. Changes may progress from peaking of the T wave as the serum potassium ion level rises (i.e., 7 mEq./liter) to ventricular fibrillation as it moves higher (i.e., 8 mEq./liter).

Hyperkalemia resulting from rapid infusion of intravenous potassium chloride may require immediate short-term therapy for the patient with borderline cardiac status. In selected situations, administration of hypertonic glucose with insulin may be prescribed to move excess potassium ions into cells rapidly, and the process lowers serum levels of the cation. The stopgap measure is useful for control of single-incident, or transient, hyperkalemia.

Hyperkalemia more frequently occurs consequent to renal tubule dysfunction. Peritoneal dialysis may be planned for removal of urea and potassium chloride from serum when renal function is compromised by acute tubule necrosis. Provision of the alternate route for removal of the electrolytes decreases the work load of the kidneys, and in many instances, nephron function improves after peritoneal dialysis has been used for a few days. Hemodialysis is required for control of electrolyte levels and maintenance of acid-base balance when patients have bilateral chronic renal failure.

Cation exchange resins. Dietary restrictions may be used to control borderline elevations of serum potassium ion levels, but cation exchange resins are employed to remove excess serum potassium ions occurring secondary to renal tubule dysfunction. When the patient has an intact bowel, cation exchange resins remove potassium ions from the serum more efficiently than does the dialysis procedure. Peritoneal dialysis clears approximately 6 to 10 mEq. of potassium ions from the serum in an hour, but cation exchange therapy can move 50 mEq. of potassium ions from the serum into the intestinal lumen in an hour.

Polystyrene sodium sulfonate (Table 7-2) is used orally or as a retention enema for removal

Table 7-2. Dosage range of drugs used to remove endogenous toxicants

Nonproprietary name	Proprietary (trade) name	Daily adult dosage range
Allopurinol	Zyloprim	Oral: 100-800 mg. ($\div$ 3)
Arginine glutamate	Modumate	I.V.: 50-75 Gm. ($\div$ 2-3)
Arginine hydrochloride	R-Gene	I.V.: 40-60 Gm. ($\div$ 2-3)
Cholestyramine resin	Cuemid, Questran	Oral: 1-16 Gm. ($\div$ 3-4)
Polystyrene sodium sulfonate	Kayexalate	Oral: 15-60 Gm. ($\div$ 1-4)
Probenecid	Benemid	Oral: 0.5-2 Gm. ($\div$ 2-4)
Sodium glutamate	Glutavene	I.V.: 25-50 Gm. ($\div$ 2)
Sulfinpyrazone	Anturan	Oral: 200-800 mg. ($\div$ 4)

of excess potassium ions from the serum. Polystyrene sodium sulfonate is a cation exchange resin that acts in the intestinal lumen by liberating its sodium ions in exchange for potassium ions. Dosage calculations are based on the ability of 1 Gm. of the drug to remove 1 mEq. of potassium ion. The aim of therapy is to lower serum potassium ion levels to 4 to 5 mEq./liter.

When administered orally, the resin acquires potassium ions in the lumen of the colon, and the new resin is excreted in the feces. Addition of a syrup to each dose of the resin increases its palatability. To avoid the high incidence of fecal impaction and constipation occurring when the resin is used, sorbitol (a sugar) is given during the period of therapy. Sorbitol (10 to 20 ml.) acts as an osmotic cathartic, and it may be given every 2 hours until 1 to 2 diarrheal stools are produced. Sorbitol also facilitates the movement of the resin along the intestinal tract, and drug effect is enhanced.

Polystyrene sodium sulfonate is often used in 150 to 200 ml. of diluent as a retention enema. Warming the solution to body temperature increases the patient's ability to retain the fluid for the prescribed period of time (30 minutes to 4 hours). The retention time is based on the level of exchange necessary to lower the patient's serum potassium ion level. Cleansing enemas are usually given before the retention enema to decrease fecal obstruction to drug contact with the cation. Removal of the resin after administration requires another enema unless the patient has diarrhea.

During therapy the potassium ion level is monitored closely to avoid hypokalemia due to excess removal of the cation. With prolonged therapy the physician will monitor blood levels of other cations (i.e., calcium, magnesium) because removal of minimal amounts of the cations over time may deplete normal serum stores.

The addition of sodium ions to the serum during therapy with cation exchange resins can be additive with frequent drug use. One gram of the drug leaves 100 mEq. of sodium ions in the intestinal tissues in exchange for potassium ions, and the exchange adds to serum levels of sodium ion. Patients on dietary salt restriction may need further limitation of foods during therapy. The chief complaints of patients during therapy are related to dislike of the oral drug, and some patients have problems with anorexia and nausea.

The action of cation exchange agents in the intestinal lumen removes the target cation from tissues and fluids lining the tract. Removal of the cation moves serum potassium ions to the intestinal tissues and fluids to equilibrate cation levels, and potassium ions continually are assessible for removal by the drug.

Urea removal. Renal failure leads to accumulation of end products of protein metabolism, and the products (urea, uric acid, creatinine) are removed by dialysis if renal dysfunction persists. Drugs may be used to control urea accumulation in blood when the patient has adequate renal function to allow excretion. Blood urea nitrogen levels may be increased by metabolic overproduction of urates or by drugs that block urate excretion. Deposition of excess urates in synovial fluids causes painful joint movement typical of gout. Although the joint collection of urates occurs in patients with metabolic overproduction of urates, gout is caused by a metabolic error related to purine metabolism, glycine conversion to uric acid, or disruption of renal tubule epithelial cell conversion of glutamine to ammonia. The particular metabolic error may not be clearly identified, but the patient with gout has synovial accumulation of urate crystals.

Blood urea nitrogen levels may be increased by drugs that affect protein anabolism or catabolism. For example, the antianabolic action of tetracycline on bacteria and on some body proteins may increase the catabolism of unused amino acids, with consequent elevation in urea production. Accelerated catabolism of body proteins caused by glucocorticoids or catabolism of malignant tissue caused by antineoplastic drugs may increase blood urea levels.

Drugs may be used to accelerate the excretion rate of urea when the patient has normal functioning kidneys. Incorporation of nitrogenous wastes and some ions (potassium, magnesium, phosphorus) into structural proteins has been demonstrated by administration of controlled parenteral feedings containing essential amino acids, 50% dextrose, and vitamins to patients with nonfunctioning kidneys.

Urate reabsorption inhibitors. Probenecid and sulfinpyrazone lower the serum uric acid level by promoting urinary excretion of uric acid or urate in treatment of patients with gout. The drugs are known as uricosuric agents because of their mode of action. They act at the renal tubule to block reabsorption of urate from the tubular urine. The decrease in serum urea levels gradually liberates urea from deposition sites (tophaceous deposits) in the body. Therapy is directed at increasing excretion of uric acid in the urine, and high levels of the urates (700 mg./24 hours) are eliminated during therapy. The quantity of uric acid can be evaluated by measuring urine specific gravity. To assure passage of uric acid with urine, it is important to provide adequate fluids and measure the quantity of urine output. Crystals may precipitate to form renal stones in the absence of adequate kidney flushing.

The elimination route of salicylates is through the binding sites for action of uricosuric drugs; therefore use of salicylates will antagonize the action of the drugs. The patient should be reminded not to take salicylates during therapy.

Uricosuric agents are sulfonamide derivatives, and they are metabolized in the kidneys to glucuronic acid. The metabolite may cause a false-positive glucose content reaction in urine tested with copper reduction tests (Benedict's qualitative reagent, Clinitest). Some hypersensitivity reactions have been reported with drug use. Patients complain of headache and gastrointestinal disturbances.

Clinical use of probenecid has been expanded to utilize its pharmacodynamic action on blocking of renal tubule binding sites to slow the excretion of drugs. It may be employed to maintain serum levels of penicillin or aminosalicylic acid. Probenecid blocking maintains therapeutic levels of the drugs in the serum with lower dosage of the drug. For example, use of probenecid during therapy with any form of penicillin can double the plasma levels of penicillin.

Alternate urate excretory pathways. Allopurinol acts on purine catabolism by inhibiting the catalyzing enzyme. It blocks *xanthine oxidase* action required for the conversion of hypoxanthine to xanthine that results in uric acid production. Allopurinol is used to decrease hyperuricemia and tophaceous deposits of urates in joints.

Allopurinol therapy decreases blood urea levels by providing an alternate metabolic pathway for excretion of purine metabolites. Allopurinol acts as a substrate for the enzyme xanthine oxidase, and the drug-enzyme action results in formation of alloxanthine (oxypurinol). Renal clearance of the more soluble oxypurines (xanthine and hypoxanthine) provides an excretion route for urea and reduces urinary uric acid levels. High levels of solute during therapy makes it necessary to increase the fluid intake of the patient to assure the presence of enough solvent for the levels of xanthine, hypoxanthine, and uric acid in the nephrons.

Some individuals have hypersensitivity reactions during therapy with allopurinol. Many patients have pruritic skin rash, fever, gastrointestinal disturbances, and malaise during the time they are receiving the drug.

Ammonia removal. Increased blood ammonia levels occur when hepatic metabolic pathways fail to convert the nitrogenous products of protein metabolism to urea. The natural process of conversion of ammonia to urea produces a metabolic product that enters renal tubule enzymatic pathways and is removed from the body as ammonium chloride. Retention of ammonia gradually disrupts vital body processes, and progressive acidosis may lead to life-threatening *hepatic coma.* Encephalopathy may be manifest as poor mentation and involuntary, jerky muscular movements when the wrists are dorsiflexed and fingers are extended (liver flap).

Primary therapeutic measures are directed at decreasing endogenous and exogenous sources of protein. Dietary restriction of protein intake may be reduced to one fourth of the *one gram per kilogram of body weight* level used as a base line for normal physiologic function.

Bacteria in the intestinal lumen enzymatically convert organic nitrogen to ammonia as a preliminary step before the products enter the

116 Drugs used to control excretion of fluid, metabolic wastes, and toxicants

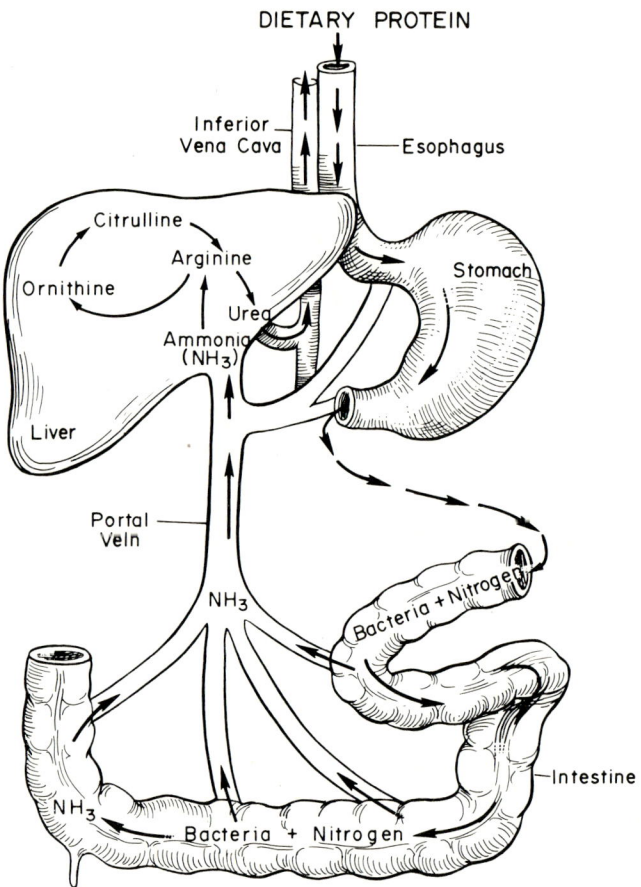

Fig. 7-2. The nitrogen component of dietary protein is enzymatically converted to ammonia (NH₃) by bacteria in the intestine. Ammonia travels via the portal veins to the liver where it is converted to urea. Venous blood leaving hepatic tissues carries urea toward the arterial circulation and the renal excretory pathway.

portal circulation and travel toward hepatic metabolic pathways (Fig. 7-2). Oral antibiotics may be used to decrease the number of the nitrogen-fixing commensals in the intestine, thereby decreasing absorption of nitrogenous products. Eradication of the bacteria may allow ingestion of adequate protein for regeneration of liver tissue. Control of sources of nitrogen is particularly important for the patient who has encephalopathy secondary to accumulation of ammonia in extracellular fluids. Frequent enemas or laxatives may be prescribed to decrease absorption of nitrogen and protein from old blood retained in the intestine (after-esophageal varicosity bleeding).

Arginine glutamate and arginine hydrochloride (Table 7-2) are components of the essential amino acid *arginine*. The hydrochloride form acts by interceding in the ammonia conversion pathways in the liver. Arginine hydrochloride provides additional arginine as a precursor to ornithine in the hepatic metabolic pathway:

Ammonia → Arginine → Ornithine →
                                     Citrulline → Urea

The process increases the conversion of ammonia to urea.

Arginine glutamate and sodium glutamate (nonessential amino acid) increase the metabolic process of amidation to increase the conversion of ammonia to urea. The drugs increase the synthesis of glutamine from ammonia or glutamate in the liver and peripheral tissues.

Each of the products used to increase the removal of ammonia are primarily natural biologic products; therefore the problems of concern to the physician in selecting an agent for ammonia removal will relate to the addition of hydrochloride or sodium components of the drug forms to the serum of acutely ill patients. Hydrochloride addition could cause acidosis, and sodium addition could cause hypochloremic alkalosis in the patient with borderline acid-base or ionic balance. Some patients have transient nausea, blushing, salivation, and an increase in respiratory depth during use of the drugs.

Bile salt removal. Obstruction in the liver or biliary tree causes retention of bile salts in the blood, and jaundice (intrahepatic cholestatic jaundice) appears. Bile acids in surface tissues irritate the nerve endings, and intense itching is present. Dryness of the skin due to the decreased fluid in superficial extracellular tissues adds to the pruritic effect of the bile acids. Contact with bedding or clothing intensifies the problem, and the patient is in acute distress.

Cholestyramine resin is an exchange resin administered orally to remove bile acids. It acts in the intestine by releasing chloride ions in exchange for bile acids, and the new resin complex is excreted with the feces. Removal of excess bile acids from the tissues in the intestinal lumen gradually moves additional bile acids to the area, and eventually tissue levels of the irritant decrease. Anion exchange raises fecal elimination of bile acids up to ten times normal levels.

The drug is given at least an hour after other drugs are administered to avoid interference with drug absorption. Resins may bind acids or absorb neutral drugs (i.e., digoxin).

Patients resist taking the mixture because of the unpleasant odor. The powder can be mixed with juices, applesauce, or crushed pineapple to disguise the odor. When mixed with carbonated beverages, the powder particles promote the liberation of carbon dioxide, and excessive foaming occurs. Gentle application of the powder to the surface of the beverage and slow stirring after wetting of the powder decrease the problem.

Long-term therapy may interfere with the absorption of fat-soluble vitamins (A, D, E, K), and the physician may plan replacement therapy to avoid interference with physiologic processes dependent on the vitamins. Patients complain of nausea, heartburn, and diarrhea during therapy with the anion-exchange resin.

TISSUE FLUID AND DEBRIS

Localized collections of fluids or proteins disrupt the normal physiologic processes of tissues containing the residual products. Isolated internal collections of protein materials (intravascular clots) prevent passage of blood through the vessel, and areas distal to the clot are partially or totally shunted off from the general circulation. Collections of tissue fluid around joints distend the tissues, immobilize the joints, and impinge on blood circulation in the area. Natural physiologic processes gradually phagocytize and remove clots and lymph drainage removes fluid accumulations, but during the slow reparative process functional problems continue.

Pharmacodynamics

With the exception of adenosine phosphate, each of the drugs given to remove tissue debris or fluid is an enzyme (Table 7-3). Some of them are familiar representatives of the enzymes or preenzyme substrates naturally produced by the pancreas (i.e., amylase, trypsin, chymotrypsin). Pharmacotherapeutic use of the enzymes is a planned transposition of their normal function in the digestive process to control physiologic problems.

Intravascular clot removal. The proteolytic enzymes, bromelains, chymotrypsin, fibrinolysin, papin, streptokinase, and trypsin (Table 7-3) are used to convert protein to peptides and amino acids. They are employed systemically to enzymatically degrade and disintegrate intravascular clots. The effect is accomplished by breakdown of the fibrin network and entrapped cells to make a pathway for blood to travel through the debris. Topical or intracavity use accomplishes a similar enzymatic degradation of protein components of necrotic tissues or exudates.

Intravascular clots can be life-threatening when occlusion of a major vessel is involved. Clinical trials been conducted to study the effectiveness of proteolytic enzymes on intravascular clot degradation. The effect of streptokinase and another enzyme, urokinase, when injected in large dosage directly into clots in the pulmonary arteries, showed x-ray evidence of dissolution of the clot and reinstitution of blood flow. The clinical trial method of injecting large doses directly at the clot site solves one of the major problems in the use of proteolytic enzymes. The drugs are nonselective in their action on protein, and prompt delivery directly to the action site enhances their effect at the target area (i.e., clot) with minimal effect on normal body proteins.

Parenteral and buccal routes of administration are utilized to move the drugs promptly to the effector tissue. Use of buccal tablets increases the speed with which the drugs are absorbed into the vascular system because the oral mucosa is richly supplied with blood vessels. When the patient holds the drug in his mouth without swallowing, the drug diffuses readily into the capillary bed and enters the venous circulation.

Parenteral use of the proteolytic enzymes carries with it the hazard of hypersensitivity reactions, and pretests for individual hypersensitivity are planned prior to administration of the intramuscular forms of the drugs. Patients complain of pain at the site of injection after intramuscular drug is administered.

Fibrinolysin is the only member of the group that is administered intravenously, and it often produces a febrile reaction that may appear up to 8 hours after the infusion is given. Intravenous administration frequently precipitates the adverse effects common to the group of proteolytic enzymes (i.e., dizziness, headache, nausea, and hypotension).

Necrotic tissue removal. Proteolytic enzymes are used primarily for debridement of necrotic tissue from wounds or decubitus ulcers. Drug effect on removal of tissue debris is enhanced when there is a plan for periodic flushing and removal of nonadherent tissue to

Table 7-3. Dosage range of drugs used to remove tissue debris or fluid

Nonproprietary name	Proprietary (trade) name	Daily adult dosage range
Adenosine phosphate	Cardiomone, My-B-Den	Subl.: 40-140 mg. ($\div 1$-7) I.M.: 20-100 mg. ($\div 1$-3)
Alpha amylase	Buclamase, Fortizyme	Buccal: 60-80 mg. ($\div 2$-3)
Bromelains	Ananase	Oral: 200,000-400,000 U. ($\div 4$)
Chymotrypsin	Chymar, Cytolav, Enzeon	Buccal: 40,000 U. ($\div 4$) I.M.: 2500-15,000 U. ($\div 1$-3)
Fibrinolysin (human)	Actase, Thrombolysin	I.V.: 250,000-500,000 U. ($\div 5$)
Papain	Papase	Buccal: 60,000-120,000 U. ($\div 6$-12)
Streptokinase		Buccal: 40,000-100,000 U. ($\div 4$) I.M.: 10,000 U. ($\div 2$)
Trypsin crystallized	Parenzyme, Tryptar	Oral: 200,000-400,000 U. ($\div 4$) I.M.: 12,500-25,000 U. ($\div 1$-2)

allow contact between drug and target tissue. Some debridement occurs each time packing or gauze covering is removed from the area. Drug effect is seen as a gradual appearance of granulation tissue around the site and gradual decrease in the depth of the crater as deeper tissues generate new cells. Heat lamps and air exposure may be planned between scheduled applications of the drug to promote drying and increase the blood supply of the tissues. Oxygen saturation by inserting an oxygen catheter through a paper cup tent over decubiti has a drying effect that promotes healing.

Denuding necrotic areas may expose capillaries and cause bleeding at the site, and copious amounts of the drug may destroy healthy tissues in the area. Controlled use of the drugs is balanced with the progression of the wound or decubitus area.

When streptokinase is used topically, it is provided in combination with another enzyme as a streptokinase-streptodornase (Varidase) preparation. The enzymes are obtained from streptococcus, and many individuals have antibodies from prior exposure to streptococcus that negate the usefulness of the drugs. The combined forms of the drugs are most effective when administered for wounds or cavities where infectious processes exist.

Tissue fluid removal. Alpha amylase is a carbohydrase physiologically active in enzymatic degradation of starch to simpler sugars. Its chief pharmacotherapeutic use is for control of inflammatory and edematous conditions (i.e., around joints) when local trauma has occurred and tissue fluid is resistant to removal by the venous or lymphatic processes naturally reversing fluid collection. Topical application of heat may be planned as an adjunct to systemic use of the drug for removal of tissue fluid. Although alpha amylase may be used for selective short-term control of localized inflammation, systemic anti-inflammatory drugs are more frequently used for control of persistent inflammation.

Adenosine phosphate is a natural physiologic component of muscle. Cyclic building and breakdown of adenosine triphosphate to adenosine diphosphate to produce phosphoric acid and energy is a familiar physiologic process. The pharmacodynamic action of adenosine phosphate decreases edema, erythema, dermatitis, and pruritus associated with varicose ulcers by a vasodilating action that improves cellular function. Some patients complain of headache, dizziness, and diarrhea during the period of therapy.

Patients with joint involvement are initially encouraged to splint the part and avoid unnecessary movement. Planned schedules for mobility are liberalized as the involved tissues show improvement. The involved tissues are protected from superimposed injury during therapy. Fluid-distended tissues or surface wounds are protected from constricting bedding or clothing. Application of heat by lamps or hot packs requires careful supervision of the patient to prevent injury to affected tissues and adjacent tissues.

REFERENCES

Abel, Ronald M., Abbott, William M., and Fischer, Josef E.: Acute renal failure, Archives of Surgery **103:**513, 1971.

Andersen, Murray N., and Juchiba, Kazuo: Measurement of acute changes in liver function and blood flow, Archives of Surgery **100:**541, 1970.

Arena, Jay M.: The treatment of poisoning, Clinical Symposia **18:**3, 1966.

Bowman, F. J., and Foulkes, E. C.: Antidiuretic hormone and urea permeability of collecting ducts, American Journal of Physiology **218:**231, 1970.

Chisolm, J. Julian, Jr.: Lead poisoning, Scientific American **224:**15, Feb., 1971.

Fernandez, Pedro C., and Kovnat, Paul J.: Metabolic acidosis reversed by the combination of a resin and a cathartic, The New England Journal of Medicine **286:**23, 1972.

Fisher, Alan E.: Chemical stimulation of the brain, Scientific American **210:**60, June, 1964.

Frieden, Earl: The biochemistry of copper, Scientific American **218:**102, May, 1968.

Hardy, Harriet L., Chamberlain, Richard I., Maloof, Clarence C., Boylen, George W., and Howell, Mary C.: Lead as an environmental poison, Clinical Pharmacology and Therapeutics **12:**982, 1971.

Janicki, R. H., and Goldstein, L.: Glutamine synthetase and renal ammonia metabolism, American Journal of Physiology **216:**1107, 1969.

Lin-Fu, Jane S.: Undue absorption of lead among children—a new look at an old problem, The New England Journal of Medicine **286:**702, 1972.

Merrill, John P.: Acute renal failure, Journal of the American Medical Association **211:**289, 1970.

Neurath, Hans: Protein-digesting enzymes, Scientific American **211:**68, Dec., 1964.

Orten, James M., and Neuhaus, Otto W.: Biochemistry, ed. 8, St. Louis, 1970, The C. V. Mosby Co.

Regan, Patricia A.: The nursing care of a patient with Wilson's disease, Journal of Neurosurgical Nursing 3:15, 1971.

Reilly, Mary Jo, editor: American hospital formulary service, vol. 2, sect. 40:00, 44:00, 64:00, Washington, D. C., 1973, American Society of Hospital Pharmacists.

Robischon, Paulette: Pica practice and other hand-mouth behavior and children's developmental level, Nursing Research 20:4, 1971.

Schubert, Jack: Chelation in medicine, Scientific American 214:40, May, 1966.

Steele, T. H.: Control of uric acid secretion, The New England Journal of Medicine 284:1193, 1971.

Stewart, Richard D.: Poisoning from chlorinated hydrocarbon solvents, American Journal of Nursing 67:85, 1967.

8
Enteric elimination

Constipation
    Pharmacodynamics
    Patient care
Diarrhea
    Pharmacodynamics
    Patient care

In the human body the synchronized physiologic processes for digestion of foods, absorption of nutrients, and movement of residue toward the anal exit are controlled by the parasympathetic nervous system. Ingestion of foods or fluids provides the stimulus that triggers the physiologic processes.

Movement of the waste products into the rectum stimulates nerves in the intestinal wall, and afferent impulses travel to the sacral segments of the spinal cord. Efferent impulses to the lower intestinal tract segments (descending colon, sigmoid colon, rectum) initiate mass movements of intestinal contents. Concurrent neural inhibition of the internal sphincter completes the involuntary neural controls that prepare for evacuation. In most individuals the stimulus to defecate occurs regularly, and completion of the process requires only that they arrange for relaxation of the external sphincter. Most individuals accomplish evacuation with little concern for the process that provided the stimuli.

At either end of the age continuum, considerably more attention is directed to ingestion of foods and elimination of the gastrointestinal tract contents. Changes in the frequency and consistency of her infant's stools are a concern to the mother. Elderly individuals plan ritualistically for continuance of the elimination patterns they consider to be necessary to health, and they become very concerned with disruption of established patterns. Although bowel evacuation has been a concern of the elderly throughout history, modern advertising media intensify the focus. Television viewers see constipation depicted as a socially crippling disorder naturally occurring after 40 years of age and middle-aged health as being dependent on regular use of laxatives.

Folklore and advertising emphasize a terminal event without consideration of the steps that can be taken to maintain the natural physiologic processes preceding the natural evacuation process. An increase in residue-producing foods, adequate fluid intake, and planned physical activity contribute to natural gastrointestinal function and decrease the need for regular use of laxatives or enemas.

CONSTIPATION

Constipation is seldom a simple problem for the patient. High levels of physical energy are expended in attempting to expel a dry, massive stool, and the patient is exhausted after completion of the task. Continued pressure on veins in the lower intestinal tract may precipitate bleeding of distended hemorrhoids.

Straining at stool is singularly undesirable for the acutely ill patient or the patient with a cardiac problem. The increase in intrathoracic pressure concurrent with physical effort to increase compression of the abdominal viscera (Valsalva maneuver) impinges on the great vessels in the thoracic cavity. At the termination of compression there is a sudden influx of venous blood into the heart. The physiologic effect of straining to evacuate has caused sudden death in cardiac patients.

Pharmacodynamics

In many situations the patient is considered a prime source of information about the agents that are most effective in control of bowel evacuation. There is an increasing practice of allowing the hospitalized patient to choose the particular laxative that he desires to use and to elect to use it as needed. Factors intrinsic in care of the patient with gastrointestinal pathology or abdominal surgery place some limits on the practice, but for patients with other problems (i.e., cardiac surgery) individual choice is allowed by many physicians during hospitalization.

Intestinal lubricant. Mineral oil (liquid petrolatum) is the most innocuous of the agents listed with cathartics (Table 8-1). The relatively nonabsorbable oil simply acts to lubricate the gastrointestinal tract and decrease dehydration of feces. Continued use of mineral oil may interfere with absorption of bile and the fat-soluble vitamins (A, D, E, K) and precipitate problems related to decreased physiologic levels of the vital substances. Continued use also causes anal leaking of the oil and soiling of clothing and bedding.

Most patients have difficulty taking the oily preparation. Even when the liquid is immediately followed by a citrus fruit drink, patients complain of the residual oily taste in their mouths.

Mineral oil is employed as a retention enema when the patient has a large mass of hard stool in the rectum. Retention of the oil for 20 to 30 minutes softens the stool, and a cleansing enema may be given to allow evacuation of feces.

Fecal softeners. Dioctyl calcium sulfosuccinate, dioctyl sodium sulfosuccinate, and poloxalkol (Table 8-1) act in the colon to lower the surface tension of fecal contents. Decreased surface tension allows water and fats to penetrate the fecal material, and there is gradual softening of the intestinal contents. The drugs are used to produce stools that are easy to evacuate. Dioctyl calcium sulfosuccinate and

Table 8-1. Dosage range of cathartics

Nonproprietary name	Proprietary (trade) name	Daily adult dosage range (oral)
Intestinal lubricant		
Mineral oil		15-30 ml.
Fecal Softeners		
Dioctyl calcium sulfosuccinate	Doxical, Surfak	150-240 mg.
Dioctyl sodium sulfosuccinate	Aquatyl, Colace, Diovac, Doxinate, Doxol, Molofac, Regutol	50-480 mg.
Methylcellulose	Cellothyl, Cologel, Hydrolose, Melozets, Methylose, Premocel, Syncelose	1-1.5 Gm.
Poloxalkol	Magcyl, Polykol	400-800 mg.
Psyllium hydrophilic mucilloid	Metamucil, Mucilose, Serutan	4-7 Gm.
Sodium carboxymethylcellulose	CMC cellulose gum	6 Gm. (÷2)
Irritant cathartics		
Aloin	Alophen	15-30 mg.
Bisacodyl	Dulcolax	10-15 mg.
Cascara sagrada	Peristaltin, Peristim	300 mg.
Castor oil	Neoloid	15-60 ml.
Danthron	Dorbane, Istizin	75-300 mg.
Oxyphenisatin acetate	Isocrin, Lavema, Prulet	5 mg.
Phenolphthalein	Phenolax	60 mg.
Senna	Senokot	0.5-2 Gm.
Sennosides A and B	Glysennid	12-24 mg.
Saline cathartics		
Magnesium citrate		200-300 ml.
Magnesium hydroxide		15-30 ml.
Magnesium sulfate		15 Gm.
Sodium biphosphate		0.5-1 Gm.
Sodium phosphate		2-8 Gm.

dioctyl sodium sulfosuccinate are used primarily for adult patients who are immobilized for long periods of time, and poloxalkol is employed primarily for infants and children. The age designation reflects common usage, but drug action is comparable in the varying age groups. Routine use of the drugs improves regularity and ease of bowel evacuation.

Methylcellulose, sodium carboxymethylcellulose, and psyllium hydrophilic mucilloid (Table 8-1) soften the stool and increase the bulk of stools by addition of a gel to the intestinal contents. Stools acquire a gelatinous consistency, and they are easily evacuated. The drugs are given in a full glass of water to assure passage into the intestinal tract because the gelatinous materials swell and become bulky enough to cause obstruction of the esophagus when small amounts of liquid are given.

Increased bulk in the intestinal lumen stimulates normal propulsive movements by pressure on the mucosal lining. Dietary intake of bran, which contains 20% cellulose, provides a natural bulky stool comparable to that produced by bulk-forming cathartics because the indigestible residue becomes distended with water in the intestinal lumen.

Colon irritants. The irritant cathartics (Table 8-1) stimulate peristalsis as a reflex response to irritation caused by drug contact with the mucosa of the intestinal lumen. Onset time of cathartic action varies, and the responsiveness of the individual's intestinal tract influences the effectiveness of the drugs in producing peristalsis. Increased peristalsis may cause cramps between the time of administration and completion of evacuation. Nursing infants may have diarrhea when the mother takes an irritant cathartic.

Castor oil is probably the best known cathartic. Use of the drug is restricted to daytime hours, since castor oil causes evacuation within 3 hours of the time it is administered. The rapid onset of action is an outcome of the unique effect of the drug and its metabolic product (ricinoleic acid), which stimulates motor activity in the small intestine. Castor oil is frequently administered to assure evacuation of the intestinal contents (including gas) prior to x-ray examinations of the abdomen.

Castor oil has a taste that most patients find very offensive, but serving the chilled drug with orange juice, lemon juice, or coffee may disguise the taste. Patients are asked to drink it quickly to decrease the distasteful spread of the oil on oral mucosa. Emulsions of the drug are somewhat more palatable.

Bisacodyl, oxyphenisatin acetate, and phenolphthalein stimulate peristalsis by their irritating effect on colon mucosa. Bisacodyl is the most frequently used drug of the group classified pharmacologically as *diphenylmethane* cathartics. Bisacodyl is insoluble in an alkaline medium; therefore oral dosage should be planned to avoid concurrently scheduled antacid administration by an hour. The drug is often employed as a suppository, and rectal use may produce evacuation in 15 to 60 minutes.

Absorption of small amounts of bisacodyl and phenophthalein from the small intestine presents no physiologic problems, but absorption of oxyphenisatin acetate from inflamed or ulcerated areas of the intestine may cause hepatitis and jaundice. Renal excretion of phenophthalein causes reddish discoloration of alkaline urine, and feces may be red tinged when alkalinity is increased by use of a soapsuds enema. The drugs are generally administered before the patient retires because the 6- to 8-hour action period provides an early morning defecation stimulus.

Cascara sagrada, danthron, senna, and sennosides A and B are known pharmacologically as *anthraquinone* cathartics. The drugs act primarily on the large intestine to increase peristalsis by direct contact with the intestinal wall or by action of the drug that returns to large intestine sites after absorption from the small intestine. Drug action may take 6 to 24 hours; therefore scheduling for bedtime use allows undisturbed sleep.

Aloin is another member of the anthraquinone cathartic group. Aloin is very irritating and its use is limited to individuals with chronic constipation and minimal peristaltic activity (i.e., patients with advanced multiple sclerosis).

Saline cathartics. Saline cathartics act by increasing the osmolality of the contents of the intestinal lumen. The resulting high-level water content rapidly moves the feces through the intestine, and evacuation may occur in 1 to 3 hours. Magnesium citrate, magnesium sulfate, sodium biphosphate, or sodium phosphate (Table 8-1) are used when rapid results are desired, but they are not used for routine control of bowel evacuation.

The effectiveness of the drugs in emptying intestinal contents produces copious amounts of watery stool, and there may be considerable flatus expelled with fecal contents. The patient should be warned that the urge to defecate may occur suddenly. Catharsis empties the bowel, and 2 to 3 days may elapse before food residue again provides the stimulus to defecation.

Magnesium hydroxide (commonly known as milk of magnesia) is frequently used for its smooth laxative effect. The drug is available in commercial preparations as an emulsion containing mineral oil. The emulsion is stored at room temperature because chilling causes the colloids of the mixture to aggregate. The larger-sized particles are less effective in the intestinal tract. Patients find the drug more palatable if it is given with fruit juice. Magnesium hydroxide is also employed in antacid preparations. Frequent use of the antacids containing magnesium hydroxide may cause diarrhea and necessitate change to an antacid preparation without the laxative component.

Patient care

Elimination patterns vary among individuals. Regularity for one individual may be daily defecation, whereas for another person it may be every 3 days. Constipation exists when the elimination pattern is lengthened or stools are hard and of insufficient quantity to indicate waste elimination. In some situations frequent passage of small amounts of liquid stools seems to indicate the patient has diarrhea, but the basic problem is leaking of feces around a large bolus of fecal material in the rectum. Cathartics will be ineffective until the fecal material is manually removed by digital manipulation. Mineral oil may be used as a retention enema before or after removal of the fecal impaction to soften the contents in the rectum.

Bisacodyl or glycerin suppositories are often used to stimulate the urge to defecate as part of a bowel training program in patients who have decreased bowel tone with weak peristaltic activity (i.e., patients with neurologic problems). To increase the stimulatory effect of the drug-containing suppository, it is gently moved from side to side in the rectum to make contract with the mucosa. Regularly scheduled use of suppositories is essential to reestablishment of daily defecation patterns.

Drugs are not a panacea for control of chronic problems with constipation. Individuals should be assisted to improve their dietary habits and to eradicate factors that are contributing to the problem. Well-balanced meals that include bulk-containing foods and an intake of fluids adequate to hydrate the intestinal contents are necessary to maintain regular bowel activity. Regular exercise and responsiveness to the urge to defecate are important components of a constipation prevention plan.

Many elderly people have established patterns for ingestion of a particular food or liquid (prune juice, prunes, hot water) early in the morning that stimulates their *gastrocolic* and *duodenocolic reflexes* and consequent successful bowel evacuation. Continuance of established practices and positioning the patient comfortably in a secluded area may help to maintain near-normal elimination patterns during illness.

A source of discomfort for the patient with constipation is the distention of the proximal bowel with flatus. The problem can be intensified by emotional stressors that increase the tendency to swallow air (aerophagia). The tense, distended abdomen is uncomfortable for the patient. Aerophagia may decrease peristalsis and aggravate or increase the retention of fecal material. Modification of the problem may be possible by encouraging ambulation and massage of the abdomen while walking. Stethoscopic examination of the abdomen aids in determining whether peristaltic activity improves with increased physical activity. Sedatives may be required when aerophagia is persistent.

Good health practices may prevent regular use of cathartics, but the drugs are necessary to relieve constipation when it exists. Whenever the opportunity presents itself, it is important to help individuals use cathartics (or any easily obtained drugs) intelligently and to seek medical advice if problems persist. It is important for the public to know that a physician should be consulted if intense abdominal pain occurs. There have been many children treated with cathartics at home for suspected constipation when appendicitis was present. Stimulation of intestinal motility by cathartics can cause an inflamed appendix to rupture.

DIARRHEA

The onset of diarrhea in infants and elderly individuals presents problems that are specific to the age groups. The hydration status in either age group is easily disturbed. Persistent diarrhea moves intestinal fluids, electrolytes, and nutrients from the body, and general physiologic imbalances may occur. The potential for acidosis, dehydration, and nutritional deficiencies necessitates prompt control of the intestinal hypermotility causing recurrent rapid emptying of the intestine.

Pharmacodynamics

Drugs may be used to control acute episodes of diarrhea, or they may be used as one aspect of a therapeutic program to control diarrhea secondary to organic disease in the intestine. Diarrhea may persist or reoccur when bacterial infection, parasitic invasion, or irritation of intestinal tissues continues to stimulate peristalsis. Antidiarrheal drugs slow peristaltic movements, and fluid and electrolyte losses are decreased. The drugs may be used for interim periods of control when an organic problem exists.

The factor precipitating acute diarrhea may be readily evident if the patient is participating in a drug therapy program, since diarrhea is an adverse reaction to many drugs. Anti-infective drugs change or suppress bacterial flora, and infants or young children frequently have diarrhea while taking antibiotics. For example, the young child receiving penicillin for control of staphylococcus-induced otitis media may have loose stools after the fourth day of therapy. Discontinuance of the antibiotic may be necessary, but careful evaluation of the stool patterns and possible precipitating factors in the child's environment are evaluated by the physician before antibiotic therapy is discontinued.

Drugs used for control of diarrhea (Table 8-2) include agents that soak up intestinal liquid (adsorbents), replace bacterial flora, or suppress intestinal motility.

Fluid adsorbents. Adsorbents are prepared from clay or a similar product that is processed to increase the surface area available for adsorption of intestinal fluid. Activated attapulgite, bismuth subcarbonate, and kaolin and pectin (Table 8-2) are given primarily for their adsorptive properties. The drugs act within the gastrointestinal tract and are not absorbed into the circulation. The agents are taken after each loose bowel movement until control is established. Removal of excess water produces bulkier, formed stools.

Pharmacologic differences between the agents may extend their usefulness beyond intestinal adsorption. For example, bismuth subcarbonate has a mild antacid action that decreases the stomach irritation found with prolonged gastrointestinal problems. The bismuth component acts to protect the irritated intestinal mucosa.

Kaolin and pectin is frequently used for control of diarrhea. Carbohydrate (pectin) added to the clay or silicate is minute (0.15 gram/15

Table 8-2. Dosage range of antidiarrheal drugs

Nonproprietary name	Proprietary (trade) name	Adult dosage range (oral)
Attapulgite, activated	Claysorb, Pharmasorb	2-4 Gm.
Bismuth subcarbonate		0.5-4 Gm.
Diphenoxylate hydrochloride	Lomotil	5 mg.
Kaolin and pectin	Kaopectate	15-30 ml.
Lactobacillus acidophilus and *L. bulgaricus*		3-4 tabs.
Opium (tincture)		5 ml.

ml.), and pectin affects the action of kaolin without adding appreciably to the caloric intake of the patient.

Bacterial replacement. Prolonged administration of antibiotics may suppress the normal bacterial growth in the intestine. Replacement bacteria are supplied when the diarrheal problem results from loss of the normal flora and overgrowth of pathogenic bacteria. *Lactobacillus acidophilus* is a natural commensal in the human intestine. Although *Lactobacillus bulgaricus* is not a natural intestinal inhabitant, the commercial preparations (tablets, granules) containing both *L. acidophilus* and *L. bulgaricus* are used to enhance production of lactic acid from carbohydrates in the intestine. The resulting acidity of the lumen contents suppresses pathogenic bacterial overgrowth. The patient may complain of increased expulsion of flatus, but the foul odor of the bowel movements subsides. Administration of the granules is simplified if they are sprinkled on food, although they may be mixed in milk or tomato juice.

Motility suppressants. Diphenoxylate hydrochloride and tincture of opium (Table 8-2) increase the tone of the intestinal musculature, ileocecal valve, and anal sphincter to slow expulsion of intestinal contents. Slowing of peristalsis allows water to be absorbed from the intestinal lumen, and a more normal stool is formed. Tincture of opium used in combination with kaolin and pectin has an additional adsorbent effect in decreasing the intestinal fluid content.

Morphine content of the two forms of tincture of opium differs. Camphorated opium tincture contains 0.04%, and opium tincture contains 1% morphine. The tinctures turn a milky color when water is added. Diphenoxylate hydrochloride is a synthetic opiate-like drug. For a child or debilitated individual, the rest provided by cessation of diarrhea and by the slight sedative effects of the drug is most desirable. The drugs potentiate the effect of other central nervous system depressants.

Use of the agents carries with it the possibility of addiction if continued large doses are taken. Diphenoxylate hydrochloride preparations have a minimal amount of atropine added to discourage use of the drug for its narcotic-like properties. The combination makes the preparation more desirable than the opium products for long-term control of diarrhea. Although the morphine content of tincture of opium is very low, the drug has been used by addicts as an interim source of narcotic.

Patient care

Changes in foods, sources of water, or emotional stressors may cause transient diarrhea in susceptible individuals. A primary factor in control of acute diarrhea is cessation of food ingestion. Any food entering the stomach causes additional stimulation of intestinal motility and perpetuates the basic problem. Sugar-containing water or similar innocuous clear liquids are absorbed from the stomach without entering the bowel, and clear liquids taken in small amounts may satisfy thirst, prevent dehydration, and supply a minimal number of calories. Alternate methods for fluid and electrolyte replacement (i.e., parenteral fluids) are necessary for the severely dehydrated patient with persistent diarrhea.

Chronic or organic disease–related diarrhea causes problems of perianal skin excoriation, emaciation, exhaustion, and depression, which must be considered in planning care. For example, concurrent with attempts to decrease frequent bowel movements, plans are made for replacement of nutrient and electrolyte losses. Readily available sources of carbohydrate (i.e., apple) and potassium ions (i.e., banana), may be utilized to replace materials for energy needs and electrolyte balance. Specific replacement therapy and care of the patient are dependent on the status of the individual patient.

During antidiarrheal drug therapy, the patient should be asked to note carefully and describe the consistency, odor, and color of stools, since the information is helpful in defining progress. For example, a greenish, mucus-containing foul-smelling stool appears with emergence of putrifying bacteria in the intestine, and therapy can be planned to correct the problem.

The drugs purport to halt diarrhea, and in accomplishing that purpose, they may overshoot and cause constipation. The problem cannot be allowed to persist, but a short waiting period may result in reinstitution of bowel movements. Stimulation of the bowel by laxatives is undesirable immediately after an episode of diarrhea.

REFERENCES

Christensen, J.: The controls of gastrointestinal movements: some old and new views, The New England Journal of Medicine **285:**85, 1971.

Grady, George F., and Keusch, Gerald T.: Pathogenesis of bacterial diarrheas, part 2, The New England Journal of Medicine **285:**891, 1971.

Hill, Margaret L.: The myelodysplastic child: bowel and bladder control, American Journal of Nursing **69:**545, 1969.

Kirschen, Martin M.: Constipation, American Journal of Proctology **13:**291, 1962.

Reilly, Mary Jo, editor: American hospital formulary service, vol. 2, sect. 56:00, Washington, D. C., 1973, American Society of Hospital Pharmacists.

Sherbaniuk, Richard W.: The physiology of diarrhea, Canadian Medical Association Journal **91:**1, 1964.

Staas, William E., Jr., and DeNault, Phyllis M.: Bowel control, American Family Physician **7:**90, Jan., 1973.

Stitcher, Joseph E., and Roth, James L. A.: The aerophagic patient, American Journal of Nursing **66:**1014, 1966.

Texter, E. Clinton, Chou, Ching-Chung, Laureta, Higino C., and Vantrappen, Gaston R.: Physiology of the gastrointestinal tract, St. Louis, 1968, The C. V. Mosby Co.

Wangnel, A. G., and Deller, D. J.: Intestinal mobility in man. III. Mechanism of constipation and diarrhea with particular reference to the irritable colon syndrome, Gastroenterology **48:**69, 1965.

Williams, Sue Rodwell: Nutrition and diet therapy, ed. 2, St. Louis, 1973, The C. V. Mosby Co.

Wood, J. D., and Perkins, W. E.: Mechanical interaction between longitudinal and circular axes of the small intestine, American Journal of Physiology **218:**762, 1970.

9
Emesis

Vomiting center response
Chemoreceptor trigger zone
Emetic stimuli
Pharmacodynamics
Patient care
Emesis induction
Pharmacodynamics
Patient care

Emesis, or vomiting, is a physiologic protective mechanism for rejecting or removing noxious materials from the stomach. Excess ingestion of food or drink may also stimulate the series of impulses that cause vomiting.

Vomiting center response

Distention of the stomach or intense irritation of the gastric mucosa initiates stimulatory afferent impulses (sympathetic, parasympathetic) that travel to the medullary *vomiting center.* Neural impulses from the distended stomach may be decreased by assuming the recumbent position to lessen pressure of adjacent organs and allow expansion of the stomach.

Afferent impulses that arrive at the right or left vomiting center stimulate interneurons between the bilateral centers. An intense stimulus will activate the motor fibers controlling the physical responses involved in rejection of stomach contents. The soft palate closes to occlude and protect the nasopharynx, and the epiglottis covers the glottis to occlude the respiratory passages. Diaphragmatic descent concurrent with abdominal muscle constriction increases the pressure on the stomach. As intragastric pressure rises, the pyloric sphincter closes tenaciously, but the cardiac sphincter relaxes, and contents of the stomach are forcefully propelled upward through the esophagus. Evacuation of contents from the distended stomach may terminate the problem.

Subthreshold impulses from the gastrointestinal structures to the vomiting center cause the uncomfortable sensation of nausea. Maintenance of the stimulus at the subthreshold level stimulates autonomic nervous system–induced salivation, cold sweat, bradycardia, and hypotension. Swallowing of secretions and air suppresses the vomiting reflex but introduces mucus and air, which distends the stomach. Distention-initiated impulses raise the neural impulses above the threshold, and vomiting ensues.

Chemoreceptor trigger zone

Persistent nausea or vomiting may be precipitated by stimulation of an area called the emetic *chemoreceptor trigger zone,* located below the floor of the fourth ventricle (Fig. 9-1). Stimulation or irritation of the chemoreceptors relays impulses to the adjacent vomiting centers in the medulla, and the sequence of events leading to vomiting are mobilized.

Projectile vomiting is precipitated via direct compression of the chemoreceptor trigger zone by increased intracranial pressure. Nausea occurring with *vertigo,* or *motion sickness,* is a manifestation of chemoreceptor trigger zone responses to a secondary stimulus from the labyrinth of the inner ear. Changes in the ear structures or movement of the perilymph in

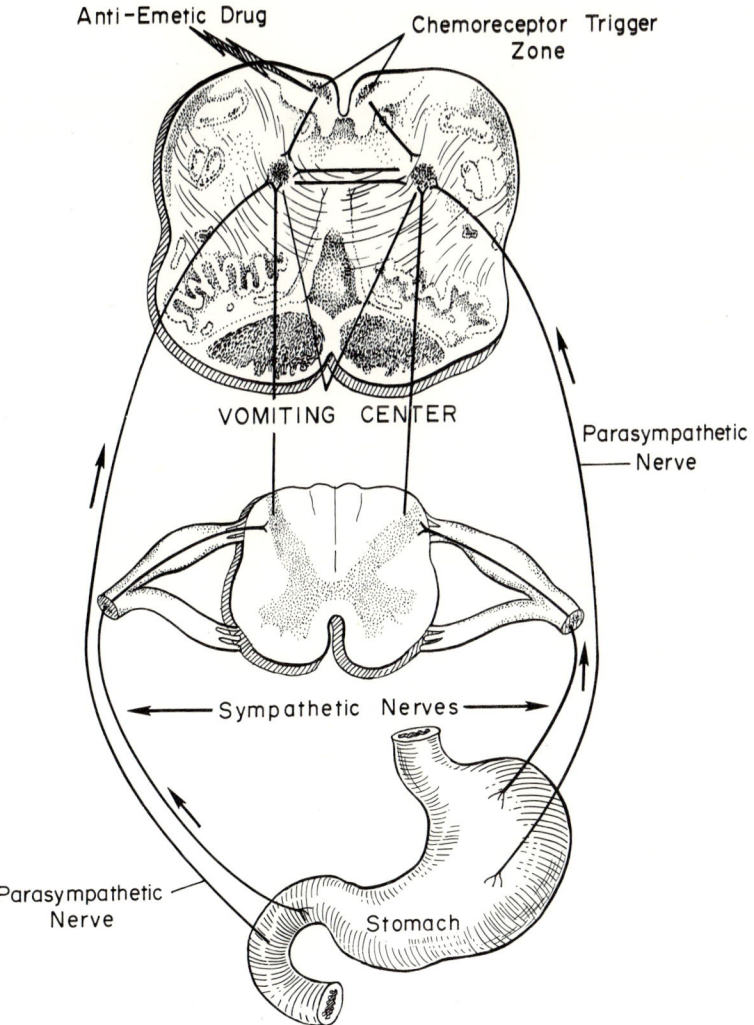

Fig. 9-1. Autonomic afferents from the stomach may stimulate the vomiting centers, or substances in the circulating blood may stimulate the chemoreceptor trigger zone to induce vomiting. Antiemetic drugs act at the chemoreceptor trigger zone to raise the threshold for emetic stimuli.

sensitive individuals initiates neural stimuli that are relayed to the chemoreceptor trigger zone. The most frequent stimuli to the centers are drugs, and it is chemoreceptor trigger zone stimulation by chemicals that causes some of the problems of nausea and vomiting during drug therapy.

Emetic stimuli

Vomiting may occur with excitation of either or both of the centers of control. For example, a patient may have intractable vomiting during radiation therapy of a malignant tumor in the intestinal tract. The edema occurring during therapy may cause areas of intestinal obstruction or distention, which stimulate the vomiting center. Release of high levels of protein from malignant tissue breakdown may provide the chemical stimulation (ammonia, urea) that excites the chemoreceptors. The two-pronged stimuli make the problem difficult to control.

The source of emetic stimuli determines the type of therapy that may be effective. Distention of organs (i.e., stomach, intestines, uterus, bladder, kidney pelvis) may initiate afferent impulses that stimulate the vomiting centers, and relief of the distention may decrease nausea and vomiting. For example, vomiting or insertion of a gastric tube empties the stomach and decreases neural stimulation of the vomiting center. Desensitization of the chemoreceptor trigger zones is the pharmacodynamic action desired in control of emesis or nausea.

Pharmacodynamics

Drugs are used to control nausea and vomiting when the occurrence of the problems is predictable and cannot be avoided, or when the problems have arisen and the stimulus cannot be removed. For example, an individual who is sensitive to fast movement (motion sickness) may take drugs to decrease the incidence of nausea and vomiting during a period of travel. A patient with cancer may be given antiemetic drugs to decrease nausea and vomiting occurring directly from stimulation of the chemoreceptor trigger zone by antineoplastic drugs or chemicals released by neoplastic tissue.

Many drugs that act on the reticular system of the cerebral tissues to modify emotional responses also have an effect on the chemoreceptor trigger zone. Patients receiving tranquilizers may have a concurrent decrease in problems with emesis. However, the sedative action of many tranquilizers makes them undesirable for selective control of emesis. The action of tranquilizers is presented in Chapter 17.

Antiemetic action site. Drugs used to control emesis (Table 9-1) act primarily on the chemoreceptor trigger zone to diminish sensitivity to irritants, and they are quite specific in their effect on the center. Oral or rectal forms of the drugs are easily managed by individuals while continuing their usual patterns of living. The chief problem for the ambulatory individual using oral forms of the drugs is the occurrence of drowsiness.

Adverse effects. The incidence of adverse effects of the drugs relates primarily to the proximity of the medullary sites for control of vital functions and the sites of antiemetic drug action. Parenteral use of any of the agents increases the incidence of adverse effects during therapy. For example, during use of the antiemetic drugs the adjacent vasomotor control centers may be affected, and the overt evidence will be a transient or slight decrease in blood pressure and a consequent period of dizziness. The problem is most evident in the individual maintaining a low blood pressure level and may be decreased by lying down for 15 minutes after taking the drug.

The drugs have an anticholinergic effect that

Table 9-1. Dosage range of antiemetics

Nonproprietary name	Proprietary (trade) name	Daily adult dosage range
Cyclizine hydrochloride	Marezine hydrochloride	Oral: 150 mg. (÷3)
Cyclizine lactate	Marezine lactate	I.M.: 150-200 mg. (÷3-4)
Dimenhydrinate	Dramamine	Oral: 50-250 mg. (÷3-4) I.M.: Same as oral I.V.: 50 mg./single dose
Diphenidol hydrochloride	Vontrol	Oral: 150-300 mg. (÷6) I.M.: 120-240 mg. (÷6) I.V.: 20 mg./single dose
Meclizine hydrochloride	Bonine	Oral: 25-50 mg.
Pipamazine	Mornidine	Oral: 5 mg./single dose
Promethazine hydrochloride	Phenergan, Remsed	Oral: 50-150 mg. (÷4-6) I.M.: Same
Pyrathiazine hydrochloride	Pyrrolazote	Oral: 75-150 mg. (÷3)
Thiethylperazine maleate	Torecan	Oral: 10-30 mg. (÷1-3) I.M.: Same
Trimethobenzamide hydrochloride	Tigan	Oral: 0.25-1 Gm. (÷1-4)

causes dryness of the oral mucosa and blurring of vision in some individuals. Other problems that occasionally are bothersome to the patient are slight incoordination, tinnitus, fatigue, and headache. The patient should be informed that taking analgesics for headache or other pain during therapy with antiemetics may cause unusual drowsiness and affect his travel, work, or social plans.

Parenteral use of promethazine hydrochloride and thiethylperazine maleate (Table 9-1) causes hypotension more frequently than do the other agents in the group. The two drugs are potent antihistaminic agents and are classified pharmacologically as *phenothiazine derivatives.* Although the phenothiazines generally cause sedation, use of promethazine hydrochloride or thiethylperazine maleate sometimes precipitates central nervous system stimulation, seen as restlessness, or extrapyramidal tract irritation, seen as jitteriness and fine tremors of the extremities.

Vestibular stimulus depression. Cyclizine hydrochoride, dimenhydrinate, diphenidol hydrochloride, and meclizine hydrochloride (Table 9-1) are useful oral agents for control of motion sickness. The drugs decrease labyrinthine excitability and the conduction of vestibular-cerebellar stimuli. Although most frequently employed for motion sickness control, the effectiveness of the drugs for decreasing chemoreceptor trigger zone sensitivity allows their use for any problem stimulating the vomiting center.

The onset of drug action is between 10 and 30 minutes after oral use. An individual taking the tablets 30 minutes before the inciting incident may proceed through the experience without occurrence of emesis or nausea. Meclizine hydrochloride provides effective control for 24 hours, although there is some individual variation. If the experience is extended (i.e., travel by bus, plane, ship), the shorter-acting drugs are taken before meals and at bedtime to prevent onset of nausea or emesis. Cyclizine hydrochloride and meclizine hydrochloride are not administered to young females in the child-bearing years or to women during the first trimester of pregnancy because the drugs have produced teratogenic effects in animals.

Patient care

During therapy with antiemetic drugs many measures enhance drug effect and decrease the stimulus to emesis. For example, the pregnant woman may modify eating patterns to avoid the high fat content of foods and to maintain a low-level buffer against accumulation of gastric acids. Frequent small amounts of dry carbohydrate foods taken without water (i.e., unsalted popcorn) may decrease the irritation of the gastric mucosa that is stimulating the vomiting center. When weight control limits snacks, antacids may be used to decrease gastric acidity.

Avoidance of peritonsillar pillars and uvula stimulation while brushing the teeth prevents gag reflex stimulation of gastric contraction. Removal of materials and odors that are noxious to the individual may help decrease nausea. Individual sensitivities determine the specific factors that constitute a stimulus and measures required to decrease stimuli.

The chief concern during persistent vomiting episodes is the losses of fluids, nutrients, and electrolytes. Gastric levels of potassium ions are ten times that of serum levels, and loss of the essential cation contributes to electrolyte imbalance. Metabolic alkalosis is also a concern when hydrochloric acid is continually emptied from the stomach by vomiting. Replacement of the potassium, hydrogen, and chloride ions is an essential aspect of the therapeutic plan for the patient with intractable vomiting.

Food and fluid replacement of electrolytes and calories can be planned as soon as antiemetic drug effect becomes evident, or parenteral replacement may be planned if a gastric tube has been inserted. The palatability and acceptability of oral liquids to the nauseated patient is variable. Coca-Cola syrup over cracked ice may be received enthusiastically by one patient and refused in preference to warm tea by another.

Heavy sedation, anesthesia, or decreased sensitivity of the neurons controlling closure of the glottis allows entrance of food into the trachea. The patient who has an incomplete closure of the glottis during vomiting may aspirate some of the material into the tracheobronchial passages. Coughing may be stimulated, or silent aspiration may occlude segments of the lungs without immediate overt problems.

Positioning of the vomiting patient must be planned to protect the unconscious patient from aspiration of vomitus. A side-lying position and close observation provide some protection to the patient.

Aspiration of vomitus may cause immediate respiratory distress or insidious changes in respiratory rate or chest expansion that decrease the ventilatory capacity of the patient. An elevated body temperature may provide the clue to atelectasis, since a low-grade temperature elevation is often seen with diffuse small atelectatic areas in the lung fields. The patient's respiratory status should be discussed with the physician when the slightest changes occur after a vomiting episode.

Ambulatory patients using antiemetic drugs should be informed that drowsiness may occur during therapy. Decreased alertness may affect the safety of the patient while driving a motor vehicle, doing hazardous work, or accomplishing tasks requiring fine motor control. Activities may be planned to avoid the maximum action period of the drug.

EMESIS INDUCTION

Removal of gastric contents can be accomplished simply by stimulation of the sensitive gag reflex at the uvula, peritonsillar pillars, or posterior oropharynx. Digital stimulation of the areas is a common emergency practice of mothers when an infant chokes or swallows any of the multitude of things found in the home.

Removal of intentionally or accidentally ingested poisons or toxic agents from the gastrointestinal tract may be accomplished by use of emetics, and drug use is planned as promptly as possible to avoid absorption of the toxic substance into the systemic circulation. Drugs employed for stimulation of emesis are only one aspect of systemic poisoning prevention. Concurrent measures are used after careful definition of the ingested substance and evaluation of the clinical status of the patient. Lavage is necessary when the ingested material is a central nervous system depressant, since emesis in the drowsy patient would cause aspiration of the stomach contents.

Pharmacodynamics

The drugs used for stimulation of emesis (Table 9-2) cause ejection of gastric contents by an irritating effect in the stomach that increases stimuli to the vomiting center or by a direct stimulatory action at the chemoreceptor trigger zone. Drugs are given to produce emesis shortly after administration of a single dose, and further use of the emetic requires consultation with the physician.

Dual center stimulation. Ipecac (Table 9-2) acts as a gastric irritant and as a stimulant of the chemoreceptor trigger zone to initiate vomiting. Although relatively slow in action, the dual center stimulation produces forceful vomiting in 30 to 60 minutes. To assure adequate fluid content in the stomach to raise the gastric material, the drug is taken with a large glassful of water. Physical activity enhances the emetic effect, and patients are encouraged to walk or move about after drug administration.

Ipecac is an effective emetic particularly useful immediately after accidental ingestion or suspected intentional ingestion of tablets or liquids. Because an emetic is frequently needed for home use after children have ingested toxic substances, community drugstores provide cost-free vials of ipecac. During National Poison Control Week, pamphlets on poison pre-

Table 9-2. Dosage range of emetics

Nonproprietary name	Proprietary (trade) name	Adult dosage range
Apomorphine hydrochloride		S.C. 5-10 mg.
Cupric sulfate		Oral: 250-500 mg.
Disulfiram	Antabuse	Oral: 125-500 mg.
Ipecac		Oral: 8-15 ml.
Mustard, black		Oral: 10 Gm.

vention and a vial of ipecac are distributed to parents of young children in the community. Parents are advised to contact the local poison control center immediately when a child accidently ingests a poisonous substance, drugs, or substances with unknown ingredients.

Ipecac is also used in lower dosage (about one eighth of the emetic dose) to produce expectoration of copious secretions when children have *tracheobronchitis*. The amount of mucus produced after use of the drug is startling. Because of its emetic effect, the drug or compounds containing ipecac are not given near mealtime.

Vomiting center stimulation. Black mustard (Table 9-2) increases the formation of an irritating volatile oil in the stomach. The conversion of the glycoside is dependent on enzymatic action, and warm water provides the catalyst. Hot water inactivates the enzyme and negates the effect of the drug. Gastric irritation causes afferent impulses to travel to the vomiting center to initiate ejection of stomach contents.

Cupric sulfate (Table 9-2) is an oxidizing agent that is administered in warm water. It acts rapidly as a stimulant to the vomiting centers by irritation of the gastric mucosa. The speed of effect decreases the time that the poison is in contact with the gastric mucosa. Cupric sulfate is most frequently used after phosphorous ingestion, and it forms a protective covering of copper over the poison to prevent absorption. When emesis does not occur after administration, the metals are removed by a mechanism for aspiration of the stomach contents (i.e., stomach pump).

Chemoreceptor trigger zone stimulation. Apomorphine hydrochloride (Table 9-2) is a potent emetic that acts directly on the chemoreceptor trigger zone to stimulate emesis within 10 to 15 minutes after subcutaneous administration. It is a synthetically prepared morphine derivative. A single dose is used because repeated dosage would result in respiratory depression.

Alcohol sensitizer. Disulfiram is an indirect-acting emetic employed to initiate vomiting when alcohol is ingested subsequent to administration of the drug. Therapy is instituted only with consent of the patient, and his consistent use of the drug is necessary for control of chronic alcoholism. The drug inhibits the formation of the liver enzymes necessary to degradation of alcohol, and acetaldehyde blood levels are increased. After using the drug, alcohol intake precipitates a violent vomiting episode. The episode may be accompanied by severe hypotension and extreme discomfort and occurs within 30 minutes after drinking alcohol.

The drug-alcohol relationship makes it necessary to screen all drugs given to the patient for their alcohol content (i.e., tinctures) and to avoid the use of alcohol-containing solutions for back rubs. Patients participate voluntarily in the control program, and when they are injured or hospitalized, they usually report their hypersensitivity to alcohol. An identification card is carried by patients using disulfiram to prevent administration of paraldehyde or any form of alcohol if they are treated in an emergency situation.

The drug causes some problems during administration. Patients complain of drowsiness and easy fatigability. The drug initially causes a metallic or garliclike taste in the mouth, although the problem subsides gradually. Impotence, headache, skin eruptions, and peripheral neuritis occur during therapy with disulfiram.

Patient care

Use of emetics for induction of vomiting is an emergency measure. A child or adult may have taken fewer tablets than originally calculated, but plans for emesis induction are carried out promptly. Careful search for dropped tablets for specific calculation of the number of missing tablets can await drug administration and emesis. The quantity, color, and contents of vomitus may provide clues to the amount of ingested material and the adequacy of removal of the substance.

Physical comfort during the 30-minute waiting period will decrease the drain on the patient's emotional and physical resources. A procedural guide can be based on a sample of a typical situation in the home when a child swallows a large number of tablets. After administration of the emetic prescribed by the physician or the poison control center, the child may be placed on the edge of the kitchen sink with outer clothing removed. A receptacle in the sink and handy face cloth are the equipment assembled for the emetic event. Relaxed interaction between the mother and child decreases the emotional trauma and allows the warmth of caring and concern to surface.

The question most often asked, "Could the incident have been prevented?", can await removal of the toxic substance. After emesis is completed, the individual is usually tired, and children may fall asleep promptly after the experience.

Continued observation for residual effects of the ingested substance will depend on the particular agent involved. Concurrent therapeutic measures are dependent on the physiologic status of the patient. Destruction of vital organ function may result from accidental or intentional ingestion of toxic, irritating, or caustic substances. A single incident may affect the life pattern of the individual.

REFERENCES

Cummins, Alvin J.: Nausea and vomiting, American Journal of Digestive Disorders **3:**710, 1958.

Davenport, Horace W.: Why the stomach does not digest itself, Scientific American **226:**86, Jan., 1972.

Downs, Howard S.: The control of vomiting, American Journal of Nursing **66:**76, 1966.

George, J. D.: Gastric acid and mobility, American Journal of Digestive Diseases **13:**376, 1968.

Guyton, Arthur C.: Textbook of medical physiology, ed. 4, Philadelphia, 1971, W. B. Saunders Co.

Hunt, J. N., and Knox, M. T.: Control of gastric emptying, American Journal of Digestive Diseases **13:**372, 1968.

Jordon, Paul H.: Clinical aspects of gastric secretions and gastric analysis, Medical Clinics of North America **52:**1305, 1968.

Kimmel, Mary E.: Antabuse in a clinic program, American Journal of Nursing **71:**1173, 1971.

Reilly, Mary Jo, editor: American hospital formulary service, vol. 2, sect. 56:20, Washington D. C., 1973, American Society of Hospital Pharmacists.

Silverstein, Herbert: The dizzy patient—diagnosis and treatment, part 2, Resident-Intern Consultant **1:**39, Nov., 1972.

Sleisenger, Marvin H., Jr.: Some implications of current research in gastroenterology, Medical Clinics of North America **52:**1269, 1968.

Wolfson, Robert J., Myers, David, Schlosser, Woodrow D., and Winchester, Richard A.: Vertigo, Clinical Symposia **17:**99, 1965.

10

Gastric acidity and intestinal motility

Sympathetic nervous system controls
Parasympathetic nervous system controls
Response to stressors
Ileal barrier
Gastric hyperacidity
    Pharmacodynamics
    Patient care
Hypermotility and secretion control
    Pharmacodynamics
    Patient care
Hypomotility
    Pharmacodynamics
    Patient care

Physiologically effective anabolic activity of the gastrointestinal tract requires the liberation of glandular secretions and the rhythmic contractions of the abdominal viscera. The parasympathetic division of the autonomic nervous system provides the stimuli required for digestive processes. Maintenance of the normal feed and breed functions provides nutrients for replenishment, recuperation, and reproduction of body tissues. Integration of autonomic function at the level of the hypothalamus can be interrupted by interceding psychic stimuli that change the patterns of gastrointestinal activity.

Sympathetic nervous system controls

Glandular release of digestive secretions and motility of the gastrointestinal organs are controlled by both the parasympathetic and sympathetic nervous system in response to the living and survival needs of the individual. When an individual is facing a threatening life situation or when the psychic interpretation of threat is internalized, the sympathetic nervous system shunts the major blood supply to peripheral muscles, the liver, the brain, and adrenal glands to provide nutrients and oxygen required for defense. The process (flight or fight response) decreases the activity of the gastrointestinal tract during the period of preferential movement of blood to vital organs. Sympathetic nervous system impulses to the gastrointestinal tract cause decreased motility and tone of the stomach and intestines, inhibition of gastric secretions, and contraction of internal sphincters (i.e., ileocecal, internal anal sphincters). During a fear-producing episode, digestion and absorption of nutrients are at a minimal level because the sympathetic nervous system stimuli inhibit the normal physiologic processes controlled by the parasympathetic nervous system.

Parasympathetic nervous system controls

The parasympathetic nervous system is the master controller of gastrointestinal activity. Parasympathetic neural stimuli increase the motility and tone of the entire digestive tract and relax junctional sphincters to allow movement of foods and residue along the enteric pathway. Mucus and enzymes are provided by concurrent neural stimulation of glands in the upper digestive tract.

Neural transmission. Vegetative or anabolic activities of the digestive tract are regulated by sensory and motor impulses carried by the vagus nerve. Afferent impulses to the medulla and integrating centers in the hypothalamus supply the information that influences the emission of efferent impulses to neuroeffector sites along the gastrointestinal tract. Vagus nerve contacts with muscle and glandular control sites are dispersed throughout the tract, but there is a higher concentration of neuroeffector sites at the proximal and distal aspects of the digestive tract.

Acetylcholine is the chemical mediator of nerve impulse transmission at preganglionic and organ effector sites in the parasympathetic nervous system. The word acetylcholine provides the basis for description of the parasympathetic nervous system activity as cholinergic activity. Acetylcholine mediates neural conduction at the preganglionic site, and the physiologic stimulatory action of acetycholine is often compared to the action of *nicotine*. Drugs that stimulate conduction at the preganglionic site are described as having a *nicotinic action*.

The terminal myoneural junction structure of the parasympathetic nervous system is a simplistic naked nerve–muscle contact site. Mediation of neural transmission at the organ effector sites is stimulated by the release of acetylcholine, and the action is often compared to the stimulatory action of *muscarine* (toxic alkaloid found in toadstools) on smooth muscle and glands. Drugs providing comparable stimulatory impulses are described as having a *muscarinic action*.

Efferent impulses mediated by the vagus nerve activate acetylcholine at the axon ending. Acetylcholine is liberated from storage sites by the enzyme acetylcholinesterase, which breaks the acetate linkage of the stored neurotransmitter. Diffusion of acetylcholine to the neuroeffector increases the permeability of the membrane to sodium ions. The action of acetylcholine converts chemical energy to electrical energy, and electric transmission of the nerve impulse follows the acetylcholine-induced sodium ion shift. Continued arrival of impulses at the axon are required for sustained release of acetylcholine because the neurotransmitter substance is rapidly cleaved by the enzymatic action of cholinesterase in axon and tissue sites. Cholinesterase-induced hydrolysis of acetylcholine releases the less active products choline and acetic acid.

Response to stressors

Stressors encountered in day-to-day living provide psychic impulses to the hypothalamic integrating centers. Efferent impulses mediated through the vagus nerve pathways have a marked stimulatory effect on glandular secretions and motility of the gastrointestinal tract. Psychic stimuli cause increased salivation and increased turgor, hyperemia, and hypersecretion of the gastric mucosa. Although it appears that psychic stimuli simply speed the digestive process and elimination of residue, protective mechanisms within the tract safeguard it against autodigestion and erosion by rapid movement of enzymes and acidic gastric contents into structures inadequately protected against their presence.

Ileal barrier

The ileocecal valve provides a physical barrier to movement of contents from the ileum. Movement of intestinal contents may proceed until the cecum becomes distended, but entrance of additional residue is halted by neural stimuli from the cecum, which cause reflex contraction of the ileocecal sphincter. The sphincter provides a natural protective barrier that assures adequate time for food breakdown and absorption before chyme enters the less absorptive colon surfaces. Protection against nutritional losses is an outcome of sphincter resistance during stress-induced digestive tract hypermotility.

Parasympathetic nervous system hyperactivity of psychic origin can be modified by inhibition of the cerebral-hypothalamic pathways of transmission. Tranquilizers or sedatives may be used to modify the stimuli and allow continuation of the balanced integration of parasympathetic neural controls. Dietary modification, antacids, or anticholinergic drugs may be included in the therapeutic plan to prevent pathology of the digestive tract or nutritional problems occurring secondary to prolonged disruption of digestive processes.

GASTRIC HYPERACIDITY

Gastric discomfort may be caused by hyperacidity, and over-the-counter antacid preparations are a popular item on the patent medicine market. Individuals use various antacid preparations to modify discomfort after overeating or to decrease epigastric pain and gaseous distention occurring as a consequence of missed or hurried meals.

Mucus secreted by the glands in the gastric mucosa protects the epithelial lining of the stomach from the proteolytic activity of hydrochloric acid and pepsin. Drug-induced alteration of the mucus barrier exposes the stomach lining to the proteolytic activity of digestive juices. Salicylates and glucocorticoids are the drugs most frequently indicted as *ulcerogenic agents*. Emotional stressors stimulate endogenous glucocorticoid release, which contributes to alteration of the mucus protection of gastric epithelium.

Antacids are frequently prescribed to prevent erosion of gastric epithelium when stress-induced parasympathetic activity causes hyperacidity or large dosage of drugs causes irritation of the stomach lining. Ulcer formation is a complex process that is not clearly understood, but the contribution of either drugs or emotions to epithelial erosion by acids clearly indicates a need for protection of the stomach lining from self-destruction.

Antacids neutralize the gastric hydrochloric acid and provide a protective layer of drug on the stomach lining. An additional benefit accrues during antacid therapy because stomach contents at lower acid levels move more readily into the duodenum. When large amounts of acidic chyme enter the duodenum, protective contraction of the pyloric sphincter (enterogastric reflex) causes retention of stomach contents, and the individual experiences discomfort from the acid-containing distended organ. Neutralization of stomach acids improves emptying time and allows continuation of digestive processes.

Pharmacodynamics

Complete neutralization of gastric hydrochloric acid would require excess ingestion of antacids. Gastric hyperacidity is modified by consistent frequent-interval administration of small amounts of the antacids to maintain gastric contents at approximately pH 4.0. Pepsin is synthesized from pepsinogen below pH 3.5; therefore maintenance of a slightly higher pH during gastric antacid therapy maintains activity of the proteolytic enzyme necessary to protein digestion. Antacid coating of the gastric lining decreases pain (often described as heartburn), distention, and intolerances to food.

Gastric antacids. The drugs used as gastric antacids (Table 10-1), with the exception of sodium bicarbonate, are aluminum, magnesium, or calcium combinations with minimum absorptive tendency. The drugs are widely employed as prophylactic agents administered concurrently with ulcerogenic drugs or as therapeutic agents for patients with gastric ulcers or ulcer diathesis.

Sodium bicarbonate acts as a local antacid in the stomach, but it also is absorbed into the systemic circulation. The drug neutralizes hydrochloric acid on contact, and liberation of

Table 10-1. Dosage range of gastric antacids

Nonproprietary name	Proprietary (trade) name	Daily adult dosage range (oral)
Aluminum carbonate gel, basic	Basaljel	300 ml. ($\div 6$)
Aluminum hydroxide gel	Alkajel, Al-U-Creme, Amphojel, Creamalin, Vanogel	30-360 ml. ($\div 6$-12)
Aluminum hydroxide with magnesium trisilicate	A-M-T, Gelusil, Magsal, Milk of Trinesium, Tri-Creamalate, Trisogel	30-360 ml. ($\div 6$-12)
Aluminum and magnesium hydroxides	Aludrox, Maalox	30-360 ml. ($\div 6$-12)
Aluminum phosphate gel	Phosphaljel	180-360 ml. ($\div 4$-12)
Calcium carbonate, precipitated		3-6 Gm. ($\div 3$)
Dihydroxyaluminum aminoacetate	Alminate, Alzinox, Dimothyn, Doraxamin, Robalate	2-24 Gm. ($\div 4$-12)
Magaldrate	Riopan	3.2-9.6 Gm. ($\div 4$-24)
Magnesium carbonate		1.5-6 Gm. ($\div 3$)
Magnesium oxide		750 mg. ($\div 3$)
Magnesium trisilicate	Magmasil, Trinesium, Tri-Sil	3-12 Gm. ($\div 3$)
Sodium bicarbonate		1.2-8 Gm. ($\div 4$)

carbon dioxide ensues. Patients taking sodium bicarbonate in liquid form have a short period of eructation (belching) after ingestion of the antacid. The rapid action of sodium bicarbonate tends to increase post-use excess hydrochloric acid (rebound acidity) in the stomach. Absorption of sodium from the gastrointestinal tract limits the use of the drug for patients on sodium-restricted diets. Excess use of the common household powdered form (baking soda) may lead to systemic alkalosis.

The basic components of the antacids vary, and the differences affect the incidence of diarrhea or constipation occurring during therapy. For example, aluminum hydroxide combines with hydrochloric acid in the stomach to free water, and the chloride ions combine with the aluminum ion component;

$$Al(OH)_3 + 3HCl \rightleftharpoons AlCl_3 + 3H_2O$$

Aluminum chloride (or calcium chloride) exchanges the chloride ions for phosphate ions in the lower intestinal tract. Fecal content of the insoluble molecules causes constipation. Aluminum hydroxide gel, aluminum phosphate gel, precipitated calcium carbonate, and dihydroxyaluminum aminoacetate may cause constipation. Combination of the foregoing drugs with magnesium carbonate, magnesium oxide, or magnesium trisilicate decreases the problem of constipation, since the magnesium component tends to cause mild diarrhea.

Magaldrate (Table 10-1) is a formulation containing aluminum and magnesium trisilicate. Because magnesium trisilicate causes diarrhea less frequently than does magnesium oxide, antacid formulations with the trisilicate may be used for longer trouble-free periods. Magnesium trisilicate also has a greater adherent effect that protects the stomach lining.

The drugs are frequently used, and they are relatively innocuous agents, with adverse effects limited to occurrence of constipation or diarrhea. In common with other drugs, continued close scrutiny for individual responses is important during therapy.

Absorption of oral forms of some drugs may be decreased by the concurrent administration of antacids. For example, absorption of tetracyclines is decreased when antacids containing aluminum, calcium, or magnesium are used. Scheduling of antacid administration is planned to avoid interference with absorption of the antibiotic when the drugs are prescribed concurrently.

Patient care

Patients with ulcer or ulcer diathesis are observed carefully for onset of bleeding from gastrointestinal erosion sites. Periodic testing of stools and vomitus for gross or microscopic blood content, evaluation of blood pressure and pulse, and assessment of changes in physiologic status are important to identification of problems at their onset. The patient's vague statement that there is something wrong may provide the earliest clue to emerging problems (i.e., gastric bleeding). His subjective evaluation provides the alert for reevaluation of vital parameters. Investigation for abdominal distention, stethoscopic determination of bowel activity, and assessment of vital organ function determine whether the problems the patient perceives are reflected in objective measurements. The emotional trauma occurring with his uneasy perception may contribute to extension of gastritis or endogenous ulcerogenic activity. Concerned attention to his problem may lower his anxiety level.

Hydrochloric acid secretion from chief cells in the gastric lining increases during the *rapid eye movement* (REM) stage of sleep; therefore the patient may awaken with gnawing gastric pain and nausea. Administration of an antacid or milk usually relieves the symptoms. The predictability of the problem is an indication that a supply of the antacid should be at the bedside for rapid administration of the drug and minimal sleep disturbance. Patients receiving sleep-inducing drugs during hospitalization may have less pain-induced sleep disturbance than do patients at home, since many hypnotics reduce REM sleep periods.

Antacids are usually taken at 1- or 2-hour intervals to maintain a gastric coating and lower gastric acidity. Chewable tablets may provide in-transit drug for the patient who travels. One ingenious individual used a 2-ounce swivel-top plastic dispenser to squeeze liquid antacid into his mouth when pain occurred while he was in commuter traffic. Utilization of a comparable device may avoid the unsightly chalky coating on teeth and lips when antacid use is required during social contacts.

Use of antacids is an integral part of an ulcer therapy plan. Repair of ulcers in the upper gastrointestinal tract requires careful instruction of the patient in aspects of therapy that are his responsibility (i.e., food, activity restrictions). Patients can maintain a trouble-free plan when they understand the rationale for limitations and the problems that require reevaluation or modification of the therapeutic program. Consistent use of antacids is an essential component of gastric mucosal protection during ulcer-inducing states or when upper digestive tract erosion has been identified.

HYPERMOTILITY AND SECRETION CONTROL

Gastric acidity, distention, irritation, or ulceration can provide afferent stimuli to the medullary and hypothalamic centers and consequent efferent impulses that increase gastroenteric motility. Visceral hypermotility can be modified by drugs that alter acetylcholine activity. Parasympathetic effector impulses arriving at the neuroeffector sites are dependent on acetylcholine to facilitate the relay of electrical impulses from nerves to the effector organ.

Pharmacodynamics

Cholinergic blocking agents. Anticholinergic drugs are used to block the action of acetylcholine at gastrointestinal tract effector sites. The drugs decrease motility and production of secretions. Modification of secretions in the digestive tract lessens afferent stimuli mediated through the vagus nerve and consequent efferent stimuli to motility of the tract.

Anticholinergic drugs employed for control of secretions and motility of the digestive tract have specificity for the particular neuroeffector sites. The drugs differ structurally from agents that block acetylcholine action at preganglionic effector sites of the sympathetic or parasym-

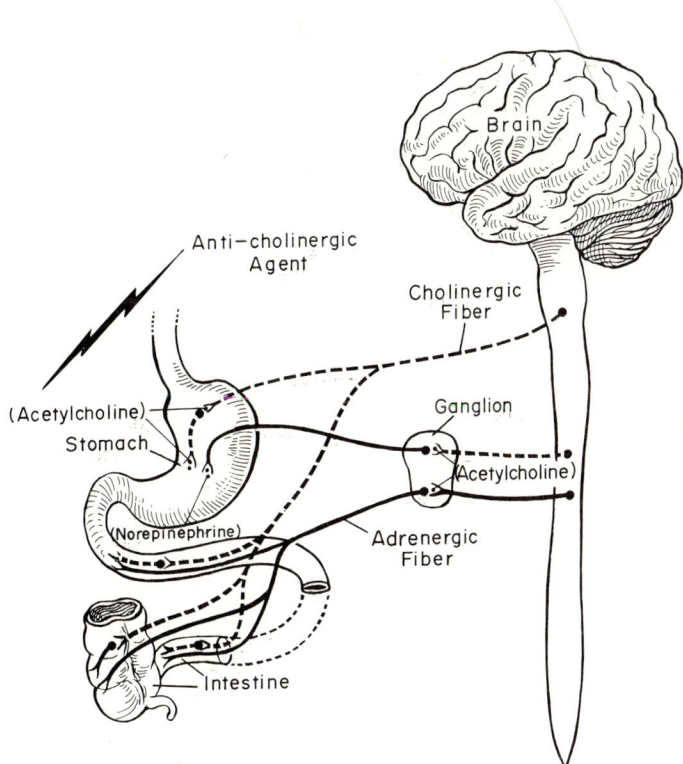

Fig. 10-1. Adrenergic (sympathetic nervous system) fibers and cholinergic (parasympathetic nervous system) fibers innervate the gastrointestinal tract. Anticholinergic agents block acetylcholine action on smooth muscle.

pathetic neural pathways (Fig. 10-1). Dosage adjustment influences the effect of the anticholinergic drugs at effector sites on smooth muscle or glands.

Anticholinergic drugs are used more frequently for control of parasympathetic nervous system–induced problems in the gastrointestinal tract than for control of hypermotility of other abdominal viscera. Eructation, abdominal distention, and vacillating pain sites in the abdomen constitute a symptom complex that can be called the primary disease of the American pace of life.

Inhibition of acetylcholine by anticholinergic drugs decreases gastrointestinal tract motility, as well as sebaceous, salivary, gastric, and pancreatic secretions. The therapeutic aim is to maintain activity of the viscera at a level that allows physiologic digestive processes to continue.

Production of saliva is one of the parameters monitored during therapy. Therapeutic dosage maintains a low-level dryness in the mouth, and dosage is reduced or elevated according to the patient's statement of discomfort. Hyposecretion of saliva is considered to be a fair indicator of suppression of gastric secretions because gastric secretions respond less readily to anticholinergic drug action than do salivary glands. Concurrent therapeutic measures for relief of gastrointestinal hypermotility include dietary modification and the use of antacids and sedatives as part of the control program.

Atropine sulfate provides a prototype or standard for definition of the specific effects of anticholinergic agents. The action of atropine sulfate in blocking acetylcholine activity is useful in preparation of patients for anesthesia induction and surgery. Parenteral administration provides prompt blocking of acetylcholine action, and suppression of gastrointestinal motility and secretions of the salivary glands provides evidence of drug action.

Atropine sulfate (Table 10-2) is administered with a sedative preoperatively, and atropine sulfate also has a slight sedative action. The anticholinergic drug decreases sweating, and the patient feels warm and complains of thirst. The typical patient continually seeks to wet his lips with a dry tongue while he is in transit to surgery. Secretions could be aspirated by the unconscious patient; therefore limitation of mucus is protective. Decreased motility of the gastrointestinal tract decreases the hazard of vomiting during surgery. The appearance of the patient provides a vivid picture for recall of the anticholinergic action of other members of the pharmacodynamic group. Close examination reveals dry, warm, slightly flushed skin and slightly dilated pupils. Although atropine sulfate dilates the pupils, the concurrent administration of a narcotic may decrease dilation. The composite picture is one of aberration of the functions controlled by the parasympathetic nervous system.

Details of effect vary among members of the anticholinergic drug group, but the action sites of the drugs are comparable to those of atropine sulfate. The effects of atropine sulfate seen in the preoperative patient would decrease the functional ability of an individual taking the anticholinergic drugs while he continues to carry on with his usual living patterns. For example, continued decreased gastrointestinal motility causes abdominal distention and constipation. Dilated pupils cause blurred vision. Decreased motility of the bladder causes urinary retention. Each of the functional problems is an adverse effect when it occurs during use of anticholinergic drugs. Atropine sulfate and scopolamine hydrobromide are exceptions because both agents are employed chiefly for their prolonged antisecretory action in preliminary preparation of the patient for anesthesia induction.

Scopolamine hydrobromide (Table 10-2) has the same effects on peripheral function as are demonstrated by atropine sulfate, and the former has a sedative effect that produces *twilight sleep*. Patients receiving scopolamine hydrobromide have amnesia for experiences occurring after drug administration. Scopolamine hydrobromide is administered with an analgesic prior to a pain-inducing experience (i.e., predelivery); the drug causes delirium in the presence of pain unless an analgesic is given.

High dosage of anticholinergic agents causes blocking of acetylcholine action at widely distributed neuroeffector sites of the parasym-

Table 10-2. Dosage range of anticholinergic drugs

Nonproprietary name	Proprietary (trade) name	Daily adult dosage range	Nonproprietary name	Proprietary (trade) name	Daily adult dosage range
Anisotropine methylbromide	Valpin	Oral: 30-40 mg. (÷3-4)	Methscopolamine bromide	Lescopine, Pamine, Proscomide	Oral: 12.5-30 mg. (÷4) I.M.: 0.75-4 mg. (÷3-4)
Atropine sulfate		Oral: 0.75 mg. (÷3) I.M.: 1.6-3.6 mg. (÷4-6) I.V.: Same as I.M.	Methylatropine nitrate	Metropine	Oral: 6-20 mg. (÷6-8)
Belladonna leaf, tincture		Oral: 0.6-9 ml. (÷2-3)	Oxyphenonium bromide	Antrenyl	Oral: 20-200 mg. (÷4) I.M.: 4-8 mg. (÷4) I.V.: 2-4 mg. (÷4)
Diphemanil methylsulfate	Prantal	Oral: 0.4-1.2 Gm. (÷4-6) I.M.: 2 mg./kg. (÷4)	Pentapiperide methylsulfate	Quilene	Oral: 30-80 mg. (÷3-4)
Glycopyrrolate	Robinul	Oral: 2-6 mg. (÷2-3) I.M.: 0.3-0.8 mg. (÷3-4) I.V.: Same as I.M.	Penthienate bromide	Monodral	Oral: 15-40 mg. (÷4)
			Pipenzolate bromide	Piptal	Oral: 20 mg. (÷4)
			Poldine methylsulfate	Nacton	Oral: 10-30 mg. (÷4)
Hexocyclium methylsufate	Tral	Oral: 100 mg. (÷4)	Propantheline bromide	Pro-Banthine	Oral: 75-240 mg. (÷4) I.M.: 120 mg. (÷4) I.V.: Same as I.M.
Homatropine methylbromide	Mesopin, Novatrin	Oral: 7.5-15 mg. (÷3)			
Isopropamide	Darbid	Oral: 10 mg. (÷2)	Scopolamine hydrobromide		Oral: 0.9-4 mg. (÷3-4) I.M: 0.3-0.6 mg./single dose
Mepenzolate bromide	Cantil	Oral: 100-200 mg. (÷4)			
Methantheline bromide	Banthine	Oral: 250-400 mg. (÷4) I.M.: 200 mg. (÷4) I.V.: Same as I.M.	Tricyclamol chloride	Elorine, Tricoloid	Oral: 0.5-1 Gm. (÷4)
			Tridihexethyl chloride	Pathilon	Oral: 100-400 mg. (÷4) I.M.: 40-80 mg. (÷4)

pathetic nervous system. Intense drying of the mouth or blurring of vision are early uncomfortable signs of dosage excess that alert the patient and stop drug use; therefore overdosage is rarely seen.

Oral administration is planned to provide therapeutic drug levels prior to the ingestion of food when the problem is related to gastrointestinal tract spasms or hypermotility. Onset of drug action is between 30 and 60 minutes; therefore administration is planned to assure relaxation of the viscera prior to mealtime.

Dicyclomine hydrochloride, methixene hydrochloride, oxyphencyclimine hydrochloride, and thiphenamil hydrochloride (Table 10-3) have a direct effect on smooth muscle action, in addition to their anticholinergic effect. Depression of smooth muscle contraction is due to the local anesthetic properties of the drugs. Thiphenamil hydrochloride has minimal anti-

Table 10-3. Dosage range of anticholinergic drugs with local anesthetic activity

Nonproprietary name	Proprietary (trade) name	Daily adult dosage range (oral)
Dicyclomine hydrochloride	Bentyl	60-160 mg. ($\div$3-4)
Methixene hydrochloride	Trest	3-6 mg. ($\div$3)
Oxyphencyclimine hydrochloride	Daricon, Setrol, Vio-Thene	20-50 mg. ($\div$2)
Thiphenamil hydrochloride	Trocinate	0.8-1.2 Gm. ($\div$4)

Table 10-4. Dosage range of direct-acting smooth muscle relaxants

Nonproprietary name	Proprietary (trade) name	Daily adult dosage range
Adiphenine hydrochloride	Trasentine	Oral: 225-600 mg. ($\div$3-4) I.M.: 50 mg./single dose I.V.: Same as I.M.
Alverine citrate	Gamatran, Profenil, Spacolin	Oral: 120-360 mg. ($\div$1-3)
Flavoxate hydrochloride	Urispas	Oral: 300-800 mg. ($\div$3-4)
Piperidolate hydrochloride	Dactil	Oral: 200 mg. ($\div$4)

cholinergic effect, and its therapeutic usefulness is related to decreasing the motility of smooth muscle in the lower digestive tract.

The chemical structure of each of the drugs influences the intensity of effectiveness in control of motility of abdominal viscera. Adverse effects of the drugs include suppression of cholinergic function in other organs with parasympathetic efferent neurons (that is, occasionally tachycardia occurs). Each of the drugs is available in forms for oral administration two to four times a day (Table 10-3).

Anticholinergic drugs are given in diverse situations in which parasympathetic responses interfere with the individual's ability to function. It is easy to envision the use of anticholinergic agents to decrease hypersalivation in a public speaker or to prevent diaphoresis in an actress working under intense lighting conditions. At low dosage range the drugs may be prescribed to provide single-dose effect on either salivation or perspiration. The drugs are available in varied dosage forms and in combinations with other drugs to provide maximum relief of acetylcholine-initiated problems.

Direct-acting muscle relaxants. Drugs used for selective suppression of organ hypermotility or spasm act directly on the visceral smooth muscle. The drugs have a local anesthesia-like effect that decreases the permeability of muscle membrane to the transfer of sodium ions and slows conduction.

Adiphenine hydrochloride, alverine citrate, and piperidolate hydrochloride (Table 10-4) have some anticholinergic effect, in addition to their direct effect on muscle. In contrast to atropine-like drugs, they do not decrease internal gland (gastric and pancreatic) secretions. Dryness of the mouth and throat, constipation, and blurred vision occur less frequently during therapy than they do with anticholinergic agents, but the patient may have one or more of the problems. The drugs produce a relaxant effect on the smooth muscle of viscera in 20 to 30 minutes; therefore they are administered orally 30 minutes before meals when the gastrointestinal tract structures are the target sites of therapy.

Flavoxate hydrochloride (Table 10-4) has an analgesic and antihistaminic effect, in addition to the local anesthetic-like effect on smooth muscle. It most frequently is used for control of the broad spectrum of problems occurring with bladder irritation or inflammation (i.e., dysuria, incontinence, urgency, frequency). Onset of effect after oral administration is longer (2 hours) than that obtained with other drugs in the group of direct-acting muscle relaxants. Elderly patients receiving flavoxate hydrochloride may become confused, and many patients complain of dizziness and headache during therapy. Annoying problems for some patients during therapy are pruritus and diaphoresis.

Patient care

It is always hazardous to guess about the factors in the individual's environment that have contributed to a particular problem, although it is probable that poor health practices have preceded the onset of gastrointestinal symptoms. Erratic schedules for meals and overeating at the evening meal before sitting for hours in a comfortable chair contribute to the rebellion of the gastrointestinal tract that compels the patient to seek medical assistance. The physician's assessment of pathophysiologic causation includes physical examination and diagnostic testing (i.e., gastrointestinal x-ray series). Many patients benefit from the physician's prescription for a revised living pattern and an antispasmodic drug. With periodic reevaluation during clinic or office visits, the individual may be able to maintain a normal living pattern.

The therapeutic plan will vary according to the site and extent of pathology, but each patient can participate in implementation of the therapeutic plan. Concurrent measures for control of the basic problem are implemented during drug therapy.

Assessment of drug effect necessitates establishment of base-line function against which progress can be measured. For example, initial persistent epigastric pain, end-of-day abdominal distention, or food intolerances may be the problems presented by the patient. Relief of symptoms during therapy is an indication of drug effect in relieving the hypersecretion-hypermotility–related problems, although not necessarily correction of the underlying cause.

The patient's knowledge of predictable drug effect will assist in defining progress and problems occurring during therapy with anticholinergic drugs. For example, the patient with bladder spasms should know that he is expected to have an increased bladder capacity with less frequent voiding. It is important for him to know that occurrence of bladder distention, difficulty in initiating urination, or a sensation of fullness after voiding are adverse effects of the drug requiring the attention of the physician. When problems occur, the pharmacotherapeutic plan may be modified to provide the drug at a level that controls spasm or subdues hypermotility without producing adverse effects.

HYPOMOTILITY

Decreased peristalsis causes distention of the intestine that is uncomfortable for the patient. Manipulation of the intestines during surgery is one of the chief contributing factors, and measures that decompress the intestine are used to relieve distention. Gastrointestinal decompression, insertion of a rectal tube, or ambulation aid in emptying the intestine of retained gases. Cholinergic substitutes have been employed in the past to improve motility of the intestine, but the only drug in current use is bethanechol chloride (Urecholine).

Pharmacodynamics

There is a close structural relationship between acetylcholine and bethanechol chloride, which acts as a substitute for the cholinergic neurotransmitter. The drug is capable of stimulating the abdominal viscera when atony exists, but widespread parasympathetic stimulation causes concurrent dilation of the bronchi, dilation of blood vessels, and slowing of impulse transmission in the heart. The diversity of effect depends on the frequency of administration and the length of time the drug is used.

Bethanechol chloride has a specific effect on the urinary bladder; it relaxes the sphincter and increases contraction of the detrusor muscle. It acts at the myoneural junction to add to acetylcholine effect within 30 minutes after the oral tablet is taken by the patient. Daily oral adult dosage is 30 to 120 mg., divided into 3 to 4 doses. Excess stimulation of parasympathetic function seldom occurs after oral administration, but subcutaneous use may cause hypermotility of the gastrointestinal and urinary tract (bladder spasm), hypersecretion of glands, bronchial spasm, generalized vasodilation, and decreased cardiac conduction.

Patient care

Prior to institution of therapy with the subcutaneously administered drug, the pharmacodynamic effect is carefully evaluated by administration of a test dose and gradual modification of the dosage for therapeutic response with generalized parasympathetic nervous system effect. The patient is observed for increasing parasympathetic activity in vital organ systems throughout parenteral therapy. The drug is administered (2.5 to 10 mg.) while the patient is recumbent to decrease the effects of vasodilation. He is asked to remain in bed for an hour after drug administration. Because increased peristalsis may cause diarrhea and bladder contraction may cause a sudden, urgent need to void after drug administration, a bedpan must be at hand to assure that the patient will remain in bed if the problems arise during the hour-long period of recumbency. Atropine sulfate is used to counteract excess acetylcholine release during subcutaneous administration of bethanechol chloride.

REFERENCES

Christensen, J.: The controls of gastrointestinal movements: some old and new views, The New England Journal of Medicine **285**:85, 1971.

DiCara, Leo V.: Learning in the autonomic nervous system, Scientific American **222**:30, Jan., 1970.

Goth, Andres: Medical pharmacology, ed. 6, St. Louis, 1972, The C. V. Mosby Co.

Held, Richard: Plasticity in sensory-motor systems, Scientific American **213**:84, Nov., 1965.

Hendrix, T. R., and Bayless, T. M.: Digestion: intestinal secretion, Annual Review of Physiology **32**:139, 1970.

Ingelfinger, Franz J.: Gastrointestinal absorption, Nutrition Today **2**:2, March, 1967.

Koelle, George B.: Acetylcholine—physiology, pharmacology and medicine, The New England Journal of Medicine **286**:1086, 1972.

Mountcastle, Vernon B., editor: Medical physiology, ed. 13, vol. 2, St. Louis, 1974, The C. V. Mosby Co.

Reilly, Mary Jo, editor: American hospital formulary service, vol. 1, sect. 12:00, Washington D. C., 1973, American Society of Hospital Pharmacists.

Spellberg, Mitchell A.: Antacids and anticholinergics: rationale of their use in peptic ulcer, Modern Medicine **39**:100, 1971.

Texter, E. C.: The control of gastrointestinal motor activity, American Journal of Digestive Disorders **9**:858, 1964.

Weinstein, Ronald S., and McNutt, N. Scott: Current concepts: cell junctions, The New England Journal of Medicine **286**:521, 1972.

UNIT THREE
DRUGS USED TO CONTROL HEMODYNAMICS

11 Cardiac output

12 Cardiac arrhythmias

13 Vascular tone

14 Vascular constriction

15 Blood coagulation

16 Red blood cell deficiency

11

Cardiac output

> Myocardial blood supply
> Neural controls
> Stroke volume output
> Conduction pathway
> Contraction force
> Cardiac chamber distention
> Pharmacodynamics
> Patient care

The heart and blood vessels form a closed hemodynamic system that provides tissues with nutrients and oxygen and removes metabolic wastes. A complex sequence of neural, hormonal, and physical stimuli effect cardiac and vascular responses to physiologic changes. Cardiac output is a key factor in maintaining hemodynamic equilibrium. The heart acts as a pump, ejecting the blood it receives and slowing or accelerating its activity to meet changing tissue needs.

Myocardial blood supply

The heart pumps about 4 to 6 liters of blood through its chamber each minute. Activity increases appreciably the amount of blood that must be directed forward. When its work load is increased, heart muscle requires additional amounts of blood to supply the oxygen and nutrients necessary for increased myocardial activity. Blood is supplied to the myocardium by the coronary arteries that branch off the aorta just above the aortic valves. The efficiency of left ventricular ejection of blood affects the quantity of blood flowing through the coronary arteries to myocardial tissue.

Neural controls

The heart is powerfully influenced by sympathetic nerves, which stimulate its activity; by parasympathetic nerves (principally the vagus nerve), which depress heart activity; and by the catecholamines *epinephrine* and *norepinephrine,* which reach the cardiac tissues by way of the bloodstream. Nervous and hormonal influences are in turn triggered by various receptors elsewhere in the circulatory or central nervous system.

Cardiac adaptations to physiologic requirements of the body during rest and exercise represent a balanced interaction of parasympathetic and sympathetic nerve impulses. Parasympathetic tone maintains the cardiac output during rest. To meet the gradually increasing demands of moderate activity, a decrease in parasympathetic tone allows increased cardiac response. Sympathetic neural responses provide the stimulus for increased cardiac output during periods of high metabolic activity.

Sympathetic nerve control. Psychologic or physiologic stressors stimulate sympathetic nerve–mediated cardiac responses. Integrated physiologic stimuli gear cardiac activity to meet anticipated needs of the body during periods of stress. The quality of the adaptive response is dependent on the frequency of stimuli, functional status of myocardial tissue, and integrity of neural conduction tissue. Cardiac adaptation to physiologic demands is necessary to survival.

During exercise or work, sympathetic nerve stimulation accelerates the cardiac rate, conduction velocity, and contractile force to meet metabolic requirements for oxygen and nutrients. Sympathetic nerve fibers (adrenergic fibers) initiate the adaptive response by stimulation of receptors in the sinoatrial (S-A) and atrioventricular (A-V) nodal tissue and adrenergic receptors scattered throughout myocardial tissue. Liberation of the transmitter substance norepinephrine from the adrenergic fibers initiates cardiac responses necessary to increase cardiac output during activity.

A great deal of physiologic preparation begins as soon as the individual senses that work, exercise, or danger is imminent. The sense organs send impulses to the cerebral cortex in response to perceptions of the external world. Hypothalamic control pathways activate sympathoadrenal mechanisms. The sympathetic nervous system becomes active, and the adrenal glands release the hormones epinephrine and norepinephrine into the bloodstream. The pulse quickens, the heart muscle contracts more forcibly, and the output of the heart begins to increase slightly. Breathing is deeper, and the respiratory rate may be faster. Voluntary muscles become tense. Blood is diverted to muscles, and blood flow through the coronary arteries increases.

Light exercise may increase coronary blood flow up to one and a half times that of rest levels. Some of the required blood supply is obtained by physiologic diversion of blood from the endocardial tissues to epicardial tissues, and the process may cause some ischemia of the endocardial tissues during periods of high metabolic activity.

Sustained levels of nervous and hormonal stimulation are as hazardous as the sharp peaks of resources mobilized in response to a single stress situation. Excessive demands on the heart may be decreased by modification of the source of stress (i.e., fear, anger, pain, activity).

Parasympathetic nerve control. Cardiac output during periods of rest or moderate physical activity is maintained by parasympathetic nervous system impulses. Stimulation of the vagus nerve slows pacemaker conduction when the neural impulses arrive at sinoatrial and atrioventricular node receptor sites. Afferent and efferent impulses transmitted by the vagus nerve maintain the balanced integration of the parasympathetic nervous system necessary to the feed and breed functions of the body.

The normal heart has adequate reserve function to maintain cardiac output when vegetative demands of other systems cause concurrent increase in parasympathetic nervous system impulses to cardiac tissue. However, the patient with borderline cardiac compensation may be adversely affected when prolonged periods of vagus nerve stimulation are required for physiologic functions. For example, the heart rate may be reflexly slowed or nodal conduction may be disrupted during periods of vagus nerve stimulation of gastrointestinal function. Vagus nerve stimulation is required for digestive processes, and a large meal may require sustained parasympathetic nerve activity. Afferent impulses from the full digestive organs to the integrating centers in the medulla are followed by efferent impulses that stimulate gastrointestinal tract motility and digestive gland secretion. Concurrent transmission of efferent vagus nerve impulses to cardiac nodal tissue receptors causes slowing of conduction through pacemaker tissue. Comparable vagus nerve–initiated slowing of cardiac action may occur when afferent vagus nerve endings are stimulated at widely distributed organ sites. A distended bladder, enemas, rectal thermometers, and cold or iced drinks can initiate vagus nerve stimulation that reflexly slows cardiac conduction.

Reflex slowing of cardiac conduction can also occur when blood distends the carotid and aortic arteries. Distention of these arteries stimulates pressor receptors in the arterial walls, and vagal afferent impulses travel to medullary integrating centers, which then send vagal efferent impulses to cardiac nodal tissue. The physiologic mechanism decreases arterial filling by slowing conduction and subsequent cardiac contraction. In some sensitive individuals external pressure on the carotid artery initiates a sequence of events comparable to those occurring when internal pressure from fullness of the artery stimulates the pressor receptors. Pressure over the carotid artery while shaving or a tight collar could cause dizziness or fainting secondary to decreased blood flow to cerebral tissues when vagus slowing of conduction decreases cardiac output.

Stroke volume output

Cardiac output is the product of stroke volume output times the cardiac rate. Stroke volume output describes the quantity of blood pumped from each ventricle with each contraction. Although no devices are in general use for measurement of the stroke volume output, contraction force can be evaluated, and it provides an indirect measurement of the stroke volume output. Measurement of the systolic blood pressure and auscultation of the heart allow definition of the cardiac contraction force. Assessment of the cardiac rate includes definition of the frequency, quality, and regularity of the heartbeat. Changes in either contraction force or rate reflect cardiac compensatory activity in adjusting output to meet changing body requirements.

Extracardiac factors or cardiac valvular obstruction may decrease the amount of blood entering the heart or the efficacy of contractions in moving blood forward. Correction of the causative factor may be elective, but intensive therapy is necessary to maintain cardiac output when a deficit occurs.

Conduction pathway

Cardiac tissue is composed of separate functioning cells that have an inherent ability to contract independently. Each myocardial cell is capable of excitation and can initiate or relay neural impulses. The normal conduction pathway consists of specialized pacemaker tissue that carries the stimulus for cardiac contraction. The impulse travels from the sinoatrial node initiation point, through the atria to the atrioventricular node, and through the bundle of His and Purkinje fibers to the ventricles.

The rhythmic impulse initiating depolarization in the normal heart arises in the cluster of nodal tissue located in the posterior wall of the right atrium. The sinus node has an emission rate of 60 to 100 impulses/minute; therefore the node initiates conduction before other myocardial cells can initiate depolarization. Impulses from the node spread radially throughout the atrium, causing the atria to contract and eject their contents into the ventricles. Some of the impulses travel to the A-V node, where there is a brief delay before the electrical wave is relayed to conduction tissue beyond the node. Impulses from the A-V node spread over the right and left bundles to activate the interventricular septum, right ventricular wall, and left ventricle. An impulse travels the entire conduction pathway in less than one half of a second.

Electrocardiographic recording (EKG) of conduction shows atrial depolarization as the P wave and ventricular depolarization as the QRS complex. Cardiac contraction follows the transmission of impulses. Atrial contraction occurs at the summit of the P wave and ventricular contraction at the summit of the R wave. The impulse travels through the atrial muscle and reaches the A-V node approximately 0.04 second after its origin in the S-A node. Delay in transmission at the A-V node allows the atria to empty blood into the ventricles before ventricular contraction begins. About 58% of the impulse travel time is spent in passage through the A-V node. On electrocardiographic recordings the P-R interval shows the time taken for the impulse to reach the ventricles and initiate ventricular depolarization. Completion of the cardiac conduction cycle includes repolarization of conduction tissue. The S-T segment of the electrocardiographic recording represents the period between completion of depolarization and repolarization, and the T wave represents the recovery phase after conduction.

Disruption of the conduction pathway results in slowing, speeding, or irregularity of conducted impulses. Conduction pathway disturbances affect the emptying of cardiac chambers and deprive vital organs and peripheral tissues of blood.

Contraction force

Rapid or irregular stimuli from myocardial tissue (i.e., ectopic beats, atrial fibrillation) may cause incomplete emptying of the ventricles during systole. Retention of blood from one contraction to the next distends the cardiac chambers and reduces contraction force. Up to a certain optimal length of the muscle fibers, increasing the end-diastolic fiber length increases the energy of cardiac muscle contraction. Beyond the optimal fiber length, the energy of contraction diminishes. For example, exercise in an athlete increases the quantity of venous blood entering the heart during diastolic filling. Blood entering the right atrium in the quiescent period increases the initial length of the cardiac muscle fibers. The healthy heart, distended with entering blood, will contract more forcefully during systole. In the individual with atrial fibrillation, increased blood returning to the atrium will overburden the heart that has been working at a borderline capacity to empty its distended chambers. The heart will be distended beyond the point of optimal activity, and muscle contraction will be diminished. In the first situation the individual will have a ready supply of oxygen and nutrients to continue physiologic activity, but in the second situation the individual will be unable to continue activity.

CARDIAC CHAMBER DISTENTION

Increased cardiac chamber pressure obstructs entrance of blood from the vena cava and the pulmonary veins. It is predictable that there will be an accumulation of blood in the peripheral and pulmonary veins when cardiac contraction ineptly removes blood from heart chambers. The disruption of normal pressure relationships that maintain fluid in the vascular system gradually causes the fluid from distended veins to extravasate into tissue spaces. When the work burden exceeds the ability of the myocardium to respond, compensatory mechanisms fail to maintain chamber emptying, and manifestations of congestive heart failure occur. Most patients with long-standing cardiac problems who enter the hospital with acute congestive failure provide a history of recent traumatic experiences involving psychologic or physiologic stressors. The precipitating factors may vary, but in the acute situation intensive therapy is required to reinstitute cardiac output.

Therapy is directed at reducing the amount of blood returning to the right atrium and increasing the efficacy of cardiac contractions in moving blood forward. Pulmonary edema requires prompt use of emergency measures: potent diuretics for rapid removal of excess fluid, application of tourniquets to trap blood in peripheral areas (rotating tourniquets), use of a positive pressure respirator assistor to improve oxygenation and create resistance to alveolar capillary transudation of fluid, administration of a narcotic analgesic to decrease metabolic activity, and a cardiotonic to improve cardiac contraction. During the life-threatening episode the patient receives each of the foregoing emergency measures almost simultaneously, and the results can be rapid reversal of an acute episode of pulmonary edema. In less urgent situations the use of a potent diuretic and a cardiotonic during a planned period of physiologic rest may adequately reduce circulating or sequestered fluid volume and improve cardiac output.

Pharmacodynamics

Drugs used to regulate cardiac output concurrently improve blood supply to the myocardium. Control of cardiac conduction problems (arrhythmias) and contraction problems has a positive effect on perfusion of peripheral tissues. The chief drugs employed specifically for control of cardiac muscle action are digitalis glycosides (Table 11-1).

Use of digitalis for its effect on cardiac output and life-threatening edema is recorded as early as the sixteenth century. The purified derivatives prescribed today are direct descendents of the foxglove plant extracts originally used for treatment of dropsy.

Digitalis glycosides are widely prescribed for their cardiotonic action, but the precise mechanism of action is not clearly understood. The glycosides are thought to affect cardiac muscle contraction by increasing the permeability of the muscle membrane to cations required for muscle action. Diffusion of calcium and sodium to the inside of the membrane improves the interdigitation of myosin and actin fibrils necessary to muscle contraction. Digitalis glycosides increase contraction force, and cardiac chambers empty more completely. The decreased end-diastolic muscle fiber length during digitalis therapy is an important factor in maintaining cardiac output.

Forceful systolic contraction empties the cardiac chambers more completely, and additional blood can enter during the diastolic filling period. Predictable outcomes of the improved cardiac function are a decrease in pulmonary and peripheral venous pressure and an increase

Table 11-1. Dosage range of digitalis glycosides

Nonproprietary name	Proprietary (trade) name	Daily adult dosage range
Acetyldigitoxin	Acylanid	Oral: 0.1-0.2 mg.
Deslanoside	Cedilanid-D	I.M.: 0.4 mg. I.V.: Same
Digitalis	Digalen, Digicardium, Digifolin, Digifortis, Diglusin, Digitol	Oral: 100 mg.
Digitoxin	Cardigin, Crystodigin, Digisidin, Digitaline Nativelle, Myodigin, Purodigin	Oral: 0.05-0.3 mg. I.M.: Same as oral I.V.: Same as oral
Digoxin	Davoxin, Lanoxin, Saroxin	Oral: 0.25-0.75 mg. I.M.: Same as oral I.V.: 0.75-1.5 mg.
Gitalin (amorphous)	Gitaligin	Oral: 0.25-1.25 mg.
Lanatoside C	Cedilanid	Oral: 0.5-1.5 mg.
Ouabain		I.V.: 0.3-0.4 mg./single dose

in arterial blood supply to tissues. The overall effect for the patient is a gradual increase in activity tolerance.

Digitalis glycosides also have an effect, mediated through the vagus nerve, on the sinoatrial node and the atrioventricular node. Digitalis stimulation of vagus nerve control slows the firing rate of the S-A node and the transmission rate through the A-V node. When the patient is in atrial fibrillation, digitalis has no effect on the erratic stimulatory pattern of atrial tissue, but many of the atria-initiated impulses bombarding the A-V node are blocked by the slower transmission rate of the node. The decreased rate of ventricular response may result in a sharp decrease in ventricular beats (i.e., from 200 beats/minute to 90 beats/minute). It is possible that the increased strength of contraction (stroke volume output), coupled with the decreased rate of contractions, may not appreciably increase the total cardiac output. Reduction of cardiac work will improve cardiac dynamics and assure that adequate amounts of blood are available for tissue metabolism.

Digitalis therapy is instituted with an initial loading dose, and a lower dosage level is used for maintenance therapy. *Digitalization* is the term used to describe the period during which large amounts of the glycoside are given for acute effect on the enlarged heart. Saturation of the heart muscle tissues with the glycoside forces the muscle to contract at its maximum potential. Maintenance dosage after digitalization is planned at a level that will maintain the muscle tone and contraction force necessary for cardiac output.

Age, size, physiologic status, and previous use of digitalis all affect digitalis use. Newborn and premature infants require intensive observation and dosage titration because immaturity of hepatic and renal function decreases their tolerance to digitalis glycosides.

Digitalis is distributed in myocardial, intestinal, liver, and skeletal muscle tissue. Digitalis crosses the placental barrier and is found in the milk of nursing mothers. Most of the digitalis preparations are metabolized in the liver. The primary route of excretion is the kidneys, although inactive metabolites are found in the feces.

The normal half-life of digitalis is lengthened from between 30 and 38 hours to 83 hours in the patient with renal failure; therefore careful assessment of the patient's renal status is important during digitalis therapy. Fine control of digitalis levels for the patient with decreased renal tubule function may include monitoring of serum drug levels and administration of the drug in liquid form to allow careful calculation of specific dosage. Dosage levels may be adjusted downward when blood urea nitrogen (BUN) levels rise to two or more times normal levels.

Digitalis glycosides. The differences between the digitalis glycosides are variations in potency, route of administration, or onset and duration of action. All digitalis glycosides have comparable actions and adverse effects in the body. Dosage used for digitalization may be four to ten times the maintenance dosage level.

The patient's cardiac status influences the physician's decision to use a 1- or 3-day period for digitalization with high dosage of the maintenance form or to use a potent form for acute effect. Each form of digitalis has a potential for improving cardiac output by modifying cardiac conduction and contraction.

Digitalis is most often used as the compressed raw product (pill) prepared with only enough additive to hold the product together. When taken orally, it is changed in the stomach to other digitalis forms (i.e., digitoxin, gitalin). It is incompletely absorbed from the gastrointestinal tract. Onset of action when administered orally is 3 to 4 hours, and when administration parenterally (liquid preparation) it is 1 to 2 hours. Elimination of a single dose from the body is complete in 2 to 3 weeks. The parenteral dose is one fifth the oral dose, and the oral maintenance dose is one tenth the digitalization dose.

Digitoxin is often used orally because it has a low incidence of gastrointestinal irritation. Onset of action when administered orally is 2 to 4 hours, and when administered parenterally it is $1/2$ to 2 hours. Elimination of a single dose from the body is complete in 2 to 3 weeks. Dosage is the same when administered orally or parenterally. The maintenance dosage by any route is one tenth the digitalization dose.

Acetyldigitoxin is similiar to digitoxin, but the former is more readily disseminated in the body. Onset of action when administered orally is 2 to 6 hours. Elimination of a single dose from the body is complete in 7 to 12 days. The oral maintenance dosage is one tenth the digitalization dose.

Digoxin when administered orally is only half absorbed from the gastrointestinal tract so that the parenteral dose is half the oral dose. Onset of action when administered orally is an hour, and when administered parenterally it is 15 to 30 minutes. Elimination of a single dose from the body is complete in 2 to 3 days. Most of the drug is metabolized in extrahepatic sites. Regardless of age, the maintenance dosage is one fourth the digitalization dose.

Gitalin when administered orally has an onset of action of 2 to 4 hours. Elimination of a single dose from the body is complete in 7 to 10 days. The maintenance dosage is one tenth the digitalization dose.

Lanatoside C is administered orally. It has a variable onset of action. A single oral dose is completely eliminated from the body in 24 hours. Maintenance dosage is one fourth the digitalization dose. Deslanoside is a derivative of lanatoside C. Onset of action is 10 to 30 minutes after parenteral administration. A single parenteral dose is completely eliminated from the body in 24 to 48 hours. Maintenance dosage is one fourth of the digitalization dose.

Ouabain is used only in emergency situations. It is a potent glycoside that is administered intravenously for digitalization. Onset of action is 5 to 15 minutes. A single intravenous dose is completely eliminated from the body in 1 to 3 days.

All forms of the digitalis glycosides must be protected from light to prevent decomposition. Solutions of the glycoside are incompatible with acids and alkali.

Adverse effects. The most frequent adverse effects of digitalis glycosides are seen as nausea and as changes in the mental status of the patient (that is, confusion, inability to concentrate, other indications of slowed mental processes). The changes are attributable to the action of digitalis on central nervous system tissues.

Almost all patients with excess serum levels of digitalis show some form of cardiac arrhythmia. The adverse effects are pathologic extensions of the therapeutic plan to slow conduction (Fig. 11-1).

Vagus nerve–mediated slowing of S-A node (sinus node) firing decreases the heart rate (bradycardia). When sinus-initiated contraction is rapid, the therapeutic effect of digitalis slows the sinus pacemaker. Digitalis glycosides effect A-V node blocking of rapid impulses, which also improves ventricular emptying. Excess digitalis causes pacemaker depression, prolongation of impulse transmission across the A-V node (prolonged P-R interval), and precarious decrease in the ventricular contraction rate. High digitalis levels may completely block A-V node transmission of impulses (complete heart block).

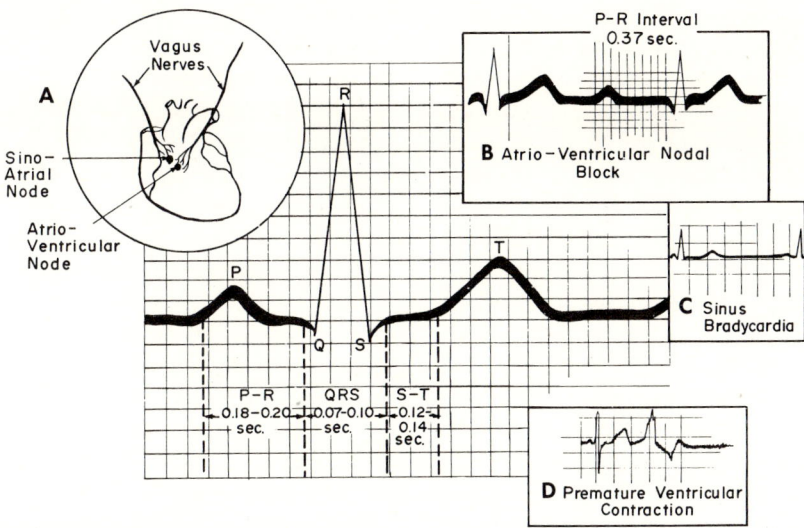

Fig. 11-1. Normal cardiac conduction intervals (center) provide a base line for EKG monitoring of drug effect. **A,** Digitalis effect is mediated through the vagus nerve–nodal tissue junction. Excess digitalis decreases the impulse transmission rate from nodal tissue; **B,** fewer impulses arise from the S-A node; **C,** impulse transmission is slowed at the A-V node; and **D,** conduction stimuli from ectopic foci in the ventricle emerge between A-V conduction intervals.

Each myocardial fiber has an ability to initiate conduction (automaticity). The S-A node is the natural pacemaker because it initiates conduction more frequently than do other myocardial fibers. Excess digitalis, by its two-pronged attack on nodal tissue, can slow the normal conduction pathway enough to allow other irritable myocardial tissue to take over pacemaker activity. The ectopic beats may be premature ventricular contractions (PVC's), premature atrial contractions (PAC's), or premature nodal contractions (PNC's). Emergence of ectopic beats is often the earliest sign of digitalis toxicity.

Evidence of the effect of excess digitalis on the ventricular rate can be obtained by taking the apical pulse. It is an established criterion that the pulse must be taken before administration of each dose of digitalis. The drug is withheld if the pulse rate drops to 60 beats/minute in an adult or 70 beats/minute in a child. Apical pulses are taken to determine the actual rate because weak ventricular contractions cannot be palpated at peripheral sites.

Most patients with irregularities in rhythm or evidence of digitalis excess are placed on cardiac monitors. The pictorial presentation of the conduction pattern makes it possible to identify changes. Prompt reporting of increased ectopic activity allows the physician to revise the therapeutic plan and may prevent progression from multiple irritable foci to the ventricular tachycardia–fibrillation–arrest sequence.

In the myocardial cell, potassium antagonizes the effect of digitalis, and dosage is planned for effective action with normal serum potassium ion levels (normal: 3.5 to 5 mEq./ml.) Low serum potassium ion levels indicate low intracellular potassium ion levels. If the serum potassium ion level falls, there is danger of overshoot of digitalis effect. The most common cause of potassium ion loss is concurrent use of diuretics for control of fluid accumulation in the cardiac patient. Prophylactic measures include ingestion of large amounts of foods high in potassium (i.e., orange juice, prunes, bananas, raisins) or administration of potassium-containing drug supplements. Peaking of the T wave on the cardiac monitor or EKG provides evidence of increasing irritability, and the physician may discontinue digitalis.

Calcium ions act synergistically with digitalis

in effecting contraction of cardiac muscle, and calcium is itself a direct cardiac muscle stimulant. Elevation of serum calcium ions above normal levels (8.5 to 10.5 mg./100 ml.) increases the sensitivity of the myocardium to digitalis effect and may unmask digitalis toxicity. Hypercalcemia is seldom a problem unless there is a markedly disrupted electrolyte balance.

The oral forms of digitalis glycosides are irritating to the gastric mucosa, and they may cause nausea and vomiting. The self-care patient should be asked to inform the physician if persistent nausea or vomiting interferes with taking his prescribed dose of digitalis. Both the omission of drug and the electrolytes lost with vomiting may adversely effect his therapeutic plan. Digitalis has a direct effect on the medullary vomiting centers so that the problem may occur when digitalis is administered by any route.

Visual disturbances often provide a clue to impending toxicity. Xanthopsia (yellow vision) is the visual disturbance most frequently described as related to digitalis toxicity. It is caused by a digitalis effect on the cones rather than the visual rods.

Glucagon. One of the newest members of the group of agents used to improve cardiac output is glucagon. The drug is a natural hormone produced by the alpha cells of the islands of Langerhans in the pancreas. It has been employed for many years to reverse the physiologic problems related to exogenous administration of excess insulin. Its use has been expanded to include administration to postoperative patients during the recovery period after cardiac surgery. When glucagon is administered (2 to 5 mg./single dose), there is improvement in myocardial oxygen extraction, increased aortic blood flow, and decreased renal vascular resistance. The positive effect on hemodynamics is partially related to accelerated enzymatic breakdown of glycogen induced by glucagon effect on the phosphorylase-glycogen sequence in the liver. Catabolism of glycogen raises the blood glucose level, and the increased glucose has a positive effect on cardiac metabolic activity. Because glucagon effect is of short duration, it is administered at intervals of an hour or less. The chief complaint of patients during administration of the drug is the occurrence of transient periods of nausea.

Patient care

Digitalis glycosides are used as part of an overall plan for maintenance of cardiac output, and each aspect of the plan is important to the effectiveness of the total plan. Long-term therapy for a patient with recurrent cardiac failure means taking digitalis daily, restricting sodium intake, modifying activity, and planning rest periods. The individual must be helped to understand the relevance of each aspect of the plan for maintaining his health status. His management of normal living pattern modifications requires self-discipline, and his understanding of the plan of therapy may keep the number of indiscretions at a minimum level.

Weight reduction is an important aspect of the program to prevent excessive cardiac work in the obese patient. The positive aspects of weight reduction should be clear to the patient. If an obese person loses 10% of his body weight, there is a decrease in resting cardiac work of 25% to 30%. For each 1% reduction in body weight there is a 2.5% to 3% reduction in resting cardiac work. Activity tolerance improves with weight reduction, and the patient's motivation to continue dietary restrictions usually improves when the positive effects on activity become evident to him.

Maintenance of digitalis serum levels requires consistent use of the digitalis glycoside. The patient should be assisted to plan a routine for taking the drug to assure that he will remember to take his medication regularly. To avoid interruption in use of the drug, he should be instructed to plan for refilling of the prescription when his supply of digitalis is low.

Periodic evaluation of his progress will be planned by the physician, and the patient must know the importance of interim contact if problems arise. Persistent fatigue, shortness of breath, peripheral edema, or gastrointestinal disturbances are some of the indications for him to seek advice from his physician.

Nursing guidelines. The patient's status will affect the amount of assistance he requires in meeting his basic needs. Tabulation of baseline data indicating his cardiac functional status will provide valuable information for defining his progress or the onset of problems. The patient's blood pressure and apical pulse provide information about his cardiac rate and contraction force. Venous distention or edema in the peripheral or pulmonary tissues indicates obstruction to venous emptying during diastole. Fullness of the venous circulation is indicated by distended neck or ankle veins; edema of the ankles, tibial, or gluteal areas; fluid sounds in the chest; or persistent productive cough. An important clue to the adequacy of cardiac output in supplying arterial blood to tissues may be the patient's statement that he is exhausted and breathless with minimal activity.

Objective measurement of the adequacy of tissue perfusion can be made by tabulating urine output; assessing activity-related changes in blood pressure, pulse, and respiration; observing skin color and temperature; and testing mental acuity. A deficit in arterial blood supply is indicated by decreased hourly urine output; pallor and coolness of the skin; tension of the neck and facial muscles; or slow, ponderous, confused responses to questions.

The availability of electrocardiograph (EKG) equipment in clinical settings makes it possible for the nurse to obtain additional evidence of the patient's cardiac conduction pattern. The complete conduction sequence can be evaluated by obtaining a lead II EKG strip, and a record of atrial activity (i.e., atrial fibrillation) can be evaluated by obtaining a V_1 EKG strip. Sample segments mounted on the patient's record provide additional graphic evidence of base-line status as a standard for comparison during the drug therapy program.

A composite profile of base-line data provides guidelines for planning measures to facilitate the movement of blood, supply needed oxygen, and reduce the work of the heart. Each of the measures is important to protect the patient's resources and support the action of drugs used to control cardiac output.

Assessment of drug effect. Changes in the patient's status are directly related to the intensity of therapy with digitalis glycosides. Dramatic changes may be seen in the patient who has received a large dose of a potent glycoside intravenously in an intensive effort to reverse life-threatening pulmonary edema. Some of the changes seen in the patient will be an outcome of measures used concurrently to reverse fluid accumulation in the lungs. Monitoring of the patient's cardiac status will provide evidence of changes in the parameters indicating improved cardiac action. Less dramatic evidence of digitalis effect is seen in the patient who is managing a daily maintenance dose of digitalis while continuing to carry out responsibilities as a family member. His ability to tolerate activity without peripheral fluid accumulation, shortness of breath, or exhaustion provides evidence of drug effect in maintaining cardiac output. Contact with either patient should include acquisition and recording of data for evaluation of the patient's progress. Changes from base-line levels provide the information necessary for revision in care plans by medical and nursing team members.

REFERENCES

Delano, Alice, Carrel, Betty, Shubin, Herbert, and Weil, Max Harry: Monitoring the acutely ill cardiac patient, Cardiovascular Nursing 7:61, 1971.

Doherty, J. E., Hall, W. H., Murphy, M. L., and Beard, O. W.: New information regarding digitalis metabolism, Chest 59:433, 1971.

Gilbo, Donna: Nursing assessment of circulatory function, Nursing Clinics of North America 3:53, 1968.

Higgins, Charles B., Vatner, Stephen F., and Braunwald, Eugene: Parasympathetic control of the heart, Pharmacological Reviews 25:119, 1973.

Jelliffe, Roger W.: Administration of digoxin, Diseases of the Chest 56:56, 1969.

Kones, Richard J., and Phillips, John H.: Glucagon: present status in cardiovascular disease, Clinical Pharmacology and Therapeutics 12:427, 1971.

Langer, G. A.: The intrinsic control of myocardial contraction, The New England Journal of Medicine 285:1065, 1971.

Littmann, David: Stethoscopes and auscultation, American Journal of Nursing 72:1238, 1972.

Mason, D. T., and Braunwald, E.: Digitalis: new facts about an old drug, American Journal of Cardiology 22:151, 1968.

Mountcastle, Vernon B., editor: Medical physiology, vols. 1 & 2, ed. 13, St. Louis, 1974, The C. V. Mosby Co.

Reilly, Mary Jo, editor: American hospital fomulary service, vol. 1, sect. 24:00, Washington, D. C., 1973, American Society of Hospital Pharmacists.

Vitti, Trieste G., Banes, Daniel, and Byers, Theodore E.: Bioavailability of digoxin, The New England Journal of Medicine 285:1433, 1971.

Warner, Howard F., Russell, Margaret W., and Spann, James F.: Heart muscle: clinical application of basic physiology and cellular anatomy, Heart & Lung 1:494, 1972.

12
Cardiac arrhythmias

Conduction-contraction sequence
Ectopic foci
Assessment
Pharmacodynamics
Patient care

Rhythm disturbances affect the responsiveness of the heart to physiologic demands, and the seriousness of an arrhythmia is determined by the body's ability to tolerate and compensate for it. Antiarrhythmic drugs may reinstitute the adaptive response by blocking stimuli, modifying conduction rate, or decreasing the irritability of the myocardial tissue. The pharmacodynamic action of a particular drug affects its use in arrhythmia control (Fig. 12-1).

Monitoring of the cardiac status of patients with myocardial infraction in coronary care units has provided statistical evidence that 90% of the patients have an arrhythmia in the early course of their recovery period. Data also indicate that 80% of the patients have some premature ventricular beats at some time during their stay in the unit. Electronic monitoring in the modern coronary care unit provides the evidence allowing identification of the particular abnormality in the heart's rhythm, and prompt therapeutic intervention has increased the survival rate of patients with acute myocardial infarction.

Conduction-contraction sequence

To understand the origin and significance of arrhythmias, it is necessary to know the electrical and mechanical activity occurring within the heart. In the normal heart, depolarization of the sinus node initiates the conduction pattern. Depolarization of the atria produces the P wave of the monitor or electrocardiographic (EKG) pattern, and atrial contraction follows conduction. The normal P-R interval (0.18 to 0.20 second) indicates the time between initiation of depolarization at the sinoatrial (S-A) node and passage of the impulse through the atrioventricular (A-V) node. Depolarization of the ventricles produces the QRS complex on the monitor or EKG, and ventricular contraction follows the 0.12-second conduction period. Completion of depolarization and repolarization of the ventricular muscle is reflected in the S-T segment. The final aspect of conduction that is commonly monitored is the phase of recovery after completion of the conduction-contraction cycle, and the interval is seen as the T wave on the monitor or EKG.

Electronic monitoring provides valuable visual evidence of cardiac conduction, but auditory evidence is available each time an apical pulse is taken. Closure of the atrioventricular valves, which produces the first heart sound, correlates with the midpoint of the ventricular depolarization wave and preparation for ventricular contraction. Closure of the aortic valve, which produces the second clearly identifiable sound at the apex of the heart, correlates with the termination of the repolarization period. Interruptions in the regularity of the heart sounds indicate erratic conduction patterns caused by interference with transmission or emergence of ectopic foci.

Ectopic foci

Each cardiac cell has the ability to conduct impulses or contract independently of other

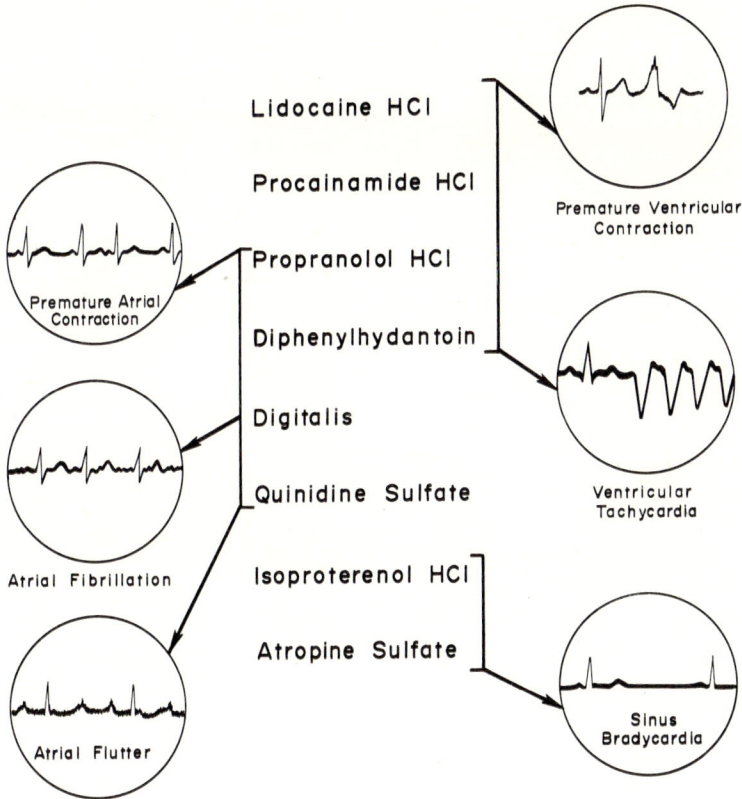

Fig. 12-1. The effector site of each drug affects its usefulness in treating cardiac arrhythmias.

cells. Initiation of depolarization by cells outside the normal conduction tissue pathway is an outcome of the property of independent conduction, or automaticity, of myocardial cells, and the impulse is described as ectopic. Excitability of myocardial sites may occur secondary to ischemia or trauma to cardiac tissue.

Atrial ectopic foci. Ectopic foci arising in atrial tissue sites may travel to the S-A node to depolarize it. Time required for the impulse to travel from the ectopic site to the S-A node causes a time lag between the new depolarization wave and the previously conducted impulse from the S-A, or sinus node. After the ectopic impulse causes depolarization of the S-A node, the depolarization pattern follows the normal conduction pathway through the A-V node, bundle of His, and Purkinje fibers. Visual evidence of the ectopic beat relates to the abnormal travel pathway of the P wave caused by depolarization from an ectopic site to the S-A node, but the remainder of the conduction pattern is unchanged. A new rhythm is established as sinus impulses again institute depolarization after the ectopic impulse–induced time lag.

Ventricular ectopic foci. Ectopic foci arising in ventricular tissue sites depolarize ventricular tissue independently. EKG patterns show bizarre widening and peaking of the QRS complex. Until completion of the ventricular depolarization-repolarization stimulated by the ectopic focus–initiated impulse, conduction from the A-V node is blocked. When the ventricular tissue is no longer refractory, impulses may again traverse the A-V node to depolarize ventricular tissue. The delay is called a *compensatory pause,* and the original conduction-contraction pattern is reestablished. In most instances, premature ventricular contractions can be identified by light tapping of the foot while listening to the basic cardiac beat. When a premature ventricular contraction emerges, continued tapping to the original rhythm will show the cardiac beat returning to the basic pattern.

Ectopic foci are indicators of irritability of the myocardium, and the chief concern is the potential for disruption of normal conduction patterns that maintain cardiac output. For example, premature ventricular contractions (PVC's) occurring before completion of cardiac filling project less blood forward. Increasing irritability of myocardial tissue indicated by frequent PVC's may precipitate a life-threatening ventricular fibrillation pattern. Drugs that act pharmacodynamically to suppress the irritable foci are usually administered when PVC's occur at a rate in excess of 5 during any minute of monitoring. Although the incidence of PVC's is an important factor, greater ventricular irritability is indicated when the ectopic beats arise from varying foci in the ventricle (multifocal PVC's). A rapid sequence of PVC's with 2 or 3 PVC's after a sinus-conducted beat (trigeminy or quadrigeminy) shows marked irritability and increases the hazard that ventricular fibrillation will be precipitated if the PVC's emerge during the vulnerable recovery period of the T wave.

Assessment

Electronic monitoring provides valuable visual evidence, but informed multisensory assessment of patients provides many vital clues to changes in physiologic function. The current practice of frequent-interval monitoring allows early identification of changes in vital parameters of patients in whom age, physical status, or acute physiologic stress increase the potential for problem emergence. When the apical pulse is taken as part of the planned subjective and objective assessment of the patient's status, it is possible to identify bradycardia, tachycardia, or ectopic beats. In selected situations the assessment can be promptly validated by taking an EKG strip to more exactly describe the problem.

Pharmacodynamics

Drugs used for control of arrhythmias provide control but seldom act on the basic cause of the cardiac irregularity. Throughout the course of therapy close observation of the patient is indicated because the drugs by their mechanism of action may themselves cause an arrhythmia.

Parasympathetic nerve effectors. Neural stimulation and blocking are useful mechanisms in arrhythmia control. Digitalis modifies ventricular response to the rapid impulses of atrial fibrillation through stimulation of the normal parasympathetic control of impulse transmission across A-V nodal fibers.

Atropine sulfate (Table 12-1) is used to abolish the parasympathetic effect on impulse conduction from the S-A node or across the A-V node. Abolition of parasympathetic nerve control increases the rate of impulse transmission. Atropine sulfate is useful for control of efferent vagus nerve impulses that cause reflex slowing of nodal conduction when carotid sinus stimulation increases (carotid sinus syndrome). Pressure receptors in the aortic or carotid sinuses respond to internal fullness of the arterial lumen by triggering a signal through the vagus nerve to slow cardiac output. In some individuals, hypersensitivity of the pressure centers causes messages to be sent with even slight internal (or external) pressure on the receptors.

Atropine sulfate also is used when patients periodically or consistently have an abnormally slow heart rate, or heart block, caused by parasympathetic nerve stimuli at the A-V node. Although nodal block may result from tissue damage or drug effect (i.e., digitalis) at or near the A-V node, it can also be precipitated as a reflex response to extracardiac vagus nerve stimulation. Atropine sulfate decreases nodal response to vagal stimuli, and impulses continue to traverse the node. The chief problem during use of atropine sulfate is concurrent depression of other parasympathetic nerve–mediated body responses (i.e., glandular secretion, gastrointestinal motility, bladder emptying).

Sympathetic nerve effectors. Sympathetic nervous system controls of physiologic activity in the cardiovascular system are mediated by norepinephrine release at receptor sites described as *alpha* or *beta receptors*. The heart has only beta receptors, and drugs used to con-

Table 12-1. Dosage range of drugs used to control cardiac arrhythmias

Nonproprietary name	Proprietary (trade) name	Daily adult dosage range
Atropine sulfate		S.C.: 2.4-3 mg. (÷6-8) I.V.: 0.5-1 mg.
Bretylium tosylate	Darenthin	I.M.: 0.4 mg. I.V.: 0.4-2 mg.
Diphenylhydantoin	Dilantin	Oral: 300 mg. (÷3) I.M.: 600 mg. (÷6) I.V.: Same as I.M.
Isoproterenol hydrochloride	Isuprel, Proternal	Oral: 30-180 mg. I.V.: 0.02-2 mg. (drip)
Lidocaine hydrochloride	Xylocaine	I.V.: 1 Gm. (drip)
Procainamide hydrochloride	Pronestyl	Oral: 2-7.5 Gm. (÷4-6) I.M.: 2-4 Gm. (÷4) I.V.: 0.2-1 Gm. (drip)
Propranolol hydrochloride	Inderal	Oral: 30-160 mg. (÷3-4) I.V: 1-3 mg./single dose
Quinidine gluconate	Quinaglute	I.M.: 3.2-4.8 Gm. (÷4-12) I.V.: 0.3-2.4 Gm.
Quinidine sulfate	Quinicardine	Oral: 2-4 Gm. (÷5)

trol sympathetic nerve responses modify norepinephrine stimulation of electrotransmission at the cardiac beta receptor sites. Norepinephrine initiates depolarization by increasing membrane permeability to sodium ions. Drugs having adrenergic beta receptor specificity also affect smooth muscles of the vasculature and the bronchi. Sympathetic nervous system–induced norepinephrine release at the extracardiac beta receptors causes dilation.

Beta receptor stimulation. Isoproterenol hydrochloride (Table 12-1) is used to stimulate sympathetic nerve activity at the A-V node when the patient has heart block. Beta receptor stimulation improves contractile force and increases the heart rate. Concurrent stimulation of beta receptors in the peripheral arteries causes dilation of the vessels and improvement of tissue perfusion. Wide distribution of the available blood supply causes hypotension.

Beta receptor blocking. Propranolol hydrochloride (Table 12-1) controls a variety of arrhythmias by its action in blocking response at the multiple sites of sympathetic fibers in the heart (Fig. 12-1). It is described as a beta-blocking agent. The physiologic effect of suppressing cardiac response to sympathetic nerve stimulation is a decrease in the adaptive response to activity or exercise. The patient taking the drug will experience symptoms of deficient blood supply during exercise (i.e., light-headedness, weakness, fatigue).

The therapeutic effect of propranolol hydrochloride on control of rapid rhythm (tachycardia) or ectopic foci is accompanied by a decrease in contractile force that decreases the metabolic rate of the myocardium. The effect can be therapeutic for the patient with coronary artery constriction or occlusion, both of which cause activity-induced pain (i.e., angina pectoris), because the drug maintains a more even blood supply–demand ratio. Propranolol hydrochloride also has a vasodilating effect on the coronary arteries that enhances the patient's exercise tolerance. The patient with borderline compensation of cardiac function, who is highly dependent on sympathetic nerve control to maintain effective output, cannot tolerate the drug. Any patient receiving propranolol hydrochloride must be observed for activity-induced decompensation resulting from cardiac chamber retention of blood. Drug dosage directly effects the level of interference with sympathetic nerve control. Dosage-related extensions of the planned pharmacodynamic action include aberrations in responses of myocardial or nodal tissue (i.e., bradycardia, asystole, cardiac arrest).

Bretylium tosylate is being used in clinical trials to test its effect on norepinephrine-

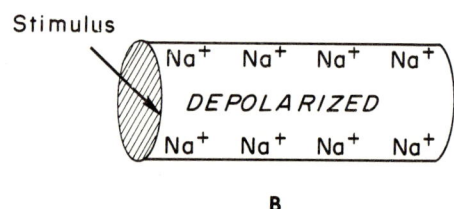
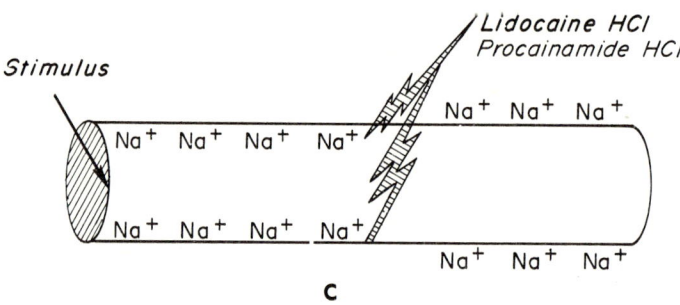

Fig. 12-2. Electromagnetic charges of sodium ions (Na⁺) effect conduction fiber activity. A, The polarized fiber is electropositive externally and electronegative internally. B, Neural stimuli initiate the depolarization necessary to fiber contraction. C, Lidocaine hydrochloride and procainamide hydrochloride decrease the permeability of the membrane to sodium shift and halt conduction.

induced cardiac arrhythmias. Reports indicate it acts by inhibiting neural fiber stimuli without blocking beta receptor sites. Use of the drug is accompanied by a decrease in compensatory control of blood ejection with postural change (postural hypotension) and by nausea or vomiting. Bretylium tosylate is administered in emergency situations when ventricular fibrillation fails to respond to other drugs.

Automaticity suppressants. Initiation of conduction requires a stimulus-associated movement of sodium ions across the membrane (Fig. 12-2). Norepinephrine release, myocardial lesions, or tissue hypoxia may initiate rapid or erratic bioelectrical activity of cardiac fibers. Drugs that interfere with the transfer of cations across the membrane fiber decrease electrical conduction. Diphenylhydantoin, lidocaine hydrochloride, procainamide hydrochloride, and quinidine sulfate (Table 12-1) suppress automaticity of myocardial fibers by decreasing membrane permeability to sodium ion influx. All the drugs have a stabilizing effect on membrane activity, but there is some specificity of effector sites among them. For example, quinidine sulfate is effective in control of atrial arrhythmias. Lidocaine hydrochloride and procainamide hydrochloride are used to control ventricular arrhythmias. Suppressants are employed in an attempt to maintain cardiac output by abolishing the automaticity of myocardial fibers. Drugs used to quell impulses from irritable foci will concurrently decrease the contractile force of the heart, and hypotension is a consequence of the decreased contractility.

Lidocaine hydrochloride is a potent drug with a local anesthetic property; it is used only in clinical situations in which the patient is under close supervision. Therapy for suppression of premature contractions arising from single or multiple ventricular foci is often initiated when the premature ventricular contractions (PVC's) appear at a rate in excess of five times a minute. Increasing PVC's indicate hyperirritability of ventricular tissue and decreasing effectiveness of contraction.

Lidocaine hydrochloride is administered either as a single, or bolus, intravenous injection (50 to 100 mg.) or by intravenous infusion (Table 12-1). Titration of the amount of drug administered by infusion with the number of PVC's requires careful monitoring of the cardiac conduction pattern. It is important to maintain a graphic record of the exact amount of drug being administered. For example: when 1 Gm. of lidocaine hydrochloride is diluted in 250 ml. of solution and the infusion delivers 60 drops/ml., there will be 1000 mg. in 15,000 drops, or 1 mg. in 15 drops. At an infusion rate of 15 drops/minute, the amount of drug the patient will be receiving is 1 mg./minute. Dosage levels above 3 to 4 mg./minute may precipitate adverse effects due to depression of inhibitory influences on motor pathways (i.e., convulsions) or depression of medullary centers (i.e., respiratory arrest). Effective therapy is dependent on careful titration of dosage with PVC occurrence and monitoring of cardiovascular status.

Procainamide hydrochloride is used for control of ventricular arrhythmias. The availability of an oral tablet makes it useful for long-term therapy. Effective suppression of ectopic beats with procainamide hydrochloride requires maintenance of consistent blood levels of the drug. Plasma values decrease to one half peak levels in $2^1/_2$ to 5 hours. The physician plans the dosage to maintain a suppressive level in the blood, and maintaining that level necessitates administration of the drug at exact time intervals. In addition to an effect on suppression of automaticity, procainamide hydrochloride has an anticholinergic (vagolytic) effect that may decrease motility of the gastrointestinal tract (paralytic ileus) or increase peripheral vasodilation, with resulting hypotension. The high incidence of hypotension makes it advisable to ask the patient to remain in a supine position for 15 to 30 minutes after drug administration. Vasopressors may be prescribed if the blood pressure falls more than 15 mm. Hg.

Diphenylhydantoin is widely prescribed for its stabilizing effect on central nervous system tissues in control of seizures. It also has a wide range of usefulness in cardiac arrhythmia control. The major problems and adverse effects during administration occur with intravenous use. It is very alkaline (pH approximately 11 to 12) and should be given in large veins, when possible. Administration in small veins causes pain and a burning sensation. The maximum rate for intravenous administration is 50 mg./minute. The few problems occurring with oral administration relate to irritation of the gastrointestinal tract. Drinking copious amounts of water with the medication decreases the problem. The most problematic adverse effects mimic the manifestations of cerebellar disease. The patient should be observed for lack of coordination and balance, and he should be asked to report the incidence of problems (i.e., ataxia).

Quinidine sulfate is used in the long-term management of patients with atrial arrhythmias. It sometimes converts atrial fibrillation to normal sinus rhythm spontaneously, and it may be employed to maintain sinus rhythm after electrical cardioversion of atrial fibrillation. Quinidine sulfate prolongs the effective refractory period of atrial tissue and slows depolarization.

The pharmacodynamic action of quinidine sulfate causes slowing of the conduction velocity in atrial, nodal, and ventricular tissue. Heart block is an adverse effect occurring during therapy and the problem is directly related to the depressant effect of quinidine sulfate on conduction through the A-V node and ventricular tissue.

Quinidine sulfate also has a vagolytic action that may cause rapid A-V node conduction and increase the potential for ventricular tachycardia. When the drug is used for control of atrial arrhythmias, digitalis glycosides are often used

162 Drugs used to control hemodynamics

CARDIAC RHYTHM RECORD

DATE	TIME	RHYTHM	RATE	COMMENTS
1/7/73	8:00 am	AF	110	Xylocaine 20 gtts/min 6 PVC's Dilantin 100 mg. p.o.
	9:00	AF	99	24 PVC's
	9:15	AF	99	30 PVC's Xylocaine 30 gtts/min Valium IM
	10:00	AF	100	20 PVC's Xylocaine 30 gtts/min
	10:30	AF	108	26 PVC's Xylocaine 30 gtts/min Catheterized 800 cc obtained
	10:45	AF	108	16 PVC's Xylocaine 20 gtts/min

Fig. 12-3. Periodic recordings of the arrhythmia patterns provide a guide for revisions of the drug administration plan. Correlation between the on-going arrhythmia, atrial fibrillation (AF), incidence of premature ventricular contractions, and drug administration rate is readily seen on the chart.

concurrently to counteract the vagolytic action of quinidine sulfate and maintain effective conduction rates. The anticholinergic (vagolytic) action of quinidine sulfate may cause peripheral vasodilation, with resulting hypotension.

Administration of quinidine sulfate with food disguises the bitter taste and decreases the incidence of problems due to gastric irritation (nausea, vomiting, diarrhea).

In some patients allergic responses have caused platelet destruction. Petechial hemorrhages in the buccal mucosa may provide an early clue to the problem, which progresses to thrombocytopenic purpura if therapy with the drug is continued. During long-term use, problems related to the cinchona tree bark origin of quinidine sulfate may appear (i.e., ringing in the ears, dizziness, skin rash, visual disturbances).

Patient care

Monitoring the progress of the patient with a cardiac arrhythmia requires astute observations and attention to detail. Regular recording of the rhythm, rate, and drug dosage on a graphic chart assures availability of data to all health team members (Fig. 12-3). The illustration shows an intensive effort to suppress PVC's by administration of two automaticity suppressants and a potent tranquilizer. Lidocaine hydrochloride (Xylocaine) at a drip rate supplying 2 mg./minute did not suppress the PVC's, and team members were deeply concerned. One nurse palpated the patient's abdomen and found the bladder was distended. The urine was removed by catheterization, and the number of PVC's decreased. The incident illustrates the complexity of problems presented by the patient with arrhythmias. Efforts were directed at decreasing sympathetic nerve stimuli (automaticity suppressants and a tranquilizer), but the distended bladder was causing reflex parasympathetic nerve (vagal) slowing of impulses through the conduction pathway. When there are 30 PVC's and the contraction rate is 99, the conduction pathway is transmitting 69 impulses/minute. Slow neural pathway conduction allows ectopic beats to emerge, or escape.

Nursing guidelines. In addition to the considerations presented earlier relative to care of the patient receiving drugs to control cardiac output (Chapter 11), there are specific considerations when monitoring the status of the patient with a cardiac arrhythmia. Drugs used to control arrhythmias, with the exception of atropine sulfate and isoproterenol hydrochloride, cause decreased myocardial contraction. There are prolongation of the P-R interval and widening of the QRS complex, but the changes are minimal. Widening of the QRS complex more than 25% above normal may indicate a pathologic extension of the pharmacodynamic effect of the drug. EKG validation of monitor patterns is essential for definition of fine change in intervals or complexes. Rhythm strips provide comparative data about the stability of the basic rhythm and the effect of drugs on the rhythm. Administration of oxygen to the patient may decrease arrhythmias because hypoxia increases the drug toxicity and arrhythmia potential of the irritable myocardium. The basic problem of the patient with a rhythm disturbance is a decrease in cardiac output; therefore his care includes measures to conserve energy and support physiologic efforts toward compensation.

REFERENCES

Amsterdam, Ezra A., Massumi, Rashid A., Zelis, Robert F., and Mason, Dean T.: Use of bretylium tosylate in the management of cardiac arrhythmias, Heart & Lung 1:269, 1972.

Arky, Ronald A.: Diphenylhydantoin and the beta cell, The New England Journal of Medicine 286:371, 1972.

Bellet, S., Roman, L., Kostis, J. B., and Fleischmann, D.: Intramuscular lidocaine in the therapy of ventricular arrhythmias, American Journal of Cardiology 27:291, 1971.

Bloomfield, Saul S., Romhilt, Donald W., Chou, Te Chuan, and Fowler, Noble O.: Quinidine for prophylaxis of arrhythmias in acute myocardial infarction, The New England Journal of Medicine 285:979, 1971.

Bogoch, Samuel, and Dreyfus, Jack: The broad range of use of diphenylhydantoin, New York, 1970, The Dreyfus Medical Foundation.

Chung, Edward K.: How to approach cardiac arrhythmias, Heart & Lung 1:523, 1972.

Davies, Robert E.: Biochemical processes in cardiac function, Hospital Practice 5:49, 1970.

Delano, Alice, Carrel, Betty, Shubin, Herbert, and Weil, Max Harry: Monitoring the acutely ill cardiac patient, Cardiovascular Nursing 7:61, 1971.

Gilbo, Donna: Nursing assessment of circulatory function, Nursing Clinics of North America 3:53, 1968.

Guyton, Arthur C.: Textbook of medical physiology, Philadelphia, 1971, W. B. Saunders Co.

James, Thomas N.: Sudden death related to myocardial infarction, Circulation 25:189, 1972.

Killip, Thomas: Management of arrhythmias in acute myocardial infarction, Hospital Medicine 7:131, 1972.

Langer, G. A.: The intrinsic control of myocardial contraction, The New England Journal of Medicine 285:1065, 1971.

Lehman, Sister Janet: Auscultation of heart sounds, American Journal of Nursing 72:1242, 1972.

Littmann, David: Stethoscopes and auscultation, American Journal of Nursing 72:1238, 1972.

Mayer, Gloria Gilbert, and Kaelin, Patricia Buchholz: Arrhythmias and cardiac output, American Journal of Nursing 72:1597, 1972.

Pitt, Bertram, and Ross, Richard S.: Beta adrenergic blockage in cardiovascular therapy, Modern Concepts of Cardiovascular Disease 38:47, 1969.

Reilly, Mary Jo, editor: American hospital formulary service, vol. 1, sect. 24:00, Washington, D. C., 1973, American Society of Hospital Pharmacists.

Warner, Howard F., Russell, Margaret W., and Spann, James F.: Heart muscle: clinical application of basic physiology and cellular anatomy, Heart & Lung 1:494, 1972.

Wenger, Nanette K.: Chemical: drugs. In Papers Presented: National Nursing Conference, Posthospital care of coronary patients, Feb. 25 and 26, 1970.

Wolf, Stewart: Central autonomic influences on cardiac rate and rhythm, Modern Concepts of Cardiovascular Disease 38:29, 1969.

13

Vascular tone

    Sympathetic nerve impulses
    Catecholamine release
    Adrenergic receptors
    Stress responses
Disrupted hemodynamic equilibrium
    Compensatory mechanisms
    Pharmacodynamics
    Patient care

Blood circulation is a closed hemodynamic system that continually makes fine adjustments to meet the demands imposed by changing environmental conditions. The autonomic nervous system maintains a balanced interaction between parasympathetic and sympathetic activity to provide the appropriate vascular responses to messages interpreted at the hypothalamus.

Sympathetic nerve impulses

The mediator substance for neural transmission at the ganglion in the sympathetic nervous system is acetylcholine. Passage of the stimulus to the postganglionic fibers causes release of the adrenergic substance *norepinephrine* at the organ effector site. Norepinephrine released by the postganglionic fibers of the sympathetic nervous system makes peripheral circulatory adjustments in response to hypothalamus-relayed stimulation.

Catecholamine release

Preaortic ganglia of the sympathetic nervous system release acetylcholine, which stimulates chromaffin cells of the adrenal medulla to produce the catecholamines *norepinephrine* and *epinephrine*. The adrenal medullary hormones control metabolic and vascular responses through natural physiologic mechanisms. Vascular responses are stimulated by either internal or external precipitators of sympathetic nervous system–induced epinephrine or norepinephrine release. Catecholamines control vascular responses by action at receptors of the peripheral vascular smooth muscle.

Release of adrenal medullary hormones provides reinforcements to maintain sympathetic nervous system responses. The neural stimulus is direct and powerful, and hormone secreted from the adrenal medulla augments the neural effect.

Adrenergic receptors

There are specific receptors at organ effector sites that are described as alpha and beta receptors for adrenergic stimulation. Arteries have both alpha and beta receptors. Only beta receptors have been identified at myocardial sites for sympathetic nervous system stimulation, and veins have only alpha receptors.

Norepinephrine acts principally at alpha receptor sites to stimulate smooth muscle of blood vessel walls, which causes constriction of arteries and veins. Each of the catecholamines acts at beta receptor sites to accelerate cardiac activity, but epinephrine has a more potent effect on heart action. Epinephrine also acts at beta receptor sites to cause bronchodilation and relaxation of smooth muscle of blood vessel walls, which causes vasodilation.

Stress responses

Stressors are natural to life activities. The sympathetic nervous system and the adrenal medullary hormones produce the physiologic

Vascular tone 165

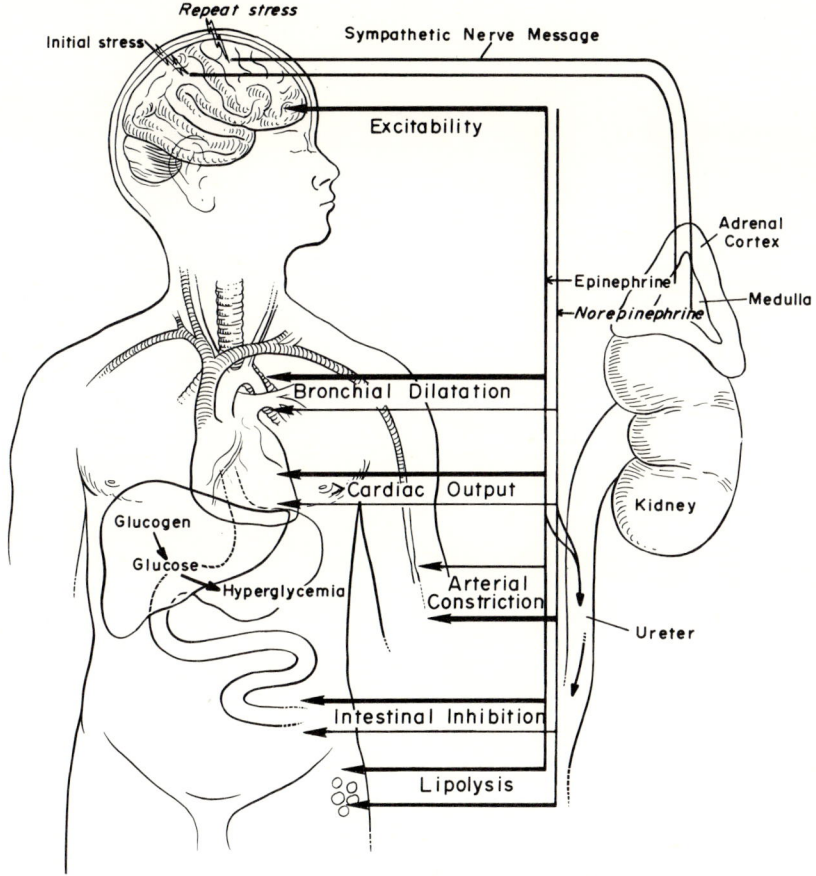

Fig. 13-1. Epinephrine and norepinephrine are liberated in response to stressors. Familiarity with the stress experience affects the catecholamine response and the physiologic events that are stimulated.

adjustments required for adaptation to varying stressors. The contribution of the catecholamines to hemodynamic equilibrium is the modification of vascular tone that maintains blood pressure levels within effective normal limits.

Norepinephrine and epinephrine produce the familiar fight or flight response. The most important role of catecholamines is the redistribution of blood flow and the increased tone of the vasculature, which results in transient elevation of blood pressure. Physiologic responses to stressors in the external or internal environment vary with stressor familiarity (Fig. 13-1).

Initial stress exposure. The first exposure to a stressor evokes release of epinephrine from the adrenal medulla, and action of the catecholamine causes central nervous system excitability, bronchial dilation, increased cardiac output, dilation of arteries, inhibition of intestinal motility, dilation of pupils, lipolysis, and mobilization of glucose from glycogen stores in the liver (Fig. 13-1).

Sudden abdominal pain or a cutting remark from a loving companion may elicit a generalized physiologic response concurrent with the stimulus. Overt signs of the physiologic impact may not be evident to the observer, but they are felt by the recipient of the physiologic changes. Acute initial stressors cause an increase in heart rate and respirations, with con-

166 Drugs used to control hemodynamics

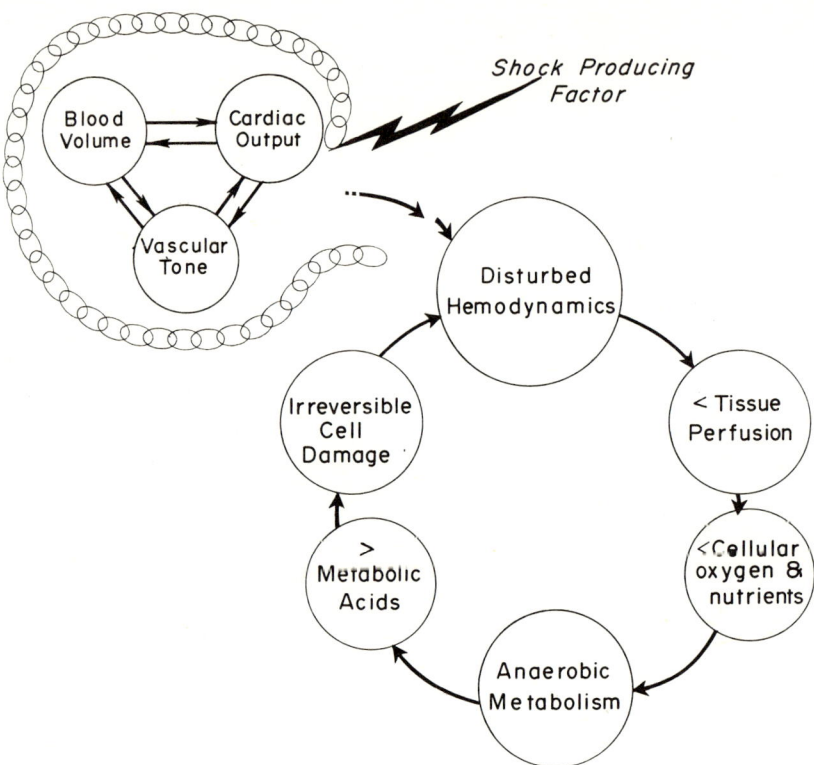

Fig. 13-2. Disruption of blood volume, cardiac output, or vascular tone by shock-producing factors affects hemodynamic equilibrium and precipitates a progression of cell-destroying events.

current metabolic changes. Cerebral stimulation causes unscreened, racing thoughts as the impact and meaning of the situation are analyzed and responses are sought.

Repeated stress exposure. Repeated exposure to a stressor builds tolerance to the stimulus as an adaptive mechanism conserving physiologic resources. Norepinephrine released in response to a familiar stressor evokes changes comparable to the natural adjustments of the sympathetic nervous system. The chief physiologic effect of norepinephrine released from the adrenal medulla is constriction of arteries. Exposure to a familiar stressor may cause slight blanching of the facial tissues, a rational stimulus-directed response, and minimal generalized metabolic reactions.

Widespread vasoconstriction induced by continued release of norepinephrine from the adrenal medulla increases peripheral arterial resistance and elevation of blood pressure in major arteries. Exhaustion of compensatory, or adaptive, mechanisms leads to a shock state.

DISRUPTED HEMODYNAMIC EQUILIBRIUM

Vascular tone has equal importance with cardiac output and blood volume in the tightly controlled chain of factors facilitating the provision of oxygen to body cells. Disruption of any one of the three factors disturbs hemodynamic equilibrium and threatens survival of body cells (Fig. 13-2). Supplies of vital oxygen molecules are rapidly depleted when tissues are deprived of replacement from circulating blood, and cells become dependent on acid-producing anaerobic metabolism to meet functional needs. Acidosis perpetuates the disturbance in hemodynamics and causes irreversible cell damage in vital organs.

Compensatory mechanisms

Disturbance in hemodynamic equilibrium mobilizes the body's adaptive mechanisms to correct the imbalance and reinstitute delivery of oxygen to cells. Physiologic adjustments are made in peripheral circulatory beds to compensate for the decreased amount of circulating fluid available. For example, a sudden deficit in blood volume (i.e., hemorrhage) initiates control measures affecting cardiac output and vascular tone to supply the necessary oxygen to tissues. Intricate control mechanisms respond to assure that available intravascular blood is supplied to vital areas of the body. Constriction of peripheral arteries decreases the blood supply to peripheral tissues, and blood is routed to the brain where oxygen and glucose supplies make the difference in survival of the organism. Other vital organs (heart, liver, lungs, adrenal glands) receive the same preferential treatment, and blood continues to be available for vital body processes. Cardiac rate accelerates to maintain the vital supply of oxygenated blood aerated at the pulmonary bed. Blood loss mobilizes the reserve blood stored in hepatic and splenic sinusoids. Tissue hypoxia stimulates the production of *erythropoietic stimulating factor,* which initiates bone marrow production of additional red blood cells.

Reinstitution of hemodynamic equilibrium necessitates correction of the precipitating factor. Pharmacotherapeutic measures are used to support the natural adaptive processes in meeting the challange of disruption and moving the organism toward equilibrium.

Pharmacodynamics

Adrenergic drugs are used to maintain vascular tone when widespread dilation of peripheral arteries compromises the blood supply to vital tissues. Adrenergic drugs may also be used to improve cardiac output as a pharmacotherapeutic approach to maintaining hemodynamic equilibrium.

Beta adrenergic effectors. Epinephrine hydrochloride is a synthetic preparation with the properties of naturally occurring epinephrine. The diversity of effect (Fig. 13-1) makes it a useful drug available for emergency situations. Epinephrine hydrochloride is employed chiefly for control of cardiopulmonary arrest or anaphylactic shock. The potent pharmacodynamic action of the drug at beta adrenergic receptors provides increased cardiac rate and contractile force in the failing heart and bronchodilation in anaphylactic shock. The general improvement in hemodynamic equilibrium includes an indirect effect on blood supply to vital tissues by acceleration of cardiac activity and dilation of peripheral arteries.

Epinephrine hydrochloride may be administered as a continuous intravenous infusion (Table 13-1), or it may be injected directly into the heart as an emergency measure during cardiac arrest. Intracardiac injection is a vital part of the resuscitative program that includes external cardiac massage and other emergency measures to reinstitute cardiac action.

Ephedrine hydrochloride, isoproterenol hydrochloride, and mephentermine sulfate (Table 13-1) are administered primarily for their pharmacodynamic action on cardiac and bronchial

Table 13-1. Dosage range of drugs used to maintain peripheral blood pressure

Nonproprietary name	Proprietary (trade) name	Adult dosage range
Angiotensin amide	Hypertensin	I.V.: 0.005-0.02 mg. (drip)
Dopamine		I.V.: 0.1-1 mg./min. (drip)
Ephedrine hydrochloride	Efedron, Ephetonin	I.M.: 25-50 mg. I.V.: 15 mg.
Epinephrine hydrochloride	Adrenalin, Adrin, Episcorb, Supranephrin, Sus-Phrine, Vasodrine	I.V.: 1-4 mg. (drip)
Isoproterenol hydrochloride	Aludrine, Isuprel	I.V.: 0.4 mg. (drip)
Levarterenol bitartrate	Levophed	I.V.: 1-5 amp. (drip)
Mephentermine sulfate	Wyamine	I.M.: 20-80 mg. I.V.: 15-30 mg.
Metaraminol bitartrate	Aramine, Pressonex	I.M.: 2-10 mg. I.V.: 0.5-5 mg.
Methoxamine hydrochloride	Vasoxyl	I.M.: 10-20 mg. I.V.: 5-10 mg.
Phenylephrine hydrochloride	Almefrin, Neo-Synephrine, Sucraphen	I.M.: 2-5 mg. I.V.: 0.2-0.5 mg.

tissues. The drugs act at beta receptors to improve cardiac rate and contractile force and dilate bronchial structures. Concurrent stimulation at arterial beta receptors improves perfusion of tissues. Dilation of the coronary arteries improves circulation of blood to the myocardium and meets the increased demands of myocardial tissue when contractile force improves.

Mephentermine sulfate has some effect on alpha receptors in arteries and veins, in addition to beta receptor action at cardiac and bronchial sites. The combined pharmacodyamic action of mephentermine sulfate improves hemodynamics by a combined effect on cardiac output and vasoconstriction in the periphery.

Dopamine (Table 13-1) is a precursor of norepinephrine biosynthesis, but the drug form acts at beta receptor sites. Dopamine improves cardiac output and causes peripheral vasodilation. The observed specificity of the pharmacodynamic action on renal arteries makes it useful for patients with compromised renal artery circulation. Increased sodium diuresis is a positive outcome occurring concurrently with improved blood circulation to the kidneys.

During the period of beta adrenergic drug administration the cardiac status of the patient is continually monitored. Stimulation of cardiac activity in a patient with subclinical coronary vessel obstruction may cause anginal pain. Pain increases as cardiac work increases the myocardial tissue demand for blood supply. Careful monitoring of the cardiac rate is planned throughout therapy with the drugs. The aim of therapy is to maintain blood pressure levels without excessive increase in cardiac rate.

Alpha adrenergic effectors. Levarterenol bitartrate, metaraminol bitartrate, methoxamine hydrochloride, and phenylephrine hydrochloride (Table 13-1) are administered to patients in shock to maintain vascular tone. The drugs act at alpha receptor sites in arteries and veins to effect vasoconstriction. Methoxamine hydrochloride is a pure alpha receptor stimulant, but levarterenol bitartrate, metaraminol bitartrate, and phenylephrine hydrochloride have some beta receptor effect on the heart.

Alpha receptor stimulators have a pharmacodynamic action comparable to that of the natural catecholamine norepinephrine (Fig. 13-1). Pharmacodynamic action causes constriction of peripheral arteries, with resulting improvement in blood pressure levels, and constriction of veins, which improves return of blood to the heart. When administered intravenously, each of the drugs has an almost immediate vasopressor effect.

Infiltration of levarterenol bitartrate or metaraminol bitartrate causes local vasoconstriction at extravenous sites. Extravasation of the drugs from infusion sites can cause extensive tissue necrosis. The drugs are often infused into large central veins via catheter to protect against infiltration.

Angiotensin effect. Angiotensin amide is a synthetic preparation that mimics the physiologic action of the natural amide angiotensin II. The natural product has been indicted as a causative factor in hypertension of renal origin because ischemic renal tissue liberates the enzyme *renin,* which converts inactive angiotensin to the active form that has a potent vasoconstrictive effect. The hypertensive effect may be desirable in selected situations in which the patient is hypotensive. The drug is infrequently used because the hypertensive action is difficult to control. Intravenous administration provides an initial therapeutic vasopressor effect in 20 to 40 seconds.

Patient care

Each of the drugs used to improve blood flow to peripheral tissues is a potent agent. Administration of the drug is titrated with the planned therapeutic response. Use of mini-drip (60 drops/ml.) intravenous equipment allows fine control of the amount of drug being administered. Placement of a second set of clamps on the tubing provides additional protection against inadvertent rapid infusion of the drug.

Prescription for the amount of vasopressor to be diluted in the infusion is explicit and usually includes the maximum systolic blood pressure desired for the patient. The figure varies as the normal for individual patients varies. The desirable blood pressure level is one that will be high enough to enhance glomerular filtration. Common ranges used as maximum therapeutic levels during intravenous vasopressor administration are 80 to 100 mm. Hg or 100 to 120 mm. Hg systolic blood pressure. Initiation of dosage requires constant observation of the patient, and blood pressure is taken every 2 minutes until stability is reached. Observation of physiologic responses and blood pressure levels are made every 5 minutes during intravenous infusion of the drug. Drug overshoot is a concern throughout therapy, since the additional burden on the heart and blood vessels consequent to a hypertensive reaction could jeopardize the progress of the patient.

Protracted periods of drug administration often make it difficult to discontinue therapy because physiologic mechanisms are slow to readapt. The vasopressors may be gradually administered as more dilute infusions while the patient's response to the change is observed carefully. The effect of position changes, including elevation of the headrest, evaluated prior to discontinuance of therapy may provide clues to the ability of physiologic sympathetic nervous system controls and pressor receptors to adapt to decreased drug levels.

When beta adrenergic effectors are administered in dilutions for intravenous infusion, the flow rate is titrated with the blood pressure and cardiac rate. Graphic records of the amount of drug being administered and tabulation of the patient's physiologic responses are useful to team members responsible for modification of plans based on the progress of the patient. For example, when 1 mg. of epinephrine hydrochloride or isoproterenol hydrochloride is diluted in 250 ml. of solution and the mini-drip equipment dispenses 60 drops/ml., there will be 1000 mcg. in 15,000 drops, or 1 mcg. in 15 drops. At an infusion rate of 15 drops/minute, the amount of drug the patient will be receiving is 1 mcg./minute. Planned periods for recording exact drug dosage, blood pressure, heart rate, mental status, and urine output provide evidence of drug effect on the hemodynamic problem.

Alpha and beta adrenergic effectors inhibit intestinal motility, and gaseous distention or constipation may occur when the drugs are administered for protracted periods of time. Long-term use of epinephrine hydrochloride necessitates plans for caloric intake to replenish glycogen stores mobilized from the liver during therapy. Blood glucose levels may produce transient hyperglycemia and positive tests for glycosuria during therapy. Central nervous system stimulation affected by exogenous epinephrine hydrochloride administration may cause headache, insomnia, and hyperexcitability.

Drug therapy is usually terminated when the patient recovers from the emergency state. The patient should be asked to report dizziness, fatigue, or drowsiness occurring after discontinuance of the drugs. Periodic evaluation of vascular responses in the immediate post-recovery period provides guides to planning care based on the patient's progress. Dramatic changes in care of patients in shock, including supportive measures to enhance blood transport and facilities for intensive care, have improved the life expectancy of patients by preventing extensive tissue destruction during hypoxic periods.

REFERENCES

Amsterdam, Ezra A., Massumi, Rashid A., Zelis, Robert F., and Mason, Dean T.: Evaluation and management of cardiogenic shock. II. Drug therapy, Heart & Lung 1:663, 1972.

Betson, Carol, and Ude, Linda: Central venous pressure, American Journal of Nursing 69:1466, 1969.

Bregman, David, and Goetz, Robert H.: Clinical experience with a new cardiac assist device: the dual-chambered intra-aortic balloon assist, The Journal of Thoracic and Cardiovascular Surgery 62:577, 1971.

Cohn, Jay N., and Luria, Myron H.: Studies in clinical shock and hypotension: hemodynamic effects of norepinephrine and angiotensin, Journal of Clinical Investigation 44:1494, 1965.

Goth, Andres: Medical pharmacology, ed. 6, St. Louis, 1972, The C. V. Mosby Co.

Guyton, Arthur C.: Textbook of medical physiology, ed. 4, Philadelphia, 1971, W. B. Saunders Co.

Levine, Seymour: Stress and behavior, Scientific American 224:26, Jan., 1971.

McGiff, John C.: Tissue hormones: angiotensin, bradykinin and the regulation of regional blood flows, Medical Clinics of North America 52:263, 1968.

Moran, N. C.: Evaluation of the pharmacologic basis for therapy of circulatory shock, American Journal of Cardiology 26:570, 1971.

Morgan, Beverly G., Abel, Francis, Mullins, Gay, and Guntheroth, Warren: Flow patterns in cavae, pulmonary artery, pulmonary vein, and aorta in intact dogs, American Journal of Physiology **210**:903, 1966.

Mundth, Eldreth D.: Postoperative care in the cardiac-surgical patient, Progress in C-V Disease **2**:229, 1968.

Reilly, Mary Jo, editor: American hospital formulary service, vol. 1, sect. 24:00, Washington, D. C., 1973, American Society of Hospital Pharmacists.

Thomas, Juergen E., and Schirger, Alexander: Orthostatic hypotension: etiologic considerations, diagnosis and treatment, Medical Clinics of North America **52**:809, 1968.

Wood, J. Edwin: The venous system, Scientific American **218**:86, Jan., 1968.

14

Vascular constriction

Hypertension
    Pharmacodynamics
    Patient care
Coronary artery constriction
    Pharmacodynamics
    Patient care
Peripheral artery constriction
    Pharmacodynamics
    Patient care

The tone of the arterial vasculature can be determined by periodic assessment of the diastolic blood pressure, and the burden placed on the vessels with each ejection of blood from the heart can be assessed by determination of the systolic blood pressure. Proximity to the initiator of the hydrostatic force determines the level of pressure impinging on the arteries with each systolic ejection of blood from the left ventricle (Fig. 14-1). Blood leaving the ventricle enters the aorta at a pressure of 120 mm. Hg, and the decrease in contents lowers the ventricular pressure to 8 mm. Hg prior to entrance of atrial blood. Pressures become steadily lower as blood moves through the hemodynamic circuit. Pressure is minimal (0 to 5 mm. Hg) at the junction of the vena cava and right atrium.

Values for normal blood pressure are predicated on the basis of systolic and diastolic pressures taken on innumerable healthy people

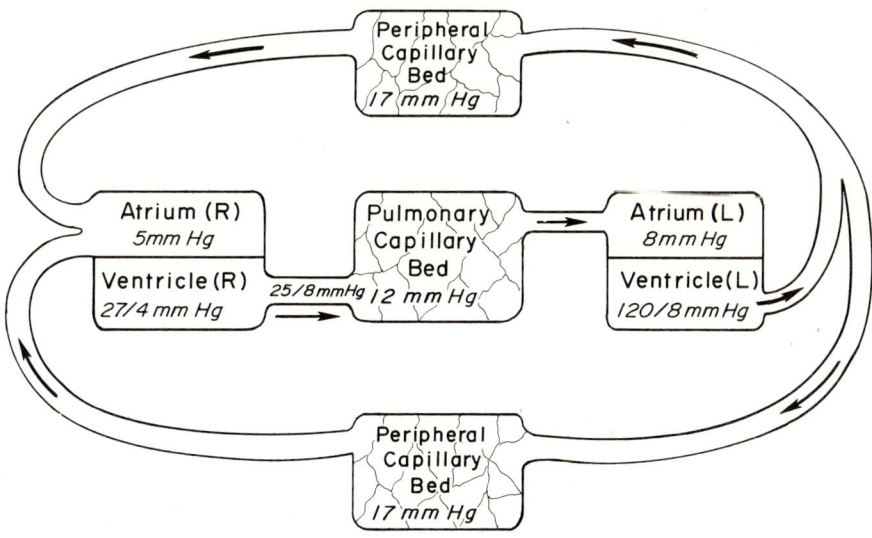

Fig. 14-1. Pressure differentials in the vascular system provide a base line for understanding hemodynamic problems. Vessel obstruction causes increased pressure backward from the blocked area and decreased pressure in vessels beyond the area of occlusion.

and reflect average blood pressure levels. The upper limits of normal are generally defined as 140 mm. Hg systolic and 90 mm. Hg diastolic pressure. The figures provide a crude guide to definition of hypertension.

HYPERTENSION

Systolic blood pressure varies with changes in cardiac output, but diastolic blood pressure reflects the steady state, or tone, of the arteries. Multiple interrelated physiologic factors affect the sustained constriction of arteries in hypertension, and varying drug groups are used to control psychologic and physiologic processes that are perpetuating the problem. Drugs are used to control the emotional reactions of the patient and to decrease psychic stimulation, both of which cause sympathetic nervous system–mediated vasoconstriction.

Diuretics are effective in controlling tissue fluid accumulation resulting from elevation of capillary pressure above normal levels. Blood volume decrease is a concurrent benefit of diuretics during therapy of patients with hypertension, and interaction between diuretics and antihypertensive drugs has a positive effect on hypertension control.

Therapeutic plans for the patient with a chronically elevated diastolic blood pressure level are comprehensive plans aimed at maintaining a pressure that supplies blood to all vital tissues and decreases the destructive effect of sustained pressure on the heart and vessels. For example, weight reduction, sodium restriction, and activity restriction may be part of the therapeutic plan.

The complexity of problems occurring with hypertension includes the presence of sustained sympathetic nervous system responses not traceable to pathology in the neural structures. The extensive adaptive mechanisms and adjustments to consistently elevated blood pressure levels are carefully evaluated by the physician as plans for use of hypotensive agents are considered.

Pharmacodynamics

Numerous agents contribute to the progress of the patient with acute or chronic hypertension. The agents specifically used for control of generalized arterial constriction act in varying ways on the sympathetic nervous system to modify vascular tone. Generalized vascular responses can be modified by drugs acting on the pressoreceptors in the carotid and aortic arteries or the multiple control sites of the sympathetic nervous system.

Catecholamine depletion

Rauwolfia alkaloids. Alseroxylon, deserpidine, *Rauwolfia serpentina,* rescinnamine, reserpine, and syrosingopine (Table 14-1) are classified pharmacologically as rauwolfia alkaloids. The drugs are known to act pharmacodynamically to deplete the neurohormone norepinephrine, thereby decreasing sympathetic nervous system stimulation at organ effector sites. The drugs are thought to prevent norepinephrine action at the receptor site by precipitous release of the amine that allows enzymatic destruction within the nerve ending. Metabolic products released at the receptor site are incapable of neural stimulation, and sympathetic nervous system responses are decreased.

Catecholamine depletion at alpha receptor sites in the vasculature decreases the vasoconstrictive effect of norepinephrine, and concurrent depletion at cardiac sites interferes with sympathetic nerve stimulation of heart rate. Slowing of the heart rate is an indicator of rauwolfia effectiveness.

The rauwolfia alkaloids cross the blood-brain barrier, and they are classified as one of the major tranquilizers. The pharmacodynamic action of rauwolfia alkaloids on central nervous system tissues includes depression of medullary vasomotor center responsiveness. The drugs have a marked sedative action that benefits the patient with hypertension, but drowsiness may interfere with activities such as driving a motor vehicle or doing tasks requiring alertness.

There is wide variation in the potency of the drugs. The more potent rauwolfia alkaloids have a cumulative tendency that allows long-term use at low dosage levels. Oral forms of the drugs have a long latent period at initiation of therapy, and it may be 2 weeks before therapeutic blood pressure levels are attained. Reserpine administered by intramuscular injection provides an effect within 2 to 3 hours.

Table 14-1. Dosage range of antihypertensive drugs

Nonproprietary name	Proprietary (trade) name	Daily adult dosage range	Nonproprietary name	Proprietary (trade) name	Daily adult dosage range
Alkavervir	Veriloid	Oral: 12-22 mg. (÷4)	Pentolinium tartrate	Ansolysen	Oral: 65-100 mg. (÷3-4) I.M.: 8-90 mg. (÷4-6)
Alseroxylon*	Koglucoid, Rau-Tab, Rautensin, Rauwiloid	Oral: 2-4 mg. (÷1-2)			
Chlorisondamine chloride	Ecolid	Oral: 12.5-200 mg.	Phenoxybenzamine hydrochloride	Dibenzyline	Oral: 10-60 mg.
Cryptenamine	Unitensen	Oral: 2-12 mg. (÷2) I.M.: 1 mg./single dose I.V.: Same as I.M.	Protoveratrine A	Protalba	Oral: 0.8-1.2 mg. (÷4)
			Protoveratrines A and B	Provell, Veralba	Oral: 1.6-6 mg. (÷4) I.M.: 0.36-2.4 mg. (÷3-6) I.V.: 0.36-0.6 mg. (÷4)
Deserpidine*	Harmonyl	Oral: 0.25-1 mg. (÷1-4)			
Guanethidine sulfate	Ismelin	Oral: 10-50 mg.	*Rauwolfia serpentina*	Raudixin, Rautina, Rautotal, Rauwistan, Rauwoldin	Oral: 150-200 mg. (÷1-2)
Hydralazine hydrochloride	Apresoline	Oral: 100-400 mg. (÷4) I.M.: 20-40 mg./single dose I.V.: Same as I.M.	Rescinnamine*	Moderil	Oral: 0.25-0.5 mg. (÷1-2)
			Reserpine*	Crystoserpine, Eskaserp, Rau-Sed, Reserpoid, Sandril, Serfin, Serpasil	Oral: 0.1-1 mg. (÷2-3) I.M.: 2-20 mg. (÷2-4)
Mecamylamine hydrochloride	Inversine	Oral: 5-25 mg. (÷2-3)			
Methyldopa	Aldomet	Oral: 0.5-3 Gm. (÷3)	Syrosingopine*	Singoserp	Oral: 0.5-3 mg.
Methyldopate hydrochloride	Aldomet ester hydrochloride	I.V.: 1-4 Gm. (÷4)	Trimethaphan camsylate	Arfonad	I.V.: 0.2-5 mg./min.
Pargyline hydrochloride	Eutonyl	Oral: 50-75 mg.			

*_Rauwolfia_ alkaloid.

Therapeutic effects of rauwolfia alkaloids decrease stimulation of vascular smooth muscle, but the absence of sympathetic nervous system balance in some tissues causes uncomfortable problems for the patient. Nasal stuffiness, continual drowsiness, and bizarre dreams are the problems identified by most patients taking the drugs.

One of the chief concerns during therapy is the tendency of the drugs to produce episodes of mental depression. The patient and his family are informed of the specific indicators of depression so that they can report changes to the physician promptly. It is most helpful if they understand the signs that discriminate between sedation or lethargy and mental depression (i.e., early morning awakening with fatigue and inability to go back to sleep, disinterest in food, depressed physiologic function).

Rauwolfia alkaloids have an ulcerogenic tendency; therefore the patient is periodically observed for evidence of food intolerances and epigastric discomfort during long-term therapy. Routine visits to the clinic or physician's office offer an opportunity to evaluate effectiveness of therapy and emergence of adverse effects of the drugs.

Guanethidine sulfate. Guanethidine sulfate acts pharmacodynamically in a manner comparable to that of the rauwolfia alkaloids to deplete catecholamine at peripheral sympathetic nerve endings. Unlike the rauwolfia alkaloids, guanethidine sulfate does not cross the blood-brain barrier. In addition to precipitating release of the neurohormone norepinephrine and destroying the amine before it is released from the nerve ending, guanethidine sulfate blocks neuronal uptake of the catecholamine.

Guanethidine sulfate dosage (Table 14-1) is increased gradually, and the patient's blood pressure is monitored regularly during the period of dosage adjustment. Drug effect is most evident when the patient is sitting or standing (orthostatic, or postural, hypotension); therefore determination of blood pressure levels is planned to correlate with the patient's arising from a supine position. Initiation of therapy usually includes a plan for monitoring both supine and standing blood pressure levels to ascertain the effective dosage of the drug. The patient is asked to seek assistance before arising to avoid falling because hypotension-related faintness or dizziness may occur with the position change.

Reduction in sympathetic neural stimuli allows increased parasympathetic nerve–controlled visceral activity. Increased gastrointestinal motility during therapy with guanethidine sulfate frequently causes uncontrollable, spontaneous defecation. The embarrassing problem may occur after eating when the gastrocolic reflex causes massive propulsive movement of intestinal contents toward the rectum. Anticholinergic drugs may be prescribed to control the problem and allow continuance of antihypertensive drug therapy.

Methyldopa. Methyldopa and methyldopate hydrochloride (Table 14-1) cause catecholamine depletion by providing the metabolite that is incorporated into the amine granule at the nerve ending. The mechanism provides a false transmitter substance that is ineffective when released from the nerve ending at the effector site. Methyldopa causes catecholamine depletion in peripheral and central nervous system sites.

Supine and orthostatic hypotension are evident in 4 to 6 hours after administration of methyldopa, and the effect persists for 24 hours. Cardiac rate is slowed for a comparable time period during therapy.

Central nervous system action of the drug causes greater sedation than that occurring with other antihypertensive drugs, but extrapyramidal signs, vertigo, and psychic depression are less pronounced.

Hemolytic anemia and liver damage occur during therapy, and these adverse effects are commonly attributed to hypersensitivity reactions. Discontinuance of drug therapy is followed by reversal of either of the problems.

Catecholamine biosynthesis deceleration. Pargyline hydrochloride (Table 14-1) is a monoamine oxidase inhibitor that accomplishes vasodilation by decelerating biosynthesis of catecholamines at cerebral and peripheral sympathetic nerve endings. There is a latent period lasting up to several days before the therapeutic effect of the drug is evident, and the hypotensive effect is chiefly orthostatic.

Monoamine oxidase inhibitors are incompatible with many foods and drugs. The patient should be asked to consult with the physician before using any drugs while taking pargyline hydrochloride. Many over-the-counter agents contain ingredients affecting pargyline hydrochloride action (i.e., antihistamines, sedatives). Foods requiring the action of bacteria or molds for their preservation or preparation (aged and natural cheese, alcoholic beverages, pickled herring, pods of broad beans) contain tyramine, which is antagonistic to the pharmacodynamic effect of pargyline hydrochloride. The ingestion of tyramine-containing foods may precipitate a sudden sharp rise in blood pressure.

Central nervous system stimulation occurs frequently during therapy with pargyline hydrochloride, and the patient may complain of insomnia, headache, or nightmares. Severe psychic depression and mood changes occur frequently, and patients and their families should understand the changes that indicate the need for reevaluation of the patient's status. Effects of the drug on gastrointestinal activity vary; some patients complain of nausea and anorexia, whereas others eat continuously and gain weight.

Direct-acting vasodilator. Hydralazine hydrochloride (Table 14-1) acts directly on the smooth muscle of blood vessels to cause vasodilation. The drug also causes cardiac stimulation, and patients complain of palpitation periodically during therapy. The adverse effects occurring during therapy are numerous. Localized collections of tissue fluid (periorbital, ankle, genital tissues) and numbness or tingling of peripheral tissues occur in many patients. Central nervous system effects include severe headache, dizziness, anxiety, and depression.

Ganglionic blocking agents. Chlorisondamine chloride, mecamylamine hydrochloride, pentolinium tartrate, and trimethaphan camsylate act at the sympathetic nervous system ganglion to interrupt acetylcholine-mediated transmission of neural stimuli. The neural transmitter substance at both sympathetic nervous system and parasympathetic nervous system ganglia is acetylcholine, and the same mediator is liberated at parasympathetic nervous system–organ effector sites. During therapy, the commonality of mediator substance affects both adrenergic and cholinergic activity, and the suppression of autonomic functions causes multiple problems. The drugs are used only in selected situations at the present time because of the difficulty in controlling adverse effects.

Adverse effects are related to the action of the drug on parasympathetic nervous system responses (i.e., dryness of mouth and throat, blurred vision, disturbances in gastrointestinal and bladder function). The diversity of adverse effects necessitates that the patient or a reliable family member understand the problems that are to be brought to the attention of the physician.

During long-term therapy a member of the family who has been instructed in the technique of blood pressure evaluation can maintain records of the patient's blood pressure. Periodic reevaluation of the patient is planned by the physician, and the records of blood pressure levels and notations of problems should accompany the patient to the clinic or office.

Pressoreceptor effectors. Pressoreceptors in the carotid and aortic sinuses respond to increased pressure or stretching of the arterial walls by sending messages through afferent nerves to the cardioinhibitory center in the medulla (Fig. 14-2). Efferent nerves slow the heart to decrease cardiac output. In hypertension the pressoreceptors seem to be reset at a higher level that allows sustained pressure to exist without appreciably slowing cardiac output.

Alkavervir, cryptenamine, protoveratrine A, and protoveratrines A and B (Table 14-1) increase the sensitivity level of the pressoreceptors in the carotid and aortic sinuses, and the receptors become responsive to sustained elevation of arterial pressure. Afferent impulses from the pressoreceptors stimulate the medulla cardioinhibitory centers, and efferent stimuli arriving at the atrial conduction fibers slow the cardiac rate and decrease cardiac output. The overall effect is a decrease in sympathetic nervous system control, with emergence of parasympathetic nervous system dominance in autonomic control of cardiac conduction.

The chief problem for the patient is persistent nausea, but the problem may be modified for some patients by administering the drug after meals. Regulation of dosage requires frequent blood pressure monitoring, since the drugs cause a high incidence of hypotension. The pharmacodynamic effect of the drugs may cause cardiac levels to slow excessively; therefore evaluation of apical pulse rate is planned during therapy.

Parenteral administration of the drugs increases the incidence of hypotension and bradycardia. Initial intravenous therapy requires monitoring of the cardiac rate and blood pressure continuously. The infusion is titrated to maintain a maximum systolic blood pressure decrease of less than 20 mm. Hg and a diastolic pressure decrease less than 10 mm. Hg.

Alpha adrenergic blocking. Phenoxybenzamine hydrochloride (Table 14-1) is the only alpha adrenergic blocking agent currently in use for control of hypertension. Other drugs with comparable pharmacodynamic action are occasionally used to block norepinephrine effect in control of peripheral vasospasm. Com-

176 Drugs used to control hemodynamics

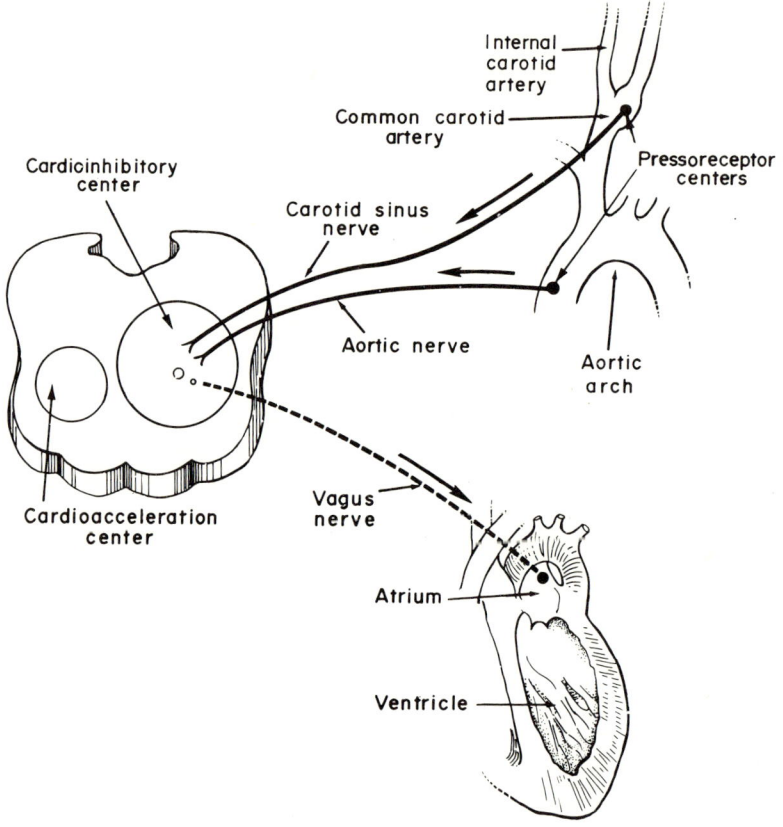

Fig. 14-2. Stimulation of the pressoreceptors in the carotid artery and aortic arch initiates afferent vagal messages to the cardioinhibitory centers. Efferent fibers act as the conduction fibers in the atrium to slow cardiac activity.

bination of phenoxybenzamine hydrochloride with the alpha receptors prevents, or blocks, the action of norepinephrine released from the sympathetic nerve ending. Blocking of norepinephrine effect allows epinephrine action at beta receptors in the arterial sites, and vasodilation ensues. In addition to orthostatic hypotension, tachycardia, hypermotility of the gastrointestinal tract, nasal congestion, and miosis occur in most patients during therapy with phenoxybenzamine hydrochloride.

Patient care

Care of the patient receiving hypotensive agents requires varied measures directed at maintaining the health status of the individual. Knowledge of the rationale for the therapeutic plan is important to informed participation in implementing the program and helping the patient understand the implications and predictable outcomes of the particular plan for his care.

Hypotensive agents are used with other agents to produce a multipronged attack on the elevated blood pressure levels of the patient, and the effectiveness of all measures is evaluated during therapy. Although it is important to determine whether the drugs have modified the cardiac and vascular status of the patient, it is also necessary to monitor the effect of changed hemodynamics on other vital functions and on problems perceived by the patient.

Pharmacodynamic effect of the drugs used to decrease vasoconstriction is accomplished by interceding at various sympathetic nervous system sites to modify neural control. The planned effect carries with it the problems of decreased reactivity to environmental (internal or external) changes. Sudden positional changes often cause postural, or orthostatic, hypotension resulting from peripheral pooling of venous blood. Drugs decreasing pressure by slowing cardiac activity (i.e., pressoreceptor effectors) may also cause dizziness during episodes of bradycardia when less blood arrives at cerebral tissues. Encouraging the patient to avoid sudden rising from a supine position by sitting on the edge of the bed before standing allows time for the redistribution of blood. Deliberate and slower movement may prevent the dizziness and loss of balance occurring with sudden movement. Application of elastic stockings or bandages from the ankle to the groin may lessen peripheral venous blood pooling and decrease hypotension.

An important factor in the pharmacotherapeutic plan for the patient is maintenance of pressure levels effective for that individual. Hypotension may exist for the patient when diastolic blood pressure drops below 90 mm. Hg. The therapeutic aim is generally to maintain the systolic level below 160 mm. Hg and the diastolic level at or below 100 mm. Hg. The condition of internal vessels is a factor in determination of the level that can effectively distribute blood to the tissues. The concept that vascular collapse exists for the patient with hypertension when the diastolic blood pressure is at a much higher level than the normal ranges of pressure is important when monitoring the effect of hypotensive agents.

Antihypertensive drugs may be used for control of acute episodes of hypertension, but the drugs are most frequently prescribed for patients with hypertension who continue with their patterns of daily living. Some individuals may need assistance to identify and modify extreme stress-producing activities and to plan specific measures within the therapeutic plan. Informed approaches to planning productive activities within the limits imposed by hypertension can increase the patient's joy in living.

CORONARY ARTERY CONSTRICTION

Elasticity and patency of the coronary arteries are necessary to supplying oxygen to meet the needs of cardiac muscle during exercise. A disproportion between supply and demand for blood limits the activity tolerance of the individual. Loss of elasticity and deposition of calcium occurring concurrently with the aging process decrease the responsiveness of coronary arteries to changing oxygen requirements of myocardial tissue. Thrombi in coronary arteries deprive myocardial tissue of blood supply in areas distal to the occlusion. The amount of blood available to nourish cardiac tissue affects the activity limits of the individual.

Oxygen requirements of the myocardium increase in a direct relationship with the intensity and duration of exercise or activity. As myocardial demands for blood exceed the supply, metabolic products are liberated (i.e., lactic acid) that irritate pain receptors in cardiac tissues and cause a classic pattern of pain perception (Fig. 14-3). Activity-related pain may be perceived in a radiation pattern including the angle of the left mandible and the left hand. Individual variation occurs, but the consistent pattern is pain that radiates to the left arm.

Pharmacodynamics

The drugs used for improvement of blood supply to the myocardium are highly specific and provide coronary vasodilation that allows activity to be resumed. Concurrent with drug use, patients with prior thrombotic occlusion of a coronary artery may participate in an exercise tolerance–building program to enhance the development of collateral circulation and supply oxygen to the tissues with minimal blood supply (ischemic tissue). The exercise program is a carefully planned progression of activities maintained below the anginal pain threshold of the patient. Weight reduction is essential for the obese patient with angina pectoris. The combined plan of therapy is directed at decreasing the number, intensity, and the duration of anginal attacks by improving the blood supply to tissues precipitating the pain syndrome.

Nitrates are used for their specific effect on dilation of the coronary arteries. Nitrates are converted to organic nitrites, and the pharmacodynamic effect is accomplished by the direct action of nitrites on smooth muscles of the cor-

178 Drugs used to control hemodynamics

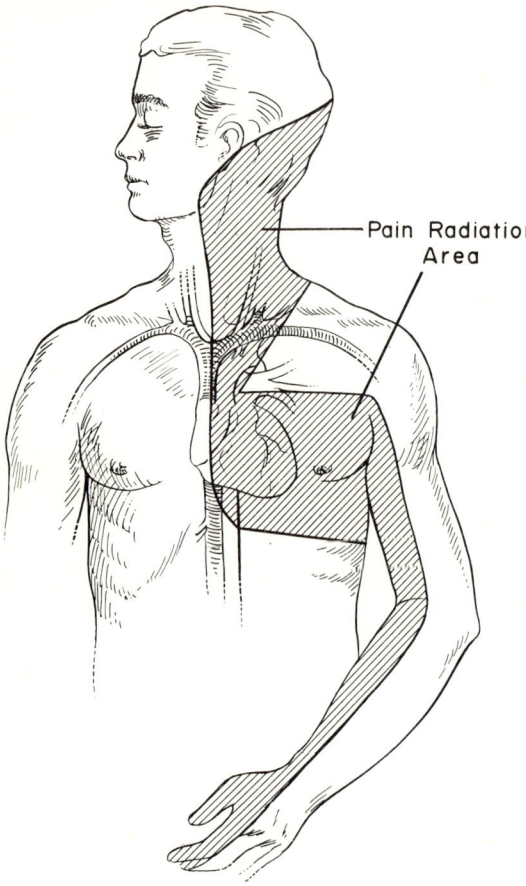

Fig. 14-3. Activity-related myocardial hypoxia produces a consistent pain radiation pattern resulting from disproportion between the demand for blood and the supply available from coronary arterial branches.

Table 14-2. Dosage range of drugs used to dilate coronary arteries

Nonproprietary name	Proprietary name	Adult dosage range
Erythrityl tetranitrate	Cardilate, Erythrol	Oral: 15-45 mg. Subl.: 15-30 mg.
Glyceryl trinitrate (nitroglycerin)		Subl.: 0.4-0.6 mg.
Inositol hexanitrate	Tolanate	Oral: 10 mg.
Isosorbide dinitrate	Isordil	Oral: 5-30 mg. Subl.: 5-10 mg.
Mannitol hexanitrate	Manicole, Maxitate, Nitranitol	Oral: 15-60 mg.
Pentaerythritol tetranitrate	Angicap, Nitrotalans, Pentritol, Peritrate, PETN	Oral: 20 mg.
Trolnitrate phosphate	Metamine, Nitretamin	Oral: 8-40 mg.

onary vasculature. Concurrent with coronary artery dilation there is vasodilation in the cerebral, splanchnic, and cutaneous vessels. The transient effect on smooth muscle of the intestine, biliary tract, and ureters is relatively innocuous during therapy, but headache and facial blushing are bothersome to the patient when high dosage of the drugs is necessary for control of periodic attacks of anginal pain.

Glyceryl trinitrate, or nitroglycerin (Table 14-2), is the drug most frequently used for control of episodic pain caused by decreased blood supply to myocardial tissue. The small sublingual tablet is allowed to dissolve under the tongue. Rapid dissolution provides nitrite effect on coronary arteries within 1 to 2 minutes.

Sublingual tablets containing erythrityl tetranitrate or isosorbide dinitrate act in a manner comparable to that of glyceryl trinitrate to dilate the coronary vessels. Isosorbide dinitrate acts within 1 to 2 minutes after the tablet is placed under the tongue. Erythrityl tetranitrate has a slower onset of action (5 to 10 minutes) when taken sublingually, but it provides a more prolonged period of effect than do the other agents.

Oral forms of the nitrates are used to provide consistent control of coronary blood supply, but patients also may require glyceryl trinitrate to control intermittent episodes of anginal pain. Administration of oral nitrates is planned before meals to provide maximum effect during eating-related work and shunting of blood to digestive organs after meals. The drugs are rapidly absorbed from the stomach in the absence of food content.

Several extended-release forms of oral nitrates are available for control of the frustrating nocturnal anginal attacks that cause the patient to waken with chest pain. The recumbent position causes hypoxia secondary to transudation of fluid into pulmonary alveolar spaces, and decreased oxygen concentrations of coronary blood precipitate anginal pain. Although some relief is provided by elevation of the mattress or pillows, the problem is resistant to positional modification in some patients. Nocturnal attacks occur most frequently during *rapid eye movement* sleep (REM), and dream recall is vivid on awakening.

Glyceryl trinitrate is occasionally used in ointment form for control of nocturnal attacks. The carefully measured layer of unguent is spread over a skin surface (usually the chest) in prescribed thickness ($1/2$ to 2 inches), and the ointment remains on the external surface to provide nightlong relief as the drug is slowly absorbed.

Fragile glass ampules containing amyl nitrite are available for emergency use by the patient. Crushing the vial in a handkerchief and inhaling the vapors provide effect in 30 seconds. Sudden, widespread dilation of arteries may cause dizziness; therefore patients are advised to be seated when taking the drug. The vapors are so noxious that the vials are distributed to young men after circumcision to control erection by reflex effect of the inhalant. A comparable coronary vasodilator with a less noxious odor, octyl nitrite (Octrite), is available in an inhaler. The convenience of use is overridden by the expense of the product, and most patients prefer the more common sublingual tablets.

Patient care

The cultural bias against taking pain-alleviating medication unless pain is present makes it difficult to communicate to the patient that sublingual forms of the drug are appropriately taken when a stress or exercise experience is forthcoming. Use of the tablets prior to the occurrence of pain-producing events decreases the incapacitation of the patient. Overdosage with the tablets is not a problem because occurrence of headache concurrent with use of several tablets causes patients to limit the number of tablets taken during any event. Patients are instructed to take additional tablets at 5-minute intervals until pain is relieved. The patient should sit in a comfortable chair when using several tablets during a short time period to avoid syncope caused by the transient hypotensive effect of the nitrites.

The frequency of drug use and the number of tablets necessary for relief of pain should be tabulated by the patient. Hospitalized patients need a supply of sublingual tablets at the bedside because immediate use is necessary for the sudden, unpredictable, intense pain. Tablets stored in a tightly stopped vial are protected against evaporation of nitroglycerin content. Deterioration of tablets decreases the therapeutic effect. Many patients benefit by a pharmacotherapeutic plan that includes both prompt-acting and extended-release forms of nitrate, and the individual plan is based on the activity tolerance of the patient.

PERIPHERAL ARTERY CONSTRICTION

The arterial blood supply to the peripheral tissues is compromised by chronic constriction of the vessels. Although aging is a common factor in causation, the problems are not limited to the aging population. Drugs are used for their direct effect on the muscles of the arterial wall to cause dilation. Many agents are capable of dilating the peripheral arteries, in addition to their effect on other organ systems. The drugs described in this section are used as primary agents for control of vasoconstriction in extremities and cerebral tissues.

Concurrent with the use of drugs to produce vasodilation, the patient is asked to increase walking exercise, cease smoking, and examine the vitamin and nutrient content of his diet. Each dimension of the therapeutic plan is directing at maximizing the potential for expansion of collateral arteries and existing arterial channels.

Pharmacodynamics

Cyclandelate, dioxyline, isoxsuprine hydrochloride, and nicotinyl alcohol (Table 14-3) act directly on the smooth muscle of the arterial vessels to cause vasodilation. Cyclandelate action is evident within 15 minutes after oral administration, and the effect lasts for 3 to 4 hours. Isoxsuprine hydrochloride tablets have a bitter taste if allowed to dissolve in the mouth. Effective levels of the drug are attained in an hour, and they last for 3 hours. Each of

Table 14-3. Dosage range of drugs frequently used to dilate peripheral arteries

Nonproprietary name	Proprietary (trade) name	Daily adult dosage range
Cyclandelate	Cyclospasmol	Oral: 0.4-1.6 Gm. (÷4)
Dioxyline	Paveril	Oral: 0.5-1 Gm. (÷3-4)
Isoxsuprine hydrochloride	Vasodilan	Oral: 30-80 mg. (÷3-4) I.M.: 5-10 mg./single dose
Nicotinyl alcohol	Roniacol	Oral: 150-600 mg. (÷3)
Nylidrin hydrochloride	Arlidin	Oral: 9-48 mg. (÷3-4) I.M.: 2.5-10 mg. (÷1-2)

the drugs is used to decrease peripheral vasospastic activity. Dioxyline is used occasionally to control constriction of coronary and pulmonary vessels.

Nylidrin hydrochloride benefits peripheral vascular circulation by an improved blood flow to the skeletal muscle, which is produced by the drug's dilating effect on small arteries and arterioles. Improved blood supply to muscle improves function and reduces anoxia-related muscle cramps or pain. Because nylidrin hydrochloride has a beta adrenergic effect (sympathomimetic) on the heart, some patients experience cardiac palpitations during therapy.

Papaverine hydrochloride (Cerespan, Pava, Pavabid, Pavadel, Vasal) is a drug traditionally used for a vasodilative effect resulting from its direct relaxant action on smooth muscle of the vasculature. It also acts on the musculature of major viscera of the abdomen, and its use has decreased as drugs with greater specificity for peripheral vessels have been formulated.

Papaverine hydrochloride is a synthetic drug prepared from opium, but it is not addictive.

Although oral forms precipitate few adverse effects, intravenous use of the drug may cause generalized vasodilation (sweating, flushed face, slight decrease in blood pressure). Papaverine is a central nervous system depressant, and lethargy, drowsiness, and malaise during therapy may be potentiated by other central nervous system depressants.

The effectiveness of the drug on compromised peripheral circulation is monitored regularly during therapy. Pedal or popliteal pulses, skin temperature, and color of the affected extremities provide clues to the effect of the drug on the vasculature.

Alpha adrenergic blocking agents that are sometimes used for their positive effect on dilation of peripheral arteries include azapetine phosphate (Ilidar); phentolamine mesylate (Regitine); and tolazoline hydrochloride (Priscoline, Tolpal). Blocking of the receptor sites prevents norepinephrine action and allows epinephrine action at beta receptors to produce vasodilation.

Patient care

The target sites for action of the drugs vary from blood vessels in the legs to arterial circulation in cerebral tissues. The effect of the drugs on the patient's problems may appear after prolonged use rather than at initiation of therapy; therefore recurrent periodic evaluation of progress by the physician is a planned part of the therapeutic program.

Peripheral pulses (radial, pedal, popliteal) indicate the status of arterial blood supply in the extremity. Comparison of the color and temperature changes in the tissues of the affected limb with those of the alternate extremity may be possible when one limb is involved, but more accurate comparison can be obtained from previous records or observations made by the patient.

Dilation of cerebral vessels may cause headache, and generalized vasodilation may lower the blood pressure at peak effect times of the drug. The patient should be aware that recurrent problems are to be evaluated with the physician to allow modification of dosage or drug form.

Self-administration of the drugs and maintenance of the plans for exercise and dietary modification are the responsibility of the patient during the long-term plan of therapy. It is important that he know the predictable effects and discomforts that may occur. His involvement in planning therapy may increase his conscientious maintenance of the plan.

REFERENCES

Benson, Herbert: How antihypertensive drugs act: a physiologic approach, Resident-Intern consultant 1:11, Feb., 1972.

Bhatia, Surindar, and Frohlich, Edward D.: The 'hypertensive' evaluation, American Family Physician 5:83, Feb., 1972.

Dustan, Harriet P., Tarazi, Robert C., and Bravo, Emmanuel L.: Dependence of arterial pressure on intravascular volume in hypertension, The New England Journal of Medicine 286:861, 1972.

Gantt, Clarence L.: Drug therapy of essential hypertension, Modern Medicine 39:94, 1971.

Goth, Andres: Medical pharmacology, ed. 6, St. Louis, 1972, The C. V. Mosby Co.

Guyton, Arthur C.: Textbook of medical physiology, ed. 4, Philadelphia, 1971, W. B. Saunders Co.

Haber, Edgar: The renin-angiotensin system in curable hypertension, Modern Concepts of Cardiovascular Disease 38:17, 1969.

Herdson, Peter B.: Some newer concepts of the fine structure of normal and diseased blood vessels, Medical Clinics of North America 51:139, 1967.

Herting, Robert L., and Hunter, Harry L.: The physiologic and pharmacologic basis for the clinical treatment of hypertension, Medical Clinics of North America 51:25, 1967.

Hollenberg, Norman K., and Adams, Douglas F.: Hypertension and intrarenal perfusion patterns in man, The American Journal of the Medical Sciences 261:232, 1971.

Indeglia, Robert A., Shea, Michael A., Griffin, Ward O., Jr., and Bernstein, Eugene F.: The importance of pulse pressure in renal hypertension, Surgical Clinics of North America 47:1395, 1967.

Jackson, Bettie Springer: Chronic peripheral arterial disease, American Journal of Nursing 72:928, 1972.

Mason, Dean T.: Control of the peripheral circulation in health and disease, Modern Concepts of Cardiovascular Disease 36:25, 1967.

Milnor, William R.: Pulsatile blood flow, The New England Journal of Medicine 287:27, 1972.

Mundth, E. D., Harthorne, J. W., Buckley, M. J., Dinsmore, R. E., and Austen, W. G.: Direct coronary artery vascularization for segmental occlusive disease, Surgery 67:168, 1970.

Page, Irvine H., editor: Symposium on hypertension, Modern Medicine 40:74, 1972.

Redwood, David R., Rosing, Douglas R., and Epstein, Stephen E.: Effects of physical training in patients with angina pectoris, The New England Journal of Medicine 286:959, 1972.

Reilly, Mary Jo, editor: American hospital formulary service, vol. 1, sect. 24:08, Washington, D. C., 1973, American Society of Hospital Pharmacists.

Russek, Henry I.: Intractable angina pectoris, Medical Clinics of North America 54:333, 1970.

Varady, P. D., and Maxwell, M. H.: Changes in diastolic blood pressure, The Journal of the American Medical Association 221:365, 1972.

Zacest, Rudolf, Gilmore, Edward, and Koch-Weser, Jan: Antihypertensive therapy with combination of propranolol and hydralazine, The New England Journal of Medicine 286:617, 1972.

15

Blood coagulation

Clot-producing factors
    Pharmacodynamics
Intravascular clotting prophylaxis
    Pharmacodynamics
    Patient care
Coagulation deficits
    Pharmacodynamics

Blood clotting is one of the body's protective mechanisms. Without this protection, large quantities of blood would spill from a small cut on the hand. There are no observable factors interrupting bleeding in the first few seconds after a laceration; then, suddenly, clotting occurs. Thrombin plays a central role as the principal autocatalyst in the clotting process. In addition to the reaction at the site of injury, other factors aid in sealing off the bleeding vessel: there is prompt local reflex vasoconstriction, clotted blood in tissues surrounding the injury compresses the vessels, and a vasoconstrictor factor is liberated from disintegrating platelets. The final physiologic seal, or clot, protects against further blood loss.

CLOT-PRODUCING FACTORS

Formation of intravascular clots disrupts normal hemodynamic relationships within the venous or arterial circulation. Venous or arterial thrombi may build to the point at which the vessel is totally occluded, or an embolus may be liberated to travel with the blood until it reaches a small vessel that stops its passage. In the arteries accumulated lipid deposits, commonly seen in patients with atherosclerosis, acquire fibrous and hyaline components and form plaques. The deposits encroach on the arterial lumen and cause irregularities that provide sites for platelet accumulation and thrombus formation.

Drugs may be used to modify factors involved in the coagulation process, as well as those contributing to clot formation. Drugs are widely used to control the formation of thrombi secondary to accumulation of lipid deposit in the arteries. Elevated serum cholesterol levels (normal: 150 to 280 mg.) are predispositional factors found in many of the 500,000 patients treated each year in the United States for acute coronary artery occlusion.

Pharmacodynamics

Dietary modification is a preliminary and important step in control of serum cholesterol levels. Long-chain saturated fatty acids cause platelet aggregation and enhance blood coagulation. The patient's diet is carefully scrutinized to seek ways to control dietary intake of fat, carbohydrate, and protein. Each of the nutrients is important to lowering serum cholesterol and lipid levels. For example, the intake of dietary fats should represent a 3:1 ratio of unsaturated fats to saturated fats to effect a reduction in serum cholesterol. Drugs may reduce hypercholesterolemia or hypertriglyceridemia during therapy, but serum levels return to pretreatment values when therapy is discontinued.

Corn oil (Table 15-1) has been used to provide unsaturated fats necessary to dietary control of fat content. Other oils have been used as dietary supplements, but patients seldom are enthusiastic with their use. The vegetable oils contain both saturated and unsaturated fatty acid glycerides, but there is a greater

Table 15-1. Dosage range of drugs used to lower blood lipid levels

Nonproprietary name	Proprietary (trade) name	Daily adult dosage range (oral)
Aluminum nicotinate	Nicalex	3-6 Gm. (÷3)
Clofibrate	Atromid-S	2 Gm. (÷4)
Corn oil		90-270 ml. (÷3)
Dextrothyroxine sodium	Choloxin	1-8 mg.
Sitosterols	Cytellin	9-36 Gm. (÷4)
Vitamin E		10-300 U.

proportion of unsaturated fatty acid glycerides in the oils. The caloric content of the oil is considered in regulation of the overall caloric intake (i.e., corn oil: 90 ml. = 540 calories).

Clofibrate is an oral tablet used to inhibit the rate of biosynthesis of cholesterol. It affects the serum levels of cholesterol or triglycerides through action on beta lipoproteins. The most frequent adverse effect is nausea, although a variety of gastrointestinal disturbances may occur during therapy. Clofibrate potentiates the effect of anticoagulants by increasing prothrombin time or platelet survival time, and by decreasing platelet adhesiveness or fibrinogen levels. The drug is used more frequently as a prophylactic measure for patients with hypercholesterolemia than for patients known to have a predisposition to clot formation.

Aluminum nicotinate decreases the biosynthesis of cholesterol by interfering with the availability of coenzyme A and increasing the catabolism and oxidation of cholesterol in the liver. The drug is taken orally with meals. The adverse effects occurring during therapy are gastrointestinal distress, flushing of facial tissues, and pruritus.

Dextrothyroxine sodium has a calorigenic effect. Oral use of the drug enhances the rate of oxidation or hydroxylation of cholesterol in the liver. Although it is a component of physiologic thyroxine, it has little effect on the metabolic rate of the individual during therapy. It reaches its maximum effect on hypercholesterolemia in 2 to 3 months when employed regularly. Its chief use is for patients having little thyroid gland activity, and in that situation the adverse effect is hypermetabolism.

Considerable interest in the value of vitamin E (tocopherols) as a hypercholesterolemic agent has resulted from reports in the news media that it rapidly reduces serum levels. Tocopherols are considered necessary components of the human diet, and there is an indication of a healthful relationship between vitamin E and polyunsaturated fat diets. The relevance of vitamin E use as a therapeutic agent for control of hypercholesterolemia is being studied, but reports of study groups are still inconclusive. Currently many individuals are benefited by changes made in dietary and activity patterns while taking vitamin E. Dietary sources of the fat-soluble vitamin are plentiful, since forms of tocopherols are found in green leafy vegetables, vegetable oils, cereals, nuts, and wheat-germ oil.

Sitosterols has been used to reduce serum levels of cholesterol. The drug acts by interfering with absorption of exogenous cholesterol and reabsorption of endogenous cholesterol. Maximum decrease in serum levels appears after sitosterols has been taken for 2 months. Adverse effects of the drug are limited to gastrointestinal disturbances.

INTRAVASCULAR CLOTTING PROPHYLAXIS

Drugs are used to prevent clot formation by interrupting the physiologic clotting process, but they have no effect on existing intravascular clots. Dissolution of existing clots is accomplished by natural physiologic processes, but it takes considerable time for the phagocytic process to remove the vascular debris.

Basically the reactions of the physiologic clotting mechanism involve formation of thromboplastin, conversion of prothrombin to thrombin, and formation of fibrin from fibrinogen (Fig. 15-1). Vitamin K is a precursor required for synthesis of several coagulation factors, and it is essential to formation of prothrombin in the liver. Vitamin K is available from many food sources, including cabbage, cauliflower, spinach, kale, cheese, tomatoes, egg yolk, fish, and liver. Bacterial synthesis of

184 Drugs used to control hemodynamics

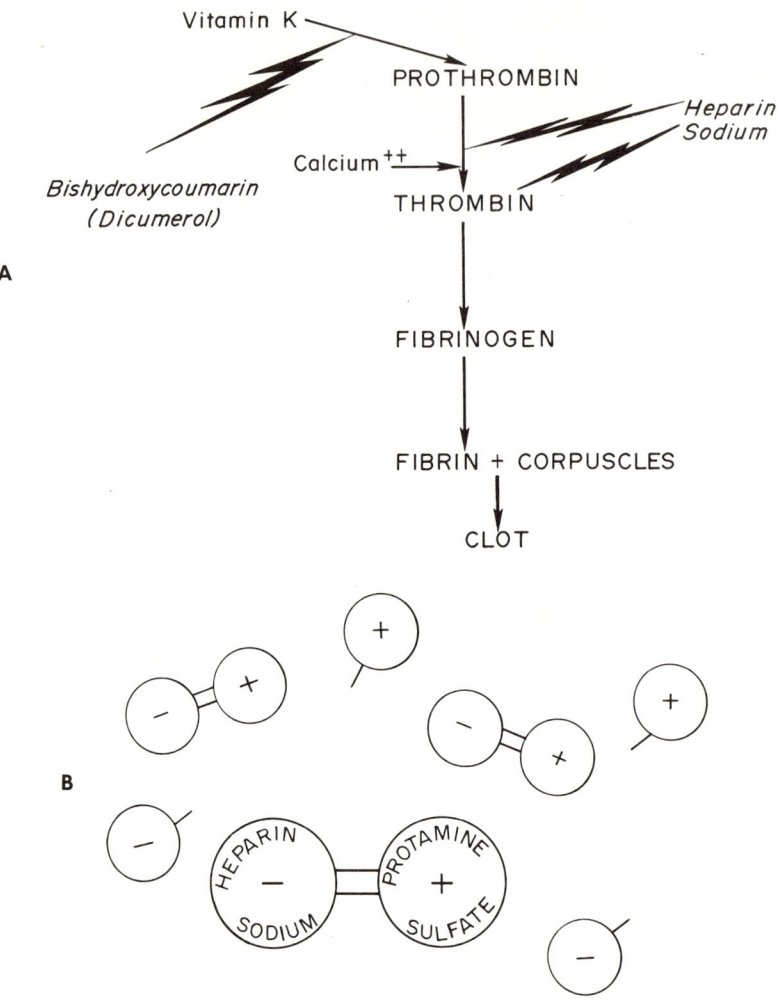

Fig. 15-1. **A,** Disruption of the normal coagulation process is accomplished as bishydroxycoumarin interferes with the prothrombin-thrombin conversion and the activity of thrombin. **B,** Administration of protamine sulfate halts the anticoagulant action of heparin sodium by uniting with the molecules and neutralizing their electroactivity.

vitamin K in the human intestine contributes to endogenous supplies necessary to maintain the coagulation process.

Pharmacodynamics

Heparin sodium and bishydroxycoumarin (Table 15-2) are examples of drugs used to interrupt the coagulation process. Hospitalized patients often receive heparin sodium intravenously as initial therapy for the prevention of clot formation. Bishydroxycoumarin may be administered orally during the time heparin sodium is administered intravenously. There is a 12- to 36-hour latent period before bishydroxycoumarin affects prothrombin formation, and at the the end of that period heparin sodium administration may be discontinued.

Inhibition of clot formation. Heparin sodium is a natural mucopolysaccharide found in the intestine. The commercial product has an effect on the clotting mechanism immediately after intravenous infusion is started (Table 15-2). Pharmacodynamic action involves interactions between heparin sodium and proteins of

Table 15-2. Dosage range of anticoagulants

Nonproprietary name	Proprietary (trade) name	Daily adult dosage range
Acenocoumarol	Sintrom	Oral: 2-28 mg.
Anisindione	Miradon	Oral: 25-300 mg.
Bishydroxycoumarin	Dicumarol	Oral: 50-300 mg.
Dipyridamole	Persantin	Oral: 100 mg. (÷4)
Heparin sodium	Bio-Heprin, Hepathrom, Lipo-Hepin, Liquaemin, Panheprin	I.V.: 5000-40,000 U. (÷4-6) S.C.: 8000-20,000 U. (÷2-3)
Phenindione	Danilone, Hedulin, Indon	Oral: 200-300 mg. (÷2)
Phenprocoumon	Liquamar, Marcumar	Oral: 0.75-30 mg.
Warfarin potassium	Athrombin-K	Oral: 5-60 mg.
Warfarin sodium	Coumadin, Panwarfin, Warcoumin	Oral: 5-60 mg. I.M.: Same as oral I.V.: Same as oral

Table 15-3. Dosage range of anticoagulant inactivators

Nonproprietary name	Proprietary (trade) name	Daily adult dosage range
Menadiol sodium diphosphate	Kappadione, Synkayvite, Thylokay	Oral: 3-24 mg. (÷1-3) I.M.: 75 mg./single dose
Menadione	Kappaxin, Kayklot, Kayquinone, Kolklot	Oral: 1-2 mg.
Menadione sodium bisulfite	Hykinone	I.M.: 0.5-2 mg. I.V.: Same as I.M.
Phytonadione (vitamin K_1)	AquaMephyton, Konakion, Mephyton, Mono-Kay	Oral: 5-50 mg. (÷2) I.M.: Same as oral I.V.: 5-25 mg.
Protamine sulfate		I.V.: 10-50 mg.

the enzyme systems to inhibit prothrombin activation and conversion to thrombin (Fig. 15-1). It interrupts the thrombokinase interaction (with calcium ions) that converts prothrombin to thrombin and blocks the enzymatic activity of thrombin necessary to fibrin formation.

Clotting time determination. Heparin sodium effect is monitored by determination of the venous clotting time. One test involves timing of the clot formation end point or the time when the clot is well formed and the test tube can be inverted without loss of blood (Lee-White method). Heparin sodium dosage is regulated to maintain the clotting time at 20 to 40 minutes (normal: below 20 minutes).

Heparin sodium inactivation. Bleeding during therapy necessitates interruption of the intravenous infusion. Circulating heparin is inactivated by administration of protamine sulfate (Table 15-3). The latter drug carries a strong positive charge, and it unites with the negative charge of heparin sodium to form an inert complex (Fig. 15-1, *B*). Protamine sulfate acts on a one-to-one basis with the dosage of heparin sodium: therefore attempts are made to calculate the amount of circulating heparin sodium. Inactivation of the anticoagulant occurs within 5 minutes after intravenous administration of protamine sulfate.

Prothrombin inactivators. Acenocoumarol, bishydroxycoumarin, phenprocoumon, warfarin sodium, and warfarin potassium (Table 15-2) are identified pharmacologically as coumarin anticoagulants. Pharmacodynamic action involves interference with the utilization of vitamin K in the liver. The anticoagulants compete with vitamin K for attachment sites in the synthesis of prothrombin.

Anisindione and phenindione (Table 15-2) act pharmacodynamically in a manner comparable to that of the coumarin derivatives. The difference in chemical derivation between these drugs and coumarin derivatives is only evident in the tendency of drug metabolites from these drugs to impart an orange-red color in alkaline urine.

The anticoagulants are oral agents used for long-term maintenance of hypoprothrombinemia. Although warfarin sodium can be given parenterally, heparin sodium is used if an anticoagulant is necessary and the patient cannot take an oral drug.

Prothrombin level monitoring. The pharmacodynamic effect is monitored by laboratory tests of prothrombin activity. The patient's prothrombin level is compared with that of an untreated individual who is his control, or guide. Daily laboratory studies are done to determine the daily dosage of the drug that will maintain the patient's prothrombin level at one and one-half to two and one-half times the control prothrombin time. Dosage is calculated on the basis of prothrombin reports each day during the drug–prothrombin level adjustment period, and administration of the drug is planned at a regular time in the late afternoon or evening to allow return of the prothrombin reports. Daily dosage prescription is the single dose needed to adjust the patient's prothrombin level to the therapeutic range. The interval between prothrombin tests is lengthened gradually as the patient's response to the drug becomes stabilized.

There are many over-the-counter drugs (including aspirin) that have an effect on prothrombin activity; therefore the patient is asked to consult with the physician before taking any medication during anticoagulant therapy. Aspirin and oral anticoagulants act at common sites in the hepatic pathway for synthesis of prothrombin, and use of the two drugs concurrently interferes with control of therapeutic levels of hypoprothrombinemia. Aspirin also has an effect on platelets that may increase bleeding potential when the patient is receiving anticoagulants.

Follow-up of the progress of the patient and determination of anticoagulant dosage are facilitated if a daily record of prothrombin values and anticoagulant dosage is maintained during therapy (Fig. 15-2). It is helpful to the physician in evaluating anticoagulant response if the patient maintains a similar record for review during periodic visits to the clinic or physician's office. Patients carry identification cards indicating the type of anticoagulant taken and the appropriate measures to use if accidental bleeding or injury occurs.

Excess prothrombin level effect. When massive bleeding or hemorrhage occurs during use

ANTICOAGULANT CHANGE 2: COUMADIN										
COAGULANT CONCENTRATION			DOSE PRESCRIBED (mg)							SIDE EFFECTS
Date Blood Drawn	Result	Control	S	M	T	W	T	F	S	
4/4/73	13.6	12.5							5	
4/5	15.7		2							
4/6	20.7			0.5						
4/7	19.9				0.5					
4/8	16.5					1.5				
4/9	11.0						1.5			
4/10	15.4							2.5		
4/11	14.2								2.5	
4/12	15.9		2.5							
4/13	14.4			5						
4/14	13.4				7.5					
4/15	17.0					7.5				
4/16	22.2					0				

Fig. 15-2. Graphic records are maintained to show the progress of anticoagulant therapy. Correlation of warfarin sodium (Coumadin) dosage with prothrombin tests is shown by daily recordings on the anticoagulant chart.

of any anticoagulant, control of the bleeding is a primary factor, and blood or plasma may be used to replace blood loss. Discontinuance of the anticoagulant is a second step, and inactivation of physiologic levels of the drug follows.

Lowering of the normal circulating prothrombin (normal: 300 to 375 units/100 ml. plasma) below the therapeutic level (normal: 10% to 30%) may result in petechial or gross hemorrhage. Bleeding that occurs during therapy with drugs acting to compete with vitamin K in the formation of prothrombin may be controlled with the administration of vitamin K.

Changes in prothrombin activity occur within 4 hours after administration of vitamin K by either intravenous or oral route. Excessive prolongation of the prothrombin time (or hemorrhage) may necessitate the use of an intravenous form of the vitamin to rapidly accelerate production of prothrombin. Menadione sodium bisulfite and phytonadione (Table 15-3) are the vitamin K preparations used parenterally. In the absence of bleeding, oral administration of menadiol sodium diphosphate or menadione may be given to return hypoprothrombinemia to the therapeutic range. The oral drugs are also used to increase the available vitamin K prior to procedures that cause excessive bleeding (i.e., tonsillectomy) or to replace deficits of the vitamin when food or bacterial sources are unavailable.

Platelet aggregation effectors. The accumulation of platelets is necessary to formation of intravascular clots, and measures preventing their aggregation can control clot formation. Endogenous physiologic levels of heparin maintain a clot-free vasculature in normal circumstances. When predisposition to clot formation is high, exogenous supplies of heparin or other prophylactic agents are needed.

One of the simplest therapeutic programs for interrupting aggregation of platelets in tiny arterioles is the consistent use of aspirin. Therapy is based on an observation that aspirin decreases the adhesiveness of platelets. Patients participating in the pharmacotherapeutic program (i.e., patients with transient blindness secondary to recurrent emboli in retinal arterioles) are delighted with the simplicity of the plan that controls their problem without extensive drug use or other therapy.

Dipyridamole (Table 15-2) is used chiefly to control platelet aggregation in patients with surgery of cardiac valves. Inhibition of glucose utilization by platelets slows aggregation in the vessel lumen. Concurrent administration of an oral anticoagulant provides a dual attack in decreasing the incidence of intravascular clots. The use of bishydroxycoumarin decreases the production of precursors to clot formation by interceding in the coagulation process, and dipyridamole decreases the aggregation of platelets and their liberation of thrombin at tissue sites. Dipyridamole is taken $1/2$ hour before or 2 hours after meals, and bishydroxycoumarin is taken in the evening during the indefinite period when the patients require the drugs as prophylaxis against clot formation.

Patient care

Immobility is a factor in stasis of blood that predisposes to clot formation in venous branches. Individuals with jobs that necessitate standing or sitting for long periods have a high potential for distortion of veins in the legs (varicosities). Exercise of the legs should be planned during periods of immobility to increase the flow of blood through the veins. Simple rotation of the ankle with extension and flexion of the leg increases the milking effect of the muscles on the deep veins and prevents stasis of blood in the veins.

The patient taking an anticoagulant is instructed to consult with his physician immediately if injury, unusual bleeding, or bruising occurs. He must understand the importance of reporting nosebleed, blood in the urine, black or bloody stools, or severe headaches. The same observations are planned while the patient is hospitalized. Testing of stools and vomitus for microscopic blood may provide early evidence of gastric bleeding.

Food-drug interactions. Excessive ingestion of foods rich in vitamin K will antagonize the effect of the anticoagulant. Discussion of dietary habits with the patient will provide clues to whether restrictions are necessary.

Drugs used concurrently with anticoagulants may affect the therapeutic program adversely by disrupting the stability of the drug-coagulation relationship necessary to prevent intravascular clot formation or hemorrhage. Potentiation of anticoagulant effect may occur with drugs that impair platelet function, anticoagulant degradation, albumin binding of the anticoagulant, or absorption of vitamin K from the intestine. Inhibition of anticoagulant effect may be caused by drugs that stimulate anticoagulant-degrading enzymes in the liver or decrease other clotting factors.

The following examples of drug interactions show some of the problems that are considered when anticoagulants are used for control of prothrombin formation. Drugs taken concurrently may potentiate the anticoagulant effect by impairing platelet function (i.e., salicylates, chlorpromazine); impairing anticoagulant degradation (i.e., tolbutamide, chloramphenicol); interfering with albumin binding of the anticoagulant (i.e., sulfisoxazole, phenylbutazone, indomethacin, clofibrate); or decreasing absorption of vitamin K from the intestine (i.e., cholestyramine resin). Drugs administered concurrent with anticoagulants may inhibit action by stimulating enzymes that degrade the anticoagulant (i.e., barbiturates, chloral hydrate, glutethimide) or decreasing other clotting factors (i.e., oral contraceptives). The diversity of categories makes it a herculean task to memorize all the drugs that fit within the classifications.

The most meaningful instructions for the patient are that he consult his physician before taking any medication that is not included in the current anticoagulant program. Additional protection is afforded by specifically telling the patient that aspirin and vitamin preparations containing vitamin K may affect the amount of drug necessary to maintain the therapeutic effect of the anticoagulant. The specific definition of the two products is necessary to demonstrate that agents the patient usually does not consider as drugs may affect control of coagulation. In a recent tabulation it was found that there are in excess of 400 readily available over-the-counter products that contain salicylates.

Schedule planning. Definition of a specific schedule for taking the drug may assure regularity of use. When patients have taken drugs on a regular basis for chronic problems, they probably will remember to take the anticoagulant each evening. Additional reminders or ritualistic schedules are necessary for the novice in drug taking. Providing the patient with a calendar and instructions for recording the amount of drug taken each day may improve recall patterns. The schedule for periodic prothrombin tests done at a laboratory near his home can be included on the calendar.

The stability of the therapeutic plan is significant. The patient should know the importance of arranging for prothrombin tests during travel and the necessity for regularly scheduled visits to the clinic or physician's office for evaluation of progress. To avoid trauma-related hemorrhage or prescription of drugs interfering with the anticoagulation plan, the patient should inform his dentist and other physicians involved in planning his care that he is taking an anticoagulant.

COAGULATION DEFICITS

Inherited or acquired deficiencies of the multiple factors necessary to blood coagulation predispose the individual to external or internal

Table 15-4. Dosage range of drugs used for antihemorrhagic effects

Nonproprietary name	Proprietary (trade) name	Daily adult dosage range
ϵ-Aminocaproic acid	ϵ-Amicar	Oral: 5-30 Gm. ($\div$4-8) I.V.: Same
Antihemophilic factor (human)	Hemofil	I.V.: 10-20 ml.
Carbazochrome salicylate	Adrenosem, Adrestat	I.M.: 4-20 mg. ($\div$4)
Factor IX complex (human)	Konȳne	I.V.: 2 U./kg.
Fibrinogen (human)	Parenogen	I.V.: 1-6 Gm.
Plasma, antihemophilic (human)		I.V.: 100 ml.
Thrombin		Oral: 10,000 U.

hemorrhage (i.e., joints, body cavities). Although fresh whole blood provides replacement, identification of the specific missing factors makes it possible to use selected agents to replace the deficit without blood volume overload.

Pharmacodynamics

Coagulation factor replacement. Antihemophilic factor, factor IX complex, and antihemophilic plasma (Table 15-4) are obtained from human sources. The agents are used for replacement of deficient coagulation factors.

Antihemophilic plasma maintains a normal clotting time for from several hours to 2 days after administration. Because it contains 60 times more factor VIII than blood plasma, it is used for temporary control of bleeding when the patient has deficient levels of the coagulation cofactor. Patients with hemophilia have plasma antihemophilic factor values of less than 5% of normal, and administration of antihemophilic factor will raise plasma antihemophilic activity by 2%. The concentrated preparation containing antihemophilic factor VIII allows low volume therapy to raise the antihemophilic factor level to that necessary to provide hemostasis in the presence of hemorrhage (30%).

Factor IX complex (human) contains factors II, VII, IX, and X in concentrations twenty-four times as high as those of normal plasma. Administration is planned to raise the level of each of the factors to that necessary for hemostasis (i.e., factor II = 20%, factor VII = 10%, factor IX = 15%, factor X = ?).

The specificity of use makes it important to review guides to the use of each of the agents before assisting with administration in an emergency situation. The patient and family are generally the most informed members of the health team when the basic problem is hemophilia-related hemorrhage. Their exposure to the problems and control patterns over the years has prepared them to handle many situations that are unfamiliar to other members of the health team. Therapeutic plans recently have been expanded to include preparation of the patient or a member of his family to administer the antihemophilic factor intravenously when bleeding occurs. Self-therapy has decreased the number of hospitalizations and increased job stability of individuals with hemophilia.

Clotting factor replacement. Provision of materials for the meshwork necessary for terminal steps in the clotting process could be as simple as placing a dry gauze over an open surface lesion. The gauze provides the framework, comparable to that of fibrin, that collects platelets, blood cells, and other plasma products, and a clot is formed. Drugs are used to improve local dynamics necessary to clot organization.

Epsilon-aminocaproic acid (Table 15-4) is known by the initials representing its composition—EACA. The pharmacodynamic action is accomplished by inhibition of the enzyme required for destruction of formed fibrin. The outcome of administration is increased fibrinogen activity in clot formation. The drug is used in any situation in which hyperfibrinolytic activity causes hemorrhage. It is employed after surgery requiring the use of cardiopulmonary bypass (i.e., cardiac surgery) because fibrinogen levels are decreased during passage of the blood through the heart-lung machine. Administration is planned to maintain a plasma level (130 mcg./ml.) effective for inhibition of systemic hyperfibrinolysis.

Fibrinogen (Table 15-4) is obtained from human sources, and it is used to maintain plasma fibrinogen levels necessary to provide the material for clotting (above 100 mg./100 ml.). Thrombin (Table 15-4) also supplies physiologic levels of the natural material. It is often used for control of superficial bleeding sites, and it may be applied as a spray or as a wetting material in a gauze matrix. Blood is removed from wounds before use of topical thrombin because the drug tends to form clots on the surface debris and bleeding may continue underneath the covering.

Carbazochrome salicylate (Table 15-4) is used for control of capillary bleeding. The pharmacodynamic effect is comparable to that of epinephrine, of which it is an oxidative product. Local vasoconstriction controls persistent oozing from terminal arterioles and capillaries (i.e., mucosa in nasopharynx).

REFERENCES

Berkowitz, Donald: Treatment of hyperlipidemia with clofibrate, The Journal of the American Medical Association **218**:1002, 1971.

Boston Collaborative Drug Surveillance Program: Interaction between chloral hydrate and warfarin, The New England Journal of Medicine **286**:53, 1972.

Evans, Geoffrey: Clinical applications of the platelet aggregation–release reaction to vascular disease, Current Concepts of Cerebrovascular Disease (Stroke) **7**:25, 1972.

Fillmore, Sidney J., and McDevitt, Ellen: Effects of coumarin compounds on the fetus, Annals of Internal Medicine **73**:731, 1970.

Geske, Cheryl S.: Anticoagulant therapy in acute myocardial infarction, Heart & Lung **1**:639, 1972.

Gotto, Antonio M., Jr.: Recognition and management of the hyperlipoproteinemias, Heart & Lung **1**:508, 1972.

Griffith, George C.: The life cycle of coronary artery disease, Heart & Lung **1**:63, 1972.

Haferkorn, Virginia: Assessing individual needs as a basis for patient teaching, Nursing Clinics of North America **6**:199, 1971.

Koch-Weser, Jan, and Sellers, Edward M.: Drug interactions with coumarin anticoagulants, The New England Journal of Medicine **285**:487, 547, 1971.

Lewis, Jessica H., and Bayer, William L.: Therapy in coagulation defects, Medical Clinics of North America **51**:1241, 1967.

McKusick, Victor A.: The royal hemophilia, Scientific American **213**:88, Aug., 1965.

Meyer, Ovid O.: Treatment with anticoagulants, Cardiovascular Nursing **4**:11, 1968.

Mountcastle, Vernon B., editor: Medical physiology, ed. 13, vol. 1, St. Louis, 1974, The C. V. Mosby Co.

Mustard, J. Fraser: Platelets and thrombosis in myocardial infarction, Hospital Practice **7**:115, 1972.

Reilly, Mary Jo, editor: American hospital formulary service, vol. 1, sect. 20:12, Washington, D. C., 1973, American Society of Hospital Pharmacists.

Sergis, Elaine, and Hilgartner, Margaret W.: Hemophilia, American Journal of Nursing **72**:2011, 1972.

Spain, David M.: Atherosclerosis, Scientific American **215**:48, Aug., 1966.

Sullivan, Jay M., Harken, Dwight E., and Gorlin, Richard: Pharmacologic control of thromboembolic complications of cardiac-valve replacement, The New England Journal of Medicine **284**:1391, 1971.

Zucker, Marjorie B.: In vitro studies of the platelet aggregation-release reaction, Current Concepts of Cerebrovascular Disease (Stroke) **7**:21, 1972.

16
Red blood cell deficiency

Erythropoiesis
    Pharmacodynamics
Hemoglobin production
    Pharmacodynamics
Plasma expansion
    Patient care

Plasma provides the vehicle for hemoglobin-laden red blood cells that carry oxygen to meet the functional needs of cells. As red blood cells move slowly through the tiny vessels at organ capillary sites, oxygen is released to areas of low oxygen concentration. The body employs a great mass of control mechanisms in adjusting hemodynamic factors to provide a continual supply of oxygen for cellular function.

Natural adaptive mechanisms of the body provide for correction of deficits in blood volume, and adjuctive therapeutic measures vary according to the extent of the deficit. Loss of copious amounts of blood requires replacement by transfusion of whole blood. In acute situations, plasma or intravenous fluids may be administered to provide adequate distribution of red blood cells to meet cellular oxygen requirements throughout the body. Drugs are used to support erythrocyte construction and hemoglobin synthesis in less acute situations in which the quality or quantity of erythrocytes is inadequate to meet physiologic needs.

ERYTHROPOIESIS

Red blood cells have a longer life-span than the leukocytes, their companions in the bloodstream, but their nonnucleated status allows only 100 to 125 days of physiologic activity.

The biologically useful hemoglobin carriers have progressed through several stages of development by the time they are released from production sites in spleen and marrow tissue.

Endothelial cells develop into large, multinucleated megaloblasts ready to divide and produce erythroblasts. At this stage of division, *deoxyribonucleic acid* (DNA) and *ribonucleic acid* (RNA) control the reproduction and structure of protein for new cells. Both vitamin B_{12} and folic acid are essential cofactors in DNA biosynthesis of nucleotides. Reproduction of the protein framework of erythrocytes is dependent on the presence of the cofactors and protein precursors for building structurally sound cells. Emerging erythroblasts and consequent red cell forms (normoblasts, reticulocytes, erythrocytes) are dependent on the careful construction of the cell framework at the initial major step of protein synthesis. The life-span of the spongy, colorless framework (stroma) is described as normocytic when the final product represents a cell produced with all the necessary components. Macrocytic or microcytic cells result from inadequate building supplies at the megaloblast division process.

Vitamin B_{12} is readily available in foods (cheese, eggs, meat, milk), and folic acid is available in green leafy vegetables, liver, and yeast. Both vitamins are synthesized by the nonpathogenic bacteria inhabiting the human intestine. Deficiencies of folic acid or vitamin B_{12} occur when the patient has gastrointestinal surgery or intestinal malabsorption that affects either food intake or intestinal bacterial action. The mucous glands of the stomach produce mucoprotein (intrinsic factor) that is necessary for the absorption of vitamin B_{12}; therefore

Table 16-1. Dosage range of drugs used as hematopoietic agents

Nonproprietary name	Proprietary (trade) name	Daily adult dosage range
Cyanocobalamin (vitamin B_{12})	Berubigen, Betalin 12, Bevatine-12, Bevidox, Biopar, Crystamin, Docibin, Dodecavite, Dodekroid, Redisol, Rubramin, Sytobex	I.M.: 0.007-1 mg. twice weekly I.V.: same
Ferrocholinate	Chel-Iron, Ferrolip	Oral: 1 Gm. (÷3)
Ferrous fumarate	Bidtinic, Eldofe, Firon, Fumasorb, Fumeron, Ircon, Toleron, Tolferain	Oral: 600-800 mg. (÷3-4)
Ferrous gluconate	Fergon, Irox, Nionate	Oral: 0.6-1.8 Gm. (÷3)
Ferrous lactate	Ferro drops	Oral: 375-750 mg. (÷3)
Ferrous sulfate	Feosol, Fer-in-Sol, Ferralyn, Sulferrous	Oral: 0.35-1.5 Gm. (÷3)
Folate sodium	Folvite Sodium	I.M.: 0.1-40 mg. I.V.: Same
Folic acid	Folvite	Oral: 0.1-40 mg.
Hydroxocobalamin (vitamin B_{12})	AlphaRedisol, Ducobee-Hy, Rubramin OH, Sytobex-H	I.M.: 0.015-0.05 mg. twice weekly
Iron dextran injection	Imferon	I.M.: 50-250 mg.
Iron sorbitex	Jectofer	I.M.: 1.5 mg./kg.
Liver injection	Pernaemon, Reticulogen	I.M.: 2 ml.
Liver injection, crude	Campolon	I.M.: 1-2 ml.
Thiamine hydrochloride (vitamin B_1)	Betalin S, Betaxin, Thiamintol, Thibex	Oral: 5-90 mg. (÷1-3) I.M.: 100 mg. (÷2)

congenital inactivity of the mucous glands (pernicious anemia) or surgical removal of large portions of the stomach deprives the patient of the vitamin from food sources.

Pharmacodynamics

Cyanocobalamin, hydroxocobalamin, liver injection, and crude liver (Table 16-1) are the drugs used to supply vitamin B_{12} for red blood construction. Liver injection was the only drug source of vitamin B_{12} for many years, but development of the naturally occurring forms of the vitamin, cyanocobalamin and hydroxocobalamin, has decreased the use of liver injections. The chief difference between the currently popular forms of vitamin B_{12} is that hydroxocobalamin tends to produce sustained, higher blood levels that require less frequent administration. An oral form of vitamin B_{12} with intrinsic factor (Bevidoral, Bifacton, Intrinase) is available for use when natural intrinsic factor also is decreased or absent. The product is expensive, but it offers the advantage of self-administration to the patient who needs long-term therapy.

Administration of both vitamin B_{12} and folic acid (Table 16-1) may be necessary for the patient with nutritional deficiency, gastrointestinal surgery, or malabsorption. The patient with decreased function or absence of gastric mucous glands that produce intrinsic factor requires vitamin B_{12} replacement to assure production of mature erythrocytes.

Administration of vitamin B_{12} to the patient with pernicious anemia has a positive effect on the neuritis occurring concurrently with deficiency of the vitamin. Neural RNA requires vitamin B_{12} as a cofactor, and within a few weeks neural function improves. Folic acid deficit may mimic deficiency of vitamin B_{12}, but administration of folic acid does not correct vitamin B_{12} deficiency–related neuritis. Therapy with folic acid may mask the more serious vitamin B_{12} deficiency; therefore definition of the specific deficiency is a planned part of the pretreatment plan.

Administration of the vitamins results in decreased production of macrocytic red blood cells and gradual production of mature cells that raise the erythrocyte pool of viable cells to the normal range (4 to 5 million/mm.³). The vitamins are renal threshold substances; therefore excesses of the vitamins from food or drugs are excreted by the kidneys. Transient central nervous system stimulation has occurred with high dosage of folic acid.

HEMOGLOBIN PRODUCTION

The gradual change in the color of red blood cells occurring after erythroblast formation is due to the addition of large amounts of pigment by hemoglobin. Iron enters the cycle as the development of cells continues through the erythrocyte series (normoblasts, reticulocytes, erythrocytes) to fully mature structures. Cells examined for hemoglobin content are described as *hyperchromic* or *hypochromic*, depending on whether hemoglobin content is high or low. The descriptions are useful guides to the oxygen-carrying capacity of the red blood cells.

Red cells are comprised largely of hemoglobin and water inside a semipermeable membrane. The oxygen-carrying capacity of blood depends on the total circulating hemoglobin mass. Each red blood cell contains millions of hemoglobin molecules, and each hemoglobin molecule is capable of uniting with oxygen at each of the four iron atom attachment sites. Attachment of oxygen forms a new substance, oxyhemoglobin. A comparable attachment mechanism occurs in muscle tissue where myoglobin picks up oxygen from hemoglobin to transport it to cytochrome effector sites. Cellular cytochromes handle oxygen within the body cells. The iron-containing cytochromes assist in combining oxygen with hydrogen ions to release energy from nutrients. Although the number of cytochromes in each cell is minimal, they are essential intracellular carriers.

The human body contains approximately 7 grams of iron in various tissues and storage sites. Physiologic processes accomplish the recycling of iron to maintain a closed system of iron conservation (Fig. 16-1). Cleavage of the porphyrin ring releases iron from the heme portion of hemoglobin, and the released iron is moved by transferrin to storage sites for ferritin. Globin released in the process is reused to build proteins, and the disrupted pigmented prophyrin ring is excreted with bile.

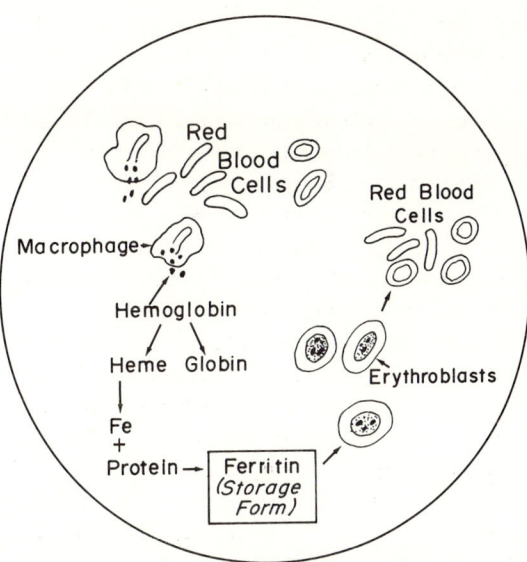

Fig. 16-1. Fragile red blood cells are broken down by macrophages in the liver, bone marrow, and spleen. The liberated iron is stored and reused for hemoglobin formation when erythroblasts synthesize new red blood cells.

Food sources of iron (ferric hydroxide) are plentiful, and they are available to replenish body stores after conversion by acids to the ferrous form, which is absorbed through the mucosa of the stomach and small intestine. Replacement of circulating storage iron is planned when hemoglobin levels fall (normal: males, 13 to 16 grams/100 ml.; females, 12 to 14 grams/100 ml.). The rate of assimilation of exogenous iron depends on the deficit in the body, and iron content of drugs appears in the hemoglobin 4 to 8 hours after oral administration.

Pharmacodynamics

The route used for iron replacement depends on the ability of the patient to take oral agents. The variety of oral forms available (Table 16-1) reflects individual tolerances to the iron products. Ferrous sulfate is the least expensive form, but many patients have gastrointestinal problems while taking it (nausea, constipation, diarrhea). Gastric irritation may be decreased by administration of the drug with meals. Children tolerate ferrous lactate best, but they may benefit from vitamin-iron mixtures that meet the growth and development needs of their bodies.

Drug replacement for correction of iron deficiency in a young child often provides rapid change in hematologic status and behavior. Absorption of iron at 25 mg./day raises the hemoglobin 1%/day in the acute iron deficiency occurring commonly at the 6-month, 12-month, and 2-year age level of children. The immediacy of effect may, within a few days, change an irritable, anoretic, pale, lethargic child to one with more manageable and more tolerable behavior. Replacement of iron continues beyond the time when red blood cells show improved hemoglobin content to assure replenishment of body stores of ferritin.

Liquid forms of iron preparations discolor the teeth; therefore the diluted liquid should be taken with a straw. Ascorbic acid preparations or citrus fruit juices provide the acid-reducing substance for ferrous iron and facilitate absorption of the drugs. Dilution of liquids or use of fruit juice as the vehicle for swallowing tablets enhances drug effect. Conversely, concurrent administration of antacids may slow absorption. Ideally the drugs are given before meals, but food may increase the individual's tolerance to the drug by decreasing gastric irritation.

Iron dextran injection or iron sorbitex (Table 16-1) is used when the individual is unable to take oral forms of iron. Intramuscular injection causes staining of the tissues that lasts for a short period. The manufacturers suggest a Z-tract method for injection. Circulars accompanying the drug describe the method of applying tension on gluteal tissue before administration of the drug. Subsequent release of the tissues occludes the injection tract and prevents leak of the discoloring drug into surrounding tissues. Changing the needle after aspiration of drug from the vial provides additional protection against tissue staining.

Some hypersensitivity reactions have occurred with the use of iron dextran injection, and sensitivity tests with partial dosage may be performed prior to administration of the drug on a regular dosage schedule. Gastrointestinal discomfort occurs after administration of either of the injection forms. The chief discomfort for the patient who is able to take some oral foods or liquids is the transient loss of taste perception. Patients taking iron preparations should be told that a dark green stool is expected while taking iron preparations as excess iron is excreted in the feces.

Thiamine hydrochloride (Table 16-1) has little direct effect on hemoglobin production, but deficiency of thiamine decreases the production of hydrochloric acid in the stomach (achlorhydria), and the conversion of food sources of iron may be affected. Replacement of thiamine is usual when severe nutritional deficiencies occurring secondary to gastrointestinal surgery or pathology jeopardize the patient's muscle and nerve function. Indirectly thiamine deficiency affects blood volume secondary to a dilating effect on cardiac muscle and peripheral vasodilation that spreads available blood over a wide body area.

PLASMA EXPANSION

In the presence of normal levels of blood proteins and excess tissue fluid, dextran osmotic agents may be used to improve blood volume. The chief advantage of the agents is the improvement of capillary blood flow without an increase in exogenous administration of fluids. Dextran 40 (Rheomacrodex) is used for volume expansion in treatment of shock or after surgery with cardiopulmonary bypass. The planned pharmacodynamic action of dextran 40 is a decrease in the stasis of blood and red blood cell aggregation in minute capillaries occurring with borderline or interrupted circulating blood volume. Expanded blood volume improves cardiac output and contributes to reinstitution of hemodynamic equilibrium.

Patient care

Changes in the volume and composition of blood affect the functional ability of the individual. Although problems range from borderline normal levels of hemoglobin, hematocrit, cell count, and volume to frank evidence of shock, there are commonalities in the problems that influence care plans. For example, modification of activity is indicated when the oxygen-carrying capacity of blood cells is limited. Both the anemic patient and the patient in shock will benefit by decreased physical activity. The level of oxygen deficit will influence therapeutic plans, and oxygen will be administered to the patient in shock to meet his greater need.

Albumin replacement and plasma expansion are usually single-incident therapy planned after definition of depleted volume in an acutely ill patient or in one convalescing from an acute illness. A concern during administration is maintenance of blood pressure at a level low enough (maximum, 85 mm. Hg) to avoid hemorrhage from trauma sites.

Drug effect can be assessed by comparison of blood values before and after drug administration and by objective measurement of vital parameters (blood pressure, pulse, respiration). Subjective evidence of improvement closely follows early improvement of the hemodynamic status (i.e., increased energy, interest in the environment, participation in self-care). Physical evidence of change is often slower to appear. Increased blood volume may be seen as warmth of skin surface long before surface desquamation of epithelial tissue exposes changes in turgor, moisture, or color in tissues other than those with high superficial capillary supply (i.e., mucous membranes, nail beds, ear lobes).

Problems of malnutrition continue. Concern with balanced diets has improved the nutrient content of foods ingested by many Americans, but realistic nutrition instruction remains a rich contribution that can be made while patients are receiving drugs to support physiologic erythropoiesis (and other problems).

REFERENCES

Boggs, D. R.: Homeostatic regulating mechanisms of hematopoiesis, Annual Review of Physiology **28:**39, 1966.

Cooper, Richard C., and Shattil, Sanford J.: Mechanism of hemolysis—the minimal red-cell defect, The New England Journal of Medicine **285:**1514, 1971.

Finch, Clement A., and Lenfant, Claude: Oxygen transport in man, The New England Journal of Medicine **286:**407, 1972.

Freedman, Michael L.: Treatment of crisis in sickle cell anemia, The American Journal of Medical Sciences **261:**305, 1971.

Gurski, Barbara M.: Rationale of nursing care for patients with blood dyscrasias, Nursing Clinics of North America **1:**23, 1966.

Lugliani, Robert, Whipp, Brian J., Winter, Benjamin, Tanaka, Kouichi R., and Wasserman, Karlman: The role of the carotid body in erythropoiesis in man, The New England Journal of Medicine **285:**1112, 1971.

McCurdy, Paul R.: Urea therapy in sickle cell disease, American Family Physician **5:**86, April, 1972.

Mountcastle, Vernon B., editor: Medical physiology, ed. 13, vol. 1, St. Louis, 1974, The C. V. Mosby Co.

Nathan, David G.: Thalassemia, The New England Journal of Medicine **286:**586, 1972.

Pochedly, Carl: Sickle cell anemia—recognition and management, American Journal of Nursing **71:**1948, 1971.

Reilly, Mary Jo, editor: American hospital formulary service, vol. 1, sect. 20:00, Washington, D. C., 1972, American Society of Hospital Pharmacists.

Shohet, Stephen B.: Hemolysis and changes in erythrocyte membrane lipids, The New England Journal of Medicine **286:**577, 638, 1972.

Solomon, Arthur K.: The state of water in red cells, Scientific American **224:**88, Feb., 1971.

Spigelman, Auri, and Warden, James M.: Surgery in patients with sickle cell disease, Archives of Surgery **104:**761, 1972.

Wilson, Patience: Iron-deficiency anemia, American Journal of Nursing **72:**502, 1972.

Zuckerkandl, Emilie: The evolution of hemoglobin, Scientific American **212:**110, May, 1965.

UNIT FOUR
DRUGS USED TO CONTROL ACTIVITY AND PAIN

17 Emotional responses

18 Cerebrocortical activity

19 Skeletal muscle contraction

20 Sleep patterns

21 Anesthesia

22 Pain

17
Emotional responses

Emotional response centers
Catecholamine biosynthesis
Psychotropic drug therapy
Psychic depression
    Pharmacodynamics
    Patient care
Anxiety states
    Antipsychotic drugs (major tranquilizers)
        Pharmacodynamics
        Patient care
    Antianxiety drugs (minor tranquilizers)
        Pharmacodynamics
        Patient care

As a social being each man strives to maintain relationships with his fellow man to accomplish both personal and social goals. Loss of ability to function within his personal social sphere disrupts the individual's ability to enjoy and contribute to the social relationships of his world.

The effect of disrupted emotional responses on physiologic function makes it vividly apparent that separation of emotional problems from physical problems is artificial. For example, more than half the individuals with endogenous depression complain of sleep disturbances and functional problems in major body systems (that is, cardiovascular: *palpitation, peripheral edema;* gastrointestinal: *constipation, nausea, decreased appetite with weight loss;* genitourinary: *urinary frequency, impotence;* neuromuscular: *weakness, fatigue, dizziness, headache, peripheral parethesias;* respiratory: *dyspnea*). Modification of emotional responses has a positive effect on the disrupted physiologic responses of the individual.

The patient who complains of emotional problems as disruptive to continuance of daily living activities may benefit by counseling and the physician's prescription for a drug to modify emotional responses. There are many individuals with problems in their social sphere that temporarily cause an emotional burden exceeding their ability to cope with the situation.

On the alternate end of the continuum are patients with psychiatric problems temporarily, intermittently, or consistently out of touch with reality who require the assistance of pharmacotherapeutic agents as part of an overall plan to modify emotional and somatic responses. Drug therapy enables them to respond to psychotherapy and to reestablish contacts within their small social sphere. The united efforts of many health team members are necessary to maintain the functional status of the individual.

Drugs modify emotional responses by interceding in the production or utilization of norepinephrine, dopamine, acetylcholine, or serotonin in central nervous system tissues. The role of serotonin as a synaptic transmitter in the central neuronal network is less clear than that of the catecholamines (norepinephrine, dopamine) and acetylcholine, but drugs affecting levels of each of the transmitter substances modify emotional responses.

Catecholamines have a stimulatory effect on central nervous system tissues, and acetylcholine has a depressant effect. Modification of the interaction, or balance, between the neural transmitter substances is the aim of drug therapy for control of emotional responses. The drugs act at central nervous system sites to modify physical activity and responsiveness to environmental stimuli.

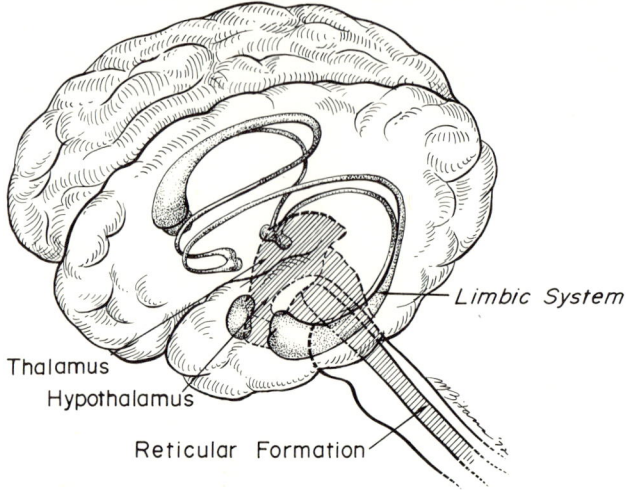

Fig. 17-1. The limbic system, thalamus, hypothalamus, and reticular formation are the effector sites of drugs used to control emotional responses.

Emotional response centers

The chief control sites for emotional responses are centered in the limbic system, thalamus, hypothalamus, and reticular formation (Fig. 17-1), but the interrelationship between cortical, subcortical, and peripheral nervous system stimuli is inseparable. The balanced relationship between the neural hormones is comparable to that exercised on other body processes, and drugs that attenuate activity of the neurohormones in the central nervous system also have some effect on functional control of the neurohormones in other areas of the body. Conversely, drugs administered to modify the liberation of neurohormonal transmitter substance in other body systems may effect the transmitter substance in the central nervous system if they are capable of crossing the blood-brain barrier. Specificity of effect is related to the particular chemical composition of the drug. Systemic effects occurring concurrently with drug action at central nervous system target sites may be modified by dosage adjustment or by concomitant administration of drugs to control adverse effects.

Catecholamine biosynthesis

Concentrations of the catecholamines are highest in the deep brain structures. Dopamine levels in the *putamen, caudate nucleus,* and *substantia nigra* are high, but the concentration of norepinephrine is highest in the anterior hypothalamus and dorsal medulla. Concentrations of the catecholamines are considerably less in the cerebral tissues.

The vital catecholamines are synthesized from *tyrosine* in a pathway that requires enzymatic action:

Tyrosine
   ↓← Tyrosine hydroxylase
Dopa
     ↓← L-Aromatic amino acid decarboxylase
   Dopamine
      ↓←Dopamine beta-oxidase
    Norepinephrine

Although the precursors, enzymes, and catecholamines are vital to controlled emotional responses, they also play an important role in peripheral responses that are integrated in brain centers. For example, low levels of dopa at the substantia nigra produces the problems of incoordinate movements and dominance of parasympathetic responses at central and peripheral sites seen in Parkinson's disease.

Psychotropic drug therapy

The pharmacotherapeutic aim is to provide a better-organized emotional response of the patient to the environment. Drugs are used to elevate or depress the level of response, and the physician's decision to use a particular agent is based on the symptom complex and behavior demonstrated by the patient. *Antidepressants* and *tranquilizers* are the chief agents used for control of emotional responses. The specific mode of action of some of the drugs is incompletely understood, but overt effects indicate particular action modality.

PSYCHIC DEPRESSION

Drugs used for mental depression of exogenous or endogenous origin act to improve mood, increase mental activity, and restore vitality. The depression of physiologic activity concurrent with depressed emotional responses necessitates the use of measures to maintain physiologic function during therapy. Disrupted organ function may potentiate emotional problems and place limits on the patient's physiologic progress.

Pharmacodynamics

The depressed patient or his family may identify the problems of hopelessness, sadness, fatigue, sleeplessness, irritability, or anorexia as requiring attention, but the problems persist until the depressed state improves. Antidepressants may be used to improve the patient's readiness for psychotherapy and relieve functional problems occurring as manifestations of his depressed state. The pharmacodynamic action of each of the antidepressants increases the level of norepinephrine at subcortical neuroeffector sites controlling emotional responses.

Monoamine oxidase inhibitors. Norepinephrine is released at the sympathetic nerve ending, and its action at the effector site initiates a tissue response. Some of the norepinephrine is recycled at the nerve ending by a mechanism described as an amine pump. The mechanism conserves catecholamine and allows continued transmission. Action of monoamine oxidase (MAO) in the axoplasm metabolizes norepinephrine, and drugs that inhibit enzymatic activity of MAO elevate levels of norepinephrine in brain tissues.

Monoamine oxidase inhibitors (MAOI) are potent agents with a cumulative effect and 2-day to 3-week latent period before therapeu-

Table 17-1. Dosage range of antidepressant drugs

Nonproprietary name	Proprietary (trade) name	Daily adult dosage range
Amitriptyline hydrochloride*	Elavil	Oral: 75-300 mg. I.M.: 80-120 mg. (÷4)
Desipramine hydrochloride*	Norpramin, Pertofrane	Oral: 50-200 mg. (÷2-3)
Doxepin hydrochloride*	Sinequan	Oral: 25-300 mg. (÷3)
Imipramine hydrochloride*	Tofranil	Oral: 50-300 mg. (÷3) I.M.: Same
Isocarboxazid†	Marplan	Oral: 10-30 mg.
Lithium carbonate	Eskalith, Lithane, Lithonate	Oral: 0.9-1.8 Gm. (÷3)
Methylphenidate hydrochloride	Ritalin	Oral: 20-60 mg. (÷2-3)
Nialamide†	Niamid	Oral: 12.5-100 mg.
Nortriptyline hydrochloride*	Aventyl	Oral: 20-100 mg. (÷2-4)
Phenelzine sulfate†	Nardil	Oral: 15-45 mg. (÷1-3)
Pipradrol hydrochloride	Meratran	Oral: 7.5-15 mg. (÷3)
Protriptyline hydrochloride*	Vivactil	Oral: 15-60 mg. (÷3-4)
Tranylcypromine sulfate†	Parnate	Oral: 20-30 mg. (÷3)

*Tricyclic compounds.
†Monoamine oxidase inhibitors.

tic action is demonstrated. Isocarboxazid, nialamide, phenelzine sulfate, and tranylcypromine sulfate (Table 17-1) are the drugs currently in use. The high potency of tranylcypromine sulfate has limited its use to hospitalized patients to assure continual supervision of depressed patients' responses.

The monoamine oxidase inhibitors are often described as *psychic energizers.* Each of the drugs has an effect on psychomotor retardation and morbid preoccupation seen in the depressed patient, but there is variation in individual responses.

Adverse effects. Adverse effects during therapy include many disturbing problems related to alterations in neurohormone levels at systemic organ sites. Patients often identify problems that may be attributed to decreased cholinergic activity (i.e., dry mouth, constipation, urine retention, transient impotence, anorexia, nausea).

Peripheral edema, orthostatic hypotension, and central nervous system stimulation (headache, restlessness, insomnia) also occur frequently. The adverse effects reflect generalized inhibition of monoamine oxidase and resultant dominance of norepinephrine activity in central and peripheral tissues.

Although each of the preceding problems is important to the patient and to his perception of progress, the most disturbing problem during therapy is the potential for monoamine oxidase inhibitors to potentiate or be potentiated by numerous drugs and foods. The dependability of the patient or those supervising his implementation of the therapeutic program is important to maintaining a problem-free course of therapy.

Drug interactions. Monoamine oxidase inhibitors potentiate the effects of alcohol, barbiturates, anesthetic agents, antihistamines, narcotics, corticoids, anticholinergic, and sympathomimetic drugs. Extreme hyperthermia may occur when meperidine hydrochloride is administered to a patient who is receiving a monoamine oxidase inhibitor. The diversity of drug interactions makes it mandatory that the patient avoid self-medication with over-the-counter preparations because many decongestants contain antihistaminic substances or sympathomimetic agents. He should be told that the physician is to be consulted before using any previously prescribed or stocked drugs from his medicine supply.

Food interactions. Foods with high tyramine content may increase the production of norepinephrine and precipitate a tyramine-related syndrome, including occipital headache, palpitation, stiffness of neck muscles, emesis, sweating, photophobia, and changes in cardiac rate. The tyramine-related syndrome has been precipitated when patients taking monoamine oxidase inhibitors have eaten cheese. The devastating effect of ingestion of foods with high tyramine content has also caused sudden hypertension with vascular rupture. The absence of monoamine oxidase for metabolization at a time when the precursor (tyramine) is present in excessive amounts causes the acute hypertensive episode. Excess amounts of norepinephrine remain free to affect blood pressure levels.

Tyramine-containing foods. Knowledge of the adverse effects occurring with ingestion of tyramine-containing foods is essential to preventing problems. Tyramine is present in foods that require action of bacteria or molds for their preservation or preparation (i.e., pickled herring, alcoholic beverages, pods of broad beans, chicken livers, and aged or natural cheese). There is an inconsequential amount of tyramine in cream cheese, processed cheese, and cottage cheese; therefore intake of these products need not be restricted. A written list of tyramine-containing foods will assist the patient or the person responsible for his care to maintain limitations or restrictions. A reference list is useful when questions arise during planning of meals or snacks for the patient.

Norepinephrine blockers. Amitriptyline hydrochloride, desipramine hydrochloride, doxepin hydrochloride, imipramine hydrochloride, nortriptyline hydrochloride, and protriptyline hydrochloride (Table 17-1) accomplish their pharmacodynamic effect by blocking the reuptake and storage of norepinephrine in the axonal cytoplasm so that higher levels of norepinephrine are available at the effector sites. Concurrent with their effect at central nervous system tissues, the drugs have an anticholinergic effect produced by blocking specific receptors in the periphery. They potentiate the effect of anticholinergic drugs, and they also potentiate the central nervous system depression of alcohol. Amitriptyline hydrochloride produces a higher tranquilizing effect in patients than do the other members of the group. The comparable chemical derivation or composition of the drugs has led to their pharmacologic classification as *tricyclic compounds.*

Many adverse effects of the drugs occur during therapy, but there are few serious problems. Blocking of cholinergic nerve impulses may cause drowsiness, dry mouth, blurred vision, constipation, urinary retention, and tachycardia. Central nervous system stimulation occurs most frequently in elderly patients, and the problems include excitement, restlessness, incoordination, and fine tremor. Orthostatic hypotension and skin rash occur, but other problems occurring during therapy should be screened against the patient's prior complaints of fatigue, insomnia, headache, and anorexia to determine whether the problems are manifestations of adverse drug action or the depressive state of the patient.

Norepinephrine release stimulators. Methylphenidate hydrochloride and pipradrol hydrochloride (Table 17-1) improve productivity by decreasing psychomotor activity or response to environmental stimuli. The drugs are cerebral stimulants, rather than true antidepressants. The pharmacodynamic effect is believed to be accomplished by increasing norepinephrine release and utilization by limbic and reticular tissues. The therapeutic effect probably results from restoration of the norepinephrine-acetylcholine balance in the neural control centers. The pharmacodynamic effect on the limbic and reticular structures relays stimuli to the cerebral cortex. Therapy with the drugs reduces the hyperactivity of children, and higher concentration levels have a positive effect on the learning level of children in the classroom. Learning ability per se is not affected, but improved attention span affects performance. Adults doing monotonous or complex tasks requiring keen focus of attention over long periods of time have increased alertness and concentration during drug therapy.

Methylphenidate hydrochloride is available for parenteral administration, but oral use is planned for long-term therapy. Few adverse effects occur with use of the drugs, but hyperexcitability, irritability, and restlessness occur in some patients. Headache, palpitation, dizziness, and drowsiness occur during therapy, but the incidence is low.

Norepinephrine storage enhancer. Lithium carbonate (Table 17-1) is extensively used to prevent recurrence of manic states and episodes of depression. Lithium carbonate is thought to maintain norepinephrine levels in the brain by accelerating uptake of the catecholamine by the amine pump. Similarity between the drug and physiologic action of sodium ions is thought to contribute to the effectiveness of lithium carbonate in accelerating the sodium ion–dependent amine pump because the drug substitutes for the sodium ion.

Therapy with lithium carbonate is initiated in controlled situations to allow evaluation of serum levels of the drug. The therapeutic aim is to maintain serum levels between 1.5 and 2 mEg./liter to avoid toxic effects occurring above that range. Patients tolerate higher dosage levels during manic states than when in remission.

Lithium carbonate interferes with sodium reabsorption at renal tubule sites, and hyponatremia may occur during therapy. The drug is also believed to move across cellular membranes during depolarization and to remain as an unnatural intracellular component. Because the drug is not removed from the cell by the sodium pump, it blocks potassium transfer into the cell.

Restricted sodium intake increases the incidence of lithium carbonate substitution for the vital electrolyte. Adverse effects include nausea, vomiting, diarrhea, and muscle fasciculations, and more devastating effects occur as serum lithium levels rise (stupor, convulsions, coma, death). Lithium carbonate is teratogenic; therefore it is not administered to young women of child-bearing age or during the first trimester of pregnancy.

Recent studies have shown that more than 30% of the patients taking lithium carbonate complain of excessive voiding and extreme thirst. The problems are thought to occur consequent to drug suppression of antidiuretic hormone (ADH) function. Interference with ADH action causes excess water excretion, and thirst is overt evidence of dehydration.

Patient care

An important concern when drugs are prescribed for the patient who is depressed is whether he actually is taking the drug. The sequestration of tablets by hospitalized patients or neglect of self-care by patients in the home makes it necessary to supervise or seek supervision of drug therapy. Dosage schedules must be explicit for the patient who is depressed, and written instructions are helpful. Effectiveness of the drugs may not become apparent for some time after initiation of therapy, and the patient's understanding of the time lag may increase his commitment to continued use of the drug. When improvement is demonstrated, it is important to encourage the patient to continue taking the drug for the prescribed therapeutic period. Cultural bias against drug-taking and individual interpretations of mental health affect the pharmacotherapeutic program and the continuance of therapy.

Drug effect may be evident as a decrease in psychomotor retardation and morbid preoccupation with details of selected topics. Mood elevation, prolonged attention span, and interest in personal grooming and environmental activities are changes that gradually move the patient into participation in the activities in the world around him.

Throughout therapy individual physiologic problems require attention. The depression of gastrointestinal activity causes retention of feces, and plans appropriate to the patient's individual problem should be implemented. Nourishment and rest are at a minimal level, but maximizing the caloric content of the foods acceptable to the patient at the times he is known to take nourishment may decrease weight loss occurring during depressive states.

Concern for the emotional state of the patient and the effectiveness of therapeutic measures directed at modifying the basic problem sometimes overshadow the physiologic problems occurring as adverse effects of the drugs the patient is receiving. For example, many of the patients taking lithium carbonate complained of excessive thirst and frequent urination. The complaints were attributed to the patients' emotional state until recent studies revealed that the drug affects fluid balance by interfering with antidiuretic hormone function. Validation of the reality of patients' complaints can prevent comparable problems from occurring during drug therapy. The multiplicity of agents provided for patients with other than clear-cut depression further confuse the situation.

To avoid emergence of problems at a level hazardous to the patient, specific plans for observation of concurrent adverse effects are made while planning observations of progress. The patient in the chaos of depression has poor memory and concentration ability, and he will need assistance to participate in his care. His feelings of worthlessness and futility make it difficult to define whether problems are emerging. It is always possible that he will secrete information about physiologic problems as he perceives they are deserved punishment for his guilt.

The astute observer, using the entire acumen of measures for evaluation of function, can discern whether autonomic nervous system imbalance or other known adverse effects of the drug exist. The importance of changes that affect the safety of the patient makes each observation a necessary part of planned care. For example, blurred vision increases the hazard of falling, and dizziness accompanying hypotension increases the accident hazard.

Throughout therapy it is important that the patient perceive through verbal and nonverbal communication that those in contact with him care about him and are concerned for his well-being. Improvement in depressive states carries with it a high potential for suicidal attempt, and the patient requires protective supervision. The patient may not be aware of improvement as early as it is evident to family members. When the patient becomes less apathetic and begins to interact with those around him, family members relax their supervision, and opportunities for a suicide attempt increase. During the depressive state the patient is too apathetic to organize a suicide attempt, but as his condition improves, ability to plan and implement a suicide scheme increases.

Drugs are only part of the total plan of therapy for the patient, and concurrent psychotherapy supports the pharmacotherapeutic plan. Many health team members are involved in planning measures to provide maximum protection for the patient who is depressed.

ANXIETY STATES

The current tranquilizers were introduced at the midpoint of the twentieth century, the Age

Table 17-2. Dosage range of the antipsychotic drugs

Nonproprietary name	Proprietary (trade) name	Daily adult dosage range	Nonproprietary name	Proprietary (trade) name	Daily adult dosage range
Acetophenazine maleate	Tindal	Oral: 40-80 mg. (÷3)	Methoxypromazine maleate	Tentone	Oral: 0.05-1.5 Gm.
Butaperazine maleate	Repoise	Oral: 15-100 mg. (÷3)	Perphenazine	Trilafon	Oral: 12-64 mg. (÷2-4)
Carphenazine maleate	Proketazine	Oral: 75-400 mg. (÷3)			I.M.: 5-30 mg. (÷3)
Chlorpromazine	Thorazine suppository	P.R.: 150-400 mg. (÷3-4)			I.V.: 5 mg./single dose
Chlorpromazine hydrochloride	Thorazine	Oral: 0.03-1 Gm. (÷2-4)	Piperacetazine	Quide	Oral: 20-160 mg. (÷2-4)
		I.M.: 0.1-2.4 Gm. (÷4-6)	Prochlorperazine	Compazine suppository	P.R.: 50 mg. (÷2)
		I.V.: 25-50 mg./single dose	Prochlorperazine edisylate	Compazine	Oral: 15-150 mg. (÷3-4)
Chlorprothixene	Taractan	Oral: 30-600 mg. (÷3-4)			I.M.: 5-40 mg. (÷3-4)
		I.M.: 75-200 mg. (÷3-4)			I.V.: Same as I.M.
Droperidol	Inapsine	I.M.: 2.25-10 mg.	Thiopropazate hydrochloride	Dartal	Oral: 15-100 mg. (÷3)
		I.V.: 0.22-0.275 mg./kg.	Thioridazine hydrochloride	Mellaril	Oral: 20-800 mg. (÷3-4)
Fluphenazine enanthate	Prolixin enanthate	I.M.: 25-100 mg./every 2 wk.	Thiothixene	Navane	Oral: 6-30 mg. (÷3)
Fluphenazine hydrochloride	Permitil, Prolixin	Oral: 1-20 mg.	Trifluoperazine	Stelazine	Oral: 4-30 mg. (÷2)
		I.M.: 2.5-10 mg. (÷3-4)			I.M.: 4-10 mg. (÷4-6)
Haloperidol	Haldol	Oral: 1-15 mg. (÷2-3)	Triflupromazine hydrochloride	Vesprin	Oral: 20-150 mg. (÷2-3)
		I.M.: 3-15 mg. (÷3-6)			I.M.: 60-150 mg. (÷2-3)
Mesoridazine	Serentil	Oral: 30-400 mg. (÷3)			I.V.: 2-8 mg./single dose
		I.M.: 25-200 mg.			

of Anxiety. Early use was fraught with problems of adverse effects, but regulation of dosage and experience with the drugs have made them helpful agents for control of emotional problems. Tranquilizers are used to raise the threshold for emotional responses to environmental stimuli or to modify avoidance behavior. In either instance the objective is to improve the functional ability of the patient.

The designation major or minor tranquilizer is one intended to describe the primary therapeutic use of the agents. Major tranquilizers are frequently used to control acute or chronic psychotic states when the patient's uncontrolled behavior is destructive to himself or to others in the environment. Minor tranquilizers are used for treatment of patients with high anxiety levels (including neuroses) that make them incapable of coping with environmental stressors and accomplishing life activities. The terms are most helpful in general patient care situations to divide the group of drugs into those with the more extreme effects and adverse effects and those with more moderate effect and fewer disruptive responses during therapy.

ANTIPSYCHOTIC DRUGS (MAJOR TRANQUILIZERS)
Pharmacodynamics

The antipsychotic drugs, or major tranquilizers (Table 17-2), have comparable pharmacodynamic effects, although there is a difference in their chemical derivation. Chlorprothixene and thiothixene are classed pharmacologically as *thioxanthenes*, and droperidol and haloperidol are classified as *butyrophenones*. The remaining drugs represent derivatives of *phenothiazines*.

There are different indications for clinical use and for concurrent adverse effects of the phenothiazines that make it useful to know the drugs included in each of the three subgroups of phenothiazines:

ALKYLPIPERIDYL PHENOTHIAZINES
  Mesoridazine
  Piperacetazine
  Thioridazine hydrochloride
PROPYLPIPERAZINE PHENOTHIAZINES
  Acetophenazine maleate
  Butaperazine maleate
  Carphenazine maleate
  Fluphenazine hydrochloride
  Perphenazine
  Prochlorperazine
  Thiopropazate hydrochloride
  Trifluoperazine
PROPYLAMINO PHENOTHIAZINES
  Chlorpromazine
  Methoxypromazine
  Triflupromazine hydrochloride

The specific chemical structure of the major tranquilizers guides the physician in selection of a drug that will produce the desired effect with minimum adverse effects during therapy of a particular patient. For example, each of the major tranquilizers produces manifestations of extrapyramidal tract irritation, but problems occur more frequently during therapy with propylpiperazine and propylamino derivatives of the phenothiazines.

Children more frequently show incoordination of voluntary muscle action (dyskinesia) during therapy with propylpiperazines. Use of the drugs may cause problems with speech, swallowing, and tongue and facial muscle control and may cause clonic contractions of the neck and shoulder muscles.

Use of the propylamino derivatives of phenothiazine frequently precipitates parkinsonian-like symptoms in elderly patients on long-term therapy. Shuffling gait, masklike facies, drooling of excessive saliva, rigid muscles with continual tremor subsiding on intentional movement, and pill-rolling movements of the fingers present a pseudoparkinsonian syndrome (Fig. 17-2). Antiparkinsonian drugs may be prescribed to control symptoms and allow tranquilizer therapy.

The major tranquilizers have antiemetic properties that make them useful for control of emesis and emotional responses. Parenteral use of the drugs during the preoperative or postoperative period provides greater readiness of the patient for a relatively stress-free pro-

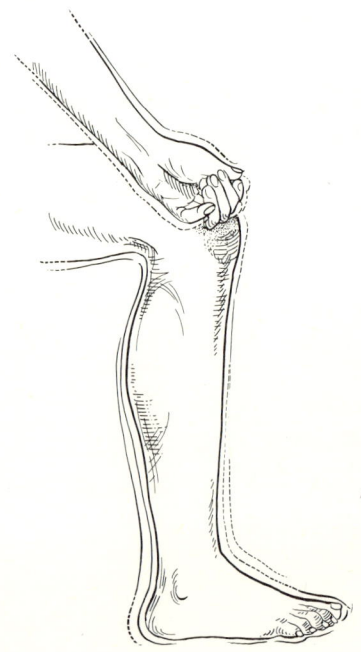

Fig. 17-2. Parkinsonian-like tremor of the extremity and pill-rolling movement of the fingers are produced by drug effect on extrapyramidal tracts.

gression of his surgical experience. The sole use of droperidol is to facilitate the induction and maintenance of anesthesia, and within 3 to 10 minutes of parenteral administration it produces an antiemetic and sedative effect.

Each of the drugs has anticholinergic and alpha-adrenergic properties that produce concurrent physiologic changes during therapy. Parenteral administration or long-term use increases the incidence of generalized autonomic nervous system effects. Observations during therapy are planned to allow revision of the therapeutic plan when disruption of function presents a hazard to the patient's progress.

The drugs are frequently used for short-term control of emesis or emotional responses, but they are regularly used for short- and long-term control of psychotic episodes. Major revisions in the care of psychiatric patients have resulted from drug-induced changes in the functional ability and environmental involvement of patients in psychiatric institutions. The effectiveness of pharmacotherapeutic control is most evident in the increasing numbers of psychiatric patients who are able to function in the community.

Patient care

The specific behavioral problem of the individual receiving the prescribed drug will influence the manifestations of drug effect. Progression of the pharmacotherapeutic plan is observed readily when the patient is hospitalized, but supervision is less intense when the patient is taking the potent tranquilizers during periods of adjustment to community living. The patient or his family need information to help them understand the pharmacotherapeutic plan because interpretation of the usefulness of the drug affects maintenance of the planned drug-use schedule. It is important to identify drug-taking schedules and provide specific instructions for observations of effects or adverse effects of the drug. Schedules for reevaluation of the patient's progress are planned, and it is important to communicate to the patient and his family that problems arising in the interval between scheduled visits to the clinic or physician's office should be reported promptly.

Many patients may safely take a holiday from drug taking when they are on long-term therapy, but the decision should be based on the physician's evaluation of psychiatric problem control, rather than on progress evaluation made by the patient or his family. Interrupted pharmacotherapeutic plans have caused patients to revert to pretreatment behavior that necessitated return to the hospital. The major tranquilizers are palliative rather than curative, and regularly scheduled drug use maintains a behavior level that makes it possible for the patient to remain in a familiar environment.

Assessment of drug effect. The major tranquilizers are used to modify behavior, and definition of effect is dependent on pretreatment base-line behavior and evolving behavioral changes during therapy. As important as change is the persistence of the behavior because consistency in responses is necessary to continued involvement with environmental activities. Concurrent plans for psychotherapy are part of the total therapeutic program, and each may support the other in moving toward control of emotional responses.

Assessment of drug adverse effect. The drugs cause a nonhypnotic sedative effect during the initial days of therapy, and the patient usually benefits from the decrease in activity. Drowsiness occurring after the first 2 weeks of therapy probably indicates a need for modification of drug dosage, and the physician should be consulted if the problem persists. Concurrent use of central nervous system depressants will add to the sedative effect of the drugs. The major tranquilizers have a selective central depressant effect, and even an overdose does not cause respiratory depression.

Throughout therapy the patient is observed for responses indicating excess anticholinergic or alpha-adrenergic blocking activity. Hypotensive responses result from peripheral blood pooling consequent to alpha-adrenergic blocking of norepinephrine activity in the arterial and venous circulation. Careful monitoring of the blood pressure and tabulation of the frequency of orthostatic hypotensive episodes during the first few weeks of therapy are useful in planning measures to protect the patient from falling. Dizziness may be lessened by avoiding sudden position changes or remaining recumbent immediately after taking the drugs. Physiologic tolerance to the blood shifts builds gradually, and the problem decreases. When the drugs are administered parenterally, there is a predictable sudden drop in blood pressure requiring that the patient remain in a supine position for an hour to allow equilibration of blood in the circulation.

Anticholinergic effects of the major tranquilizers have minor significance in patients who can relay messages about problems to those concerned with their care, but the psychiatric patient may have profound problems of gastrointestinal function before he relays information. Constipation, urinary retention, and anorexia are problems occurring secondary to decreased parasympathetic nervous system activity, and plans for observation and control of related functional changes are a necessary part of planning for the patient's care.

Planned observations for the onset of symptoms indicating irritation of the extrapyramidal tracts include planned assessment of control of fine movements. It is possible to observe the movements of facial and peripheral muscles while conversing with the patient, and the movement used by individuals to support verbal statements may reveal problems of voluntary muscle control. Evidence of dyskinesia or of a parkinsonian-like syndrome (discussed earlier in the chapter) are initially seen as motor muscle incoordination or clumsy movement. Specific observations are planned, and changes in muscle control can be evaluated with members of the nursing and medical team to plan protective measures and modification of drug dosage appropriate for the patient.

Hypersensitivity reactions are the other major group of adverse reactions occurring during drug use. The responses range from tissue fluid accumulations to light-source sensitivity reactions. Localized tissue fluid accumulations (angioedema) or peripheral and respiratory tract edema is comparable to that caused by the histamine release common to allergic responses. There have been incidences of anaphylactoid reactions with life-threatening cardiopulmonary arrest during therapy with the major tranquilizers.

Edema of the structures of the biliary tract has caused cholestatic jaundice. Observation of the sclera during the time the patient is taking the drugs may provide an early clue to the problem, and the patient's family can be asked to make periodic observations while the patient is taking the drugs at home. Obstruction to bile entering the intestinal tract progressively decreases the brown color of feces as bile content lessens.

Light-source sensitivity occurs in some patients, and the manifestations are phototoxic or photoallergic reactions. (Fig. 17-3). The reactions are seen most frequently in patients receiving chlorpromazine for long periods of time, but the incidence of reaction in these patients may be related to the large number of psychiatric ambulatory patients taking chlorpromazine. Sensitization causes a heat- or light-induced reaction. Exposure to heat (i.e., sunlight) causes an alteration of the cell membrane or cytoplasm that results in a reaction inappropriate to the length of exposure to the heat source. The patient may have a deep red sunburn after a very short period of time outdoors on a sunny day. However, light-source reactions can occur with long exposure to ultraviolet lighting. The alternate type of light-source sensitivity occurs as an allergen-antibody response leading to extensive skin eruptions. Patients who require the drug but demonstrate light exposure sensitivity reactions can use protective clothing, sunshades, or an umbrella when out in the sunshine.

Spillage of chlorpromazine solution on skin surfaces cause dermatitis, and nurses who are sensitive to the drug wear rubber gloves while preparing it. Placing a new needle on the syringe after aspiration of the drug may protect the patient from unnecessary exposure to the irritant and decrease the hard tract nodules found with continual intramuscular administration of the drug.

The major tranquilizers are not innocuous agents, but their benefits usually outweigh distressing to some patients. Impotence, blockade of ovulation, or cessation of menses are some of the manifestations of drug effect on the reproductive processes.

The major tranquilizers are not innocuous agents, but their benefits usually outweigh

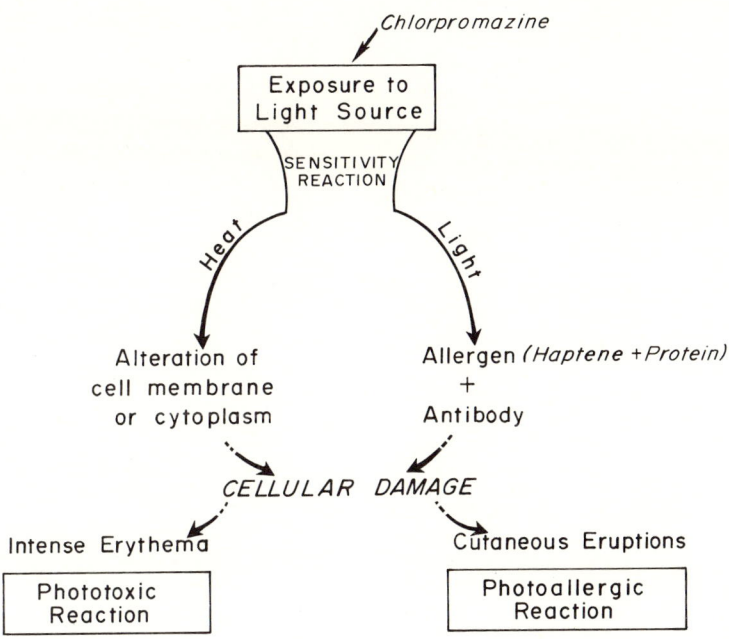

Fig. 17-3. Chlorpromazine increases sensitivity to strong light sources. Short periods of exposure to moderate sunlight may lead to intense sunburn (phototoxic reaction) or severe skin eruptions (photoallergic reaction).

problems occurring concurrently with use. The high incidence of adverse reactions requires that team members continually observe the progress of the patient's pharmacotherapeutic plan. Persistent problems may necessitate modification of the therapeutic plan, but it benefits the patient if stability of therapy can be maintained through careful planning by health team members.

ANTIANXIETY DRUGS (MINOR TRANQUILIZERS)
Pharmacodynamics

Alcohol is the oldest and most frequently used tranquilizer, and moderate use provides emotional calm in a turbulent society. Drugs commonly used for treatment of patients with high anxiety levels produce an emotional calmness that improves the individual's ability to participate in activities of daily living. The drugs may be prescribed for control of anxiety states in individuals requiring assistance for a short time period while personal emotional control is insufficient to cope with life situations. More frequently, the drugs are prescribed for long periods of time as supportive treatment for patients whose consistently high anxiety levels interfere with ability to function.

Dependence and overdosage are problems occurring with use of the antianxiety agents. Increasing concern about the high incidence of both problems has led to the practice of prescribing fewer tablets so that the individual must return for a new prescription. Closer evaluation of the individual's emotional state and periodic evaluation of progress is possible when frequent physician contact is established. The patient who manages to be supplied with drugs by diversity of physician contact is deprived of concurrent counseling or psychotherapy necessary to emotional equilibrium. The chronic drug user is an individual seeking help with problems he is unable to manage without assistance. Both physician and nurse may assist the individual by defining factors contributing to the chronic anxiety state and measures that may have a positive effect on the patient's ability to cope with life's problems.

Emylcamate, mebutamate, meprobamate, phenaglycodol, and tybamate (Table 17-3) are

Table 17-3. Dosage range of the antianxiety drugs

Nonproprietary name	Proprietary (trade) name	Daily adult dosage range
Benactyzine hydrochloride	Phobex, Suavitil	Oral: 3-10 mg. (÷3)
Buclizine hydrochloride	Softran, Vibazine	Oral: 50-150 mg. (÷1-3)
Chlordiazepoxide	Libritabs	Oral: 15-300 mg. (÷3-4)
Chlordiazepoxide hydrochloride	Librium	I.M.: 75-300 mg. (÷4-6) I.V.: Same
Diazepam	Valium	Oral: 4-40 mg. (÷3-4) I.M.: 4-90 mg. (÷3) I.V.: 5-15 mg./single dose
Emylcamate	Striatran	Oral: 600-800 mg. (÷3-4)
Hydroxyzine hydrochloride	Atarax	Oral: 75-400 mg. (÷3-4) I.M.: 100-600 mg. (÷4-6)
Hydroxyzine pamoate	Vistaril	Oral: 75-400 mg. (÷3-4)
Mebutamate	Capla	Oral: 0.9-1.2 Gm. (÷3-4)
Meprobamate	Equanil, Meprospan, Meprotabs, Miltown	Oral: 1.2-2.4 Gm. (÷3-4)
Oxazepam	Serax	Oral: 30-120 mg. (÷3-4)
Phenaglycodol	Ultran	Oral: 0.8-1.8 Gm. (÷4-6)
Tybamate	Solacen	Oral: 0.75-2 Gm. (÷3-4)

closely related chemically and are classified pharmacologically as the *propanediol series*, or as relatives of meprobamate. The relaxation of skeletal muscle occurring during use of the drugs is thought to result from the pharmacodynamic effect on interneurons. The drugs are frequently used as antianxiety agents or to decrease centrally induced stimuli to sympathetic nervous system activity (i.e., hypertension). During therapy some patients have persistent hypotension resulting from the depressive effect of the drug on vasomotor centers in the medulla and spinal cord, although vasomotor conduction at the hypothalamic level may also be involved. Complaints of headache or insomnia often make it necessary for the patient's pharmacotherapeutic plan to be revised. The frequency of therapeutic use of the drugs indicates effectiveness in control of anxiety states, but occasional hypersensitivity reactions occur during therapy.

Chlordiazepoxide, diazepam, and oxazepam are chemically related as *benzodiazepines*. The drugs produce a significant relaxant effect on skeletal muscles by depression of the polysynaptic reflex arcs of the spinal cord. Parenteral administration of diazepam has been used effectively for central control of intractable clonic contractions of skeletal muscles in patients with central nervous system trauma. The anticonvulsant action provides good control of the violent convulsions of *status epilepticus* and *alcohol withdrawal*. The large intravenous anticonvulsant dose causes mental confusion. Parenteral use is accompanied by hypotension. Oral administration is generally planned for ambulatory patients. Hypotension is minimal with oral use, and it is usually limited to the initial days of therapy.

Buclizine hydrochloride and hydroxyzine hydrochloride are antihistamines with less potent effect than that of the phenothiazines. During therapy the patient is observed carefully for anticholinergic, alpha-adrenergic, and hypersensitivity reactions comparable to those of the phenothiazines. The incidence of adverse effects is lower, but problems arise when the patient is on long-term therapy. Mild sedation occurs, and the drugs potentiate the action of other depressants (i.e., alcohol, barbiturates). Buclizine hydrochloride and hydroxyzine hydrochloride have teratogenic effects, and so they are not used for women in the child-bearing years or during the first trimester of pregnancy.

Benactyzine hydrochloride has antihistaminic effects, and it is an anticholinergic drug. Therapy is usually planned on the basis of the patient's need for tranquilizer effect concurrent with modification of parasympathetic activity.

Patient care

Drug use by individuals capable of maintaining self-care and social activities in their natural environment decreases the frequency of contact with health team members. Initiation of therapy and return visit contacts provide opportunities for evaluation of the particular needs of the patient, and the opportunities can be used to assist the patient to maximize effective use of the drugs.

Oftentimes the schedule for drug taking is left to the patient's discretion with intervals between dosage as the only rigid guide. The anxious patient is not always able to concentrate or think logically during an anxiety state; therefore written suggestions provide better references than oral instructions unless there is a family member or dependable friend with the patient during the clinic or office visit.

The drugs have varying levels of effect on the emotional responses of patients. The low incidence of adverse effects during drug use is an important asset when the patient is receiving the agents without close supervision. Initial use of the drugs causes drowsiness that interferes with the individual's ability to function, and the patient should know that driving a motor vehicle or doing tasks requiring coordination or fine control may be hazardous during the early period of drug therapy.

Drowsiness, hypotension, muscle relaxation, and decreased ability to concentrate may each contribute to the patient's inability to participate in environmental activities during the initial days of therapy. The patient should be helped to understand the predictability of lethargy and the frequent desire to rest until tolerance to the new drug regimen is established. For the individual who is responsible for care of young children, it is helpful if the assistance of an adult is available during the adjustment period. It is often helpful to discuss schedules for drug use that allow accomplishment of necessary activities when there is the least hazard of ataxia, incoordination, or drowsiness.

Hypersensitivity reactions occur in some patients during therapy, and the patient is asked to report any unusual changes to the physician before continuing with the therapeutic plan. Tolerance to alcohol is decreased during therapy, and patients who find it impossible to avoid drinking at a social event should plan to omit the drug prior to the occasion.

The oral agents provide an effect within 30 minutes of the time of ingestion. The patient will manage therapy best if he understands the therapeutic aim in modifying emotional responses. Drug use should not cause physical immobility or out of contact tranquillity. Consistent use of the drugs may reestablish equilibrium in the patient's environment by modifying the behavior pattern that has disrupted his interpersonal relationships.

REFERENCES

Ayd, Frank J., Jr.: Recognizing and treating depressed patients, Modern Medicine **39**:80, 1971.

Baldessarini, Ross J.: Interactions of drugs and amines in the brain (editorial), The New England Journal of Medicine **286**:542, 1972.

Benter, Beverly A.: Mood swings, Nursing '72 **2**:28, 1972.

Bey, D. R., Chapman, R. E., and Tornquist, K. L.: A lithium clinic, The American Journal of Psychiatry **129**:468, 1972.

Daniels, Farrington, Jr., van der Leun, Jan C., and Johnson, Brian E.: Sunburn, Scientific American **219**:38, July, 1968.

Frohman, Lawrence A.: Clinical neuropharmacology of hypothalamic releasing factors, The New England Journal of Medicine **286**:1391, 1972.

Goodman, Louis S., and Gilman, Arthur, editors: The pharmacological basis of therapeutics, ed. 4, New York, 1970, The Macmillan Co.

Goth, Andres.: Medical pharmacology, ed. 6, St. Louis, 1972, The C. V. Mosby Co.

Guyton, Arthur C.: Textbook of medical physiology, ed. 4, Philadelphia, 1971, W. B. Saunders Co.

Hollister, Leo E.: Drug therapy: mental disorders—antianxiety and antidepressant drugs, The New England Journal of Medicine **286**:1195, 1972.

Hollister, Leo E.: Drug therapy: mental disorders—antipsychotic and antimanic drugs, The New England Journal of Medicine **286**:984, 1972.

Kline, Nathan S., and Davis, John M.: Psychotropic drugs, American Journal of Nursing **73:**54, 1973.

Martin, W. R., Sloan, J. W., Sapira, J. D., and Jasinski, D. R.: Physiologic, subjective, and behavioral effects of amphetamine, methamphetamine, ephedrine, phenmetrazine, and methylphenidate in man, Clinical Pharmacology and Therapeutics **12:**245, 1971.

Reilly, Mary Jo, editor: American hospital formulary service, vol. 1, sect. 28:00, Washington, D. C., 1973, American Society of Hospital Pharmacists.

Schuckit, M., Robins, E., and Feighner, J.: Tricyclic antidepressants and monoamine oxidase inhibitors, Archives of General Psychiatry **24:**509, 1971.

Spensley, James, and Rockwell, Don A.: Psychosis during methylphenidate abuse, The New England Journal of Medicine **286:**880, 1972.

Stewart, Mark A.: Hyperactive children, Scientific American **222:**94, April, 1970.

Stockwell, Martha L.: Depression: an operational definition with themes related to the nurse's role. In Zderad, Loretta T., and Belcher, Helen C.: Developing behavioral concepts in nursing, vol. 1, Atlanta, 1968, Southern Regional Education Board.

Weiss, Jay M.: Psychological factors in stress and disease, Scientific American **226:**104, June, 1972.

Wyatt, Richard J., Fram, David H., Buchbinder, Rona, and Snyder, Frederick: Treatment of intractable narcolepsy with a monoamine oxidase inhibitor, The New England Journal of Medicine **285:**987, 1971.

18

Cerebrocortical activity

Seizures
    Grand mal seizures
    Petit mal seizures
    Psychomotor seizures
    Pharmacodynamics
    Patient care
Parkinsonism
    Pharmacodynamics
    Patient care

Bioelectrical activity in brain tissue is comparable to that occurring in all body tissues. Central nervous system electrical activity differs only in the multiplicity of physiologic functions dependent on maintenance of open circuits between neuronal connections and interconnections. Disruption of transmission pathways within the cerebral tissues or in major tracts leaving the control areas triggers malfunction manifest at a distance from the originating source in brain tissue.

Periodic or persistent stimuli emerging in cerebrocortical or subcortical sites can stimulate discharge of efferent neurons to cause convulsive movements or sustained rigidity of peripheral muscles. High dosage or chronic use of some of the drugs discussed in preceding chapters cause convulsions or a parkinsonian-like syndrome resulting from disruption of neural electrical transmission at central cortical or extrapyramidal tract sites. Residual drug in tissues may continue the disruption for a short period of time after discontinuance of drug therapy.

Pharmacotherapy may be planned to decrease electrical activity of cerebral tissues or to maintain the balance between the central neurohormonal transmitter substances. The characteristics of the inciting stimulus affects whether the pharmacotherapeutic plan is for acute or long-term use of the drugs.

SEIZURES

Hyperexcitability of cerebrocortical neurons may result from irritable foci or drug-induced electrical hyperactivity. There is a safety level, or threshold, that governs the level of disruption required to precipitate seizures. The threshold level of an individual affects his predisposition to seizures (seizure proneness or diathesis) in response to a stimulus. For example, elevation of body temperature is a stimulus to seizures in young children with low convulsive thresholds. When two infants have a similar elevation of body temperature (i.e., 104° F.), one of the infants may have convulsions whereas the other remains convulsion-free. Intensive measures to reduce the body temperature of the convulsing infant may terminate the problem, and subsequent control of high temperature elevation may prevent future above-threshold stimulus to convulsions.

Epilepsy is the Greek word for seizures, but the term is most often employed to describe chronic seizure diathesis. Brain trauma (i.e., injury, neurosurgery), cerebral hypoxia, or endogenous toxic substances (i.e., drugs, metabolic wastes, or bacterial toxins) may produce seizures. Specific characteristics of the precipitating factor influence the peripheral manifestations of seizure activity. Specifics of the seizure pattern and electroencephalographic (EEG) tracings guide the physician in selection of the therapeutic program for the individual. The source of disruptive electrical activity affects consequent uncontrolled peripheral paroxysm or interruption in function. Foci from subcortical sites (i.e., thalamus, hypothalamus) may pass to the cortex and cause a widespread distortion of electric transmission and widespread convulsive activity in the periphery. Seizures are described as *grand mal, petit mal,* or *psychomotor* on the basis of the manifestations of electrical disruption. Patients have amnesia for events occurring during their seizures.

Grand mal seizures

Grand mal seizures follow a fairly consistent pattern of generalized activity: initiating signal (aura, outcry); loss of consciousness; fall to supine position; tonic contractions followed by clonic contractions of the musculature of the extremities, trunk and head; urinary or fecal incontinence; and deep sleep. Episodes may last from 1 to 10 minutes. There is a period of refractoriness to a second seizure and the interval is called *postictal depression.*

Petit mal seizures

Petit mal seizures are subclassified into three types on the basis of events manifest during the seizure. During the *short-stare type* of petit mal seizures there is clouding of consciousness, vacuous stare, and head bobbing or blinking of the eyelids. The *akinetic type* of petit mal seizures is manifest as a loss of consciousness and muscle tone (falling if the patient is erect) and sudden involuntary jerks of trunk and limbs. The *myoclonic type* of petit mal seizures is manifest as involuntary contractions of trunk, head, or extremity muscle groups (generalized, limited) and a fall to supine position (dependent on limbs involved). Petit mal seizures generally last only 5 to 30 seconds, and a second episode may occur within a short period of time.

A focus in any cerebral lobe causes manifestations of disruption, or peripheral movements characteristic of function control areas involved. Initial seizure activity may be limited, with gradual progression to generalized, or grand mal, convulsive movements. A focus at the motor strip on the anterior ridge of the cortical central gyrus causes a sequence known as *Jacksonian seizures.* Electrical disruption radiates along the motor control sites from the focal point in a consistent travel pathway. Peripheral manifestations of the travel route taken by the electric stimulus relates directly to the sites of motor control. For example, excitation at a focus at the lower portion of the motor tract may first be manifest by convulsive movements of the tongue, lips, and adjacent structures. Travel upward along the motor strip next involves upper parts of the face, thumb, hand, and finally the lower extremities as the impulse traverses the pathways of motor control to the upper ridge of the central gyrus.

Psychomotor seizures

Psychomotor seizures usually originate from foci in the temporal or frontal cortical lobes. The disruption causes purposeful behavior that may be irrelevant to the particular environment or circumstances at the time of the seizure. The 3- to 5-minute episodes include a brief loss of consciousness. Automatic, purposeless disjointed movements and sounds may occur during the seizure period.

Pharmacodynamics

Drugs may be prescribed to modify generalized or focal seizure activity. Anticonvulsants are used to control acute or chronic seizure diathesis, or they may be employed to abort a convulsive episode. Prophylactic use of anticonvulsants after neurosurgery is a common practice, and long-term use of drugs is necessary for prevention of periodic recurrent seizures. The aim of therapy is to protect the patient against the physical and emotional disruption of seizures.

Anticonvulsants are used to modify bioelectrical activity and raise the threshold response to stimuli. Combinations of drugs are often prescribed to manage the complex problems of seizure control. Sedatives are used to decrease response to psychic stimuli constituting seizure precipitants (anxiety, excitement, fear), whereas specific agents may be used concurrently to modify electrical activity.

Most of the drugs given to modify seizure diathesis cause dizziness and drowsiness. The effect of central nervous system depressants

Table 18-1. Dosage range of anticonvulsant drugs

Nonproprietary name	Proprietary (trade) name	Daily adult dosage range
Diphenylhydantoin*†	Dihycon, Di-Lan, Dilantin, EKKO	Oral: 300-600 mg. (÷3)
Diphenylhydantoin sodium*†	Convul, Danten, Denyl, Dihycon sodium, Dilantin sodium, Diphenylan sodium	Oral: 300-600 mg. (÷3) I.M.: 300-800 mg. (÷3-4) I.V.: 300-500 mg. (÷2)
Ethosuximide‡	Zarontin	Oral: 0.5-1.5 Gm. (÷2)
Ethotoin*†	Peganone	Oral: 1-5 Gm. (÷4-6)
Magnesium sulfate, 50%*		I.M.: 6-12 ml.
Mephenytoin*	Mesantoin	Oral: 0.1-1.8 Gm. (÷1-4)
Mephobarbital*	Mebaral	Oral: 200-800 mg. (÷1-2)
Metharbital*	Gemonil	Oral: 100-800 mg. (÷1-3)
Methsuximide‡	Celontin	Oral: 0.3-1.2 Gm.
Paramethadione‡	Paradione	Oral: 0.9-2.1 Gm. (÷3)
Phensuximide‡	Milontin	Oral: 1-3 Gm. (÷2-3)
Primidone*†	Mysoline	Oral: 0.25-2 Gm.
Trimethadione‡	Tridione	Oral: 1-2 Gm. (÷3)

*Grand mal seizure control.
†Psychomotor seizure control.
‡Petit mal seizure control.

administered concurrently is potentiated by anticonvulsant drugs. Patient safety is dependent on use of measures to protect him from injury if coordination or balance are affected during drug therapy. Many patients complain of nausea and anorexia during initial days of drug therapy, but the problems subside with continued use of most of the drugs. Skin rash occurs in some patients receiving anticonvulsant drugs, and the patient is asked to bring the problem to the attention of a health team member as soon as it is observed.

Magnesium sulfate, 50% (Table 18-1), acts pharmacodynamically as a central nervous system depressant. Rapidity of action after administration provides relief of tetanic contractions by a combined effect on central nervous system activity and interference at peripheral neuromuscular junctions. Magnesium sulfate, 50%, is used for abolition of acute continuous convulsive episodes (status epilepticus). Depressant effect on central nervous system tissues includes the vital medullary centers, and cardiac and respiratory depression may occur concurrently with seizure control. Onset of medullary center depression can be reversed by administration of calcium salts, which compete with magnesium ions and prevent progression of magnesium ion–initiated depression of vital centers.

Mephobarbital, metharbital, and primidone (Table 18-1) as well as phenobarbital modify cerebrocortical activity and response to psychic stimuli at a level that provides protection against generalized seizure activity. Each of the drugs acts as a barbiturate. Primidone, although unrecognizable as a barbiturate by its nonproprietary name, is metabolized endogenously to a barbiturate form. Patients are sometimes irritable and complain of headache during therapy with the drugs.

Ethosuximide, methsuximide, and phensuximide (Table 18-1) are oral agents used to raise the seizure threshold and decrease motor cortex response to stimuli. The drugs are chemical relatives *(succinimides);* therefore effects and adverse effects are comparable between the drugs. Apathy, nervousness, headache, or blurred vision have occurred during therapy with the drugs. Albuminuria occurs during initial therapy; therefore regular urinalysis is usually planned.

Paramethadione and trimethadione (Table 18-1) unlike other anticonvulsants, are specific depressants, and sedative effects do not occur during therapy. The two drugs are chemical relatives, and both cause depression of leukocytes. The patient is asked to bring to the attention of the physician any evidence of swollen glands or persistent cutaneous eruptions during long-term therapy. Blurring of vision in bright light (hemeralopia) and photosensitivity occur during therapy, and the patient should be advised of protective measures to guard against injury. Tolerance of bright light may be improved by wearing dark glasses. Photosensitivity may be decreased by using protective covering (i.e., umbrella, sunshade) if sunlight exposure is unavoidable.

Phenacemide (Phenurone) is a highly toxic drug used only when other drugs fail to control convulsions because it has a potential for causing blood cell destruction. Anemia, agranulocytosis, or thrombocytopenia may occur during drug therapy; therefore regularly scheduled evaluation of the hematologic status of the patient is planned. Changes in activity tolerance, persistent infections, cutaneous bleeding, persistent bleeding from wounds, fever, or sore throat are the manifestations providing clues to hematologic problems. The patient is advised of the necessity for contacting the physician when problems occur between planned contact periods.

Diphenylhydantoin, diphenylhydantoin sodium, ethotoin, and mephenytoin (Table 18-1) are closely related anticonvulsant drugs. Diphenylhydantoin is the most frequently prescribed drug for prophylactic, short-term, or long-term control of grand mal seizures. The drugs decrease the voltage, frequency and spread of electrical discharges within the motor cortex.

Dosage adjustment is individualized to provide the drug at a level effective for seizure control with minimal adverse effects. The high incidence of diphenylhydantoin use has provided a clear definition of the many adverse effects and drug interactions occurring during therapy. Each of the related drugs carries the potential for causing comparable problems with long-term therapy. The patient's understanding of effects and adverse effects may increase the effectiveness of the pharmacotherapeutic plan.

Metabolism of diphenylhydantoin is inhibited by many drugs, and the total drug regimen of the patient is carefully planned by the physician throughout the therapeutic period. Diphenylhydantoin potentiates the anticoagulant action of coumarin derivatives. When the pharmacotherapeutic plan includes use of an anticoagulant, the prothrombin level is evaluated regularly during initiation and withdrawal of the anticoagulant. The pharmacodynamic peak of orally administered diphenylhydantoin is 6 to 9 days, and problems occurring during therapy that lead to discontinuance of the drug may continue for a comparable period (6 to 9 days) beyond the pharmacotherapeutic interval.

Alkalinity of diphenylhydantoin (approximate pH = 12) makes it irritating to tissues when administered by any route. Gastric irritation can be lessened by administration of the drug with large amounts of water or with food. Although alkalinity makes the injection of diphenylhydantoin sodium painful, rapidity of pharmacodynamic action (5 to 20 minutes) makes the drug an ideal agent for control of acute convulsive states. Various formulations (suspensions, capsules, solutions) make the drug available for all age groups. Extended-release forms are also available for control of nocturnal seizures.

Intravenous injection of the drug is planned to run at a slow rate to avoid local irritation of the vein. Acute respiratory and cardiovascular depression occur when the drug is administered rapidly.

The drug is distributed in all body tissues and it crosses the placental barrier and enters the milk of nursing mothers. Although monitoring for adverse effects is necessary in either situation, the infant is protected by the low level action of the drug on normal neural transmission. Diphenylhydantoin does not alter normal excitation and response of neurons.

Adverse effects during therapy with diphenylhydantoin are frequent and varied. The drug's inhibition of dietary folic acid absorption may precipitate anemia (megaloblastic anemia). The reported incidence of anemia and other blood dyscrasias occurring with *hydantoin* derivatives necessitates periodic hematologic studies and careful evaluation of the patient's status.

Central nervous system manifestations of adverse effect include incoordination, ataxia, bumping into inanimate objects, and falling. Concurrent central effect of the drug on extrapyramidal fibers may cause fine tremor and clumsiness in performing manual tasks.

During long-term therapy, diphenylhydantoin causes gingivitis and hyperplasia of the gums. The characteristic redness and overgrowth can be modified by scrupulous oral hygiene. Hyperplasia of the gums may necessitate surgical removal (gingivectomy) by an oral surgeon when the condition of the gingiva becomes cosmetically offensive to the individual. Heavy growth of hair (hirsuitism) is another cosmetic problem occurring in adolescents taking diphenylhydantoin for long-term therapy.

Patient care

Prior to or during drug therapy the patient may have a seizure episode, and the observations made during the event are important to his continued therapy. Seizures are usually self-limiting, although in rare instances the continual convulsive movements known as *status epilepticus* persist for an indeterminate period of time. The classifications and ensuing events of seizures offer broad guidelines in consideration of measures appropriate to care of the patient. Mixed seizures often occur, and a rigid definition of seizures is inappropriate.

Preplanning for protection of the patient with grand mal seizure diathesis in the hospital situation includes measures to protect against injury during uncontrolled movements that may result in bruised tissues or fractured bones. Placing padded cushions on side rails provides readily mobilized protectors for the bed patient during a seizure. Football helmets are used for young ambulatory patients to protect against head injury from falls at seizure onset. Restraints are unnecessary and they may provide an added stimulus to the convulsive state. Eyeglasses and dentures are usually removed during initial seizure control periods.

A rubber or plastic airway, padded throat sticks, and suction equipment at the patient's bedside provide emergency equipment to maintain a patent airway. Insertion of an airway is accomplished prior to the tight closure of the mouth occurring in the tonic state. Attempts to insert the airway after that point may cause injury to the oral tissues or teeth. Forceful exhalation causes accumulation of secretions in the tightly closed mouth, and cyanosis or respiratory difficulty may be lessened by suctioning excess secretions to reinstitute a patent airway. Operational equipment in a state of readiness at the bedside provides protection to the patient in the sudden emergency of seizure onset.

Sudden loud noises or bright lights may provide sensory stimulus to seizures in some patients. The flickering light of a distorted television picture or a child with a piercing cry may provide a stimulus. Modifying environmental factors to lessen stimuli may decrease seizure incidence.

It is important to recognize a seizure and objectively tabulate the events occurring during the episode. The duration of the seizure and specific description of the sequence of events, observed before and during the incident, provide clues to precipitating factors. Movement of the head, fixation of the eyes, and progression of tonic or clonic movements of the extremities are important observations. A graphic record of onset time, duration, and events provides guidelines for all team members planning patient care.

Seizures may occur at any time or place, and the initiate often finds it difficult to leave the individual's thrashing arms and legs unhampered during the episode. Protection of the patient from injury and maintenance of a patent airway are the two objectives during a seizure, and measures appropriate to the objectives are employed. For example, the individual who is in an erect position when the aura occurs may be gently eased to the ground. Placing any available clothing or cushioning material under his head will protect against injury from banging of the head against the hard ground surface. A rolled handkerchief placed between the teeth prior to tonic closure of the jaw will help maintain an open airway and protect the tongue from being bitten. Rolling the individual to his side during the deep sleep state after the seizure allows secretions to drain from the mouth.

At the termination of a grand mal seizure the patient usually recognizes that the environment has changed. Awareness that a seizure has occurred is disturbing to the patient. It is important to protect the patient from vivid descriptions of events that occurred during the seizure state. The incident is emotionally traumatic to the patient, and he has the right to protection from the prying eyes of curious onlookers during and after the episode. Lurid tales are told by people who observe a seizure. Current ignorance of epilepsy as a health problem can be propagated by fables told by onlookers at the seizure scene.

The preceding discussion has focused on grand mal seizures, but other forms of seizure activity may occur. Uncontrollable twitching of the tongue and perioral muscles occurring several times during a short period of hours may be the manifestations of focal seizure activity in a patient with head injury or neurosurgery. Prompt sharing of the observations with members of the nursing and medical team makes it possible to plan protective measures for the patient and modify the therapeutic regimen on the basis of the incident.

Control of seizures may be primarily dependent on the pharmacotherapeutic plan, and the patient is usually sincerely interested in attaining control. Measures to increase the effectiveness of drugs while avoiding the emergence of adverse effects are a necessary component of therapy.

Initial therapy may be accompanied by drowsiness, dizziness, ataxia, or vertigo that endangers the patient's safety. Use of ambulatory aids (i.e., walker, stair rails) may prevent falls. The physically healthy individual is interested in returning to usual living patterns, and restrictions are generally limited to the patient's particular problems. The patient who understands the necessity of limiting hazardous situations when unsteadiness jeopardizes safety can plan to postpone some activities or reschedule them to accomplish tasks when the problems are absent. Driving a motor vehicle, or climbing ladders requires concentration and steadiness, and the patient must consider these and comparable situations as contraindicated when drowsiness or unsteadiness occurs during drug therapy.

Long-term use of the drugs necessitates periodic evaluation of drug effect in controlling seizures, and the patient is also observed periodically to ascertain whether there is concurrent drug effect on vital organ function. Evaluation of hematologic status and renal and hepatic function usually are planned at the time of clinic or office visits. The patient should be encouraged to contact a health team member when any new health problem arises between planned contact periods.

Injury- or toxin-induced seizures may be treated by removal of the causative factor. Removal of a clot or lesion that is impinging on cerebral tissues or discontinuance of a toxic drug precipitator may terminate the problem. Planned observations for seizure activity are continued after removal of the etiologic factor to assure the protection of the patient until the effect of therapy is established.

Epilepsy is a chronic health problem, and the patient has the same adjustment to knowledge of the diagnosis and therapy requisite to health maintenance as do patients with other chronic health problems. Each contact that helps interpret the sincere concern and acceptance by professionals is a step forward for the patient who is trying to accept a problem that is poorly understood in our culture.

PARKINSONISM

Motor activity is controlled by many interrelated brain centers. Feedback circuits between subcortical and cortical structures maintain the balanced movements automatically accomplished in response to clues from the central cortical sites. Disruption of the subcortical centers or depletion of their neurohormonal mediators causes loss of the gross movements usually accomplished without concentration and planning.

The close anatomic relationship between components of the basal ganglia (caudate nucleus, globus pallidus, putamen) and other subcortical structures concerned with motor functions (red nucleus, substantia nigra, subthalamus, thalamus) provides an intercommunication system for movement. Control circuits between the subcortical, cortical, and reticular structures comprise the complex network for control of motor function.

Neural transmission is accomplished by transmitter substances, and in the brain the activity of *serotonin, acetylcholine,* and *norepinephrine* provides the hormonal stimulus to activity. *Dopamine* as one of the precursors of norepinephrine is vital to maintenance of the balance of hormonal excitation and inhibition controlled by central sites. Inhibition of dopamine liberation or production has an adverse effect on automatic movements by depressing the centers controlling peripheral muscle responses. Acetylcholine activity is uninhibited when dopamine levels are insufficient to maintain neurochemical balance in the brain.

Dopamine production in the substantia nigra provides some of the hormonal transmitter necessary to neural activity in the brain. Some of the drugs presented in preceding chapters interfere with dopamine receptors (i.e., chlorpromazine and haloperidol) or deplete dopamine supplies in brain tissue (i.e., reserpine). Dopamine depletion or block induces a syndrome described as pseudoparkinsonism. Parkinson's disease is the pattern on which description of the syndrome is based. Although the manifestations are comparable, Parkinson's disease is a chronic health problem that results from lack of dopamine production in the substantia nigra.

Coordinated neural stimuli to muscles provide contraction or relaxation of extensor and flexor muscles necessary to accomplish movement. Extrapyramidal tract controls of small muscle groups provide the coordination required for complex muscle activity.

At central cortical motor sites efferent inhibitory impulses of the extrapyramidal tract travel through the basal ganglia en route to skeletal muscles. Rigidity and spasticity of muscles occur when the level of dopamine is insufficient for neurotransmission at the basal ganglia. Absence of inhibitory impulses that naturally decrease extensor tone and increase flexor tone allows dominance of efferent pyramidal tract neurons from the cerebral cortex motor area. Dominance of the facilitatory fibers of the pyramidal tract increases tone of the extensor muscles and decreases tone of the flexor muscles. Absence or deficiency of dopamine also causes problems of acetylcholine dominance in central and peripheral sites.

It is difficult to envision the problems related to Parkinson's disease or pseudoparkinsonism, but analysis of a few automatic movements may help to assemble a visual image. For example, the student reading a textbook periodically turns the pages, sips a refreshing liquid, brushes away the unruly lock of hair, and changes position. The events occur with only minimal distraction from the initial task. If each movement and each act required strict attention of the student, the initial task would be abandoned to allow concentration on basic needs. The entire episode would be tiring enough to necessitate rest on completion of the components of the previous short action sequence.

Patients with Parkinson's disease (or pseudoparkinsonism) must plan voluntary control of each muscle movement required to accomplish a task. Thought processes are unimpaired by the depletion or blocking of dopamine activity, but conscious control of each dimension of movement requires attention and concentration. There is an absence of nonverbal clues naturally used by individuals to reinforce verbalization during a conversation. Smiling, frowning, or concurrent hand motions are prohibitive when verbal interaction requires concentration on forming the words rather than on planning movement of extraneous muscles. Speech is slow and studied. The monotonous progression of words and masklike facies demonstrate the muscle control necessary to conduct conversation.

Contraction of opposing muscle groups in the extremities maintains the arms and legs in a tense spastic position (akinesia). Most patients have tremors described as nonintention tremors, which are present in the resting state, but lessened when the patient moves the extremity. Rigidity and tremor affect mobility, and disruption of the motor controls for forward progression when walking adds an additional problem. Propulsion gait occurs when the patient walks. Braking the forward walking motion is difficult, and forward progression continues beyond the intended distance or goal. The patient may walk into a wall or other obstacle in his path.

Absence of muscle control affects visceral function. Constipation, incontinence, and decreased sexual capacity are common problems. Excess saliva (sialorrhea) and tears concurrent with the decreased ability to automatically swallow or blink makes secretions a frustrating problem for the patient.

Control of pseudoparkinsonism may be accomplished by withdrawing the causative agent (i.e., phenothiazine drug) but control of Parkinson's disease requires lifelong therapy. Pharmacotherapy is planned to maintain the neurohormonal balance and reinstitute equilibrium between brain centers for motor control. Drugs may improve the functional status of the patient by acting at brain sites to inhibit acetylcholine activity or replace dopamine.

Pharmacodynamics

Dopamine replacement. Knowledge of the etiology of Parkinson's disease led to specific drug therapy to stimulate synthesis of the missing neurotransmitter, dopamine. The drug used for replacement—L-dopa, or levodopa (Table 18-2)—is converted in the basal ganglia to dopamine and utilized in neural functions. L-Dopa has only been available in the last decade, and long-range results are being observed with cautious optimism. L-Dopa is no simple panacea for the patient with Parkinson's disease. Therapy is protracted and fraught with problems of adverse effects, which make the initial period of therapy a sequence of dosage adjustments to provide the drug while protecting the physical and psychic state of the patient.

The patient seeking therapy with levodopa is usually one who desperately seeks reversal of the pathologic process that makes every day of his life a series of planned, studied movements. The patient and his family approach therapy with optimistic plans for the future, and it is important that they be allowed to retain hope. Guarded statements by professional contacts may maintain realistic progress evaluation and prevent some of the depression when short-term reversals occur during therapy.

As the dosage tolerance of the patient increases, attempts are made to raise dosage gradually to the maximum level (8 Gm./24 hours). The patient's willingness to tolerate

Table 18-2. Dosage range of Parkinson disease–specific drugs

Nonproprietary name	Proprietary (trade) name	Daily adult dosage range
Benztropine mesylate	Cogentin	Oral: 1-18 mg. ($\div$2-3) I.M.: Same as oral I.V.: Same as oral
Biperiden hydrochloride	Akineton	Oral: 3-8 mg. ($\div$3-4)
Biperiden lactate	Akineton lactate	I.M.: 8 mg. I.V.: 5-10 mg.
Chlorphenoxamine hydrochloride	Phenoxene	Oral: 150-400 mg. ($\div$3)
Cycrimine hydrochloride	Pagitane	Oral: 7.5-25 mg. ($\div$3-5)
Ethopropazine hydrochloride	Parsidol	Oral: 40-600 mg. ($\div$4)
Levodopa	Dopar, Larodopa	Oral: 0.5-8 Gm. ($\div$6)
Orphenadrine citrate	Disipal citrate, Norflex citrate	I.M.: 120 mg. ($\div$2) I.V.: Same as I.M.
Orphenadrine hydrochloride	Disipal, Norflex	Oral: 150-400 mg. ($\div$3)
Procyclidine hydrochloride	Kemadrin	Oral: 7.5-60 mg. ($\div$3)
Trihexyphenidyl hydrochloride	Artane, Pipanol, Tremin	Oral: 1-15 mg. ($\div$3-4)

adverse effects makes it necessary to evaluate objectively the effect of concurrent drug-induced nausea, anorexia, vomiting, or weakness on caloric intake and consequent energy level.

Therapy with levodopa carries with it the hazard of psychic disturbances (hallucinations, emotional changes), orthostatic hypotension, and hypersexuality. The latter problem was highly exaggerated to provide the base for a movie production. News media carried stories of miraculous recovery from Parkinson's disease when the drug was introduced. At the present time neither hypersexuality nor sudden miraculous recovery is a significant outcome of therapy. Current reports of patient progress after long-term drug therapy indicate repression of symptoms and a marked increase in functional ability in many patients. Chronic therapy is a necessity because dopamine deficiency is a lifelong problem for the patient.

Patients tend to be very selective in foods eaten and are most often disinterested in food. Chocolate, old cheese, and Chianti wine are favorite snacks for many patients, but the tyramine-containing foods suppress the production of dopamine during therapy. Tyramine content of all preferred foods should be examined. It is advisable for the patient to avoid high ingestion of any of the foods that require action of bacteria or molds in their preparation or preservation (i.e., pickled herring, alcoholic beverages, pods of broad beans, chicken livers, and aged or natural cheese) because the inhibition of dopamine effect seems related to competition at the preliminary synthesis of tyrosine to dopa (predopamine).

Pyridoxine (vitamin B_6) rapidly reverses the effect of levodopa by decarboxylation of the drug in the periphery. Vitamin preparations should be scrutinized for content of the offender, and foods high in pyridoxine are avoided. Pyridoxine is found in many foods, but patients are asked to avoid only those foods with high vitamin B_6 content: dried beans, dry milk, products containing whole grains, salmon, tuna, pork, and beef liver or kidneys.

Concurrent administration of the antiviral drug amantadine hydrochloride (Symmetrel) potentiates the effect of levodopa. The epidemiologic finding that there is a relationship between influenza virus exposure after World War I and the incidence of Parkinson's disease provides the rationale for concurrent antiviral therapy. Long-term harboring of the viral *genomes* and some unidentified precipitant that causes emergence of Parkinson's disease in individuals exposed to influenza more than fifty years earlier is the prevailing theory of the etiology of Parkinson's disease.

Levodopa causes an increase in blood sugar levels during therapy, but the predictable rise is of minor concern in most patients. Metabolites produced by drug decarboxylation in the gastrointestinal tract and liver appear in the urine. The metabolites produce false-positive reactions to ketone tests done with sodium nitroprusside reagent (Acetest, Ketostix, Labstix). When accurate analysis is needed, substitution of another test reagent is advisable.

There is a relationship between elevated plasma catecholamines and the emergence of cardiac arrhythmias during therapy. Patients treated with levodopa are monitored closely for emergence of cardiac irregularities. Most patients are over 60 years old at the time of therapy with levodopa, and care should include plans for regularly scheduled evaluation of apical pulse and blood pressure to identify changes.

Consistent evaluation of the comparative lying and standing blood pressure levels is planned as an aid in identifying the onset of orthostatic hypotension. Protection of the patient necessitates ambulatory limitation when hypotension is present. The patient's postural control is hampered by the occurrence of orthostatic hypotension during therapy. Sudden automatic movements to reach for support are not possible for the patient with Parkinson's disease, and the patient may fall.

Acetylcholine inhibition. With the exception of levodopa, all the drugs used for treatment of Parkinson's disease are anticholinergic agents (Table 18-2). They act primarily at central sites to inhibit cerebral motor impulses and block efferent impulses causing rigidity of the musculature.

Most of the drugs are used specifically for control of the spastic contraction of opposing sets of muscles. When rigidity improves, tremor often increases.

Procyclidine hydrochloride (Table 18-2) is used for control of acute incidents of extrapyramidal tract–initiated tremor, in addition to control of Parkinson's disease–related tremor. Ethopropazine hydrochloride acts to suppress major tremor by blocking ganglionic transmission. Suppression of tremor is an essential aspect of therapy to prevent exhaustion of the patient's energy reserves by continuous muscular activity. Drugs with antihistaminic and anticholinergic effect (i.e., diphenhydramine) are also used to control extrapyramidal signs occurring during therapy with tranquilizers (i.e., phenothiazines).

The drugs used for control of parkinsonism, including levodopa, have a suppressant effect on peripheral functions controlled by the parasympathetic nervous system. Drug action controls sialorrhea and excess lacrimation. Drowsiness, dry mouth, blurred vision, dizziness, nausea, central nervous system stimulation, tachycardia, and headache may occur with use of the drugs. Preplanning for the anticholinergic responses may prevent adverse effects on the patient's well-being and comfort. Unsteadiness and disinterest in food or decreased commitment to continuation of therapy may occur consequent to emergence of the adverse effects.

Hypersensitivity to the drugs is rare, but skin rash may occur during use of benztropine mesylate, orphenadrine citrate, orphenadrine hydrochloride, or trihexyphenidyl hydrochloride. Similarities in pharmacodynamic action of the Parkinson disease–specific drugs makes them comparable as therapeutic agents for control of extrapyramidal symptoms. The problems occurring concurrent with their use make it necessary to plan specific observations of the patient throughout therapy. For example, ethopropazine hydrochloride produces many adverse effects, in addition to the anticholinergic effects produced by other drugs in the grouping. Euphoria, hostility, paranoia, hypotension, and paresthesia added to the predictable problems of suppression of parasympathetic nervous system activity constitute a therapeutic course that is uncomfortable and hazardous for the patient.

The desperate need to function with greater ease makes the pharmacotherapeutic plan worthwhile to the patient. It is a frustrating situation for a thinking, feeling individual to be deprived of the ability to express himself freely through fluent speech and nonverbal communication so easily employed by other individuals. It is understandable that in such circumstances the individual is willing to take any steps that may reverse the process. The Parkinson disease–specific drugs offer some measure of symptom control, and changing from one anticholinergic drug to another may allow continued therapy when adverse effects occur.

Patient care

Maintenance of the pharmacotherapeutic plan is dependent in part on the continued willingness and ability of the patient to function while taking the drugs. Gastrointestinal disturbances (i.e., nausea, vomiting, anorexia) pose a major threat to the nutritional state of the patient. Carefully planned measures may modify the caloric deprivation. Between-meal snacks planned on the basis of patient preferences can provide nutrients when the patient's tolerance is highest. Family members may provide special treats not available in the hospital situation, and they often enjoy the opportunity to contribute in a realistic way to the patient's progress.

Accomplishment of each activity is a slow process for the patient. It is difficult to watch the patient slowly managing small bits of food, but the activity is important physically and psychologically for the patient. After the food is prepared in a manner indicated by the patient's functional ability, he should be allowed to take his time. It is a challenge to creativity to find ways to keep hot foods in a condition that makes them palatable when the patient takes a long time to eat, but the attempt to maintain food quality communicates caring and concern to the patient.

Many patients have difficulty swallowing, and they require small bits of food. Medications in liquid form are easier to swallow, and tablets crushed and placed in pureed fruit (i.e., applesauce) are managed easily. Administration of medications takes an inordinate amount of time, and the patient seems to have greater difficulty when hurried.

Exercise and physical therapy are usually part of the comprehensive plan for the patient. Muscles may be weak from previous long periods of immobility, and gradual exercise is necessary to begin a mobility program as the patient's condition improves. Ambulation is arduous, and the patient needs continual encouragement to move forward with muscle retraining.

Each of the drugs is a potent agent planned for a potent effect on the status of the patient, and it is important throughout therapy to plan observations for drug effect on all body systems. Immobility contributes to the incidence of constipation, and stiffness of joints, tremor, and spasticity contribute to problems of ambulation. Drug-induced dizziness, drowsiness, blurred vision, or mental confusion present additional hazards to safe mobilization, and occurrence of the problems may necessitate temporary limitation of activity.

Each positive outcome of therapy affects the patient's ability to function and indicates progress to him. Some of the positive effects are accompanied by problems. For example, decreased salivation obliterates a problem, but a dry mouth causes ill-fitting dentures. The frustrations are numerous, but nothing seems as important to the patient as general functional improvement.

The patient's difficulty with speech may increase his hesitancy to communicate the presence of problems unless opportunity is provided for him to take his time to relay the messages. Sitting quietly at the patient's bedside makes it evident to him that his sentences can be completed and he will be heard by someone who is concerned with his progress. The patient's intelligence is not impaired, and he can assist in tabulation of progress and adverse effects when he knows the particular assessments useful to evaluation of his progress.

Therapy with levodopa is planned to produce results in months rather than in days or weeks. Individually arranged contact with the patient at a later date may provide the opportunity to see the result of therapy. Oftentimes patient contact is limited to the acute and traumatic dosage adjustment period.

It is *hope* that helps the patient through the early days of the levodopa therapeutic regimen. All of the individuals around him hope that the future holds the same promise for him that it has for many others.

REFERENCES

Bogoch, Samuel, and Drefus, Jack: The broad range use of diphenylhydantoin, New York, 1970, The Drefus Medical Foundation.

Brokken, Bonnie, Lewis, Frances I., and Martin, William E.: Studies in clinical nursing: L-dopa—a nursing adventure, Nursing Clinics of North America 4:733, 1969.

Carozza, Virginia J.: Understanding the patient with epilepsy, Nursing Clinics of North America 5:13, 1970.

Cotzias, George C., Papavasiliou, Paul S., and Gellene, Rosemary: Modification of parkinsonism—chronic treatment with L-dopa, The New England Journal of Medicine 280:337, 1969.

Fangman, Anne, and O'Malley, William E.: L-Dopa and the patient with Parkinson's disease, American Journal of Nursing 69:1455, 1969.

Goth, Andres: Medical pharmacology, ed. 6, St. Louis, 1972, The C. V. Mosby Co.

Haber, Martha E.: Parkinson's disease: challenge to the health professions, Nursing Clinics of North America 4:263, 1969.

Howard, Frank M., Jr., Seybold, Marjorie E., and Reiher, Jean: The treatment of recurrent convulsions with intravenous injection of diazepam, Medical Clinics of North America 52:977, 1968.

Karnes, William E.: Medical treatment for convulsive disorders, Medical Clinics of North America 52:959, 1968.

Kutt, Henn, and Louis, Sidney: Untoward effects of anticonvulsants (editorial), The New England Journal of Medicine 286:1316, 1972.

Lippold, Olaf: Physiological tremor, Scientific American 224:65, March, 1971.

Loranger, Armand W., Goodell, Helen, Lee, John E., and McDowell, Fletcher: Levodopa treatment of Parkinson's syndrome, Archives of General Psychiatry 26:163, 1972.

Luria, A. R.: The functional organization of the brain, Scientific American 222:66, March, 1970.

Malherbe, Christian, Burrill, Karen C., Levin, Seymour R., Karam, John H., and Forsham, Peter H.: Effect of diphenylhydantoin on insulin secretion in man, The New England Journal of Medicine 286:339, 1972.

McDowell, Fletcher: Convulsions and cerebral atherosclerosis, Current Concepts of Cerebrovascular Disease (Stroke) 4:7, 1969.

Mountcastle, Vernon B., editor: Medical physiology, ed. 13, vol. 2, St. Louis, 1974, The C. V. Mosby Co.

Papavasiliou, Paul S., Cotzias, George C., Düby, Simone E., Steck, Andreas J., Fehling, Clas, and Bell, Margaret A.: Levodopa in parkinsonism: potentiation of central effects, The New England Journal of Medicine 286:8, 1972.

Reilly, Mary Jo, editor: American hospital formulary service, vol. 1, sect. 12:00, 28:00, Washington, D. C., 1973, American Society of Hospital Pharmacists.

Schmidt, Richard Penrose, and Wilder, B. Joseph: Epilepsy, Philadelphia, 1968, F. A. Davis Co.

Tate, Gayle: Assessment and direction of nursing care for patients with acute central nervous system insult, Nursing Clinics of North America 6:165, 1971.

Wand, Martin, and Mather, John A.: Diphenylhydantoin intoxication mimicking botulism, The New England Journal of Medicine 286:88, 1972.

Yahr, Melvin D., and Duvoisin, Roger C.: Drug therapy: drug therapy of parkinsonism, The New England Journal of Medicine 287:20, 1972.

19

Skeletal muscle contraction

Neural transmitters
Motor end-plate transmission
Cholinesterase inhibitors
Pharmacodynamics
Patient care
Motor end-plate inhibition
Pharmacodynamics
Patient care
Muscular hypertonicity
Pharmacodynamics
Patient care

Muscle contraction is dependent on the transmission of impulses through motor pathways for voluntary control and on stimuli propagated by afferent sensory endings in the periphery for both voluntary and reflex control. In addition to integrity of the anatomic nerve and muscle structures, muscle contraction requires the presence of transmitter substances, cations, and anions for electrophysiologic equilibrium. Calcium ions at the membrane surface and within the sarcoplasmic reticulum affect the contractile force of muscle response to neural stimuli. Activity or reactivity of the striated muscle affects functional and protective mechanisms in the body. Drugs can be used to control striated muscle tone by modifying the response to neural stimuli.

Neural transmitters

Acetylcholine is the chief chemical mediator of nerve transmission at the ganglion and the myoneural junction of the parasympathetic nervous system, and it is the mediator at the ganglion of the sympathetic nervous system. The myoneural junctional mediator of the sympathetic nervous system is norepinephrine. Acetylcholine is also the chief chemical mediator of nerve transmission at the myoneural junction in the skeletal musculature.

The presence of acetylcholine at the junctional sites in both branches of the autonomic nervous system and in skeletal muscle motor end-plate sites affects the action of drugs used for control of acetylcholine activity. Pharmacodynamic action can be controlled partially by use of drugs with high selectivity for particular sites, or by dosage regulation, but at high dosage it is predictable that effects of the drug will be observed in tissues other than target action sites.

Motor end-plate transmission

There is a structural difference between visceral and skeletal muscle receptors. The structure of the visceral myoneural junction is a simplistic naked nerve–muscle contact, but the skeletal muscle junction is a complex motor end plate with definite receptor sites for the mediator chemical. Motor stimuli arriving at the nerve ending liberate acetylcholine, and the chemical mediator moves to the motor end plate to initiate muscle polarization (Fig. 19-1). The enzyme cholinesterase at the motor nerve ending and motor end plate site inactivates acetylcholine. The prompt action of the enzyme cleaves acetylcholine to acetate and choline.

Drugs can be used to affect acetylcholine activity at the motor end plate by inhibiting cholinesterase activity, substituting for acetylcholine, or blocking receptor sites for acetylcholine. Understanding of the mechanisms of neuroeffector transmission simplifies analysis

Skeletal muscle contraction

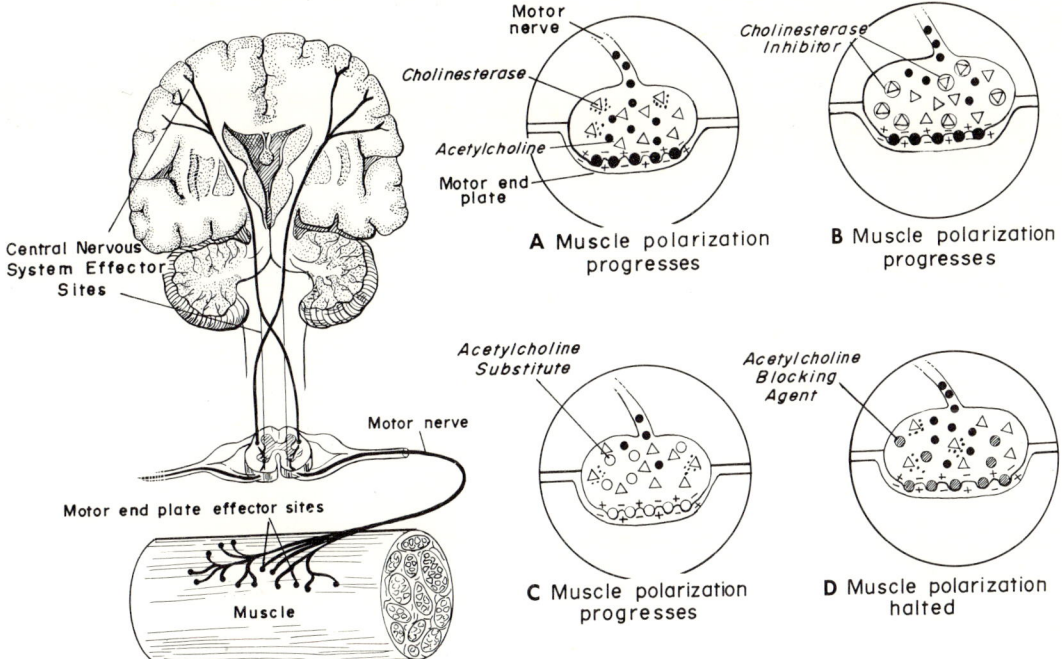

Fig. 19-1. Central and peripheral effector sites of drugs used to modify skeletal muscle activity. Schematic inserts show motor end-plate effector sites. **A**, Acetylcholine released at the nerve ending moves to the end plate to initiate depolarization of the muscle. Cholinesterase destroys acetylcholine at the contact site. **B**, Cholinesterase inhibitor prevents destruction of acetylcholine. **C**, Acetylcholine substitute provides additional acetylcholine-like activity. **D**, Acetylcholine blocking agent prevents muscle depolarization at the end plate.

of effects of drugs used to alter skeletal muscle polarization cycles.

CHOLINESTERASE INHIBITORS
Pharmacodynamics

Preventing the activity of cholinesterase in enzymatic conversion of acetylcholine to acetate and choline permits the level of the physiologic mediator at the myoneural junction to build up. Elevated levels of acetylcholine result in a higher level stimulus to muscle contraction.

Each of the drugs identified as cholinesterase inhibitors (Table 19-1) acts to improve muscle tone by decreasing the enzymatic destruction of acetylcholine. Neostigmine bromide and neostigmine methylsulfate are the only members of the group used for stimulation of smooth muscle contraction in abdominal viscera (i.e., uterus, bladder). For example, the drug may be administered parenterally for prevention of postoperative atony of the urinary bladder or ileus. Drug-induced contraction of either organ improves elimination after surgery and increases the patient's comfort.

The drugs are used principally to improve transmission at the myoneural junction of skeletal muscles and of small muscle groups innervated by motor tracts of the cranial nerves. Pa-

Table 19-1. Dosage range of cholinesterase inhibitors

Nonproprietary name	Proprietary (trade) name	Daily adult dosage range
Ambenonium chloride	Mytelase	Oral: 15-200 mg. (÷3-4)
Neostigmine bromide	Prostigmin bromide	Oral: 45-90 mg.(÷3)
Neostigmine methylsulfate	Prostigmin methylsulfate	I.M.: 1-2 mg. (÷4-6)
Pyridostigmine bromide	Mestinon	Oral: 0.36-1.5 Gm.

tients with the symptom complex known as *myasthenia gravis* require the anticholinesterase drugs for survival. The situation of these patients presents a vivid example of the necessity of acetylcholine for myoneural transmission. Ptosis of the eyelid or decreased responses of the facial muscles are tolerable, but atony of the muscles controlling respiration and swallowing are life threatening.

Timing of drug administration depends on the pharmacotherapeutic plan. The patient receiving neostigmine methylsulfate may be given it preoperatively to prevent postoperative atony, or he may receive the drug only postoperatively when atony occurs. The patient with myasthenia gravis is dependent on the drugs for myoneural transmission and must receive the drugs at regular intervals around the clock. Extended-release tablets are available to provide pharmacodynamic effect on transmission without disturbing the sleep of the patient during the night.

Few drugs demonstrate as vividly the pharmacodynamic action seen when a cholinesterase inhibitor is administered to a patient with myasthenia gravis. Ability to sustain a squeezing grip on an object in the hand increases dramatically. Depth of respirations improves as contractile strength of respiratory muscles increases, and improved vital capacity allows the patient to project air over the vocal cords more forcefully to produce a more audible voice.

Short-term use of the drugs may produce evidence of excess acetylcholine activity at the myoneural junction, but problems more often are related to long-term use of the drugs. Excess acetylcholine effect can be controlled by anticholinergic drugs. The predictability of atropine sulfate effect makes it the drug of choice to counteract the effect of cholinesterase inhibitors.

Patient care

Either underdosage or overdosage of drugs presents complex manifestations when the status of the patient with myasthenia gravis changes. Important clues for the nurse observer who may find the patient in an extremely weak condition and barely breathing in the middle of the night is the presence of parasympathetic-related problems. Patients may have excess tearing, copious secretions in the nose and mouth, profuse perspiration, and incontinence of feces or urine. Concurrent signs of excess acetylcholine transmission are seen in skeletal muscle. Muscle membrane remains depolarized as a consequence of continual stimuli that prevent repolarization. The drugs are used for control of peripheral muscle function, but the commonalities of mediator substance in skeletal and smooth muscle cause an effect in those functions controlled by both peripheral muscle and the parasympathetic nervous system when excess cholinesterase-inhibiting drugs are used. Evidence of increased acetylcholine activity is an indication that pharmacodynamic activity of the cholinesterase inhibitor is at a high level, and relief of the patient's symptoms requires use of an anticholinergic drug. Conversely, when the patient is in acute distress (extremely weak and barely breathing) and there is no evidence of increased acetylcholine activity, administration of the cholinesterase inhibitor is required to reinstitute acetylcholine activity at the myoneural junction.

The patient with myasthenia gravis takes the drugs for long-term inhibition of cholinesterase. He must understand that emergence of gastrointestinal disturbances or changes in voiding patterns are indicative of overaction of the drugs. Careful directions for immediate protective measures and prompt contact with the physician are essential during institution of the therapeutic plan. The multiple problems of the patient with myasthenia gravis necessitate investigation of all aspects of the disease entity in planning care of the patient. Myasthenia gravis is often described as a pharmacologic disease, and drug dosage regulation is an important aspect of the therapeutic plan.

MOTOR END-PLATE INHIBITION
Pharmacodynamics

Several agents intercede at the myoneural junction to interfere with acetylcholine transmission of nerve impulses. The drugs block the action of acetylcholine at the muscle junction by competitively binding to the receptor sites. Pharmacodynamic action causes paralysis of the muscles in a predictable and orderly progression, with return of function following a reversal of the initiation pattern.

Decamethonium bromide (Syncurine) and succinylcholine chloride (Anectine, Quelicin, Sucostrin) have a competitive effect at the receptor site comparable to that of excess acetylcholine. They cause depolarization and an initial contraction but prevent subsequent contractions by preventing repolarization. Dimethyl tubocurarine iodide (Metubine), dimethyl tubocurarine chloride (Mecostrin), gallamine triethiodide (Flaxedil), and tubocurarine chloride act by a different mechanism to prevent depolarization. They move rapidly to the myoneural junction where they act at the end plate and muscles remain in a relaxed state. The latter group is described as *curariform* drugs.

The potent drugs are administered intravenously by the physician for control of convulsions or for abolition of muscle activity during surgery (i.e., thoracic surgery). Within 3 minutes after the intravenous infusion is started, the patient's eyelids feel heavy, and swallowing and talking become difficult. Progression of muscle weakness follows a consistent pattern: extremities, neck, trunk, spine, intercostals, and finally diaphragm. An endotracheal tube is inserted as the oropharyngeal responses decrease, and artificial ventilation is started as muscles controlling respiration weaken.

Succinylcholine chloride administration is often accompanied by use of hexafluorenium bromide (Mylaxen) to prolong the action time of the former drug. Succinylcholine chloride is rapidly hydrolyzed by cholinesterase to choline and succinic acid. Prolonged and smoother action is accomplished by concurrent administration of an anticholinesterase that suppresses enzymatic hydrolysis, but curariform drugs generally are used to attain prolonged periods of muscular relaxation (i.e., during cardiac surgery).

Edrophonium chloride (Tensilon) is used to antagonize the effect of the curariform drugs. It acts as an acetylcholine substitute and displaces the drug from the motor end-plate. Administration of edrophonium chloride reinstitutes muscle contraction in response to neural stimulation.

Patient care

Knowledge of the progression and reversal of the order of muscle function return is important to the nurse responsible for the patient's care during the immediate period after administration when observation of muscle function is intense. The information frequently is useful to the nurse responsible for the preparation of the patient for his surgical experience. The anesthetist meets with the patient prior to surgery to explain planned approaches to the particular anesthesia program. Accompanying the physician during the visit allows orientation to the patient's anxiety level during the discussion and his understanding of the specific plan. The patient's subsequent questions about the discussion can be clarified best if the specific plan is understood by the nurse.

Many patients use a trust approach in the preoperative period, but some want to know what measures are involved in their specific surgical experience. The patient is preparing himself for a stressful situation. He can be supported in his efforts when team members work in a united manner to keep communication clear and relevant to his needs and level of readiness for information sharing.

MUSCULAR HYPERTONICITY

Hypertonicity of muscles may occur secondary to disruption of sensory or motor nerve control centers, or it may occur with injury or trauma to muscles or their articulations. Pain stimuli from a locus at the muscle site send afferent messages to the spinal reflex arcs, and efferent stimuli cause contraction of muscles in the area. Protective splinting by contraction of adjacent muscles causes pain that intensifies reflex contraction, and a vicious cycle of spasm-pain-spasm is instituted.

The sequence may occur after excessive use of a muscle or muscle group for prolonged periods. For example, the first attempt at strenuous sports (i.e., tennis, bowling) may initiate muscle splinting. Accumulation of acidic products, or metabolic wastes, in the muscle initiates reflex splinting that becomes painful and induces further splinting. The sequence of events may cause immobility or painful function of the part for many hours.

Localized application of heat or warm baths

improves circulation and relieves the pain by interrupting the cyclic contraction of muscle in response to pain. Heat or massage mobilizes inhibitory fibers to block pain impulses, and muscle contraction decreases. A vivid example is the effectiveness of harsh massage of a stubbed toe that gradually relieves the pain by mobilizing inhibitory fibers.

Electronic nerve stimulators for the control of intractable pain operate on a similar principle. When pain occurs (i.e., trigeminal neuralgia), the patient turns on the pocket-size control device that electronically stimulates nerve endings through implanted electrodes in the affected area. Increased stimuli mobilize inhibitory responses that halt the excruciating pain.

Muscle spasm, or hypertonicity, may continue until the pain stimulus is removed. Metabolic products causing cyclic spasm are removed by venous drainage from the muscle bed within a short time, but anatomic or physiologic disruption may require surgical correction or use of pain-alleviating drugs.

Many tranquilizers cause relaxation of skeletal muscle by inhibiting central interneural pathways, but the agents used specifically for relaxation of the voluntary muscle have less central effect than the drugs generally used for tranquilizer, or antianxiety, activity. Muscle relaxants interrupt the multisynaptic pathways involved in propagation of impulses between the periphery and the spinal cord. Many muscle relaxants have a concomitant effect on interneurons at higher levels that affects pain interpretation areas in the cerebral cortex. Drugs also are used to halt the transmission of neural stimuli at the myoneural junction by affecting acetylcholine activity. Decreasing the levels of neural transmitter substance slows muscular activity, and pain is decreased.

Pharmacodynamics

Central interneuron inhibition. Drugs given for relaxation of skeletal muscle are part of a therapeutic plan to reduce spasm and increase the motion of adjacent structures by concurrent use of heat, massage, therapeutic exercise, and drugs to relieve pain. Muscle relaxants (Table 19-2) differ somewhat in their chemical derivation, but each of the agents acts in a comparable manner at varying levels on the multisynaptic neural pathways in the spinal cord and subcortical areas to interrupt transmission of reflex stimuli causing hypertonicity of the muscle. The drugs often affect higher interneuronal sites and cause some analgesia, but drowsiness is seldom a problem with oral forms of the drugs. When lassitude and weakness of noninvolved muscle groups

Table 19-2. Dosage range of skeletal muscle relaxants

Nonproprietary name	Proprietary (trade) name	Daily adult dosage range
Carisoprodol	Rela, Soma	Oral: 1.4 Gm. (÷4)
Chlormezanone	Trancopal	Oral: 300-800 mg. (÷3-4)
Chlorphenesin carbamate	Maolate	Oral: 1.6-2.4 Gm. (÷4)
Chlorzoxazone	Paraflex	Oral: 1.5-3 Gm. (÷3-4)
Mephenesin	Daserol, Dioloxol, Mepherol, Mephson, Myanesin, Myoxane, Oranixon, Prolax, Relaxar, Sinan, Thoxidil, Tolhart, Tolosate, Tolserol, Tolulox	Oral: 1-3 Gm. (÷3-5) I.V.: 50-150 ml./single dose
Mephenesin carbamate	Tolseram	Oral: 1-3 Gm. (÷3-5)
Metaxalone	Skelaxin	Oral: 2.4-3.2 Gm. (÷3-4)
Methocarbamol	Robaxin	Oral: 4-9 Gm. (÷4) I.M.: 1.5-3 Gm. (÷3) I.V.: 1-3 Gm./single dose
Phenyramidol hydrochloride	Analexin	Oral: 200-400 mg./single dose
Promoxolane	Dimethylane	Oral: 0.75-1 Gm./single dose
Styramate	Sinaxar	Oral: 200-400 mg./single dose

limits the functional ability of the patient, the physician may modify dosage of the drug.

Mephenesin and methocarbamol (Table 19-2) may be used parenterally for their effect on interneurons at the junction of upper and lower motor neurons to decrease hyperexcitability, tremor, or spasm of peripheral skeletal muscles. Intravenous administration of the drugs produces an effect within 10 minutes, but patients complain of pain at the injection site when methocarbamol is infused. Mephenesin has a short duration of action; therefore its use is limited to acute situations.

Patient care

Prolonged hypertonicity of muscles with continual splinting gradually causes muscle atrophy. Drug-instituted relaxation of muscle provides an opportunity to mobilize the affected structures. Prior application of moist heat or warm baths may enhance muscle relaxation and allow wider range of motion.

Plans for physical therapeutic procedures should be clear to the patient and to each member of the nursing team to assure continuance of measures for mobilization and protection of the musculoskeletal structures. Knowledge of interim exercises, mobilization techniques, and appropriate methods for use of appliances are important for a consistent approach to the patient's care. Timing of drug administration to correlate with planned periods of exercise has a positive effect on the readiness of the musculature for therapy. Measures that decrease discomfort may make the patient more amenable to the exercise plan.

Planned observations of drug effect on muscle relaxation are accompanied by assessment of the effect of immobility on adjacent tissues. Immobility affects muscle strength or tone and it may affect blood circulation in an involved extremity. Fluid accumulates in distal parts of an extremity that remains immobilized in a dependent position.

Observations of the patient's activity level include assessment of alertness and coordination because drowsiness, incoordination, and weakness of muscles occur in some patients during drug therapy. Drug effect on central interneurons may potentiate the action of other sedatives or central nervous system depressants.

Hypersensitivity reactions (i.e., dermatitis, hepatotoxicity) have occurred with use of the muscle relaxants, and planned observation for skin rash or yellowing of the sclera may provide early evidence of adverse drug effect. Metaxalone therapy is usually limited to a 10-day period because drug administration beyond that time has caused hepatotoxicity and bone marrow depression in some patients.

Metabolites of chlorzoxazone sometimes produce an orange or purple-red color in the patient's urine, and the urine may show a false-positive test for bile when the test solution is a ferric chloride reagent. Metaxalone produces a reducing agent that causes a false-positive reaction for glycosuria when Benedict's qualitative reagent or Clinitest is used. Test procedures using test tapes for analysis of glucose content are unaffected by the reducing agent.

REFERENCES

Corbin, Kendall B.: Common neurologic brachial pain problems, Medical Clinics of North America **52:**773, 1968.

Goodman, Louis S., and Gilman, Arthur, editors: The pharmacological basis of therapeutics, ed. 4, New York, 1970, The Macmillan Co.

Goth, Andres: Medical pharmacology, ed. 6, St. Louis, 1972, The C. V. Mosby Co.

Guyton, Arthur C.: Textbook of medical physiology, ed. 4, Philadelphia, 1971, W. B. Saunders Co.

Irving, Laurence: Adaptations to cold, Scientific American **214:**94, Jan., 1966.

Koelle, George B.: Acetylcholine-physiology, pharmacology, and medicine, The New England Journal of Medicine **286:**1086, 1972.

Liverani, Louise, and Osserman, Ruth Sue: Myasthenia gravis: a nursing care plan, Nursing Clinics of North America **7:**185, 1972.

Margaria, Rodolfo: The sources of muscular energy, Scientific American **226:**84, March, 1972.

Merton, P. A.: How we control the contraction of our muscles, Scientific American **226:**30, May, 1972.

O'Connor, Carol T.: Curare in patient care, American Journal of Nursing **72:**913, 1972.

Orten, James M., and Neuhaus, Otto W.: Biochemistry, ed. 8, St. Louis, 1970, The C. V. Mosby Co.

Reilly, Mary Jo, editor: American hospital formulary service, vol. 1, sect. 12:00, Washington, D. C., 1973, American Society of Hospital Pharmacists.

Walts, Leonard F., Levin, Norman, and Dillon, John B.: Assessment of recovery from curare, Journal of the American Medical Association **213:**1894, 1970.

Weinstein, Ronald S., and McNutt, N. Scott: Current concepts: cell junctions, The New England Journal of Medicine **286:**521, 1972.

20

Sleep patterns

Sleep cycles
Sleep disruption
Pharmacodynamics
Patient care

The vitality of an individual and his enthusiasm for involvement in living are dependent on a balance between activity and rest. Sleep contributes to the psychosomatic equilibrium that makes each day a new beginning. Inability to sleep depletes the psychic and physiologic reserves of the individual. Sleep studies indicate that the quality of sleep is as important as the length of time the individual sleeps.

Sleep cycles

A natural sleep is preceded by a latent period lasting 30 to 60 minutes after retiring. The combined effect of muscle relaxation, self-hypnosis, and neurohormonal action gradually moves the individual out of contact with the environment, and he is asleep. Natural sleep is a rhythmic progression through stages that provide physical rest and psychic equanimity.

Stages I and II are light sleep periods that allow easy arousal. Stage III is a transition from the lighter to deeper state of sleep. Stage IV is a deep sleep state. The deep sleep period is longest in the first sequence of sleep stage progression when physical fatigue causes deep relaxation. The low metabolic state of Stages I, II, III, and IV is interrupted by a period known as *rapid eye movement sleep* (REM). Vivid, colorful dreams, increased metabolic activity, and multidirectional eye movements occur during REM sleep. Periodically throughout the rhythmic sleep sequence there are short intervals of awakening (Fig. 20-1).

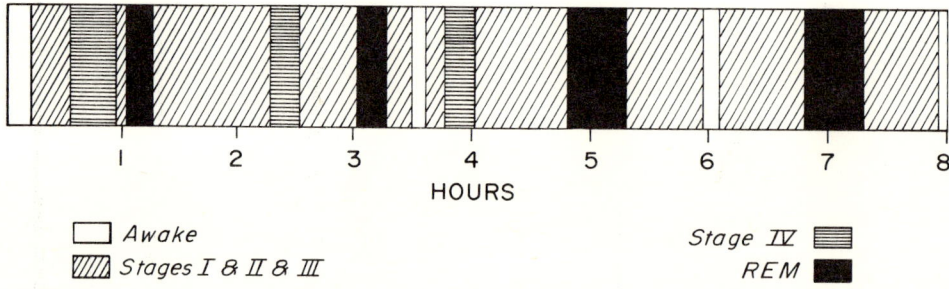

Fig. 20-1. Predictable progression of sleep stages in a normal individual during an 8-hour period (diagrammatic).

Sleep disruption

Anxiety, pain, environmental noise, physical exhaustion, and drugs are protagonists to normal sleep patterns. Anxiety causes an insomnia demonstrated by an increase in sleep latency, nocturnal awakenings, and a decrease in total sleep time. Environmental stimuli or forced awakening (i.e., for physical assessment of the patient's status) also contribute to the disruption of sleep patterns and consequent decrease in total sleep time. Disruption of sleep affects the natural awakening behavior patterns of the individual.

Extreme physical fatigue after hours of heavy work lengthens Stage IV sleep and decreases REM time. Most of the drugs used for sleep control decrease Stage IV sleep and REM time. Drug-induced deprivation of Stage IV sleep may not adversely affect the physically inactive hospitalized patient, but decreased REM time lessens psychic release and may increase anxiety, tension, and irritability.

Pharmacodynamics

Control of sleep patterns can be accomplished by various drugs (Table 20-1) that move the patient gradually through levels of consciousness to progressively decrease responsiveness to environmental stimuli. Periodic use of small dosage of some sleep-inducing (hypnotic) drugs provides daytime sedation of the hyperactive individual. Larger dosage provides the hypnotic and muscle relaxant effect requisite to sleep induction and maintenance. Beyond the dosage necessary to sleep control, drugs move the patient further into an unconscious, or anesthetic, state. Higher levels of the drug cause coma or death. Up to the end point, the patient's status may be reversible at any interval along the continuum:

Sedation ⇌ Hypnosis ⇌ Sleep ⇌ (Stage IV) ⇌ Anesthesia ⇌ Coma → Death

High dosage levels of central nervous system depressants may be administered to increase pharmacodynamic action to the anesthesia level. Progression through the continuum also occurs with accidental or intentional overdosage of drugs that depress the central nervous system (i.e., barbiturates).

Sleep induction and maintenance. The most common pharmacotherapeutic use of sedative-hypnotic agents is to induce sleep. The specific action sites of hypnotics are unclear, although the result produced by the drugs suggests an effect on suppressing interneuronal activity between the thalamus and the cerebral cortex. The drugs raise the arousal threshold to stimuli and reduce motor activity. Subcortical sites of action include the reticular and limbic formations.

Neurohormones act on the pontile reticular formation to stimulate metabolic activity and eye movements during REM time of natural sleep. Partial inhibition of norepinephrine, or its precursors tyrosine and dopamine, decreases the incidence of REM sleep during therapy with most of the hypnotic drugs.

The aim of therapy with hypnotic drugs is to produce nearly natural sleep from which the patient can be roused without difficulty. During therapy with any of the agents employed to induce and maintain sleep, patients occasionally complain of headache or nausea after use of the drugs. Initial therapy may occasionally cause a period of hyperactivity, hyperexcitability, and compulsive talking. There is considerable variation in individual responses to the drugs used for sleep production. A patient may become hyperactive with one drug but have restful sleep with another. Discussion of drug-related problems with the physician allows change to another agent that provides sleep.

Chloral hydrate has been used as a hypnotic since 1869, and it is still considered to produce sleep closely resembling a natural pattern. There is some decrease in Stage IV sleep, but other patterns follow a natural time sequence. Chloral betaine and petrichloral (Table 20-1) are converted to *trichloroacetic acid,* which is also the active form of chloral hydrate. The drugs act within 30 minutes after oral administration, and sleep may last up to 8 hours. The drugs are particularly useful for elderly patients, causing less mental confusion and disorientation than do other hypnotics.

Administration of chloral hydrate close to the time of alcohol ingestion concocts endogenous knockout drops. Patients responsible for self-administration of the drug at home should

Table 20-1. Dosage range of drugs used for sedative-hypnotic effect

Nonproprietary name	Proprietary (trade) name	Daily adult dosage range	Nonproprietary name	Proprietary (trade) name	Daily adult dosage range
Amobarbital sodium*	Amytal sodium	Oral: 40-200 mg. (÷1-3) I.M.: Same as oral I.V.: 0.25-1 Gm./single dose	Paraldehyde		Oral: 4-15 ml. I.M.: 5-10 ml.
			Pentobarbital sodium*	Isobarb, Napental, Nembutal, Pental	Oral: 45-120 mg. (÷3-4) I.M.: Same as oral I.V.: 200-500 mg. (÷2-6)
Aprobarbital*	Alurate	Oral: 60-160 mg. (÷3)			
Barbital*	Barbitone, Veronal	Oral: 130-500 mg. (÷2-3)	Petrichloral	Periclor	Oral: 300-600 mg.
Barbital sodium*	Medinal	Oral: 130-500 mg. (÷2-3)	Phenobarbital sodium*	Luminal sodium	Oral: 30-650 mg. (÷2-4) I.V.: 300 mg.
Butabarbital sodium*	Bubartal sodium, Butisol sodium	Oral: 24-240 mg. (÷3-4) I.M.: Same	Probarbital sodium*	Ipral	Oral: 150-390 mg. (÷3)
Chloral betaine	Beta-Chlor	Oral: 0.75-2 Gm. (÷3)	Promazine hydrochloride†	Sparine	Oral: 0.1-1 Gm. (÷4-6) I.M.: Same as oral I.V.: 50-300 mg.
Chloral hydrate	Felsules, Lorinal, Noctec, Somnos	Oral: 0.75-2 Gm. (÷3)			
Ethchlorvynol	Placidyl	Oral: 0.2-1 Gm. (÷2-3)			
Ethinamate	Valmid	Oral: 0.5-1 Gm.	Propiomazine hydrochloride†	Largon	I.M.: 20-60 mg. (÷2) I.V.: 40-60 mg. (÷2)
Flurazepam hydrochloride	Dalmane	Oral: 15-30 mg.			
Glutethimide	Doriden	Oral: 0.375-1 Gm. (÷3)	Secobarbital sodium*	Evronal, Seconal sodium	Oral: 45-200 mg. (÷3-4) I.M.: Same as oral I.V.: 250 mg./single dose
Hexobarbital*	Sombucaps, Sombulex	Oral 0.5-1.5 Gm. (÷2-3)			
Methaqualone	Quaalude, Sopor	Oral: 150-300 mg. (÷4)			
Methaqualone hydrochloride	Parest, Somnafac	Oral: 200-400 mg.	Sodium bromide		Oral: 2-4 Gm. (÷2-4)
Methotrimeprazine hydrochloride†	Levoprome	I.M.: 2-120 mg. (÷4-6)	Talbutal*	Lotusate	Oral: 60-150 mg. (÷2-3)
			Triclofos sodium	Triclos	Oral: 1.5 Gm.
Methyprylon	Noludar	Oral: 15-400 mg. (÷3-4)	Vinbarbital*	Delvinal	Oral: 90-200 mg. (÷3-4)

*Barbiturates.
†Antihistamines (phenothiazines).

know the hazard of drug-alcohol combination.

Chloral hydrate is irritating to the gastric mucosa, and the irritant effect stimulates peristalsis in some patients. Serving the drug with water, fruit juice, milk, formula, or ginger ale provides dilution of the drug adequate to decrease gastric irritation. Suppositories are available for patients who have gastric intolerance to oral forms of the drug.

Glucuronide metabolites of trichloroacetic acid may cause a false-positive reaction to Benedict's qualitative reagent test for glycosuria. Use of tape tests can be substituted, since they are unaffected by the metabolites.

Triclofos sodium (Table 20-1) has a hypnotic effect comparable to that of chloral hydrate. The metabolic product *trichloroethanol* produces the pharmacodynamic effect, and sleep stages are similar to those of normal sleep. The chief advantage over chloral hydrate is the lower incidence of gastrointestinal disturbances induced by triclofos sodium.

Paraldehyde (Table 20-1) has also been used for many years. Although it produces a hypnotic effect within 10 to 15 minutes, use of the drug is limited to control of acute alcoholism, convulsions, or comparable problems. One of the reasons for the limited use of paraldehyde is the pungent odor and taste of the liquid. The odor permeates the air for many feet around the patient when the drug is administered by any route. Paraldehyde is metabolized by the liver and excreted from the lungs. The air pollution results from the drug liberated with each exhalation of the patient.

Paraldehyde is more palatable for the patient when served in milk or iced fruit juice, although alcoholics tolerate ingestion of the undisguised drug fairly well. Paraldehyde is dispensed in rubber-stoppered bottles because air exposure converts it to toxic acetic acid. In addition to oral or deep intramuscular administration, the drug is sometimes prescribed as a retention enema. A drug-oil mixture in a 1:2 ratio is used to decrease mucosal irritation.

Methotrimeprazine hydrochloride, promazine hydrochloride, and propiomazine hydrochloride (Table 20-1) are pharmacologically classified as antihistamines of the *phenothiazine series*. The high sedative-hypnotic effect of the drugs makes them primarily useful for induction of sleep in anxious patients. The absence of respiratory depression when high doses are administered makes the drugs very useful. Intramuscular injection of the drugs produces an effect within 30 minutes that lasts up to 4 hours. There is a decrease of REM time during drug therapy. The short action time of the drugs necessitates repeated administration if the patient wakens or is agitated at the end of 4 hours.

Concurrent antihistaminic and antiemetic properties provide additional relief of physiologic problems and expand the usefulness of the drugs. Patients complain of dizziness, dry mouth, and cardiac palpitation during therapy, but the chief problem is the emergence of hypotension. Promazine hydrochloride and propiomazine hydrochloride cause postural hypotension most frequently when administered parenterally, but the decrease in pressure levels is moderate. The patient may compensate for the problem by remaining recumbent for a short period after receiving the drug and modifying the speed of positional changes.

Orthostatic hypotension occurring with intramuscular administration of methotrimeprazine hydrochloride may persist for 4 to 12 hours; therefore the drug is administered only when the patient can remain supine for 6 to 12 hours. The pronounced adverse effect on hemodynamic equilibrium limits use of the drug to nonambulatory patients. The total period of drug use is limited to 30 days because of the adverse action on hemodynamics.

The drugs have produced extrapyramidal tract irritation, with consequent parkinsonian-like symptoms (i.e., tremor of the extremities that is relieved with voluntary movement, masklike facies, excess salivation, propulsion gait). Planned observations for changes in motor coordination are indicated throughout therapy.

Other adverse reactions to the drugs include cholestatic jaundice and agranulocytosis. Contact with the patient offers an opportunity to observe the sclera to ascertain whether icterus is present. Observations of the stool color provide overt evidence of bile content because clay-colored feces occur in its absence.

Hematologic studies are usually planned by the physician if drug therapy is protracted. The patient's complaints of sore throat, mouth lesions, or fever often provide the first clues to emerging problems. Onset of the symptoms is brought to the attention of the physician, since they may be the result of leukocyte depression.

Ethchlorvynol and ethinamate (Table 20-1) produce a hypnotic effect in $1/2$ hour after oral administration that lasts for 4 to 5 hours. The drugs lessen REM sleep time. Ethinamate causes few problems during therapy, but ethchlorvynol may cause morning drowsiness, blurring of vision, and transient hypotension. Most patients taking the drugs complain of morning hangover.

Methaqualone, methaqualone hydrochloride, and methyprylon (Table 20-1) produce a hypnotic effect in approximately 30 minutes that lasts up to 8 hours. Methaqualone hydrochloride and methyprylon depress REM sleep time, but methaqualone allows normal REM time. Morning drowsiness and gastrointestinal disturbances occur during therapy with each of the drugs.

Flurazepam hydrochloride produces a hypnotic effect in 20 to 45 minutes that lasts for 8 hours. Decreased Stage IV sleep occurs during therapy, but normal REM time occurs in sleep patterns. Dizziness, tachycardia, and gastrointestinal disturbances are the chief complaints of patients during therapy.

Glutethimide (Table 20-1) induces sleep in 15 to 30 minutes that lasts for 4 to 8 hours. The drug depresses REM and Stage IV sleep time. Glutethimide has an anticholinergic action, in addition to its hypnotic effect. Distribution of the drug is highest in lipoid tissue, but it enters all body tissues.

The high lipid affinity of glutethimide makes it possible to dialyze excess drug by using a dialysate high in lipids. The method has been employed in clinical trials to treat patients with overdose of glutethimide. Dialysis offers hope that intoxication with the drug can be controlled.

Glutethimide acts synergistically with anticoagulants to lower the circulating prothrombin of patients receiving the two drugs concurrently. Adverse effects include morning drowsiness and transient hypotension. The adverse effect of greatest concern is the reported incidence of decreased pharyngeal and laryngeal reflexes in some patients receiving the drug. The problem occurs infrequently, but the incidence of the problem suggests planned observations of patients during initial therapy.

Sodium bromide (Table 20-1) is used primarily for daytime sedation. Bromides are components of numerous over-the-counter drug preparations, including effervescent antacid preparations. Sodium bromide is irritating to the gastric mucosa, and administration with milk, foods, or water may decrease gastric discomfort. The drug gradually accumulates until serum content rises to a level required to produce a sedative effect. Long-term use produces a characteristic generalized rash (bromide rash) and tremulousness of hands, lips, and tongue. Impaired mental processes, auditory and visual hallucinations, or coma may follow continued ingestion after onset of early evidence of excess levels of the drug.

Barbiturates. Barbiturates (Table 20-1) are prescribed more frequently for sedation or sleep than other drugs classified as sedative-hypnotics. Barbiturates can be recognized by the terminal-barbital in the nonproprietary name. Talbutal is the one exception to the recognition clue for barbiturates.

The onset of most barbiturate-induced hypnotic action occurs 20 minutes after oral administration. Barbital, barbital sodium, and phenobarbital sodium require 30 to 60 minutes for production of hypnotic effect.

Hexobarbital, pentobarbital sodium, and secobarbital sodium have a shorter duration of hypnotic action (4 to 6 hours) than other barbiturates (6 to 8 hours). Each of the drugs depresses REM and Stage IV sleep time. It is characteristic during therapy with barbiturates that the patient wakens feeling drowsy, and the phenomenon may be directly related to the change in sleep patterns.

Barbiturates are distributed in all body tissues, but they have a particular affinity for lipoid tissue. The drugs move into lipoid tissue from the bloodstream, and they return to the circulating fluids when lipoid attachment, hepatic breakdown, or urinary excretion lowers the blood content of drug.

Barbital and barbital sodium are excreted unchanged in the urine. Renal tubular recycling slows clearance from the bloodstream; tubules reabsorb the drug nearly as quickly as the glomeruli remove it from the capillaries. Other forms of the barbiturates are metabolized by the liver and excreted in the urine without the persistent renal tubular recycling occurring with barbital.

Some hypersensitive patients have photosensitivity and dermatologic reactions during therapy with barbiturates. Problems occur most frequently in patients with a history of allergic reactions. When reactions occur and use of the drugs is necessary to the patient's progress, protection from direct sunlight and strong ultraviolet artificial lighting may decrease the erythema or dermatitis. Patients receiving sedative dosage on a self-medication schedule should be advised of the drug–light source relationship so that they can protect against continuance of sensitivity reactions during therapy.

Barbiturates cause respiratory depression and hypotension when administered intravenously. The effects are most marked when the drugs are injected rapidly into the vein, but they may occur with therapeutic administration by any parenteral route.

Methohexital sodium (Brevital), thiamylal sodium (Surital), and thiopental sodium (Pentothal) are barbiturates administered by the physician to induce relaxation necessary for minor surgical procedures or induction of general anesthesia. Pharmacodynamic action is evident in 20 to 60 seconds after intravenous infusion is started. The rapid action in producing a hypnotic state has popularized the description of the drugs as truth serum.

The high lipophilic tendency of the drugs moves them rapidly to the finely vascularized lipid-containing cerebrocortical tissues. Subsequent movement of the drugs out of lipid tissue to equilibrate with blood levels terminates the anesthetic effect within 30 minutes after injection of a single dose of the drug. Continuous infusion may be planned to provide prolonged anesthetic action. Atropine sulfate is generally administered prior to use of the drugs to prevent parasympathetic nervous system–induced spastic adduction of the vocal cords, with consequent block of respiratory passages.

Drug overdosage. Excess amounts of any of the sedative-hypnotics cause progression of the patient through the consciousness-unconsciousness continuum and gradually produces Stage IV sleep, anesthesia, coma, or death. The progression is directly related to the quantity of drug ingested and the pharmacodynamic action of the particular drug. The wide use of barbiturates for sedation and hypnosis makes them available for accidental or intentional ingestion of excess amounts.

The lipotropic characteristic of barbiturates is a primary factor in the toxic effect of overdosage. Methohexital sodium, thiamylal sodium, and thiopental sodium overdosage may occur during administration by physician or dentist; therefore they are used only when an individual with expertise in resuscitative measures is present. Other forms of the barbiturates are available through prescriptions or any of the multiple ways people find to obtain drugs by illicit means.

Lipid affinity of the barbiturates can be viewed by separation of the drugs into groups with comparable lipotropic activity:

A. HIGH LIPOID AFFINITY
   Hexobarbital
   Pentobarbital sodium
   Secobarbital sodium
B. MODERATE LIPOID AFFINITY
   Amobarbital sodium
   Aprobarbital
   Butabarbital sodium
   Probarbital sodium
   Talbutal
   Vinbarbital
C. LOW LIPOID AFFINITY
   Barbital
   Barbital sodium
   Phenobarbital

Group A barbiturates have a high lipotropic affinity that moves them quickly to lipid tissue in the cerebral cortex after oral use. The rapidity of effect produces sudden respiratory depression and marked decrease in blood pressure when excess drug is ingested. Coma and death more frequently occur after overdosage with group A barbiturates because time-lapse between ingestion and pharmacodynamic action is too short to allow reversal of the acute respiratory and cardiovascular depression. The drugs are the most frequently misused of the barbiturate group.

Group B barbiturates have an intermediate, or moderate, lipotropic tendency. Although overdosage may produce a protracted period of sedation, the slower movement to cerebral tissues allows time-lapse for reconsideration by the individual intentionally ingesting the drug and implementation of measures to abort drug effect.

Group C barbiturates move slowly into lipid-containing tissues, and they may require up to 60 minutes for onset of pharmacodynamic action. Urinary excretion decreases blood levels, and lipid tissue drug moves to equilibrate with blood levels. Hepatic detoxification, urinary excretion, and slow lipotropic activity protects the individual from life-threatening respiratory and cardiovascular depression occurring with the agents having greater lipotropic activity.

Care of the patient with overdosage of any central nervous system depressant requires the use of measures appropriate to the symptoms presented. Immediate plans may be made for removal of residual drug from the stomach, or hemodialysis may be planned when the offending agent is diffusible. Insertion of an endotracheal tube or a tracheostomy may be needed by the patient with depression of medullary respiratory control centers. Concurrent administration of oxygen and mechanical artificial ventilation are required during prolonged respiratory depression. In the absence of equipment for artificial ventilation, mouth-to-mouth breathing by any attendant at the scene may make the difference between life and death for the patient.

Elevation of the lower extremities (Trendelenburg position) shunts available blood to cerebral tissues while drugs are administered to reverse the hypotensive state. Vascular collapse is the chief concern, but cardiac activity is monitored closely, and external massage is administered if arrest occurs.

Prolonged hypoventilation and consequent tissue hypoxia increase accumulation of carbonic acid in tissues. Resuscitative measures require concurrent administration of a systemic alkalinizer (i.e., sodium bicarbonate) to return the internal bicarbonate–carbonic acid relationship to a 20:1 ratio necessary to tissue function.

Close observation of respiratory and vascular status continues after the acute episode, and the same assessments are planned for the patient with less intense effect of the drug on physiologic function. Most drugs (except paraldehyde) are eliminated by the kidneys, and continued urine output is necessary to decrease blood levels of the drug. Measurement of urine quantity is necessary for at least 2 days, since many drugs are slowly eliminated from the body.

Patients who have intentionally ingested drugs in a suicide attempt require close supervision to protect them against repeated attempts at self-destruction. Planned close companionship of a specific staff member or a relative may prevent reoccurrence of the incident. The patient is usually encouraged to maintain contact with a psychiatrist to ascertain the therapeutic approach appropriate to the individual's problems.

Drug abuse is a major social problem, and overdosage represents a complex problem of unidentified drug interactions, rather than ingestion of one drug. The use of uppers (amphetamines) and downers (barbiturates) is fairly common practice among drug abusers, but drug taking may involve more complex formulations intended to counteract or modify the effect of drugs. In the latter situation it is difficult to determine which drug is causing the problem and measures most appropriate to inactivate or remove circulating drugs.

In many situations the drug abuser will be aware that follow-up psychiatric evaluation is a planned aspect of emergency room care. Careful supervision is planned to assure that the patient remains available, but many patients find a way to escape from the agency before arrival of the psychiatrist.

Patient care

Knowledge of sleep patterns can be assistive in ascertaining whether prolonged wakefulness (sleep deprivation) or disruption of the sleep stage sequence is affecting the performance level of patients. Sleep deprivation for prolonged periods of time causes disruption of time sense, decreased motor coordination, dulling of mental processes, and increased tension and anxiety. Distortion of time sense by disruption of daily activities and sleep patterns or sleep deprivation is the basic approach to breaking down the resistance of political prisoners. The process places the individual in a mental state allowing brainwashing because controls become disorganized.

Increased sleep latency time is a common problem of individuals who are unable to discipline their minds to halt presleep problem solving, but most of the individuals eventually find measures that lull the brain and relax muscles before retiring. In the hospital situation, sleep latency may be decreased by a relaxing back massage and a hypnotic drug.

Individuals with multiple living problems impinging on them for long periods of time are less fortunate. Insomnia leaves the anxious individual poorly equipped to face the new day. Exogenous problems that increase sleep latency, nocturnal awakenings, and early arousal eventually set a vicious cycle in motion. Sedatives or hypnotics may modify the problem, but concurrent assistance with removal of stressors increases drug effect and lessens dependency on drugs for sleep control. For example, the preoperative patient may need clarification of specific details of the forthcoming experience. Most patients really are asking who will be nearby throughout the surgical experience. Clarification of the familiar contact persons or the expertise of those who will be with him throughout the experience often allows the patient relaxation and drug-assisted sleep.

Contact with the patient in the home or hospital provides an opportunity to discuss factors contributing to persistent sleep deprivation and help the patient to decrease some of the stressors. For example, the mother of two children who is having marital problems is in a highly anxious state. Discussion reveals that the 4-month-old infant wakens four times each night, and mother rises to change his diaper and give him a bottle of milk. Her actions reveal a high level clue-response without evaluation of alternatives. Objective discussion can help her examine the possibility of allowing the child to cry without operant behavior on her part. She may be able to think of ways to modify the intensity of his alarm to make the crying less upsetting to the household (i.e., placing the crib in another room). After a predictable 2-night rehabilitation period, exogenous sleep disruption may be eliminated, and the greater rest may modify the mother's anxiety to a level at which she feels more in control.

Knowledge of sleep patterns and the effects of deprivation should serve as a guide to planning scheduled assessments that disturb the patient's sleep. It is surprising how accurately the mother of a child, by placing her hand on the child's cheek, forehead, and abdomen, can judge within 1° the child's temperature level. Elevation of the temperature increases the metabolic rate, and it is possible to gently touch superficial tissues, palpate the pulse, and count the respirations before making a judgment about whether the patient should be awakened for an exact definition of body temperature. The clinical course of the patient enters into the decision, but the point in question is whether sleep must be disturbed. Temperature taking can be planned to correlate with patient's awakenings to decrease sleep disruption and allow progression of sleep patterns. Rigid schedules place the patient's physical rest and psychic refreshment in jeopardy.

Drugs to control sleep are only effective when environmental conditions allow the patient to take advantage of drug action. Definition of drug effect includes observations of the sleep time of the patient and the patient's perception of rest. Validation with the patient allows assessment of quality of sleep in addition to quantity. The patient who consistently awakens with hangover symptoms, including headache or morning drowsiness, may elect to try sleeping without use of the prescribed drug. The many drugs available make it possible for the physician to prescribe an alternate drug that produces sleep without aftereffects.

The sedative-hypnotic drugs are habit forming. Withdrawal of the drug after long-term use may precipitate abstinence, or withdrawal, signs common to habitual drug abusers: anxiety, tremor, insomnia, confusion, perceptual distortions, agitation, and delirium. Gastrointestinal disturbances and orthostatic hypotension are additional manifestations of withdrawal of the sedative or hypnotic drug. Grand mal seizures occur in some patients, and the muscle agitation and consequent hyperthermia leads to exhaustion. Continuous seizure activity may cause cardiovascular collapse and death. Withdrawal symptoms occur with chronic or habitual use of short-acting barbiturates (group A) and other sedative-hypnotics (chloral hydrate, glutethimide, methyprylon, paraldehyde).

Initial drug dependence can be prevented by seeking ways to interrupt the routine use of sleep-inducing drugs. For example, on a night when the unit census is low, it is predictable that there will be fewer environmental noises to disturb the patient's sleep. After his backrub before retiring, he could be encouraged to relax and try to sleep. Assurance that he may have the drug if long sleep latency ensues may make it possible for him to relax and sleep.

Short-term regular use of hypnotics causes a singular problem that tends to increase drug dependency. Consistent drug-related depression of REM sleep time causes rebound when the drug is discontinued. The phenomenon increases REM time, and the high incidence of vivid dreams seems to fill the patient's sleep time. Fear of recurrence makes the patient seek the drug to produce dreamless sleep. Communicating that it is a rebound phenomenon and that compensation subsides rapidly after the first night or two may make it possible for him to discontinue use of the drug.

The gentle touch of natural sleep has no substitute. Nursing measures can be used to prepare the environment and protect the patient from disturbances so that hypnotic agents can produce some of the benefits of natural sleep.

REFERENCES

Anthony, Catherine Parker, and Kolthoff, Norma J.: Textbook of anatomy and physiology, ed. 8, St. Louis, 1971, The C. V. Mosby Co.

Bradley, P. B.: Synaptic transmission in the central nervous system and its relevance for drug action, International Review of Neurology 11:1, 1968.

Cheatham, James S.: A profile of the drug dependent patient, Southern Medical Journal 64:1354, 1971.

Done, Alan K.: The subtle overdose, Emergency Medicine 4:134, April, 1972.

Fass, Grace: Sleep, drugs, and dreams, American Journal of Nursing 71:2316, 1971.

Gardner, M. Arlene Martin: Responsiveness as a measure of consciousness, American Journal of Nursing 68:1034, 1968.

Golub, Sharon: Rapid eye movement sleep, Nursing Outlook 15:56, 1967.

Goodman, Louis S., and Gilman, Arthur, editors: The pharmacological basis of therapeutics, ed. 4, New York, 1970, The Macmillan Co.

Greenberg, Ramon, Pillard, Richard, Pearlman, Chester: The effect of dream (stage REM) deprivation on adaptation to stress, Psychosomatic Medicine 34:257, 1972.

Jouvet, Michel: The states of sleep, Scientific American 216:62, Feb., 1967.

Kales, Anthony, and Kales, Joyce: Evaluation, diagnosis, and treatment of clinical conditions related to sleep, The Journal of the American Medical Association 213:2234, 1970.

King, LeRoy H., Jr., Decherd, Jonathan F., Newton, Jerry L., Shires, Dana L., Jr., and Bradley, Kent P.: A clinically efficient and economical lipid dialyzer: use in treatment of glutethimide intoxication, The Journal of the American Medical Association 211:652, 1970.

Long, Barbara: Sleep, American Journal of Nursing 69:1896, 1969.

McFadden, Eileen H., and Giblin, Elizabeth C.: Sleep deprivation in patients having open-heart surgery, Nursing Research 20:249, 1971.

Meinhart, Noreen T., and Aspinall, Mary Jo: Nursing interventions in hypovigilance, American Journal of Nursing 69:994, 1969.

Reilly, Mary Jo, editor: American hospital formulary service, vol. 1, sect. 28:24, Washington, D. C., 1973, American Society of Hospital Pharmacists.

Williams, Donald H.: Sleep and disease, American Journal of Nursing 71:2321, 1971.

Zung, W. W.: Pharmacology of disordered sleep, The Journal of the American Medical Association 211:1533, 1970.

21
Anesthesia

Inhalation anesthesia
    Anesthesia stages
    Pharmacodynamics
    Patient care
Local anesthesia
    Topical anesthetic agents
    Hypersensitivity reactions

The physiologic status of the patient during induction and maintenance of general anesthesia is the sole responsibility of the anesthetist. Under his direction, surgery progresses or is halted to protect the patient's status. The relationship between anesthetist and patient during the surgical experience is a thing of mystical beauty. Titration of the anesthetic agent and supportive drugs with the physiologic status of the patient requires continual monitoring and fine adjustments to maintain the level of anesthesia while also maintaining physiologic equilibrium during the period of surgery.

INHALATION ANESTHESIA

The choice of anesthetic agent is based on the planned procedure and the muscle relaxation required to perform the surgery. Within this framework, administration of varying agents is balanced to provide analgesia and anesthesia within the context of the patient's status prior to and during surgery. For example, an intravenous barbiturate may be used to provide short-term anesthesia when extensive muscle relaxation is not required, and nitrous oxide may be administered concurrently to provide analgesia.

In another situation the patient with a cardiac problem requiring emergency surgery may receive a curariform drug, morphine sulfate, and nitrous oxide. The combination provides analgesia and muscle relaxation adequate to allow thoracic surgery while vasopressors and oxygen are being used to maintain the patient's physiologic status. In poor-risk cardiac patients, morphine sulfate maintains cardiac output and stimulates catecholamine release from the adrenals. The combined pharmacodynamic action of the morphine sulfate combats the tendency toward shock in the operative period.

Balanced anesthesia makes it impossible to define stages of anesthesia in the traditional four stages originally described with use of ether for anesthesia. Sophisticated methods for administering several agents concomitantly cause the anesthesia stages to overlap, or merge. Open-heart surgery may be done during Stage I that was previously thought to allow only minor surgical procedures. Highly skilled use of drugs and anesthetic agents that interact to control analgesia, consciousness, and muscle relaxation is an integral part of the anesthetist's function.

Anesthesia stages

Traditional descriptions of responses occurring with induction of general anesthesia may be observed when a single inhalation anesthetic agent is used. Induction and maintenance of anesthesia follow a predictable pattern:

STAGE I: Euphoria, gradual loss of consciousness
STAGE II: Hyperexcitement (thrashing of extremities), hyperactivity of reflexes (eyelids, swallowing), dilation of pupils

Table 21-1. Agents used for inhalation anesthesia

Anesthetic agent	Induction rate	Recovery rate	Postanesthesia concerns
Cyclopropane* (trimethylene)	Rapid	Rapid	Hypotension, depressed respiratory rate, nausea, vomiting, ventricular arrhythmias
Ether† (diethyl oxide)	Slow	Slow	Copious secretions, nausea, vomiting
Ethyl chloride†	Rapid	Rapid	Muscle spasms, arrhythmias, hepatotoxicity
Ethylene*	Rapid	Rapid	Prolonged wound seepage, prolonged clotting time
Halothane†	Rapid	Rapid	Shallow, quiet respirations; shivering; hepatotoxicity
Methoxyflurane†	Moderate	Moderate	High urine output syndrome (decreased concentrating by distal tubules, excessive thirst); hepatotoxicity
Nitrous oxide* (nitrous monoxide)	Rapid	Rapid	Short-term euphoria
Trichloroethylene† (trichlorethene)	Rapid	Rapid	Tachypnea, bradycardia, ventricular arrhythmias
Vinyl ether† (divinyl oxide)	Rapid	Rapid	Copious secretions, nephrotoxicity, hepatotoxicity

*Gas.
†Liquid with volatile vapor.

STAGE III: Depression of corneal reflex and pupillary response to light, voluntary control absent, muscle tone decreased
STAGE IV: Medullary paralysis, death

Stage I allows performance of simple procedures, and the patient has amnesia for the experience. Nitrous oxide administered for tooth extraction in the dentist's office maintains the patient at Stage I during the procedure. The popularized laughing gas causes giddiness or uncontrollable crying for a short period after use. The patient should be accompanied by a friend or relative after use of nitrous oxide because judgment and steadiness may be affected for a short time after recovery. If it is necessary for the patient to drive a motor vehicle as he leaves the clinic or office, it is appropriate to encourage a waiting period.

The predictable occurrence of Stage II during use of a general anesthetic agent makes it necessary to pre-plan measures to protect against falling from the operating table during the thrashing and moving away period of induction. Emesis or retching often occurs during Stage II. The stage is short-lived as additional anesthetic agent is administered to induce Stage III. Recovery from anesthesia occurs in reverse order through the stages followed during induction.

Pharmacodynamics

There are several liquids with volatile vapors and gases commonly used for inhalation anesthesia (Table 21-1). Inhalation of the agent causes the gases to enter the capillaries in the alveolar bed, and the agent moves to tissues in the viscera, brain, and heart where it is liberated from protein-binding sites. Muscle tissue and finally adipose tissue receive the agent from the circulating fluids. The sequence of delivery to tissues is important because it relates to the release rate. The amount of adipose tissue receiving the anesthetic agent is increased in the obese patient, and recovery from the effect of the anesthetic is slower.

When tissues become saturated with the anesthetic agent, the pharmacodynamic effect is at its maximal level for a given amount of agent. The tissues gradually release the agent, and it is liberated from the lungs. Some residual drug is detoxified in the liver and excreted via the kidneys. Control of inhaled gases is accomplished as the anesthetist halts or slows the administration rate. Rapid reversal of the effect of the anesthetic can be accomplished by administration of 100% oxygen.

Each of the agents presents problems during anesthesia induction and maintenance, but the chief problems occurring in the immediate postoperative period relate to shallow respirations, nausea or vomiting that may cause aspiration of gastric contents, or hypotension.

New anesthetics are being introduced continually, and there is no one agent that suits all purposes. Studies of the various agents currently in use have revealed a low incidence of hepatotoxicity. The appearance of jaundice 7 to 10 days after surgery may be an indication of the patient's sensitivity to the anesthetic agent. In some instances the studies showed hepatic necrosis, but the incidence was highest when there was a history of previous jaundice or hepatitis. Careful history taking prior to surgery has decreased the incidence of postoperative hepatotoxicity.

Methoxyflurane occasionally causes a self-limiting high urine output syndrome. Copious amounts of dilute urine are eliminated, and the patient complains of intense thirst. During the period of the syndrome (2 to 3 days) the amount and specific gravity of the urine are monitored.

Patient care

During recovery from anesthesia the anesthetist follows the patient closely until consciousness returns. The nurse is primarily responsible for the patient after he leaves the operating room. Observations of physiologic status, implementation of postoperative prescriptions, and tabulation and reporting of the patient's progress are aspects of the immediate recovery room care.

Primary nursing responsibilities include providing measures for the comfort and safety of the patient. Communication by touch and voice during the immediate postoperative period adds to the relaxation and smooth recovery of the patient. Patients have been found to be highly responsive to suggestions made during the Stage I and the early consciousness period. Instructions or assurances made during this period have resulted in a decreased incidence of voiding problems and a lessening of pain in the postrecovery period.

Preoperative preparation for coughing and deep breathing exercises has a direct effect on the postoperative period. The patient who has practiced preoperatively will most readily assist in the ventilation program after surgery. All general anesthetics are depressants, and shallow respirations are seen in most patients. Periodic coughing and sighing increase lung compliance and improve gas exchange.

The extent of surgical intervention and the involvement of vital organs in the surgical procedure affect the postoperative progression of the patient. Surgery constitutes a physiologic stressor, and all patients require monitoring after the surgical procedure until equilibrium is reestablished.

Prior to recovery from anesthesia, maintenance of a patent airway and positioning to prevent aspiration of secretions are primary problems. Throughout the recovery period pulmonary ventilation and hemodynamic status are monitored closely, and measures are used to protect the progress of the patient.

Intricate monitoring devices under the expert observation of nurse clinicians with educational and experiential preparation for intensive care contribute to the safety of the patient during the highly dependent state. Continuation of care in intensive units is planned for patients with extensive surgery, but patients with lesser procedures are retained in the recovery unit only until their vital signs are stabilized.

LOCAL ANESTHESIA

Administration of local anesthetics may be planned by the physician to block neural transmission causing intractable pain, or drugs may be administered at a central location to allow pain-free surgery. The chief responsibility of the nurse when patients have nerve-blocking anesthesia is to protect the involved part from injury during the period of insensitivity.

An example of local anesthetic effect is the immobility and lack of sensation in facial tissues after injection of one of the cocaine products by a dentist. Control of saliva and movement of the muscles are affected until the action of the anesthetic agent on neural endings subsides. There is danger of biting into oral mucosa and causing bleeding during the anesthetic period. The same loss of motor and sensory function in major body areas affects the patient's ability to move voluntarily or to perceive pressure or injury in desensitized tissues.

The limited area required for dental work makes it possible for the dentist to inject the local anesthetic into the tissues near the site, and the agent reaches the tiny nerve endings. The process is called infiltration anesthesia.

Infiltration anesthesia may be used in procedures requiring short-term surgery in other assessable areas (i.e., the skin). A vasoconstrictor (i.e., epinephrine) may be injected into subcutaneous tissues with the anesthetic to retard infiltration from the target area.

Local anesthetics accomplish their effect primarily by decreasing the permeability of the nerve membrane to the influx of sodium ions necessary to depolarization of the neuron. When administered by infiltration, the anesthetic acts readily on fine, small unmyelinated fibers, but administration can be planned to cause anesthesia of larger segments of the body. For example, injection of a local anesthetic into the subarachnoid space of the spinal canal allows the anesthetic agent to act on the myelinated nerves of the cauda equina to provide their anesthetic effect. The needle is introduced between the lumbar vertebrae (L_2 and L_3) for spinal anesthesia. The level chosen avoids contact with the spinal cord because its terminal tip is above the level of L_2.

Injection of a local anesthetic into the epidural space at or below the site used for spinal anesthesia (i.e., L_3 and L_4) provides regional anesthesia by drug action at large myelinated nerve trunks leaving the spinal canal. Local anesthetics have a high affinity for lipoid tissue, and they move readily to the nerves.

Caudal anesthesia is the description of desensitization in the perineal or saddle area accomplished by administration of the local anesthetic agent into the epidural space at the terminal aspect of the spinal canal. Regional block is more limited than that obtained when the anesthetic is introduced at a higher level because nerve trunks are smaller and specific for the perineal area.

Regional and spinal anesthesia are planned to block transmission of nerve impulses, and the progression of nerve blockade occurs in a predictable sequence: autonomic, temperature, touch, pain, motor, pressure and proprioception. Autonomic block may persist longer than other neural blockade; therefore the return of vascular responses is carefully monitored to ascertain when spinal or regional anesthesia effect has terminated.

Procaine is the prototype of currently used local anesthetics, and the particular agent for nerve blockade is selected by the physician or anesthetist. An important consideration for the nurse who receives the patient on the unit after nerve block is the predictable duration and extent of anesthesia.

Topical anesthetic agents

Ethyl chloride is used as a topical local anesthetic for minor incision of superficial tissues. Rapid vaporization of the fine spray causes freezing of the topical layers of tissue that blocks nerve conduction for about 1 minute. Procedures requiring lengthy probing may require subsequent infiltration of the site with a local anesthetic.

Numerous ointments and lotions used for pruritus contain small amounts of local anesthetic that add to the effect of the unguent by decreasing topical irritation. The amount of target tissue anesthesia after drug administration will depend on the proportion of the local anesthetic drug to the vehicle used for its delivery to the topical area. Dibucaine ointment (Nupercainal) is an example of an anesthetic ointment applied to topical areas.

Use of topical anesthetic-containing ointments carries with it the hazard of sensitization, and subsequent use of the local anesthetic may cause a hypersensitivity reaction. Although local anesthetics by other routes find their way into the circulation, topical application to the intact skin does not result in absorption. After use of an anesthetic-containing ointment, it is important to wash residual material from the hands to prevent inadvertent application to other tissue areas.

Lidocaine hydrochloride (Xylocaine) is frequently employed as a topical local anesthetic. For example, a viscous preparation is used to decrease the pain occurring concurrently with extensive inflammation of oral and oropharyngeal tissues. The patient is asked to gargle with the solution and expectorate the liquid. After agitation of the drug around the oral tissues, desensitization of the nerves aborts the pain and also the gag reflex. Instructions for drug use must include explicit directions for the patient to avoid eating or drinking until sensitivity of the tissues returns. Timing of fluid ingestion for the patient with inflamed tissues is a simple matter because he feels pain as the effect of the drug subsides.

A local anesthetic spray may be used prior to insertion of a bronchoscope or similar large device that would stimulate the gag reflex during the procedure. When a local anesthetic is employed to desensitize the oropharyngeal area, testing of returning sensitivity of the uvula and peritonsillar pillars is necessary before allowing oral liquids. Touching the tissues with a cotton swab assists in determination of the response to stimuli. Foods and fluids are withheld until the return of tissue sensitivity.

Hypersensitivity reactions

Systemic reactions to local anesthetics involve the cardiovascular system and the central nervous system. The reactions represent hypersensitivity to the local anesthetics. Alarming reactions involve convulsions and cardiopulmonary arrest, but reactions can include any of the common manifestations of decreased responses of the central nervous system and cardiovascular system. Allergic responses also occur, and individuals handling the drugs frequently (i.e., dentists) are particularly prone to development of allergic reactions.

REFERENCES

Bakutis, Alice: Anesthetic reactions, Nursing '72 **2:**16, 1972.

Clark, Richard B.: The case for spinal anesthesia, American Journal of Nursing **67:**294, 1967.

Covino, Benjamin G.: Local anesthesia, The New England Journal of Medicine **286:**975, 1035, 1972.

Gardner, M. Arlene Martin: Responsiveness as a measure of consciousness, American Journal of Nursing **68:**1034, 1968.

Goth, Andres: Medical pharmacology, ed. 6, St. Louis, 1972, The C. V. Mosby Co.

Greiss, Frank C., Jr.: Obstetric anesthesia, American Journal of Nursing **71:**67, 1971.

Hollenberg, Norman K., McDonald, Franklin, Cotran, Ramzi, Galvanek, Eleonora G., Warhol, Michael, Vandam, Leroy D., and Merrill, John P.: Acute renal failure: a complication of methoxyflurane anesthesia, The New England Journal of Medicine **286:**877, 1972.

Minckley, Barbara Blake: Physiologic hazards of position changes in the anesthetized patient, American Journal of Nursing **69:**2606, 1969.

Reynolds, Edward S., Brown, Burnell R., Jr., and Vandam, Leroy D.: Massive hepatic necrosis after fluroxene anesthesia—case of drug interaction? The New England Journal of Medicine **286:**530, 1972.

Rodger, Bertha P.: Therapeutic conversation and posthypnotic suggestion, American Journal of Nursing **72:**715, 1972.

Therrian, Barbara, and Salmon, James H.: Percutaneous cordotomy for relief of intractable pain, American Journal of Nursing **68:**2594, 1968.

22
Pain

Pharmacodynamics
Patient care

Pain is a common experience. Each of us can conjure up details of a particular pain episode, the personal meaning of the experience, and measures used to relieve the pain. Recall may include a vivid image of the sensation as stabbing, throbbing, or pressure, but amnesia exists for a re-feeling description of the neural stimulus. Recall of the measures effective in alleviating the pain are protective patterns used when pain recurs. Associative patterns of millions of people move them to use analgesics periodically to relieve episodes of minor pain. Some individuals use a problem-solving approach to determine whether hunger, fluid deficit, prolonged pressure, or fatigue is contributing to pain perception, and they plan to remove the cause to enhance the effect of the drug used to relieve pain.

The literature abounds with tales of stoic individuals who heroically continued with activities necessary to meet their moral commitments before collapsing with wounds received prior to or during the fray. The incapacitated individual or the hospitalized patient is disadvantaged because he cannot move away or become physically involved in activities to subordinate the painful stimuli.

Pain is a lonely experience, and health team members desiring to help the individual cope with illness can assist by using measures to communicate to the patient that he is not alone. Physical comfort measures and nonverbal communication are additives to the drugs administered for alleviation of pain. The drug administered by an individual capable of communicating that she cares can lessen the isolation, fear, anxiety, and apprehension of the patient and help him maintain resources at a level necessary to his progress or survival.

Intractable pain may require injection of local anesthetics or severing of nerves to decrease the stimulus along the pathways from the initiating source to the cortical structures. Approaches vary as neurosurgeons strive to minimize the anatomic sacrifice of other sensors closely allied with pain fibers in the routes from organ to central pathways (i.e., position, vibration, touch).

Tiny unmyelinated pain fibers travel with myelinated fibers of peripheral nerves toward the spinal cord. The nerve bundles pass through the dorsal root ganglion and synapse en route to the posterior root of the spinal cord. The fibers cross over to the spinothalamic tract on the opposite side of the cord, and the sensory stimulus arrives at the receptor sites of the thalamic and cortical centers opposite to the side of the initial stimulus. Arrival at thalamic sites precipitates vague, generalized awareness of the stimulus, and passage to cortical centers in the posterior ridge of the central gyrus allows discrimination of the specific sensory stimulus site.

Reflex actions in response to sudden pain protect the individual from injury, and secondary interpretation brings complicated conditioned reflexes into the pattern of responses subsequent to the initial reflex action. At a comparable threshold level, individual response to pain stimuli varies greatly. The challenge to nurses is to plan measures appropriate to the individual's need. It may be necessary to ascertain whether the tense muscles, anorexia, insomnia, and accelerated pulse rate are evidence of pain in the stoic individual. In contrast to care of the stoic is the need to plan measures for the demanding, restless, irritable individual that will decrease pain-induced anxiety. Although approaches differ according to the responses of the individual, the intent is to protect energy reserves and improve the health status of the individual.

Astute observations and discriminating problem solving are necessary because most pain-alleviating drugs are prescribed to be administered as needed (p.r.n) by the patient. It is important for the nurse to react to the overt or covert evidence that pain exists with an appreciation that responses to pain vary.

Analgesics may be prescribed to relieve pain and modify elevated temperature, or local anesthetics may be used topically to provide temporary desensitization of neural fibers. The predictable threshold stimulus and the patient's evaluation of intensity guide the physician in prescribing specific drugs. Prescription for a potent analgesic or a minor analgesic for relief of a patient's pain requires discrimination of the pain level. Observations of the patient and evaluation of his pain perception are important factors in selecting the appropriate drug to administer when the patient has more than one prescription for pain alleviation.

It is important in the acute situation to view pain as a natural antidote for pain-alleviating drugs and the patient in a different situation from that of the drug-user enjoying the euphoria of effect without pain interception. Cultural concern with drug abuse at the present time cannot be superimposed on the patient in acute distress. Chronic use of any drug carries with it psychic and physiologic problems quite different from those occurring with short-term use. Evaluation of the patient's pain control regimen becomes an appropriate concern of all health team members when drug therapy is prolonged.

Pharmacodynamics

Addictive analgesics. Relief of pain is the time-honored effect of the addictive analgesics. The term is descriptive of the potential for addiction occurring with long-term use of any of the agents (Table 22-1). Pharmacodynamic action relieves pain by raising the pain threshold and interfering with the pain perception centers.

The efficacy of the drugs is measured against the effect of morphine sulfate in relieving severe pain or codeine sulfate in relieving moderate pain. The analgesic action of the prototypes

Table 22-1. Dosage range of addictive analgesic drugs

Nonproprietary name	Proprietary (trade) name	Adult dosage range
Alphaprodine hydrochloride	Nisentil	S.C.: 40-60 mg. I.V.: 20-30 mg.
Anileridine hydrochloride	Leritine hydrochloride	Oral: 25-50 mg.
Anileridine phosphate	Apodol, Leritine phosphate	I.M.: 25-75 mg. I.V.: 10 mg.
Codeine sulfate		S.C.: 10-30 mg.
Dextromoramide tartrate	Palfium	Oral: 2-5 mg. I.M.: Same
Fentanyl citrate	Sublimaze	I.M.: 0.25-0.1 mg.
Hydromorphone hydrochloride	Dilaudid	Oral: 1-3 mg. S.C.: Same
Levorphanol tartrate	Levo-Dromoran	Oral: 2-3 mg. S.C.: 1-3 mg.
Meperidine hydrochloride	Demerol	Oral: 25-150 mg. I.M.: Same
Methadone hydrochloride	Adanon, Althose, Dolophine	Oral: 5-15 mg. I.M.: Same
Morphine sulfate		S.C.: 10-15 mg. I.V.: Same
Oxycodone		Oral: 4.88 mg.
Oxymorphone hydrochloride	Numorphan	Oral: 5-10 mg. I.M.: 0.5-3 mg. I.V.: 0.75 mg.
Pantopium	Pantapon	S.C.: 5-20 mg.

morphine sulfate and codeine sulfate differs, although both drugs affect the same receptors. Codeine sulfate has an incomplete analgesic action, but morphine sulfate has a more complete action and provides a higher level of analgesia.

The variation in potency of addictive analgesics from that of the prototypes is modified by dosage adjustment. Utilization of any of the addictive analgesics is planned by seeking the drug that controls the patient's pain with the lowest incidence of adverse effects.

Each of the addictive analgesics has commonalities of effect when used therapeutically for control of pain. The natural opium alkaloids codeine sulfate, morphine sulfate, and pantopium and the synthetic derivatives of opiates have consistent effects on body systems that provide guidelines for observations of the patient receiving any of the addictive analgesics.

Each of the opiates and its derivatives has an antitussive and sedative action, in addition to its analgesic action. Sedative or antitussive action may be increased or decreased by dosage modification. For example, codeine sulfate may be given at low dosage levels for control of cough without inducing sedation or analgesia. At the lower dosage range, cough suppression is provided without concurrent depressant effect on respiratory centers, which are adjacent to the cough control centers in the medulla.

There are a large number of structural derivatives of the natural opiates, but despite attempts to prepare drugs with limited adverse effects, each of the addictive analgesics produces effects that are undesirable when the drugs are used for analgesia. The drugs have a potential for respiratory depression, and the effects are profound at toxic dosage levels. Pupil constriction and slight hypothermia occur after administration, but the most problematic physiologic effect is caused by the action of the drugs on smooth muscle. The spasmogenic action of the opiates on smooth muscle causes decreased organ motility (i.e., gastrointestinal tract), and decreased peristalsis is common after administration. Each of the drugs has a comparable action on organ systems, presumably through its action on the same tissue receptors.

Codeine sulfate provides analgesia with few adverse effects when administered orally or injected subcutaneously. The only adverse effect at therapeutic dosage range is nausea. Some patients may become nauseated with any formulation containing the drug (i.e., cough syrup). Increasing the dosage of codeine sulfate produces effects and adverse effects similar to those of morphine sulfate.

Morphine sulfate produces drowsiness and euphoria concurrent with pain relief. Constriction of the pupils is an effect of morphine that can be used to evaluate the status of the patient. Pupil constriction is believed to result from a central effect of the drug and is always present when the drug is used. Constriction may persist for a major part of the 4-hour action period attributed to morphine sulfate.

Constriction of smooth muscles of the gastrointestinal tract, biliary structures, urinary tract, and bronchi presents functional problems with repeated drug administration. Use of morphine sulfate, known to cause increased tonus and constriction of smooth muscle, to patients with renal or biliary colic seems an enigma until one views the abolition of intense pain as the rationale for use of the drug. Observations during continued drug use include evaluation of organ function affected by the smooth muscle spasmogenic effect of the drug (i.e., intestinal motility, urinary output).

Emesis is relatively common with the use of morphine sulfate. The drug acts as a stimulant to the chemoreceptors controlling vomiting. Individuals differ in tolerance to the drug, and emesis may make it necessary for the physician to prescribe another analgesic for pain control when the individual continues to be nauseated. Emesis or nausea often decreases after the first few doses of morphine sulfate have been given.

Dextromoramide tartrate, hydromorphone hydrochloride, levorphanol tartrate, meperidine hydrochloride, methadone hydrochloride, oxycodone, oxymorphone hydrochloride, and pantopium (Table 22-1) provide analgesic effect within 15 to 20 minutes after oral administration that lasts up to 5 hours. The drugs are prescribed for parenteral use to provide prompt pain relief for patients in acute distress. Intravenous administration provides relief of pain in 1 to 2 minutes, but subcutaneous injection may require a longer time (8 to 15 minutes) for onset of action.

Alphaprodine hydrochloride, anileridine hydrochloride, and fentanyl citrate (Table 22-1) may be prescribed for oral use. Analgesic effect lasts approximately 2 hours when taken orally, subcutaneously, or intramuscularly.

Alphaprodine hydrochloride, anileridine hydrochloride, fentanyl citrate, and meperidine hydrochloride are classified pharmacologically as members of the *meperidine series.* The drugs have a smooth muscle–relaxant action, particularly in abdominal viscera. Consistent observations of patients receiving meperidine hydrochloride after postoperative awakening and prior to movement by stretcher to their room has revealed a high incidence of lowered blood pressure immediately after movement of the patients to their beds. Allowing equilibrium to be established before transfer of the patient prevents the hypotensive episode. Vasodilation seems to be the source of the problem because the patient's skin is warm, moist, and pink during the hypotensive incident. Although the problem arises frequently with meperidine hydrochloride, it is advisable to observe patients for comparable problems while receiving other drugs in the meperidine grouping.

Methadone maintenance. Methadone hydrochloride and dextromoramide tartrate are members of the pharmacologic grouping known as the *methadone series.* The drugs are widely used in other countries as substitute agents for individuals previously addicted to narcotics. Initial use of methadone hydrochloride in the United States was limited to a planned withdrawal program, but recent trials are based on substitution of the oral agent for one that must be injected. Although controversy exists, proponents of the plan believe that the substitute drug decreases the dependence on black market sources and decreases the hazard of hepatitis occurring with persistent shots. Conversion of addiction to methadone hydrochloride decreases the financial and physical drain on the patient's resources. Methadone dosage is calibrated according to the addiction dosage of drug when the patient seeks therapy. Coordinated efforts of many health team members are aimed at assisting the patient with rehabilitation and return to his community. Withdrawal symptoms are limited under the plan, and most patients only have occasional rhinorrhea. Drug administration at the clinic once or twice daily allows the patient to maintain living patterns during therapy.

Evaluation of drug requirement. Each of the addictive analgesics causes problems with addiction susceptibility, tolerance to analgesic effects, and respiratory depression (with overdosage of drug). Reevaluation of the patient's need for the drugs and observation of the effectiveness of the administered dose are a planned part of the pain control program. Automatic discontinuance of prescriptions for addictive analgesics is required in institutions, and the practice allows reevaluation of need at the end of each 72-hour period before the drug is prescribed for continued use for pain control.

Withdrawal signs. Tolerance to addictive analgesics decreases effective pain control over extended periods of time, but the chief concern during therapy is the addiction potential. Withdrawal of addictive drugs produces physiologic disturbances distressing to the patient and observer. The gradual progression of uncontrollable lacrimation-rhinorrhea-diaphoresis-yawning portends the beginning of withdrawal, or abstinence, symptoms. Violent gastrointestinal disturbances, muscle spasms, joint pains, and gradual evidence of increased metabolic activity appear progressively in the cold turkey of abstinence. Administration of a narcotic halts the syndrome. Substitution of any one of the addicting analgesics for another halts withdrawal symptoms. Addicts can use any of the drugs in the group to support their habit, but there are differences in potency and duration of action between the various addictive analgesics.

Respiratory depression. The addictive analgesics act at medullary centers to cause depression of respiration by increasing the threshold for carbon dioxide sensitivity. Block of the chemoreceptor sites in the medullary centers causes decreased rhythm and rate of respiratory cycles. Morphine sulfate at therapeutic dosage range may cause respiratory depression, but the problem occurs at high dosage levels with each of the addictive analgesics. Administration of morphine sulfate is contraindicated when voluntary respirations drop to 15/minute.

Respiratory depression occurring during use of addictive analgesics can be reversed by narcotic antagonists. Levallorphan tartrate (Lorfan), nalorphine hydrochloride (Nalline), or naloxone hydrochloride (Narcan) act pharmacodynamically by competing with the narcotic for receptor sites in the respiratory center to lower the threshold for carbon dioxide stimulus to respiration. Ventilation is controlled by respiratory assistors until the depressant effects of the addictive analgesic have been reversed. Specific problems of gas exchange and use of the narcotic antagonists are presented in Chapter 5.

Analgesic-antipyretic drugs. Analgesics control pain by interference with pathways within cerebral tissues. It is probable that many peripheral mechanisms contribute to the effectiveness of the drugs. Interference with the pain-stimulating effect of bradykinin released at the site of tissue injury enhances the control of trauma-related pain. Acetylsalicylic acid blocks production of hormonelike prostaglandins that precipitate inflammation, fever, and headache. The anti-inflammatory actions may account for analgesia produced by acetylsalicylic acid, but other mechanisms probably are involved (i.e., blockade of lysosomal enzyme release, blockade of kinins at receptor sites). Tracer studies and clinical trials eventually may reveal specific mechanisms of action, but widespread use of many analgesics for control of minor pain is based on empirical demonstration of effectiveness.

A large group of drugs is used for control of minor pain or elevation of body temperature accompanying infection (Table 22-2). Invasion of the body by pathogens is accompanied by an elevation of body temperature, resulting from the activity of pyrogens liberated by the leukocytes responding to the invasion. The pyrogenic substance acts on the hypothalamic heat-regulating centers to reset thermostatic controls at a higher level. Mobilization of autonomic responses to control heat dissipation results in a gradual elevation of internal body temperature. Sudden temperature elevation causes chills as the temperature moves above that of the environment. The muscular movement occurring during chills produces heat that rapidly moves the internal temperature to the hypothalamic setting.

Antipyretic drugs act by lowering the raised thermostat. Autonomic nervous system response causes vasodilation necessary to dissipate the excess heat to reduce the temperature to the lower thermostatic control level. Diaphoresis accompanying the process provides the water necessary to heat dissipation.

Acetylsalicylic acid and related salicylates—carbaspirin calcium, choline salicylate, salicylamide, and sodium salicylate (Table 22-2)—are the drugs traditionally used for control of

Table 22-2. Dosage range of analgesic-antipyretic drugs

Nonproprietary name	Proprietary (trade) name	Daily adult dosage range
Acetaminophen	Apamide, Febrolin, Fendon, Lyteca, Nebs, Tempra, Tylenol	Oral: 1.8-3.6 Gm. (÷6)
Acetophenetidin		Oral: 2.1 Gm. (÷8)
Acetylsalicylic acid	A.S.A., Aspirin, Asteric, Ecotrin	Oral: 0.9-10 Gm. (÷3-6)
Carbaspirin calcium	Calurin	Oral: 1.8-10 Gm. (÷6)
Choline salicylate	Arthropan	Oral: 8.7-14.5 Gm. (÷4-6)
Dipyrone	Dimethone, Narone, Nartate, Novaldin, Pydirone, Pyral, Pyrilgin	Oral: 1.28-6 Gm. (÷4-6) I.M.: 4-12 Gm. (÷4-12) I.V.: Same as I.M.
Mefenamic acid	Ponstel	Oral: 1 Gm. (÷6)
Salicylamide	Amid-Sal, Liquiprin, Raspberin, Salamide, Salicim, Salrin	Oral: 1.8-12 Gm. (÷6)
Sodium salicylate		Oral: 1.8-15 Gm. (÷4-8)

minor pain, elevated temperature, and chronic inflammatory responses (i.e., arthritis). Aspirin is a common household item, and there are few people who do not know the bitter taste of the drug when dissolved in the mouth. Pediatric preparations have been formulated to disguise the taste, and they are widely used for their antipyretic effect. Disguising the taste has made it an interesting product for children, and overdosage has become a problem as youngsters find the pleasant-tasting liquid or tablet accessible in the home.

As antipyretics the drugs are usually prescribed to be administered when the oral temperature rises above 102° F. A single dose of the drug lowers the temperature, which gradually rises to predrug levels. When the temperature is taken at 4-hour intervals and the drug is given for temperature elevation, the moderate peaks and valleys of the graphic record show the temperature level at a fairly consistent elevation. Marked swings in body temperature are more uncomfortable for the patient than modified higher levels of body temperature. Alternate diaphoresis and chills as the temperature falls and rises keep the patient scrambling to remove blankets or to find an adequate amount of protection against chills. With persistent temperature levels above 104° F. there is tissue and enzyme destruction by heat.

Sporadic use of salicylates creates few problems, and most individuals select a form of the drugs that provides maximum relief of problems with the least irritation to gastric mucosa. Long-term use of large amounts of salicylates carries with it problems peculiar to the group of drugs. These problems are described as salicylism: *visual disturbances, tinnitus, dizziness, mental confusion, diaphoresis, nausea, vomiting,* and *intense thirst.* The entity is an indication that serum drug levels are high, and discontinuance of drug use for a short period may provide relief. The problems of greatest concern during long-term therapy are irritation of gastric mucosa or gastric ulcer and lowering of prothrombin levels caused by the salicylates. Combined problems with gastritis and potentiation of bleeding tendency can adversely affect the patient's progress. Enteric-coated tablets or administration of the drugs with foods or antacids may minimize gastric irritation. Patients on long-term therapy are asked to observe the color of their stools and note the frequency and characteristics of digestive disturbances. They are asked to report occurrence of black or tarry stools or epigastric discomfort to the physician before continuing drug therapy.

Renal tubular excretion of salicylates utilizes available base for elimination of the drug, and additional sodium ions are lost in sweat. Depletion of available base reserves can be lessened by concurrent administration of antacids during long-term therapy.

Acetaminophen, acetophenetidin, dipyrone, and mefenamic acid are nonsalicylate drugs employed for analgesic and antipyretic effect. The drugs may be used in lieu of acetylsalicylic acid for patients with known allergy or gastric ulcers.

Acetaminophen is frequently prescribed for pain and temperature control for children or adults. Effect of the drug is seen in 15 minutes after oral use, and muscle-relaxant properties of the drug add to the patient's comfort during the 3-hour period of drug action.

Acetophenetidin is quite often a component of combinations used for pain relief. The action of the drug is cumulative, and during long-term use the physician may periodically recommend omission of one of the scheduled doses each day for a few days. Urine may acquire a dark brown to wine hue imparted by metabolites of the drug. Modification of quantity of the drug by combination with other agents has decreased the incidence of problems related to its use (agranulocytosis, anemia, hepatotoxicity, alteration of the oxygen-carrying capacity of hemoglobin by formation of methemoglobin or sulfhemoglobin).

Mefenamic acid effects last up to 6 hours after oral administration; in addition to analgesic and antipyretic effects, it also has an anti-inflammatory action. Mefenamic acid and dipyrone cause vertigo more frequently than other analgesic-antipyretic agents. Skin rash and depression of leukocyte and erythrocyte production have occurred in some patients taking the drugs: therefore periodic hematologic studies are planned during therapy. The pa-

Table 22-3. Dosage range of analgesics

Nonproprietary name	Proprietary (trade) name	Daily adult dosage range
Carbamazepine	Tegretol	Oral: 0.2-1.2 Gm. (÷2)
Cobra venom extract	Cobroxin, Nyloxin	I.M.: 0.5-3 ml.
Ethoheptazine citrate	Zactane	Oral: 225-600 mg. (÷3-4)
Indomethacin	Indocin	Oral: 50-200 mg. (÷2-3)
Oxyphenbutazone	Tandearil	Oral: 300-600 mg. (÷3-4)
Pentazocine hydrochloride	Talwin	Oral: 600-800 mg. (÷6-8)
Pentazocine lactate	Talwin lactate	I.M.: 180-240 mg. (÷6-8)
Phenylbutazone	Butazolidin	Oral: 300-600 mg. (÷3-4)
Propoxyphene hydrochloride	Darvon	Oral: 195-260 mg. (÷3-4)

tient is asked to consult with the physician if fever, chills, sore throat, or oral lesions occur during therapy, since the signs may be indicative of agranulocytosis. Reevaluation of the hematologic status is planned when the signs occur.

Analgesics. Each of the drugs in the foregoing section is capable of controlling minor pain, but concurrent antipyretic action makes them useful agents for control of either pain or hyperpyrexia. The analgesics presented in this section are used primarily for control of minor pain.

Propoxyphene hydrochloride (Table 22-3) is commonly employed for control of pain in varied body sites. The rapidity of effect (15 to 60 minutes) and long duration of action (4 to 6 hours) make it useful for control of periodic pain. Although continued use may cause constipation, drowsiness, and skin rash, periodic use of the drug alone or in combination forms containing other analgesics provides pain relief without occurrence of adverse effects. Psychic dependence has occurred with persistent chronic use of the drug.

Pentazocine hydrochloride (Table 22-3) is widely prescribed as an oral agent for control of pain. Intramuscular use of pentazocine lactate provides pain relief in 10 to 30 minutes after administration. The potent effect of the drug when administered intravenously is seen in 2 to 3 minutes. Intravenous administration increases the potential for decreased visceral motility and for the hypnotic effects of the drug.

Periodic use of pentazocine hydrochloride is relatively problem free. Continued use of the drug, particularly by patients known to be chronic drug abusers, has caused withdrawal signs when the drug was discontinued; therefore the dependence potential is a concern during long-term therapy. At therapeutic dosage ranges the drug sometimes causes depression of respirations, increased cardiac rate, and hypotension. Adverse effects are more pronounced with parenteral administration. Hypoxia secondary to depressed respirations are hazardous to the fetus when the drug is administered during labor. Administration of supplementary oxygen is indicated if respiratory depression occurs during therapy.

Ethoheptazine citrate (Table 22-3) is a mild acetylsalicylic acid–like analgesic, and it is frequently used in combination with other analgesics (i.e., propoxyphene hydrochloride). The synergistic effect causes greater analgesia than that occurring when either agent is employed alone; therefore it is probable that each of the drugs has a different mode of action.

Cobra venom extract (Table 22-3) is administered parenterally for control of intractable pain. The drug is available in combined form with formic and silicic acid and is most popular as the combination. Action peak is slow and may take up to 16 weeks, but use of the drug allows decreased use of addictive analgesics in patients requiring long-term control of intense pain (i.e., terminal cancer). Protein content of the drug necessitates skin test doses prior to use and observation for hypersensitivity reactions during therapy.

Analgesic–anti-inflammatory drugs. Acetylsalicylic acid is the drug most frequently given for control of pain and inflammation in joints, but other agents are employed in selected situations in which acetylsalicylic acid is ineffective. Salicylates are used at high dosage levels for control of joint pain, and at high levels the drugs increase excretion of uric acid by competitive action at renal tubule transport sites that blocks reabsorption of uric acid. Removal of uric acid decreases deposits in joints that cause deformity and pain.

Oxyphenbutazone and phenylbutazone (Table 22-3) are used orally for their analgesic, antipyretic, and anti-inflammatory effect in control of joint pains. The drugs produce an action peak in about 3 days that lasts for 7 days. Dietary sodium intake is restricted during therapy because the drugs cause sodium chloride and water retention by enhancing reabsorption of sodium in the renal tubules. Short-term therapy is generally aproblematic, but long-term use increases the incidence of gastric irritation and hypersensitivity reactions (i.e., skin rash, fever, edema). The drugs cause thrombocytopenia and displace coumarin-type drugs from plasma-binding sites with consequent intratissue bleeding (purpura). One half the therapeutic dosage is employed during long-term therapy to minimize adverse effects.

Indomethacin (Table 22-3) is specifically used for relief of articular pain, and it has additional effects as an antipyretic and anti-inflammatory drug. Pharmacodynamic action on inhibition of cellular exudates and suppression of vascular permeability has a positive effect on painful joints during therapy. The high incidence of gastrointestinal disturbances is somewhat modified by concurrent use of an antacid or taking the drug with or after meals. Pharmacodynamic action begins within 1 hour after administration and lasts for 4 to 6 hours. Initial therapy often provides relief of joint pain, but as therapy progresses, patients complain of increasing gastrointestinal disturbances and neurologic problems. Throbbing morning headache and disturbed equilibrium resulting from intracranial vasoconstriction often make it necessary to modify or discontinue drug therapy. Serious psychiatric disturbances and blood dyscrasias have occurred during therapy.

Colchicine (Colchin) is a specific agent used for therapy of gout. The drug has been employed since the sixteenth century as a gout-specific agent, but there is little knowledge of the specific pharmacodynamic action on the articular process. Evidence that the painful inflammatory process subsides promptly during initial therapy makes it probable that the drug has an effect on leukocytic invasion. Oral administration (4 to 5 mg./24 hours divided into 4 to 5 doses) is continued until diarrhea occurs. Onset of diarrhea is considered the end point of therapy, and abatement of articular pain and swelling usually occurs within the 12- to 24-hour period before occurrence of diarrhea.

Other agents are used to relieve the excruciating pain and inflammation of joints caused by various inflammatory processes. The corticosteroids are often injected directly into the area and provide prompt pain relief. Rapidly progressing arthritic processes may necessitate the use of gold salts to halt articular destruction and related pain. Aurothioglucose (Solganal) and gold sodium thiomalate (Myochrysine) may be administered by intragluteal injection. The patient may complain of facial flushing and vertigo, and he may become giddy during drug administration. The drugs enter tissue fluids and are retained in the liver, spleen, kidneys, and skin, in addition to direct delivery to joint articulations. The gold salts are toxic, and dermatitis, stomatitis, and destruction of blood elements may occur when the patient is receiving weekly or biweekly injections of the drugs. The retention of gold salts in the skin increases photosensitivity reactions; the patient may decrease these reactions by avoiding intense sunlight or ultraviolet light.

Central pain control. Carbamazepine (Table 22-3) is used for treatment of trigeminal neuralgia (tic douloureux) and other central pain. Carbamazepine acts pharmacodynamically by decreasing synaptic transmission in the trigeminal nucleus. Concurrent with specific effect on the excruciating pain, the drug has mild sedative, anticholinergic, and muscle relaxant effects produced by inhibition of neuromuscular transmission at the spinal level. The diversity of actions limits its use to patients with persistent pain directly related to fifth cranial nerve involvement. Dosage is regulated at the level that modifies the pain, and discontinuance of the drug is planned as soon as pain is alleviated.

Patient care

Alleviation of the pain source may be beyond the province of the nurse, but measures to increase the effectiveness of drugs are the particular armamentarium the nurse can mobilize to assist the patient to deal with pain. The clue to mobilization may be the perception of physical signs, the patient's verbal request for help, or the obvious malposition of the patient that indicates uneven muscle tension.

Judgment is necessary in timing the use of pain relieving measures. Correction of the patient's distorted position may relieve discomfort and allow continuance with activity or rest. The patient in acute distress will also benefit by measures to remove environmental or positional pain stimuli. Timing of comfort measures in relation to administration of a pain-relieving drug is a primary concern in planning care of the patient in acute distress. His needs suggest a sequence of actions differing from the previous situation. Correction of obvious positional or environmental problems may be accomplished quickly before the pain-control drug is administered. Measures to increase the comfort of the patient may be planned in the interval between drug administration and predictable onset of drug action. Planned utilization of contact time with the patient when it is meaningful to his stress level enhances the action of the drug and communicates that there is concern for his well-being.

Reality for the patient is the way he perceives the situation as the sufferer; his perception may change as he feels less isolated and more protected. Measures to increase his comfort, generously offered, may make the difference between healthful and unhealthful responses to pain.

Objective and subjective measurement of pain relief attained with use of a particular drug include assessments by the nurse and the patient. Modification of the pharmacotherapeutic plan is dependent on accurate evaluation of drug effect. The continuance of the total therapeutic plan may be dependent on whether the patient can participate in activities necessary to his progress (i.e., physical exercise, coughing exercises). Pain-alleviating drugs administered prior to the activity are planned to increase the ability of the patient to accomplish the task. Avoidance of pain is an instinct, but modification of the neural stimulus should be sufficient to move the patient toward accomplishment of the therapeutic goal. Inadequate pain relief increases the hesitancy to move forward in deference to the need to protect self from pain.

Support of the effect of drugs specifically administered for temperature control may include tepid baths or use of an automatic cooling blanket. When the body temperature rises above 104° F., intensive efforts are necessary to modify the temperature rapidly. Cooling of superficial tissues modifies internal temperature by cooling the blood circulating through surface vessels. Surface cooling lowers the temperature of the central blood pool. Rapid cooling may be accomplished by placing cool alcohol cloths in the body areas where large vessels surface, but the procedure must be accomplished without precipitation of chills because muscle work produces internal heat and negates the effect of the applications. Any measure that will cool the total body surface evenly may have a positive effect on decreasing internal body temperature. Whether procedures involve bathing, an automatic cooling blanket, or an electric fan near an open window on a cold day, the patient's status is carefully observed to assure that the measures are used below the point of shivering.

Administration of analgesics with concurrent antipyretic effect for control of hyperpyrexia over protracted time periods necessitates assessment of hydration status and planning for the replacement of fluid losses. Diaphoresis occurring after administration of the drugs may cause the bedding and bed clothing of the patient to be damp or wet, and the patient will feel exceedingly cold when the temperature begins to rise again.

Many of the drugs used for pain are ulcerogenic; therefore plans for evaluation of the effect of the drugs on gastrointestinal tissue may include periodic examination of the stools for microscopic blood content. Changes in eating patterns or the emergence of food intolerances may provide early clues to gastric irritation. Concurrent administration of antacids or food may decrease gastric discomfort.

Hypersensitivity to the analgesics ranges from simple itching of the perinasal area after administration of an opiate to generalized skin rash. Each of the drugs has a hypersensitivity potential, and the appearance of skin rash is an early warning sign of individual sensitivity to the drug. Consultation with the nursing and medical team as soon as rash appears provides opportunity for modification of the pharmacotherapeutic plan and definition of measures to decrease the pruritic rash.

Analgesics are commonly taken by members of the community. There is little concern with the adverse effect of use of the minor analgesics, and it seems unwise to impose fear of problems on the periodic user of analgesics. Larger dosages and combinations of nonaddictive drugs with addictive drugs for the patient with persistent pain introduces into the patient situation concern with effects and adverse effects. Judicious planning by health team members is necessary to prevent problems occurring during therapy with seemingly innocuous drugs and with addictive narcotics.

Pain alleviation is a patient's right. Accomplishment of the pharmacotherapeutic plan that will protect his right is the challenge to health team members.

REFERENCES

Alderman, Edwin L., Barry, William H., Graham, Anthony, and Harrison, Donald C.: Hemodynamic effects of morphine and pentazocine differ in cardiac patients, The New England Journal of Medicine **287**:623, 1972.

Bonica, John J.: Oral analgesics for chronic pain, Modern Medicine **39**:87, 1971.

Bowden, Charles L., and Maddux, James F.: Methadone maintenance: myth and reality, The American Journal of Psychiatry **129**:435, 1972.

Boyd, Eldon M.: The safety and toxicity of aspirin, American Journal of Nursing **71**:964, 1971.

Carroll, Mary Helen: Preventing newborn deaths from drug withdrawal, R.N. **34**:34, 1971.

Chambers, Wilda G., and Price, Geraldine G.: Influence of nurse upon effects of analgesics administered, Nursing Research **16**:228, 1967.

Diamond, Seymour, and Baltes, Bernard J.: Management of headache by the family physician, American Family Physician **5**:68, April, 1972.

Fink, Max, Freedman, Alfred M., Zaks, Arthur M., and Resnick, Richard B.: Narcotic antagonists: another approach to addiction therapy, American Journal of Nursing **71**:1359, 1971.

Gates, Marshall: Analgesic drugs, Scientific American **215**:131, Nov., 1966.

Goodman, Louis S., and Gilman, Arthur, editors: The pharmacological basis of therapeutics, ed. 4, New York, 1970, The Macmillan Co.

Hackett, Thomas P.: Pain and prejudice: why do we doubt that the patient is in pain? Medical Times **99**:130, 1971.

Krane, Stephen M.: Action of salicylates (editorial), The New England Journal of Medicine **286**:317, 1972.

Levine, David G., Levin, Donald B., Sloan, Ira H., and Chappel, John N.: Personality correlates of success in a methadone maintenance program, The American Journal of Psychiatry **129**:456, 1972.

Maddux, James F., and Bowden, Charles L.: Critique of success with methadone maintenance, The American Journal of Psychiatry **129**:440, 1972.

McBride, Mary A. B.: The additive to the analgesic, American Journal of Nursing **69**:974, 1969.

McCaffery, Margo, and Moss, Fay: Nursing intervention for bodily pain, American Journal of Nursing **67**:1224, 1967.

Moertel, C. G., Ahmann, D. L., Taylor, W. F., and Schwartau, Neal: A comparative evaluation of marketed analgesic drugs, The New England Journal of Medicine **286**:813, 1972.

Mountcastle, Vernon B., editor: Medical physiology, vol. 2, ed. 13, St. Louis, 1974, The C. V. Mosby Co.

Nichols, John R.: How opiates change behavior, Scientific American **212**:80, Feb., 1965.

Noble, Peter, and Barnes, Gill G.: Drug taking in adolescent girls: factors associated with the progression of narcotic use, British Medical Journal **2**:620, 1971.

Poplar, James F.: Characteristics of nurse addicts, American Journal of Nursing **69**:117, 1969.

Reilly, Mary Jo, editor: American hospital formulary service, vol. 1, sect. 28:00, vol. 2, sect. 72:00, Washington, D. C., 1973, American Society of Hospital Pharmacists.

Rogers, John G.: My opinion; a new test for pain, Resident-Intern Consultant **11**:40, Aug., 1971.

Rogoff, Bernard: Rheumatoid arthritis—after salicylates, what then? Resident-Intern Consultant **1**:13, Feb., 1972.

Storlie, Frances: Pain: describing it more accurately, Nursing '72 **2**:15, 1972.

Sweet, William H., and Wepsic, James G.: Relation of fiber size in trigeminal posterior root to conduction of impulses for pain and touch; production of analgesia without anesthesia in the effective treatment of trigeminal neuralgia, Transactions of the American Neurological Association **95**:134, 1970.

Vandam, Leroy D.: Drug therapy: analgetic drugs—the mild analgesics, The New England Journal of Medicine **286**:20, 1971.

Webb, Carolyn: Tactics to reduce a child's fear of pain, American Journal of Nursing **66**:2698, 1966.

UNIT FIVE
DRUGS USED TO CONTROL ANABOLIC-CATABOLIC BALANCE

23　Malnutrition

24　Metabolic activity

25　Glucose assimilation

23

Malnutrition

Appetite suppression
    Pharmacodynamics
Amphetamine abuse
Protein building
    Pharmacodynamics

Malnutrition continues to be a major health problem in the world. Many Americans are malnourished in the midst of plentiful supplies of food and money. A state of balanced nutrition exists when an individual ingests adequate nutrients for building and maintaining body tissues.

Parenteral hyperalimentation and minimal residue, or elemental, formulations have been developed to meet the nutritional needs of acutely ill patients. Provision of nutrients in a form easily assimilated by body cells has a profound effect on wound healing and general tissue health of the patient with long illness or extensive major surgery. Use of the formulations has decreased the extremes of cachexia formerly accompanying devastating health problems (i.e., extensive gastrointestinal surgery, malignancy).

Widespread nutritional imbalances occur with disproportion of foods ingested. Cellular growth, development, and function are chiefly dependent on nutrients supplied from dietary sources. Carbohydrates, fats, or proteins can be used to meet metabolic requirements, but proteins contain the key factor nitrogen, which is necessary to cellular growth. Excess ingestion of carbohydrate leads to deposition of surplus in adipose tissues, from which it is mobilized during periods of nutrient deprivation. Absence of reserves from glycogen or triglyceride stores necessitates breakdown of tissue protein to meet metabolic needs. Therapy for either obesity or cachexia is directed basically at modification of nutrient intake patterns.

Pharmacotherapy may be planned to support the program for dietary modification. Drugs may be used to decrease appetite for foods and increase physical activity or to maximize the utilization of available foods.

APPETITE SUPPRESSION

Drug-induced appetite suppression supports the attempts of the individual to lose weight. By decreasing food ingestion, the body becomes dependent on glycogen, triglyceride, and fatty acid stores for ongoing metabolic needs, and the process reduces body weight. The plan is only effective when the individual is sincerely interested in weight reduction. Psychologic and cultural factors are interrelated aspects in dietary excesses, and they play a significant role in weight control programs.

Drug therapy assists with weight control by decreasing the individual's desire for food. The ideal weight reduction plan includes a drug-diet program providing nutrients to meet tissue needs for vitamins, minerals, and protein throughout the weight reduction period. Sustained levels of endogenous glucose are needed by brain, retinal, and germinal epithelium to maintain function, and blood glucose content must be maintained. Dietary restrictions are carefully planned with the individual to allow scheduling of food intake within the caloric restrictions that meet metabolic needs. Realistically many individuals use the drugs to implement a minimal food intake or crash diet plan.

Denial plays a role in the resistance of individuals to weight control in the face of known health hazards attributable to obesity. Many individuals turn off when cardiac overload, respiratory work, or circulatory problems are presented as obesity-related health hazards. Factors reinforcing persistent maintenance of food restrictions often relate to signs of improvement in appearance or activity tolerance that are important to the individual. Positive feedback may provide the motivating factor necessary to success of the weight reduction plan.

Pharmacodynamics

Amphetamine use. The primary group of drugs prescribed for appetite suppression (anorexigenics) are derivatives of amphetamines (Table 23-1). The drugs produce a sustained state of activity readiness, comparable to flight or fight readiness, by stimulation of sympathetic nervous system responses. Amine oxidase inhibition in cerebrocortical and reticular-activating structures is thought to provide the central stimulation that elevates mood and increases mental acuity. As a secondary response, increased peripheral norepinephrine released from adrenergic nerve terminals accelerates physical activity levels.

Predictable effects of increased catecholamine levels in the periphery occur during therapy. The effects are those preparing the body for action: constriction of superficial blood vessels, shunting of blood to the muscles and vital organs, decreased motility of the gastrointestinal and urinary tract, accelerated cardiac and respiratory activity, and dilation of the pupils and bronchus. The readiness pattern persists throughout the period of drug therapy, and termination of drug therapy may leave the patient letdown, tired, and depressed.

Central nervous system stimulation may increase interest and involvement in environmental activities, but there is considerable variation in individual response to the drugs. A taciturn individual may become talkative, enthusiastic, and physically more active, whereas another individual may be unable to concentrate, irritable, nervous, and hyperactive.

Central nervous system stimulation is the chief contribution the drugs make to weight

Table 23-1. Dosage range of appetite suppressants

Nonproprietary name	Proprietary (trade) name	Daily adult dosage range (oral)
Amphetamine sulfate	Amphedrine, Benzedrine sulfate, Linampheta	2.5-30 mg. ($\div$1-3)
Benzphetamine hydrochloride	Didrex	25-150 mg. ($\div$1-3)
Chlorphentermine hydrochloride	Pre-Sate	65 mg.
Dextroamphetamine hydrochloride	Daro-Tab	2.5-15 mg. ($\div$1-3)
Dextroamphetamine sulfate	Amfetasul, Amphex, Amsustain, Cendex, Dexedrine sulfate, Perke-One, Zamitam	2.5-15 mg. ($\div$1-3)
Diethylpropion hydrochloride	Natorexic, Tenuate, Tepanil	75-100 mg. ($\div$3-4)
Levamfetamine succinate	Amodril, Cydril	7.5-30 mg. ($\div$3)
Levamfetamine sulfate	Ad-Nil	7.5-30 mg. ($\div$3)
Levamfetamine tannate	Elpandryl	7.5-30 mg. ($\div$3)
Methamphetamine hydrochloride	Amphedroxin Desamine, Desox-Desyphed, Dexoval, Dexstim, D-O-E, Doxyphed, Drinalfa, Efroxine, Methedrine, Norodin, Semoxydrine, Syndrox	5-15 mg. ($\div$2-3)
Phendimetrazine tartrate	Plegine	35-70 mg. ($\div$2-3)
Phenmetrazine hydrochloride	Preludin	25-75 mg. ($\div$2-3)
Phentermine hydrochloride	Wilpo	24 mg. ($\div$3)
Phentermine resin	Ionamin	15-30 mg.

control. Psychic energy keeps the individual physically active, and the increased metabolic rate gradually mobilizes body stores in adipose tissue to meet energy needs during the period of decreased food intake. Disinterest in foods concurrent with increased physical activity produces a decline in body weight. The drugs have an effect on acuity of smell and taste that enhances food disinterest. There is an urgency to the accomplishment of weight modification during the early days of therapy because tolerance to the drugs develops after a few weeks and prior overeating patterns may be reestablished.

Amphetamine derivatives have been used therapeutically to elevate depressed emotional states or as adjunctive therapy in treating patients with drug-induced respiratory depression. For many years the amphetamines were considered the drugs of choice for treatment of mental depression, but the acceleration of physical and mental processes failed to meet the objectives of therapy. The psychic energy stimulated by the amphetamine failed to provide concentration and improvement in rational thought processes. The drugs have been replaced by new *psychic energizers* that allow psychotherapy and environmental involvement to be used as part of the total therapeutic plan for control of mental depression. The pharmacodynamic actions of antidepressant drugs, or psychic energizers, are presented in Chapter 17.

Methamphetamine hydrochloride (Table 23-1) is the nonproprietary name of the drug commonly known as speed. At the present time the drug is considered too dangerous to be used for medical purposes, although it was a popular anorexigenic and psychic energizer in the past.

Accessibility of the drugs for use as uppers by drug abusers desiring the euphoria-producing properties of the amphetamines has been facilitated by availability of the drugs from individuals having prescriptions for anorexigenics. There are illicit sources ready to propagate use of the drugs for their psychic stimulation action. Therapeutic use of amphetamines has declined since abuse has become a worldwide health problem.

Excretion control. Disruption of the natural anabolic-catabolic balance to increase catabolism of endogenous adipose tissues increases the production of acidic breakdown products (ketones) in the bloodstream. Acidity of the urine during therapy with amphetamines enhances elimination of the drug. Elimination of the acidic end products requires an intake of fluid in amounts adequate to assure renal excretion. Drug abusers, cognizant that the urinary excretion of drug is greater in acidic urine, plan to take small amounts of carbohydrate periodically to prevent catabolism-related urine acidity. By modification of the urinary pH, the drug user can prolong elimination of the drug and maintain its pharmacodynamic effect for several days.

Amphetamine formulations. There is variation in potency between the amphetamines, but dosage modification minimizes the differences. Dextroamphetamine hydrochloride, dextroamphetamine sulfate, and methamphetamine hydrochloride are the more widely used anorexigenic drugs, for they produce minimal norepinephrine-mediated peripheral responses. The dextro form is an active central nervous system stimulant, but the levo form provides less effect. Many anorexogenic drugs contain mixtures of the dextro and levo forms of amphetamine.

Administration schedules. Chlorphentermine hydrochloride is only available in an extended-release form, and it is administered once a day after breakfast for daylong anorexigenic effect. Other derivatives of amphetamine are taken periodically throughout the day or as extended-release formulations. Selection of the specific derivative and the form of the drug is based on individual living patterns. Those with ready access to foods (i.e., cooks, bakers, homemakers) may need a sustained level of drug to avoid periods of appetite stimulation during the day. Other individuals may be assisted in their plan for weight control when regularly scheduled drug use reminds them of the restriction plan. The drugs usually are prescribed to be taken from $1/2$ to 1 hour before meals. The last daily dose is taken at least 6 hours before bedtime to avoid interruption of sleep patterns by the stimulatory effect of the drug.

Adverse effects. During therapy with amphetamines, the chief adverse effects are extensions of the pharmacodynamic action of the drug. Suppression of parasympathetic nervous system responses may precipitate constipation, blurred vision, or nausea and vomiting. Dryness and a characteristic metallic taste in the mouth may increase the individual's oral fluid intake. The increased liquid has a positive effect on urinary output of ketones and drug metabolites. Increased fluid intake also decreases constipation and liquifies thick, tenacious secretions that occur during therapy with amphetamines.

Large doses of the amphetamines increase the stimulation of vital parameters, and the patient must be observed for changes in respiratory and cardiac rate. At therapeutic dosage levels, patients may complain of acceleration of heartbeat, insomnia, and irritability, which may be modified by changes in dosage. These problems may necessitate discontinuance of therapy with amphetamine. Although hypersensitivity to the drugs is rare, urticaria may occur during therapy. The patient is asked to consult with the physician before continuing scheduled use of the drug if skin reactions appear.

AMPHETAMINE ABUSE

The extended periods of wakefulness produced by amphetamines has propagated use of the drugs by individuals desiring to extend physical or mental activity beyond limits tolerable to the body without exogenous stimulation. The mental acuity and wakefulness may benefit the student who plans last-minute study for comprehensive examinations, and round-the-clock physical activity may provide increased income for the worker. In each instance the protracted activity periods are accomplished at the price of depression of activity after use. Dependence on the drugs for accomplishment of tasks necessitates continued use or reuse of the stimulants when comparable situations arise in the future. Tolerance to amphetamines develops with continued use, and increased dosage is necessary to maintain the desired effect.

Task-oriented dependence on amphetamines continues to be a health problem, but widespread use of the drugs solely for their psychic stimulatory effect has increased misuse of amphetamines. Availability and low cost have expanded individual trials with amphetamines to include all age groups.

The chronic user becomes dependent on amphetamines, alcohol, or sedatives to maintain a sequence of psychic activity allowing a semblance of normal living in society. The amphetamine-induced accelerated psychic activity is enjoyed for its own sake, and there is no desire to channel the energy. The individual's mind is racing too fast to concentrate, and he savors the experience. For many individuals, termination of the experience is accomplished by use of sedatives that abolish amphetamine effect and allow return to the scheduled activities of the world. For example, the youngster may use the amphetamine-sedative sequence after school, and appear at home in time for the evening meal without providing a clue to adults in the household that the experience took place.

Sequential use of uppers (amphetamines) and downers (sedatives) may allow maintenance of societal contact during use, and some individuals continue with work obligations. The hazards of drug-induced tachycardia suddenly reversed by sedatives have caused fatal cardiac arrest in some drug abusers.

Periodic use of amphetamines with concurrent alcohol ingestion to modify the psychic elevation is a common pattern. Beer sipping during drug action periods provides some of the calories necessary to slow fat metabolism and consequent amphetamine excretion.

The abuser has amphetamine-induced pupil dilation that necessitates wearing dark glasses and avoiding direct bright light. Mobile colored lights are sometimes part of the indoor scene set to provide psychic fantasy at a high level. The individual with a light complexion shows deep periorbital reddening that is a startling addition to the bloodshot eyes.

Adverse effects of amphetamine abuse relate to the pattern of use and the neglect of physiologic needs for sleep. Amphetamines disrupt normal sleep patterns by reducing the periods of Stage IV and *rapid eye movement* (REM) sleep. Absence of REM sleep deprives the individual of the emotional release through dreams that is necessary to psychic health. Continued loss of REM sleep contributes to the emergence of hallucinations and psychotic episodes occurring with amphetamine abuse. Psychosis may persist for weeks and is accompanied by complete withdrawal from social contacts. Psychosis may occur after intensive periods of drug use or after initial use of a large dose of amphetamine. Psychotic episodes include auditory and visual hallucinations with paranoid ideation.

Current programs aimed at decreasing abuse of drugs are being conducted to orient individuals to the hazards of drug use. Many adults continue to view the problem as that of an isolated segment of the population and overlook the reality of drug use within their social sphere or household until overt problems emerge.

Prolonged use may lead to habituation and psychically induced physical dependence. In addition to the effect of chronic abuse on physiologic and psychic function, the productivity of the individual is affected as social and work relations are disrupted.

PROTEIN BUILDING

Continued deprivation of nutrients gradually depletes glycogen and triglyceride stores, and the body becomes dependent on tissue sources for amino acids to meet metabolic needs. Protein is readily converted to energy-producing carbohydrates, and the nitrogen is liberated for excretion. A catabolic state may continue to mobilize tissue stores until peripheral muscle tissue is severely depleted of protein. Obvious limits exist for catabolic destruction of vital body tissues.

Catabolism of protein may be halted by provision of exogenous sources of glucose, fats, or protein. The diversity of preparations currently available for gastrointestinal or intravenous nutrient infusion makes extreme cachexia a rarity except with extensive hepatic destruction or malignant tissue invasion. Nutrient supplements are useful in prevention of catabolism and in instituting anabolic activity necessary to rebuilding of body tissues.

Gastrointestinal feedings based on the diets used for astronauts during space flight provide nutrients in a form that requires minimal digestive activity. Nutrients from the elemental diets (i.e., Jejunal Special Dietary Food) are absorbed in the duodenum or jejunum, and they produce minimal residue. The innovation is a major breakthrough for the patient with extensive pathology or surgery of the gastrointestinal tract who previously became cachectic before food tolerance and peristaltic activity were established. Daily ingestion of pudding, broth, or beverage formulations supplies up to 1750 calories to meet the basic nutrient needs of the nonambulatory patient. Alternation of the particular form of nutrient varies the diet, and patients tolerate the feedings better than previously used blenderized formulations. Amino acids (5.9 grams), fats (1.6 grams), and carbohydrates (379 grams) make up the calories available in the daily feedings that also provide daily vitamin and electrolyte requirements. Utilization of the special dietary foods before surgery raises the patient's nutritional status to a level that has a positive effect on

Table 23-2. Dosage range of anabolic steroids

Nonproprietary name	Proprietary (trade) name	Daily adult dosage range
Ethylestrenol	Maxibolin	Oral: 4-8 mg.
Methandriol	Androdiol, Diolandrone, Drostene, Methostan, Nabadial, Neostene, Stenediol	Oral: 10-40 mg. I.M.: 7.5-25 mg.
Methandrostenolone	Dianabol	Oral: 5-20 mg.
Nandrolone decanoate	Deca-Durabolin	I.M.: 50-100 mg. monthly
Nandrolone phenpropionate	Durabolin	I.M.: 25-50 mg. weekly
Oxandrolone	Anavar	Oral: 2.5-20 mg. (÷2-4)
Oxymetholone	Adroyd, Anadrol	Oral: 5-30 mg.
Stanozolol	Winstrol	Oral: 4-6 mg. (÷2-3)

the postoperative course. After surgery the foods are continued by oral or gastrointestinal tube feedings to maintain nutrition of body tissues and promote wound healing.

Protein hydrolysate (Amigen, Aminosol, Hyprotigen, Parenamine, Travamin) are also used to provide amino acids to meet tissue maintenance needs. The basic protein content (38 grams/liter) can be administered by intravenous, oral, or gastrointestinal tube feedings. The solutions provide protein for tissue needs, and additional intake of carbohydrate serves to meet energy needs and spare protein stores. Varying forms of parenteral hyperalimentation are being tested in clinical practice, and the resultant tissue nutrition in devastating illness has improved the tolerance of individuals to extensive injury or disease.

Pharmacotherapeutic plans are aimed at inducing storage of proteins from available nutrient sources. The natural anabolic activity of male sex hormones provides the basis of pharmacodynamic action for control of body protein building.

Pharmacodynamics

Anabolic steroids. Androgens are produced by the adrenal glands in both males and females in small amounts, but they are the chief hormones produced by the male gonads. Androgens maintain sexual development and function in the male. Anabolic androgens are synthesized or purified to limit the effect on sex characteristics. Pharmacodynamic action of the anabolic androgens (Table 23-2) induces retention of nitrogen, potassium, and phosphorus necessary to tissue building.

Androgens are used when deceleration of amino acid catabolism or acceleration of protein anabolism is required for maintenance of body tissues. The effectiveness of the therapeutic plan is dependent on the availability of materials for storage; therefore protein and carbohydrate intake is provided throughout therapy. Patients experience androgen-induced weight gain, a sense of well-being, and improvement in appetite that supports anabolism during the therapeutic period.

Some of the steroids offer the advantage of long intervals between parenteral administration. Nandrolone decanoate and nandrolone phenpropionate (Table 23-2) are slowly released from parenteral depots of drug, and weekly or monthly administration supplies continued androgenic activity. There are minor differences between the androgens, but they have a comparable pharmacodynamic action. Effectiveness of therapy is difficult to evaluate: nutrient intake is necessary to drug effect, and the differentiation between food or drug effect on tissue health is somewhat controversial.

Administration of anabolic steriods to children provides the calcium, phosphates, and protein necessary to maturation of bone. The chief concern during therapy is that bone maturation may proceed faster than linear bone growth. Periodic evaluation of bone age is planned to avoid adverse effect on skeletal development resulting from premature epiphyseal closure.

Adverse effects. Long-term therapy in children or women may cause emergence of masculine characteristics: *hirsuitism, clitoral enlargement,* and *voice deepening* or *hoarseness.* The effects are usually irreversible: therefore planned observations are necessary to halt drug therapy at the earliest evidence of the problems. Long-term administration may affect sexual development and activity in either males or females. Androgen-induced sodium ion and water retention may cause fluid accumulation in tissues during therapy. Large doses or prolonged administration of anabolic androgens to females may cause emergence of male sex characteristics comparable to those caused by other androgenic drugs presented in Chapter 27.

REFERENCES

Alexander, James K.: Cardiovascular complications of obesity, Cardiovascular Nursing **5:**19, 1969.

Anthony, Catherine Parker, and Kolthoff, Norma J.: Textbook of anatomy and physiology, ed. 8, St. Louis, 1971, The C. V. Mosby Co.

Boakes, R. J., Bradley, P. B., and Candy, J. M.: Abolition of the response of brain stem neurones to iontophoretically applied d-amphetamine by reserpine, Nature **229:**496, 1971.

Carr, L. A. and Moore, K. E.: Effects of amphetamine on the contents of norepinephrine and its metabolites in the effluent of perfused cerebral ventricles of the cat, Biochemical Pharmacology **19:**2361, 1970.

Dudrick, Stanley J., and Rhoads, Jonathan E.: Total intravenous feeding, Scientific American **226**:73, May, 1972.

Gordon, Edgar S.: New concepts of the biochemistry and physiology of obesity, Medical Clinics of North America **48**:1285, 1964.

Goth, Andres: Medical pharmacology, ed. 6, St. Louis, 1972, The C. V. Mosby Co.

Meng, H. C.: Principles of parenteral nutrition, Hospital Medicine **6**:102, 1971.

Olsen, Ward A.: Current concepts: practical approach to diagnosis of disorders of intestinal absorption, The New England Journal of Medicine **285**:1358, 1971.

Orten, James M., and Neuhaus, Otto W.: Biochemistry, ed. 8, St. Louis, 1970, The C. V. Mosby Co.

Parsa, Mohamad H., Thornton, Beverly H., and Ferrer, Jose M.: Central venous alimentation, American Journal of Nursing **72**:2042, 1972.

Reilly, Mary Jo, editor: American hospital formulary service, vol. 1, sect. 28:20, vol. 2, sect. 68:08, Washington, D. C., 1973, American Society of Hospital Pharmacists.

Stokes, Shirlee A.: Fasting for obesity, American Journal of Nursing **69**:796, 1969.

Swanke, W. R.: Amphetamine abuse, The New Physician **1**:591, 1970.

Texter, E. Clinton Jr., Chou, Ching-Chung, Laureta, Higino C., and Vantrappen, Gaston R.: Physiology of the gastrointestinal tract, St. Louis, 1968, The C. V. Mosby Co.

Wiley, Loy: Hyperalimentation, Nursing '72 **2**:26, 1972.

Williams, Sue Rodwell: Nutrition and diet therapy, ed. 2, St. Louis, 1973, The C. V. Mosby Co.

Young, Vernon R., and Scrimshaw, Nevins: The physiology of starvation, Scientific American **225**:14, Oct., 1971.

24

Metabolic activity

Thyroid glandular function
    Pharmacodynamics
    Patient care
Calcium ion balance
    Calcium sources
    Hypocalcemia
    Hypercalcemia
    Calcium balance assessment
    Pharmacodynamics

The thyroid gland is dynamically involved in producing hormone levels that regulate the metabolic rate of physiologic processes. The thyroid gland and the tiny glands adjacent to it, the parathyroids, interact to control mineralization of bone as part of their role in maintaining calcium ion levels in the body.

THYROID GLANDULAR FUNCTION

Thyroid glandular activity is controlled by anterior pituitary release of the thyrotropic hormone, thyroid stimulating hormone (TSH). The thyrotropic hormone affects the uptake of iodides from the bloodstream and the activity of multiple proteolytic enzymes within the thyroid gland that produce and release hormones into the bloodstream to act on body processes (Fig. 24-1).

Foods and water provide the iodine necessary to production of thyroid hormones. Thyroxine is the only body substance carrying a significant amount of iodine; therefore the iodine-protein level in serum (normal: 3.5 to 8 mcg.%) is a test of function of the thyroid gland (protein-bound iodine, or P.B.I.). Iodine from the gastrointestinal tract is converted to the organic iodide essential to hormone synthesis.

Pharmacodynamics

Thyroid hormone control. Production of thyroxine or triiodothyronine necessary to biologic function can be interrupted by drugs that intercede at varying sites to interfere with production of the hormones (Fig. 24-1). Thiocyanates and perchlorates block the activity of the iodide trap that concentrates iodides before they enter the synthetic pathway. Thiocyanates and perchlorates have produced toxic effects (including renal necrosis); therefore they seldom are used for long-term control of thyroid function. Conversion of the iodides to iodine is blocked by inhibition of oxidizing enzymes by thiouracil derivatives, and sulfonamides inhibit formation of the storage form of thyroid hormone.

Hyperactivity of the thyroid gland affects all body systems, and the increased metabolic activity is destructive to vital organ function. Destruction of hyperactive thyroid tissue is often accomplished by use of radioactive iodide, and the radiopharmaceutical has a dramatic effect on reversal of the hyperthyroid syndrome.

Thyroid hormone inhibitors. Iothiouracil sodium, methylthiouracil, propylthiouracil, and methimazole (Table 24-1) are used to inhibit oxidation of iodides and prevent their combination with tyrosine in the formation of thyroxine. The drugs are selective for the thyroid glandular tissue, but oral administration allows passage through the placental barrier and into the milk of nursing mothers. The fetus or the

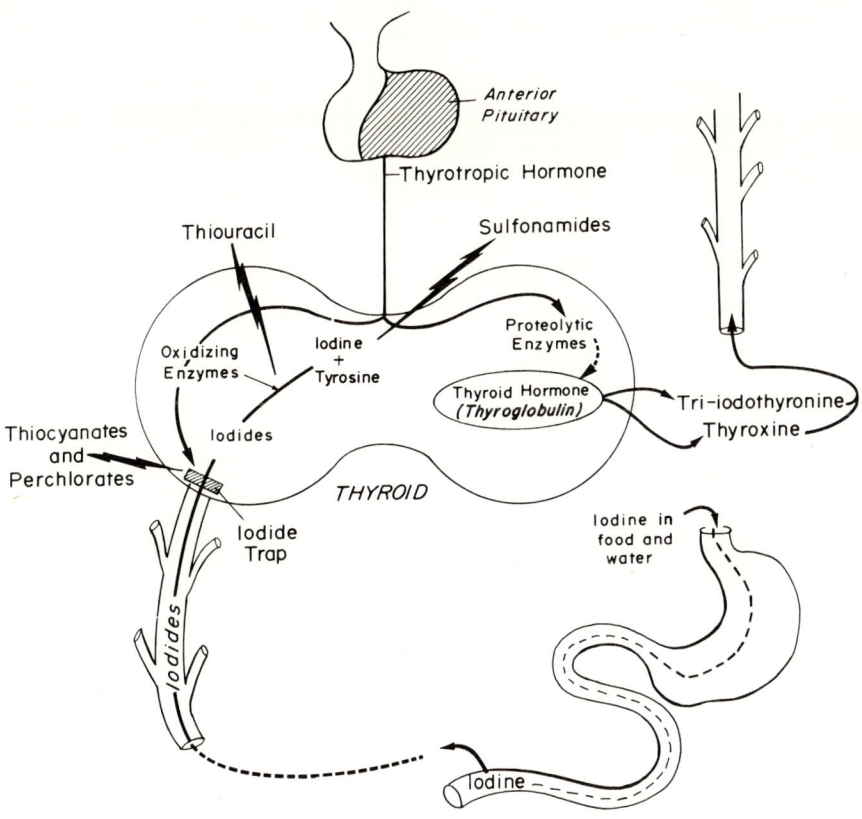

Fig. 24-1. Ingested iodine is carried by the bloodstream to the thyroid gland where it is used in the synthesis of thyroid hormone. Iodide uptake and thyroid hormone release are controlled by thyrotropic hormone. Pharmacologic agents that interfere with iodide uptake or enzymatic activity in the gland decrease thyroid hormone output.

nursing infant would have hypothyroidism if the mother received antithyroid drugs.

There is some delay in overt evidence of effect as stored thyroxine continues to be released while the drugs prevent formation of additional hormone. Thiouracil derivatives cause some adverse effects, including allergic reactions (skin rash, urticaria) and agranulocytosis, but the incidence is low. The patient is closely observed for progression of the therapeutic plan, and periodic contact allows frequent blood counts and physical examination for adverse effects. Patients are asked to consult with the physician immediately if fever or sore throat occurs during therapy because these signs precede the onset of agranulocytosis.

Thyroid hormone enhancers. Activity of the thyroid gland is dependent on the hormonal stimulation of the pituitary gland. In the presence of decreased activity of the anterior lobe of the pituitary gland, thyroid function will be affected adversely. Drug substitution is possible by intramuscular administration of thyrotropin (Table 24-1).

Deficiency of iodine in foods or water occurs in inland areas, and absence of the precursor for thyroid hormone formation deprives the body of the natural substance for physiologic activity. Iodized salt is a readily available source of iodine, but strong iodine solution may be used for replacement. Natural sources (foods, water, iodized salt) are preferable to the drug, since many individuals are hypersensitive to iodine sources (i.e., shellfish, saltwater fish). Reactions include swelling and hypersecretion of glands or largygeal edema, as well as other allergic responses.

Thyroid hormone replacement is provided

Table 24-1. Dosage range of drugs used for thyroid hormone control

Nonproprietary name	Proprietary (trade) name	Daily adult dosage range
Iodine solution, strong	Lugol's solution	Oral: 0.3-3 ml. (÷3)
Iothiouracil sodium	Itrumil	Oral: 150-300 mg. (÷1-3)
Levothyroxine sodium	Letter, Levoid, Synthroid, Titroid	Oral: 0.025-1 mg. I.V.: 0.1-0.4 mg.
Liothyronine sodium	Cytomel	Oral: 0.005-0.1 mg.
Methimazole	Tapazole	Oral: 5-60 mg. (÷1-3)
Methylthiouracil	Methiacil, Muracil	Oral: 300-600 mg. (÷3)
Propylthiouracil		Oral: 50-600 mg. (÷1-6)
Thyroglobulin	Endothyrin, Proloid	Oral: 15-200 mg.
Thyroid	Thyrar	Oral: 15-180 mg.
Thyrotropin	Thytropar	I.M.: 10-30 U.

by oral substitutes for the natural product. Levothyroxine sodium, liothyronine sodium, thyroglobulin, and thyroid (Table 24-1) are the most frequently used drugs. The similarity of the agents to natural thyroid hormone causes a feedback suppression of thyrotropin production from the anterior pituitary gland. Liothyronine sodium effect when administered orally may be apparent in 1 to 3 days, but the other agents require 1 to 3 weeks for establishment of continuous effect on metabolic activity. Observations of function of body systems are important because increased levels of hormone may be present during drug administration. The patient is observed carefully for evidence of physical hyperactivity and accelerated metabolic functions during therapy.

Patient care

Pharmacotherapy is planned to modify the physiologic activity of the patient, and the patient's response to therapy is monitored throughout the period the drugs are being taken. Base-line functional levels of the patient with decreased thyroid function (myxedema) may indicate apathy, lack of ambition, lack of interest in environmental events, and sensitivity to cold. The general lack of vitality is accompanied by depressed vital organ, bowel, and bladder function. Decreased activity of hepatic enzymatic action necessary to degradation of many drugs (i.e., sedatives, narcotics) makes the patient sensitive to many agents.

Hyperactivity of the thyroid gland causes hyperactivity of all body functions. The base-line functional levels of individual patients provide guidelines for planning care and definition of progress. The drugs used to control hyperactivity of the thyroid gland may precipitate signs of hypothyroid activity as extensions of pharmacodynamic effect beyond the planned level, whereas hormonal replacement may precipitate hyperactivity during therapy of the patient with hypothyroid function. Observations of all vital functions throughout therapy provide the evidence that is necessary to maintaining or modifying the therapeutic plan.

CALCIUM ION BALANCE

The constant interchange of bone is controlled by parathyroid hormone and calcitonin, which removes or restores calcium ions to the serum bathing the osseous tissues. Parathyroid hormone mediates the liberation of calcium phosphate from bone, and calcitonin from the thyroid tissue mediates the deposition of calcium phosphate on the collagen matrix of bone.

Calcium ion levels at nerve and muscle membranes play an important role in maintaining the passage of sodium ions necessary to conduction of neural stimuli and contraction of muscles. Calcium ions in the *sarcoplasmic reticulum* are actively involved in the meshing of *actin and myosin filaments* of the *myofibrils*. Calcium ions from reticulum sites interact with contractile proteins during contraction and are released as the filaments return to resting positions. Reticulum stores of calcium ions are involved in turning on muscle action. Sarcoplasmic calcium ions are maintained at functional levels when serum calcium ion content is within the normal range.

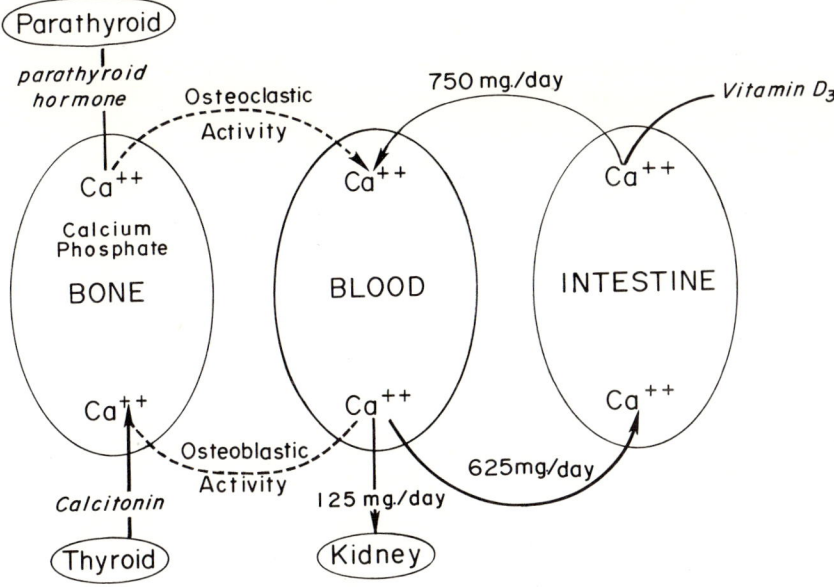

Fig. 24-2. Serum calcium ion levels are maintained by regulation of cation absorption from intestine or bone. Parathyroid hormone stimulates osteoclastic activity when calcium ion levels are low. Calcitonin provides the stimulus for storage of calcium salts in bone (osteoblastic activity) when the serum calcium ion level is elevated.

Calcium sources

Physiologic levels of serum calcium ions (normal: 8.5 to 10.5 mg./100 ml.) are obtained from food sources and from storage deposits in bone. Calcium salts obtained from foods (i.e., milk, milk products) are absorbed in the slightly acidic medium of the upper small intestine. Vitamin D_3 from liver stores is necessary for absorption of calcium ions. Movement of calcium salts from the serum to digestive enzymes, bone deposition, and renal or fecal excretion maintains serum levels of the cation (Fig. 24-2).

The constant interchange of bone is controlled primarily by parathyroid hormone and calcitonin, which remove or restore calcium ions to the serum bathing the osseous tissues. Parathyroid hormone mediates the liberation of calcium phosphate from bone, and calcitonin from the thyroid tissue mediates the deposition of calcium phosphate on the collagen matrix of bone.

Hypocalcemia

Hypocalcemia (i.e., serum calcium ion levels below 7 mg.%) increases the excitability of neural tissue by increasing the permeability of the membrane to transfer of sodium ions. The increased rate of sodium ion influx may cause a high level excitability of the neurons that maintains spontaneous firing of impulses. Sustained muscle contractions or tetanic convulsions provide evidence of extreme lowering of serum calcium ion levels. Testing of the excitability of nerves to external factors can be accomplished by a quick tap of the finger (flicking motion) on the cheek in the area of the seventh cranial nerve (facial nerve). The stimulation will cause twitching of the facial muscles in latent hypocalcemia (Chvostek's sign). A second test is done by applying pressure over a nerve (i.e., by applying a tourniquet on the forearm). In the presence of hypocalcemia the neural stimulation causes carpopedal spasm (Trousseau's sign).

Hypercalcemia

Hypercalcemia (i.e., serum calcium ion levels above 12 mg.%) blocks influx of sodium ions necessary to depolarization of the nerves and muscle. Responses become progressively

268 Drugs used to control anabolic-catabolic balance

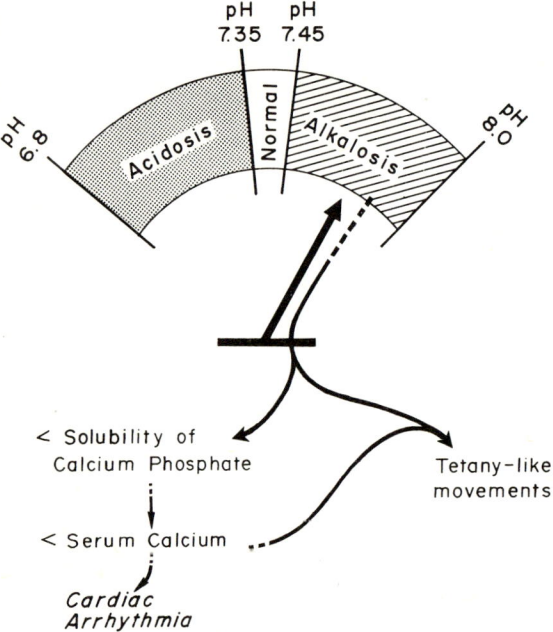

Fig. 24-3. Blood alkalinity decreases calcium absorption. The effect on membrane potentials is evidenced by hyperexcitability of cardiac and peripheral nerve tissues.

weaker, and all responses dependent on neural activity gradually become depressed.

Calcium balance assessment

The recognition of either hypocalcemia or hypercalcemia is important in many clinical situations. For example, the patient that is artificially ventilated by a respirator may become hyperreactive to touch. Fine twitching of the terminal phalanges may be observed during repositioning of the arm. For a complete interpretation of the problem, it is important to know that the solubility of calcium salts is decreased in an alkalotic state (Fig. 24-3). Immediate action is based on knowledge of the previous status of the patient, current assessment of physiologic changes, and knowledge of the relationship between mechanically induced hyperventilation, respiratory alkalosis, hypocalcemia, and hyperirritability of nerves.

Pharmacodynamics

Drugs are available to support physiologic attempts to regulate serum calcium ion levels

Table 24-2. Dosage range of drugs used to control serum calcium ion levels

Nonproprietary name	Proprietary (trade) name	Daily adult dosage range
Calciferol (vitamin D₂)	Drisdol	Oral: 0.02-0.125 mg.
Calcium gluconate		Oral: 6 Gm. (÷3)
Calcium lactate		Oral: 15 Gm. (÷5)
Dibasic calcium phosphate		Oral: 12 Gm. (÷3)
Hydrocalciferol	Hytakerol	Oral: 0.75-2.5 mg.
Parathyroid hormone	Paroidin	I.M.: 40-300 U. (÷2)
Sodium phytate	Rencal	Oral: 8 Gm.

by activity at each of the key points in the cation cycle. Pharmacotherapeutic plans are aimed at maintaining levels of the cation that enhance neural and muscular function.

Intestinal absorption inhibitor. Sodium phytate (Table 24-2) is administered to decrease absorption of calcium ions from food sources and to prevent reabsorption of the calcium component of digestive enzymes liberated into the intestinal tract. Sodium phytate acts pharmacodynamically by cation exchange in the intestinal lumen. The drug liberates sodium ions in exchange for calcium ions to form calcium phytate, which is excreted in the feces. The chief use of the drug is to inhibit calcium uptake when the parathyroid gland is hyperactive.

Intestinal absorption enhancer. Vitamin D is essential to absorption of calcium salts from the intestinal tract. The fat-soluble vitamin is stored in the liver, but when reserves are low, calciferol (Table 24-2) is administered for replenishment of vitamin D stores. Activated 7-dehydrocholesterol (vitamin D_3) is a component of many vitamin preparations prescribed for health maintenance. The most familiar source of vitamin D is sunlight, and replacement may be necessary for the institutionalized patient to assure utilization of ingested food sources of calcium salts.

Cation replacement. Maintenance of daily requirements of calcium salts when the patient is unable to ingest foods containing the cation or when losses are excessive (i.e., diarrhea) may be planned by using some of the readily absorbed forms of the cation. The daily requirements of the cation for adults is 1 gram each day, and for children the daily requirement to maintain integrity of the processes requiring calcium ions is 1 to 1.4 grams. The daily requirement for women during pregnancy or lactation is 1.5 to 2 grams daily.

Calcium gluconate, calcium lactate, or dibasic calcium phosphate (Table 24-2) may be prescribed for oral replacement of losses of calcium ions or to maintain the daily intake level. Oral agents are utilized best if the drugs are administered at least 1 hour after meals. Intravenous replacement may be planned with a calcium salt solution if the patient is unable to take oral drugs.

Osteoclastic activity control. Parenteral administration of parathyroid hormone (Table 24-2) is planned when the natural glandular product is deficient. Administration of parathyroid hormone mobilizes bone calcium phosphate. The inorganic phosphate is excreted by the kidneys, and the calcium ion remains to raise the serum levels to the normal range. Excess calcium ions are excreted by the kidneys. Repeated use of the hormone causes the production of antihormones, and hydrocalciferol (Table 24-2) may be administered orally to maintain the function usually accomplished by the natural hormone. The drug takes about 7 to 10 days for maximum effect on osteoclastic activity to maintain serum levels of calcium ions. Dosage adjustment is based on the serum levels of the cation and the amount of calcium ions excreted in the urine.

REFERENCES

Avioli, Louis V.: The diagnosis of primary hyperparathyroidism, Medical Clinics of North America **52**:451, 1968.

Bassett, C. Andrew L.: Electrical effects in bone, Scientific American **213**:18, Oct., 1965.

Fitch, Coy D.: Muscle wasting disease of endocrine origin, Medical Clinics of North America **52**:243, 1968.

Frost, H. M., Villanueva, A. R., Jaworski, Z. F., Meunier, P., and Shimizu, A. G.: Evaluation of cellular-level haversian bone resorption in human hyperparathyroid states, Henry Ford Hospital Medical Journal **17**:259, 1969.

Gillie, R. Bruce: Endemic goiter, Scientific American **224**:92, June, 1971.

Goodman, Louis S., and Gilman, Arthur, editors: The pharmacological basis of therapeutics, ed. 4, New York, 1970, The Macmillan Co.

Goth, Andres: Medical pharmacology, ed. 6, St. Louis, 1972, The C. V. Mosby Co.

Green, William L.: Guidelines for the treatment of myxedema, Medical Clinics of North America **52**:431, 1968.

Guyton, Arthur C.: Textbook of medical physiology, Philadelphia, 1971, W. B. Saunders Co.

Hagen, Garrett A.: Treatment of thyrotoxicosis with ^{131}I and post-therapy hypothyroidism, Medical Clinics of North America **52**:417, 1968.

Hershman, Jerome M., and Pittman, James A., Jr.: Control of thyrotropin secretion in man, The New England Journal of Medicine **285**:997, 1971.

Hoyle, Graham: How is muscle turned on and off? Scientific American **222**:84, April, 1970.

Kinsella, Ralph A., and Back, Donald K.: Thyroid acropachy, Medical Clinics of North America **52**:393, 1968.

Leonard, James J., and deGroot, William J.: The thyroid state and the cardiovascular system, Modern Concepts of Cardiovascular Disease **38**:23, May, 1969.

Lonsdale, Kathleen: Human stones, Scientific American **219**:104, Dec., 1968.

Loomis, W. F.: Rickets, Scientific American **223**:76, Dec., 1970.

Magaria, Rodolfo: The sources of muscular energy, Scientific American **226**:84, March, 1972.

McDougall, I. R., Greig, W. R., and Gillespie, F. C.: Radioactive iodine (^{125}I) therapy for thyrotoxicosis, The New England Journal of Medicine **285**:1099, 1971.

Merton, P. A.: How we control the contraction of our muscles, Scientific American **226**:30, May, 1972.

Orten, James M., and Neuhaus, Otto W.: Biochemistry, ed. 8, St. Louis, 1970, The C. V. Mosby Co.

Pittman, James A., Jr., Haigler, E. David, Jr., Hershman, Jerome M., and Pittman, Constance S.: Hypothalamic hypothyroidism, The New England Journal of Medicine **285**:844, 1971.

Purnell, Don C., Smith, Lynwood H., Scholz, Donald A., Elveback, Lila R., and Arnaud, Claude D.: Primary hyperparathyroidism, American Journal of Medicine **50**:670, 1971.

Raisz, Lawrence G.: Current concepts: the diagnosis of hyperparathyroidism, The New England Journal of Medicine **285**:1006, 1971.

Rasmussen, Howard, and Pechet, Maurice M.: Calcitonin, Scientific American **223**:42, Oct., 1970.

Reilly, Mary Jo, editor: American hospital formulary

service, vol. 2, sect. 68:00, Washington, D. C., 1973, American Society of Hospital Pharmacists.

Rosenberg, Isadore N.: Current concepts: evaluation of thyroid function, The New England Journal of Medicine **286:**924, 1972.

Ross, Russell, and Bornstein, Paul: Elastic fibers in the body, Scientific American **224:**44, June, 1971.

Thoma, George E., and Leightner, William F.: Dynamic clinical laboratory tests of thyroid functions, Medical Clinics of North America **52:**463, 1968.

Tronzo, Raymond G.: Bone: self-repairing, self-renewing, Resident-Intern Consultant **1:**20, May, 1972.

25

Glucose assimilation

Insulin deficiency
Insulin excess
Pharmacodynamics
Patient care

Nutrients in the bloodstream are in forms preparing them for assimilation by cells. Glucose content in the plasma bathing the pancreatic beta cells stimulates release of insulin, and the hormone provides the final factor necessary to entrance of glucose, fatty acids, and amino acids into cells. Brain tissue need not await the emergence of insulin for glucose assimilation; supplies are available by membrane diffusion that is independent of insulin activity. When cellular glucose content equilibrates with blood supplies, the excess is stored as triglycerides in adipose tissue or as glycogen in muscle and liver tissues. Insulin facilitates deposition of liver glucose by increasing the *glucokinase* necessary for processing glycogen for hepatic storage.

Fatty acids and amino acids are partially dependent on glucose for entrance into cellular, or depot, sites. Insulin mediates the preparation of glucose metabolites (i.e., alpha-glycerophosphate) that combine with fatty acids to prepare neutral fat storage forms. Amino acid transport across cell membranes is accomplished with the assistance of insulin. The process is comparable to glucose transport, with equilibration between cells and blood supplies providing the mechanism to halt transport.

Insulin deficiency

The absence of insulin affects assimilation of nutrients and deprives cells of the materials necessary for energy and building needs. Continued ingestion of carbohydrate in the absence of insulin for cellular transport raises the blood sugar level above normal limits (80 to 120 mg.%). Glucose-induced hyperosmolality of blood gradually increases the osmotic movement of fluid from tissues to dilute the concentrated vascular fluid. The effect is that of an endogenous osmotic diuretic causing increased fluid to enter the glomerular capillaries. Blood glucose levels above the renal threshold level allow spilling of glucose into the glomerular filtrate. High osmolality of the glucose-containing tubular urine osmotically holds water to produce large quantities of urine. Depletion of interstitial fluid causes generalized tissue dehydration and pruritus. Concurrent hypothalamic thirst center stimulation increases the desire to ingest large amounts of fluid.

The persistent problems of pruritus, increased urination (polyuria), and insatiable thirst (polydipsia) may cause the patient to seek medical attention. Insulin deficiency may increase hunger (polyphagia) by a combination of internal factors (i.e., cellular nutrient deprivation, osmotic emptying of gastrointestinal contents, high ingestion of rapidly digested carbohydrates). The 4-P sequence (pruritus, polyuria, polydipsia, polyphagia) is an endogenous insulin deficiency–induced problem of the patient initially diagnosed as having *diabetes mellitus*.

Insulin deficiency allows the cells to starve in the midst of plentiful supplies of nutrients. The glucose-laden blood must stand by unable to unload the nutrients without the assistance of insulin carriers.

The absence of insulin causes liberation of fatty acids from storage sites to provide alternate nutrients for metabolic needs. Ketone bodies produced by fatty acid metabolism flood the bloodstream and *metabolic acidosis* ensues. Renal excretion of the metabolites maintains ketoaciduria until the blood level of ketones is decreased. Concurrent protein catabolism provides small amounts of nutrients during the deprivation period. The process liberates urea and increases the renal pool of glucose, ketones, and urea to be excreted. Urea and glucose act synergistically as osmotic diuretics, and urine volume is sharply increased.

Acceleration of fatty acid metabolism consequent to insulin deprivation produces high levels of acidic products, and the normal carbonic acid–bicarbonate ratio moves from the 1:20 relationship of physiologic equilibrium. Protracted acid-base shift disrupts vital organ function. The immediate problem manifest with imbalance is depression of cerebral activity that proceeds to coma when the acidotic state persists.

Increased acidotic products provide the hydrogen ion stimulus to medullary centers that increases the depth and rate of respirations (hyperpnea). The body attempts to remove excess carbon dioxide to reinstitute the carbonic acid–bicarbonate ratio. The composite picture of acute hyperglycemia, or insulin deprivation, includes pruritus, polyuria, polydipsia, and polyphagia, as well as tissue dehydration, progressive weakness and lethargy, depression of mental processes, and deep forceful respirations. The slowly progressing sequence known as diabetic acidosis also includes nausea, vomiting, abdominal pain, and an acetone or nail polish remover–like odor to the patient's breath. Blood tests reveal hyperglycemia, and urine tests indicate the presence of acetones and glucose.

Continued burning of the alternate fuel (fatty acids) rather than the primary fuel (glucose) perpetuates the acidotic state. Reversal of the entity is a complex process requiring administration of insulin to institute utilization of circulating glucose for cellular metabolic activity and concurrent measures to correct the acid-base imbalance. The physiologic status of the patient at the time of therapy determines whether the process can be halted by parenteral administration of insulin without additional measures.

The critical status of a patient with diabetes mellitus who is in coma at the time of therapy requires intensive status-monitored replacement therapy. Initial administration of fluids and insulin replaces lost extracellular water and electrolytes and provides the hormone necessary to move blood glucose into the cells. Acid-base ratios are modified by administration of sodium bicarbonate or sodium lactate formulations. The intravenous solutions replace deficient base and accelerate the removal of hydrogen ions. Monitoring of blood sugar levels provides the clues necessary to determine when available blood glucose has been depleted, and additional insulin or glucose may be required for progression toward equilibrium. Excretion or storage of the free fatty acids and lipids (triglycerides, cholesterol, phospholipids) that flood the bloodstream in the absence of insulin is fraught with problems of warring factions resisting or competing for supremacy. Fatty acids interfere with glucose metabolism, and while they are in plentiful supply the battle rages. Gradual decrease in ketones in the blood and urine provides evidence that equilibrium has been reached.

Frequent recurrent acidotic states are incompatible with cellular life, and the patient with diabetes mellitus is instructed about physiologic changes that provide early warning signs. Administration of insulin when polydipsia, unsteadiness, and weakness are accompanied by positive urine acetone and glucose tests may allow the patient lifelong ignorance of the realities of *diabetic acidosis.*

Insulin excess

Glucose assimilation requires insulin for transport into cells. Excess insulin may rapidly move all available blood sugar into muscle and adipose tissue and leave the blood without reserves to supply glucose for on-going needs of cells (Fig. 25-1). Once sequestered in muscle, mobilization of the stored glycogen requires additional insulin. Hypoglycemia provides the stimulus for protective physiologic processes

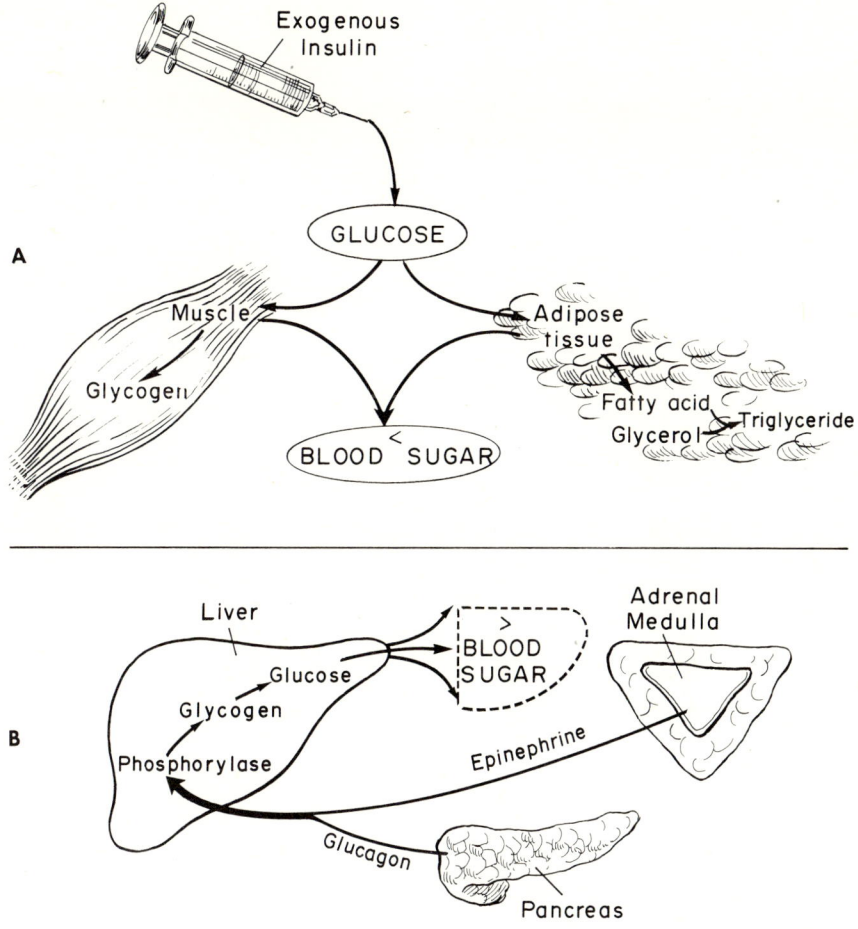

Fig. 25-1. A, Administration of insulin stimulates rapid movement of glucose into muscle and adipose tissue. **B,** Hypoglycemia stimulates epinephrine and glucagon release. The hormones act to convert glycogen to glucose. Depletion of glycogen stores halts the compensatory process.

that interact to provide a temporary increase in blood sugar. Hypoglycemic levels in tissues bathing the alpha cells of the pancreas liberate the hormone glucagon, which has an ability to liberate glucose from the storage sites in hepatic tissue. Concurrent hypoglycemia-induced excitation of the sympathetic nervous system centers in the hypothalamus stimulates release of adrenal catecholamines. Epinephrine and glucagon act synergistically to stimulate hepatic glycogenolysis. The hormones increase the activity of *phosphorylase* necessary to enzymatic degradation of glycogen to glucose and phosphate (Fig. 25-1, *B*). The process provides a temporary rise in blood sugar. Depletion of hepatic glycogen stores slows the process, although glucagon may continue to provide some glucose by stimulating glyconeogenesis in hepatic tissues. Commercial preparations of glucagon are available to assist in termination of hypoglycemia.

The physiologic struggle to provide glucose to meet metabolic needs is manifest in behavioral and functional changes. Initially cerebral glucose deprivation produces irritability or mental confusion that rapidly proceeds to more devastating problems (disorientation, convulsions, unconsciousness). Peripheral norepinephrine and epinephrine activity contribute to anxiety, tremor, tachycardia, and weakness. Constriction of superficial vessels cools the skin surface. Absence of tissue heat for evaporation of metabolically produced surface water causes the skin to be cold and covered with moisture. The patient is pale, sweating, and trembling. Headache and hunger also are attributable to the physiologic events (nutrient deprivation and hormone activity).

Ingestion of glucose supplies the material to reverse the physiologic changes occurring with insulin excess. Patients with diabetes mellitus are instructed to carry a glucose supply in purse or pocket for use when hypoglycemia results from insulin excess. A packet of sugar, glass of orange juice, or candy source adequately supplies the emergency needs of the patient. The patient's blood and urine are sugar free when excess insulin is present. Intravenous replacement of glucose is necessary in the acute state of insulin excess. Administration is titrated with blood and urine glucose content to avoid hyperglycemia.

The chief differentiating factor between the outcome of the two entities (insulin deficiency and insulin excess) is the response of brain tissue. Insulin deficiency is accompanied by high blood sugar levels, and physiologic changes progress slowly to the acidotic state. During diabetic acidosis the brain is irritated by acid products, but it is supplied with glucose to meet neuronal needs. Insulin excess removes sugar from the bloodstream, and the brain is deprived of the continual supply of glucose necessary to neuronal activity. Short periods of deprivation may cause death of neurons in the brain tissue.

Table 25-1. Dosage range of oral hypoglycemic drugs

Nonproprietary name	Proprietary (trade) name	Daily adult dosage range (oral)
Acetohexamide	Dymelor	0.25-1.5 Gm.
Chlorpropamide	Diabinese	0.1-0.75 Gm.
Phenformin hydrochloride	DBI	0.025-0.4 Gm. ($\div$3-4)
Tolazamide	Tolinase	0.1-1 Gm. ($\div$2)
Tolbutamide	Orinase	0.5-3 Gm. ($\div$1-3)

Pharmacodynamics

Endogenous insulin for nutrient utilization may be deficient or absent in the individual with diabetes mellitus. Replacement of deficiency is individualized to provide each patient with insulin supplies that meet his needs. Interrelationships between hormonal status, growth rate, activity levels, body weight, and age at the time of onset are some of the factors that affect the individualized plan.

Absence of functioning pancreatic beta cells necessitates exogenous replacement of insulin. Individuals whose insulin production is deficient but whose pancreatic beta cells are capable of producing insulin may be placed on a therapeutic plan using oral hypoglycemics.

Oral hypoglycemic drugs. Acetohexamide, chlorpropamide, tolazamide, and tolbutamide (Table 25-1) act pharmacodynamically to stimulate pancreatic beta cell production of insulin. Oral hypoglycemic drugs are used only for adults with residual pancreatic function. The mode of action is considered to be direct cell stimulation, with some increase in beta cell response to elevated blood glucose levels. The drugs are classified pharmacologically as *sulfonylureas,* and they are *sulfonamide derivatives.* The drugs are dependent on residual pancreatic islet function and are employed most often for individuals with maturity-onset diabetes.

Prescription of the particular hypoglycemic drug is dependent on remaining islet cell function, and dosage is balanced with activity, diet, and endogenous insulin production. Chlorpropamide provides a long period of hypoglycemic action (up to 36 hours). The duration of action of other hypoglycemic drugs varies: acetohexamide, 12 to 24 hours; tolbutamide, 6 to 12 hours; and tolazamide, 4 to 6 hours.

Phenformin hydrochloride (Table 25-1) acts pharmacodynamically to increase utilization of glucose at the cellular level. Its action is dependent on availability of insulin in circulating fluids, and it may be used in combination with insulin injections. Performin hydrochloride seems to facilitate entrance of glucose into anaerobic pathways that produce pyruvate and lactate, but it may also decrease the resistance of an insulin antagonist at cellular membranes.

Pharmacodynamic action begins in 1 to 2 hours and lasts up to 9 hours.

Oral hypoglycemic drugs may be used after initial diagnosis of diabetes mellitus, or the patient may be transferred to oral agents after a period of exogenous insulin therapy. During conversion from insulin to oral agents the patient is observed carefully for evidence of hyperglycemia. Urine testing for glycosuria and acetones is done three times a day during the first week or until oral agent effect is established. Patient participation in the urine testing plan allows an opportunity to practice a skill that he needs throughout his lifetime. Oral hypoglycemic agents control diabetes in patients with residual pancreatic function or cellular block to glucose transport, but they are not curative. Infection, long periods of stress, or surgery disrupt established equilibrium by precipitation of endogenous glycogenolysis or gluconeogenesis. It may be necessary to use parenteral insulin to control hyperglycemia and maintain balance. Patients using oral hypoglycemics are instructed in the technique of insulin administration to enable them to meet emergency needs for insulin.

Patients taking the oral hypoglycemic agents over long periods of time seem to have minimal problems with adverse reactions to the drugs. Periodic evaluation is necessary to assure maintenance of the therapeutic plan and to determine drug effect. Some individuals have problems with gastrointestinal disturbances that can be modified by dividing the dosage to allow smaller amounts of the drug to be taken at regularly scheduled intervals throughout the day.

Some hypersensitivity reactions occur during therapy, and the sulfonylurea group occasionally causes skin eruptions. The patient is asked to consult with the physician if skin rash, jaundice, or persistent pruritus appear at any time during therapy.

Hypoglycemia may occur as an extension of the pharmacodynamic effect of the drug; therefore patients are asked to carry a supply of a simple sugar in purse or pocket. Alcohol intolerance that occurs in some patients is accompanied by tachycardia and decrease in blood pressure. The individual appears to be in an advanced state of drunkenness with minimal alcohol ingestion. Tolbutamide and its derivatives frequently cause intolerance to alcohol.

A metallic or bitter taste in the mouth occurs with use of phenformin hydrochloride. The diversity of annoying problems (headache, weakness, paresthesias) that may occur during therapy are brought to the physician's attention, since individual reactions to the oral hypoglycemic agents vary, and another agent may be prescribed. The total pharmacotherapeutic regimen is planned carefully by the physician because many drugs interfere with the effectiveness of the oral hypoglycemic agents. For example, thiazides (i.e., some diuretics) and corticosteroids interfere with the hypoglycemic activity of the oral drugs, and higher hypoglycemic drug dosage may be necessary when the drugs are used concurrently. Sulfaphenazole, phenylbutazone, and monoamine oxidase inhibitors potentiate the hypoglycemic activity of the drugs. The extensive number of drugs affecting oral hypoglycemic drug action makes it important for the patient always to inform any physician prescribing drugs for his care that he is taking an oral hypoglycemic agent.

Insulin (exogenous). Insulin preparations for parenteral administration are comparable to the hormonal agents found in the human body, but the drug substitutes are obtained from animal sources. The variations in insulin preparations consist of additives that affect the rate of absorption. Longer-acting derivatives require less frequent administration, and they are the forms of choice as primary therapy for patients whose hyperglycemic state can be controlled with their use. When individuals require concurrent use of short-acting forms to maintain blood glucose control, the drugs are employed if urine testing shows glycosuria or acetone bodies.

The varying times of onset, peak effect, and duration of action of the insulin preparations provide active hormone during the peak activity and food ingestion times of the individual. The activity of injected amorphous insulin is shown in Fig. 25-2 (top). Impurities affect the dependability of amorphous insulin action;

276 Drugs used to control anabolic-catabolic balance

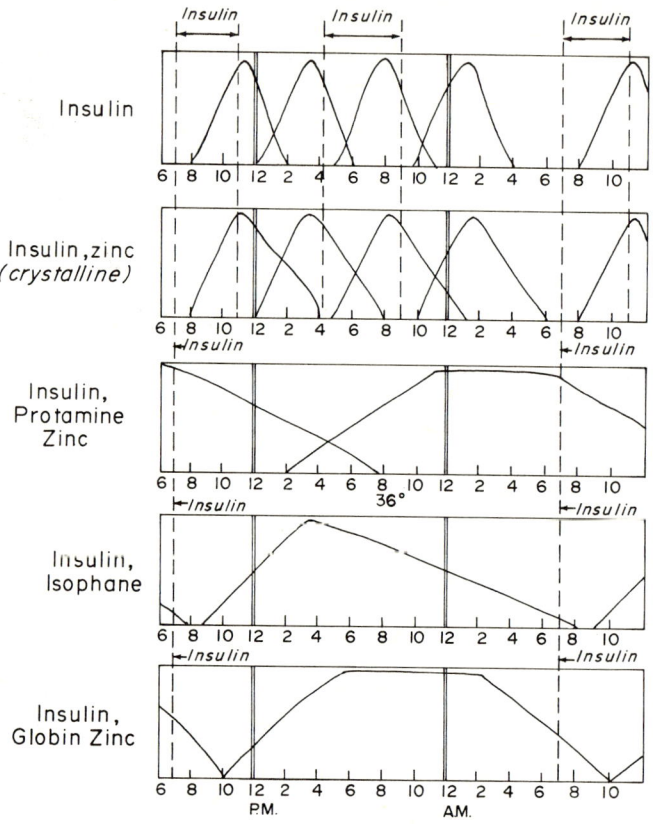

Fig. 25-2. Comparison of the onset, peak, and duration of action of insulin preparations, using the sample time of 6 o'clock in the morning for administration. Readministration of exogenous insulin is indicated when the peak of action declines.

therefore a rapid-acting insulin with a short pharmacodynamic effect is manufactured by precipitating insulin in the presence of zinc crystals. The crystalline zinc insulin (Fig. 25-2), or insulin injection (Regular Iletin), becomes available to facilitate cellular transport of nutrients about an hour after administration. The administration of insulin injection at 8 o'clock in the morning provides peak action 3 hours later. Administration $1/2$ to 1 hour before breakfast assures available insulin in the period after digestion, when blood sugar levels are elevated. The 6- to 8-hour duration of pharmacodynamic action necessitates readministration during the early afternoon.

Insulin injection provides the rapid action necessary when the patient has a hyperglycemic reaction, and injections are planned according to the blood sugar levels of the patient. Insulin is needed to control diabetic acidosis, and insulin injection is the only form that can be administered intravenously. Administration is titrated with blood sugar levels, and injections are continued until the blood sugar returns to the normal range.

Insulin injection is used most frequently for short-term control of blood sugar levels, and it may be given for interim control when the patient is receiving a longer-acting insulin preparation. Urine tests provide guides to the amount of sugar or acetone being excreted in the urine, and insulin injection may be prescribed to be administered on a sliding scale according to test results before meals or before retiring. For example:

Glycosuria test	Insulin injection
4+	12 units
3+	8 units
2+	4 units
1+	0 units

The prescription often includes directions for use of insulin injection according to the amount of acetone in the urine (i.e., "moderate to large acetone, add 4 units").

Protamine zinc insulin suspension (protamine, zinc, and Iletin) (Fig. 25-2) has a duration of action lasting 30 to 36 hours. Administration of the drug at 2 o'clock in the afternoon would provide pharmacodynamic control of hyperglycemia for the individual who works during the night hours. However, the nighttime plateau of action would cause the sleeping patient to waken with sweating and chills and gradually progressing signs of insulin excess. Insulin peak usually is planned to correlate with eating patterns, but the drug may be administered an hour before retiring to control hyperglycemia in patients with a high blood sugar in the morning, even though urinalysis before going to bed is negative.

Isophane insulin suspension (NPH Iletin) (Fig. 25-2) is available for mobilization of nutrients within 2 hours after administration. Administration of the drug at 8 o'clock in the morning provides daylong mealtime insulin, and drug action reaches its peak in approximately 8 hours. Insulin is available throughout the 24-hour period, with minimal levels as the morning administration time arrives.

Globin zinc insulin injection (Fig. 25-2) is available to reduce hyperglycemia by movement of nutrients into cells within 2 to 4 hours after administration. The illustrated action peak occurring between 6 P.M. and 2 A.M. would seem an ideal plan for the individual whose work obligations are heaviest in the evening hours. Insulin would be available for utilization of nutrients from an evening meal and for the snack after work. Initial administration schedule can be planned to allow the long period of maximum effect to meet the individual's needs.

Insulin products prepared by addition of zinc in acetate (Lente insulins) are also used for fast, intermediate, or long action. Prompt insulin zinc suspension (Semilente) action onset time is $1/2$ to 1 hour, and the pharmacodynamic effect lasts 12 to 16 hours. Insulin zinc suspension (Lente) action onset time is 1 to 4 hours, and the pharmacodynamic effect lasts 24 to 30 hours. Extended insulin zinc suspension (Ultralente) action onset time is 4 to 8 hours, and the pharmacodynamic effect lasts 34 to 46 hours. The chief advantage offered by Lente insulins is that they are mutually miscible; therefore they can be administered in various proportions in the same syringe without loss of potency.

Fig. 25-2 provides a base for viewing the living patterns of individuals in relation to the types of insulin prescribed for control of diabetes. Knowledge of the time of administration provides the information necessary to predicting the time when food should be available. Administration time and duration of effect are also important factors in control of adverse effects. For example, the long duration of action of protamine zinc insulin suspension (36 hours) may cause recurrent hypoglycemia. Sugar, orange juice, or a candy bar may control the immediate problem, but the long action peak of the drug may cause recurrence of hypoglycemia unless a longer-acting carbohydrate (i.e., bread, crackers) is eaten.

In the past carbohydrate intake was severely restricted so that insulin dosage could be kept at a minimum. The practice left a narrow margin before the body began to mobilize fats to meet nutrient needs. Currently there is considerable liberty allowed in carbohydrate content of the diabetic diet. The patient is expected to distribute the foods between meals and snacks, with consideration of action periods of the prescribed insulin.

The chief problems occurring during therapy with insulin are those described earlier as related to insulin deficiency and insulin excess. Self-therapy is gradually extended to allow the individual with diabetes mellitus to suit insulin dosage to physiologic demand. The patient must understand the entire plan of therapy, for he is primarily responsible for the long-term management of the regimen.

Patient care

Effective treatment of diabetes mellitus is dependent on the patient's willingness to follow the prescribed regimen; therefore all who participate in care of the patient during the period of intensive supervision have an obligation to involve him in the program. He must be oriented to the course that can be followed to reach the goal of optimum health, and he must understand the implications of deviation

278 Drugs used to control anabolic-catabolic balance

from the course of action. The guided learning experiences the patient has during this period will help him to realize his potential and move toward independence within the limits set by his disease.

After the initial period of supervision, the patient begins to utilize his new learning as he resumes his place in society. The mental and physical health of the individual is dependent on the successes and failures he has during the early phases of the learning process.

To the diabetic, the road he must follow to attain optimum health is precipitous, and the usual challenge of goal-directed learning is obscured by a period of grief. This is a natural reaction to the knowledge that he has a chronic health problem which will affect his life circumstantially and psychologically in varied ways. This is a crucial period for the diabetic, and whether he is "floored" by the diagnosis or adjusts to it depends on the help he receives.

The patient's anxiety about change in his life habits may interfere with his ability to participate in efforts to teach him about aspects of his care. The direction the teaching program must take is indicated by the problem that is the center of his attention.

The major problem the diabetic faces is deprivation of food. Food exchanges are an enigma to him, but with guidance in selection of meals he will begin to realize that even his idiosyncrasies in relation to foods can be accommodated.

The satisfactions the patient derives from participation in the teaching program are necessary components of the learning process. If the patient is allowed independence while being guided, his persistence in following the therapeutic regimen will be increased. Early in-

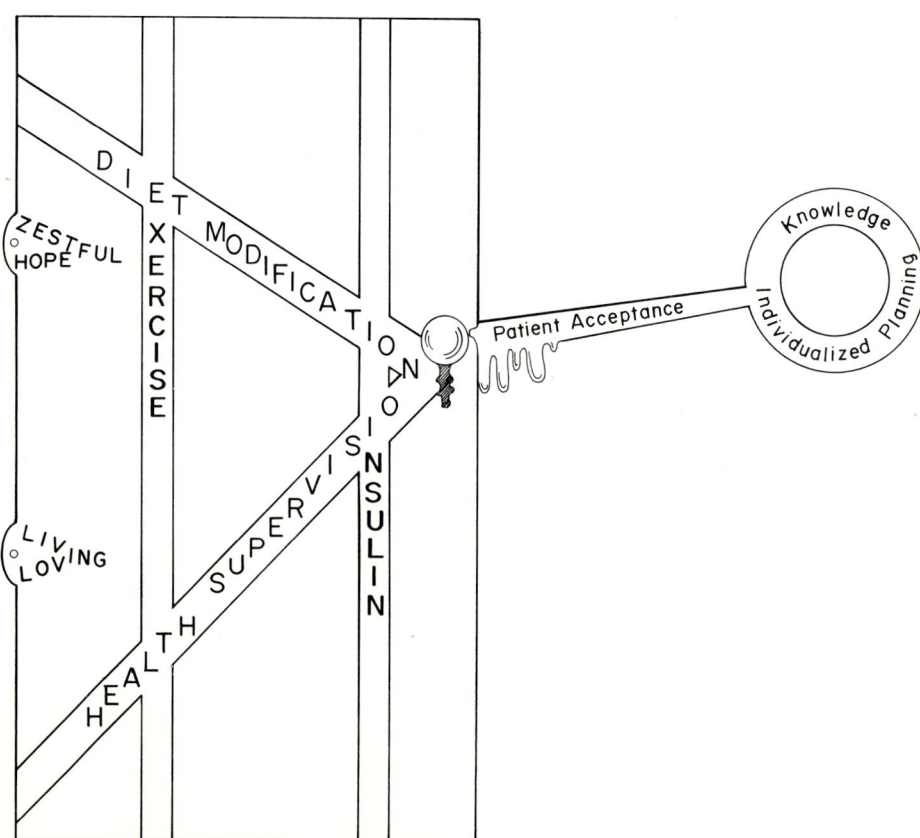

Fig. 25-3. Factors affecting the living pattern of the individual with diabetes mellitus.

itiation of the involvement of the patient allows opportunity for reinforcement of learning.

Opportunity must be provided for progressive movement toward an ability to administer insulin. Until the patient actually injects the insulin himself, he cannot safely be released from supervised care. Alternatives exist when the patient is unable to assume responsibility for injection of insulin. A family member can be taught to administer insulin, or a visiting nurse can be asked to follow initial teaching until the patient can function independently.

The institution of standardized concentrations of insulin in 1973 was a major advance in simplification of dosage calculations. Fast, intermediate, and long-acting insulins are available in standard forms containing 100 units/ml. Syringes employed for administration are calibrated to facilitate preparation of the prescribed dosage of 100 unit/ml. insulin.

The patient seeks treatment initially because some of the distressing problems related to loss of natural equilibrium are interfering with living patterns. Guiding him toward understanding of the measures utilized for restoration of equilibrium helps him to establish goals and purposes that make sense and therefore constitute motivational forces.

The goal of therapy is to help the patient continue an optimistic, forward-looking approach to life. Health team members working together can help the patient accept and understand the interrelated plan for diet modification, health supervision, exercise, and insulin control necessary to a healthful life (Fig. 25-3).

REFERENCES

Anthony, Catherine Parker, and Kolthoff, Norma Jane: Textbook of anatomy and physiology, ed. 8, St. Louis, 1971, The C. V. Mosby Co.

Arky, Ronald A., and Knopp, Robert H.: Current concepts: evaluation of islet-cell function in man, The New England Journal of Medicine **285**:1130, 1971.

Goodman, Louis S., and Gilman, Arthur, editors: The pharmacological basis of therapeutics, ed. 4, New York, 1970, The Macmillan Co.

Hornback, May: Diabetes mellitus: the nurse's role, Nursing Clinics of North America **5**:3, 1970.

Huang, Sheila H.: Nursing assessment in planning care for a diabetic patient, Nursing Clinics of North America **6**:135, 1971.

Levin, Marvin E.: Endocrine syndromes associated with pancreatic islet cell tumors, Medical Clinics of North America **52**:295, 1968.

Moore, Mary Lou: Diabetes in children, American Journal of Nursing **67**:104, 1967.

Mountcastle, Vernon B., editor: Medical physiology, ed. 13, vol. 1, St. Louis, 1974, The C. V. Mosby Co.

Muller, Walter A., Faloona, Gerald R., and Unger, Roger H.: Influence of the antecedent diet upon glucagon and insulin secretion, The New England Journal of Medicine **285**:1450, 1971.

Orten, James M., and Neuhaus, Otto W.: Biochemistry ed. 8, St. Louis, 1970, The C. V. Mosby Co.

Pastan, Ira: Cyclic AMP, Scientific American **227**:97, Aug., 1972.

Reilly, Mary Jo, editor: American hospital formulary service, vol. 2, sect. 68:00, Washington, D. C., 1973, American Society of Hospital Pharmacists.

Soeldner, J. Stuart, and Steinke, Jurgen: Insulin resistance, Medical Clinics of North America **49**:939, 1965.

Watkins, Julia D., and Moss, Fay T.: Confusion in the management of diabetes, American Journal of Nursing **69**:521, 1969.

Williams, Sue Rodwell: Nutrition and diet therapy, ed. 2, St. Louis, 1973, The C. V. Mosby Co.

Zitnik, Ruth: First, you take a grapefruit, American Journal of Nursing **68**:1285, 1968.

UNIT SIX
DRUGS USED TO CONTROL REPRODUCTION AND FERTILITY

26 Cell proliferation

27 Gonadal function and fertility

26

Cell proliferation

Pharmacodynamics
Patient care

Cancer is a descriptive term designating an uncontrolled proliferation of abnormal cells. Tissues constructed by cancer cells are poorly differentiated and unable to carry on the physiologic functions of the tissues from which they originate. The invasive malignant tissues obstruct physiologic processes and compete with normal tissues for nutrients. The high anabolic activity of cancer cells necessitates accelerated utilization of nucleic acids, and so the cells pilfer their supplies from body stores. Normal cells are deprived of the materials necessary for deoxyribonucleic acid (DNA) and ribonucleic acid (RNA) synthesis of proteins and enzymes (Fig. 26-1). Since man has no physiologic mechanism to protect him against the invasion of the disruptive, nutrient-demanding tissues, the competition for nutrients gradually decreases the growth rate of normal tissues.

The characteristic rapid reproduction patterns of cancer cells begin with mutations in the genetic system of a cell nucleus and reproduction of the mutant. Studies of tissues obtained from animal and human cancer sites indicate that the initial disruptor is a virus. Conditions that predispose the cell to viral invasion are still unclear. Recent research reports indicate that cells produce antibodies for the antigenic neoplastic tissue components during various stages of cancer tissue growth. The antigen-antibody

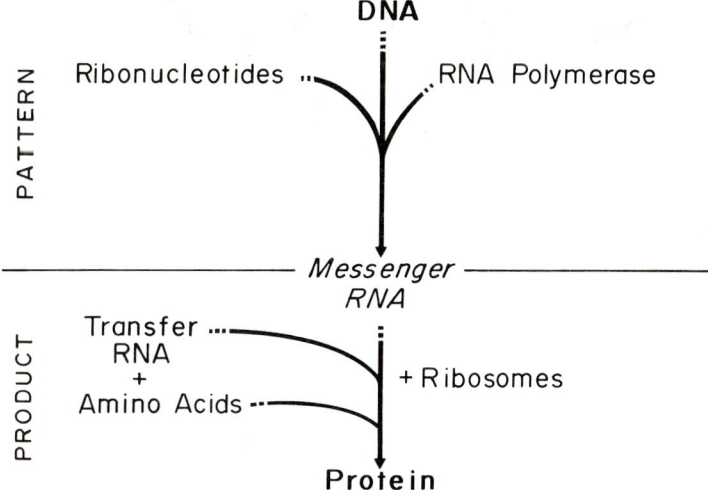

Fig. 26-1. Schematic diagram of factors involved in protein synthesis. Deoxyribonucleic acid (DNA) provides the pattern for ribonucleic acid (RNA) production. DNA-polymerase interaction leads to synthesis of messenger-RNA (mRNA). Ribosomes, amino acids, and transfer-RNA interact with mRNA in the synthesis of new protein.

sequence is a stimulus-response phenomenon and seems to have no direct effect on the progression of cancer tissue growth.

The potential for emergence of mutants exists in all body tissues, but the highest incidence is in those tissues with a rapid turnover rate. There is a direct relationship between the occurrence of mutants and the high metabolic and mitotic activity of *reticuloendothelial, intestinal, gonadal,* and *epidermal tissues.* Leukemia is an example of abnormal cell proliferation originating in the rapidly reproducing cells of the bone marrow and lymphatic tissue. In older age groups there is a high incidence of cancer of the intestines, breast, genitalia, and skin. It is possible that the aging process contributes to the emergence of mutants by changing the DNA or RNA pattern for assembly of protein building materials.

Pharmacodynamics

Studies of man's biochemical processes have led to discovery of drugs that by biologic variation or biologic antagonism exploit the differences in characteristics between cancer and normal cells. One agent, or a combination of agents, may be used in an effort to destroy the malignant tissue and to increase the specificity of action in particular tissue. Drug combinations or alternation of drugs decreases drug tolerance.

Hormones. Sex hormones have a high level specificity for gonadal sites. Administration of opposite-sex hormones causes regression of malignancies originating in the reproductive organs. Changing the hormonal balance of the patient removes the normal hormonal stimulus to growth from the affected sex organs. In the male patient with prostatic cancer, changing the hormonal balance by administering female sex hormones causes regression and shrinking of the prostatic tumor and its metastatic extensions. Castration or adrenalectomy may be required to decrease sources of androgens.

Differences in the normal hormonal balance in premenopausal and postmenopausal women influence the selection of sex hormones for treatment of malignancies of the female reproductive organs (i.e., breast cancer). The natural hormonal status in the premenopausal woman is estrogenic, and so androgens are administered to effect opposite-sex hormone regression of cancer tissue. Further depression of estrogen sources is accomplished by removal of the ovaries. Treatment aimed at changing the hormonal balance of patients who are five years postmenopause necessitates administration of estrogens because the hormonal dominance in these individuals is androgenic.

Specific problems of fertility and climacteric control for which androgens, estrogens, and progestins are used are presented in Chapter 27. The major problem for the patient receiving the large doses of sex hormones necessary to treat malignancy is the emergence of secondary characteristics of the opposite sex. Male patients develop gynecomastia, a high-pitched voice, and atrophy of the genitalia. The one problem that male patients tolerate well is the loss of beard, which decreases the need to shave daily.

Premenopausal female patients face the problem of masculinization when male hormones are administered. Typical androgenic effects include growth of facial hair, deepening of the voice, oiliness of the skin, and increased libido. With estrogen therapy, postmenopausal women may enjoy return of some of the female hormone–induced changes, with the possible exception of periodic vaginal bleeding (pseudomenstruation).

Each group of patients need assistance in accepting the change in sex characteristics. It is important for them to view the changes as directly related to the therapeutic regimen, rather than as changes in themselves.

Antineoplastic drugs. Antineoplastic drugs, with the exception of sex hormones, are used in the treatment of patients with widely disseminated cancer or with multiple metastatic lesions. Cancer that involves the blood cells or the lymphatic tissues spreads the targets so widely throughout the body that systemic drug administration is necessary to destroy the malignant tissue (Fig. 26-2). The drugs may be used alone or as adjuvants to irradiation or surgery.

A major problem in antineoplastic therapy is that normal cells, during the fragile stages of division, are also vulnerable to destruction by

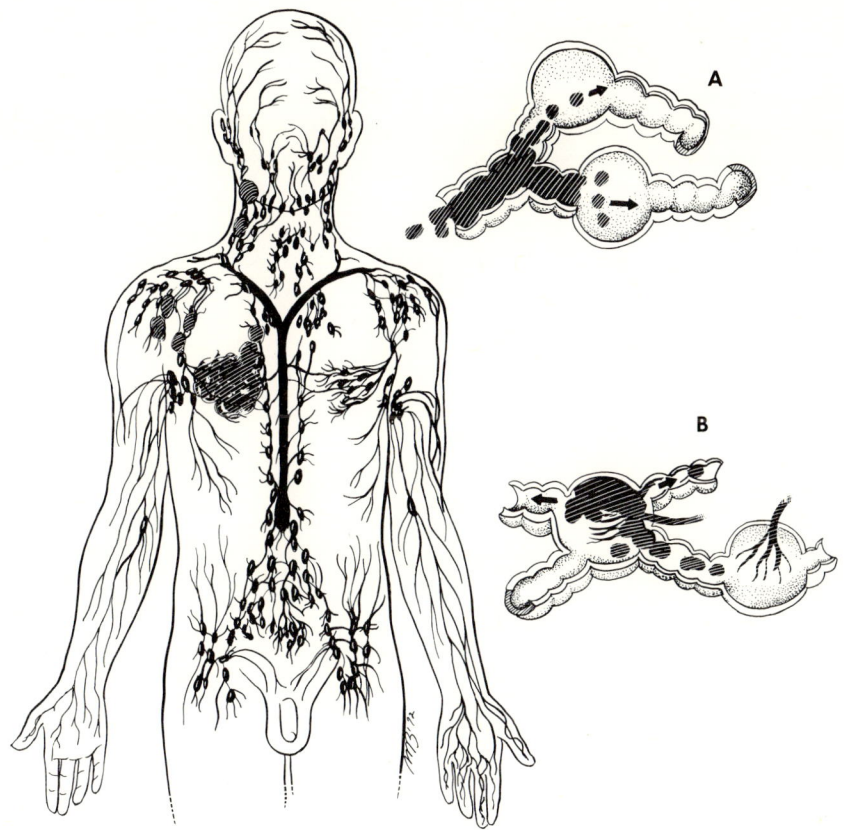

Fig. 26-2. Lymphatic vessels provide routes for extension of cancer tissue. Cancer cells (i.e., from a cancer site on the right chest wall) move into the vessels. **A,** Cancer cells move through the vessels toward the lymph nodes. **B,** Small emboli from the cancer tissue move through the lymph nodes and find easy access into distal vessels.

cytotoxic drugs. Disruption of function is predictable in organs in which metabolic activity is high. Tissues most readily affected are the gastrointestinal epithelia and reticuloendothelial tissue. The vulnerability of the gastrointestinal tissue is related to its high mitotic activity in replacing worn cells every 1 to 8 days along the entire tract. The short life-span of platelets and leukocytes (8 to 12 days) necessitates continual activity in the blood-forming organs to produce cells for physiologic processes. Although there is variation within each of the drug groups used, it is predictable that vital body processes will be suppressed by drugs whose action is to interfere with reproduction in all rapidly proliferating cells.

The potential for suppression of body processes presents problems during drug therapy, but it is also the rationale for use of the antineoplastic drugs. For example, in leukemia the malignant white blood cells crowd out other blood elements, and their destruction is necessary for survival of the patient. Antineoplastic drugs are used in an intensive effort to suppress white blood cell proliferation. The initial drop in leukocyte counts is therapeutic for the patient. When a patient who is receiving the drugs for metastatic lesions in intestinal nodes has a depression of the white cell or platelet (thrombocyte) count, it is an ominous sign. It is probable that the drug regimen will be interrupted to provide a rest period to allow blood cells time for regeneration. Periodic rest periods capitalize on the low capacity of malignant cells for repair. Correlated with the drop in blood cell counts in the foregoing situations is a change in bleeding problems. The patient with leukemia will probably have a decrease in bleeding epi-

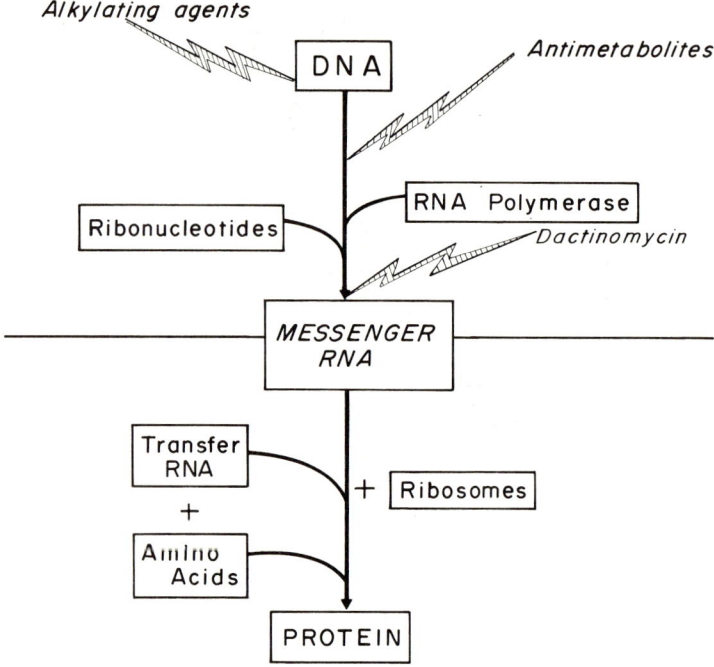

Fig. 26-3. Antineoplastic agents interrupt the DNA-RNA protein synthesis pattern. Alkylating agents interfere with the formation of DNA. Antimetabolites and dactinomycin interfere with the synthesis of messenger RNA.

sodes. The patient with intestinal cancer will be observed carefully for petechiae and evidence of internal bleeding until his platelet count returns to a normal level.

There is some specificity in drugs used systemically to destroy cancer tissue. The decision to prescribe a particular drug is made by the physician on the basis of best evidence obtained from carefully controlled clinical trials, as well as from his experience with particular drugs. The major problem with drugs specifically selected for a specific type of tissue is the potential for disruption of function in adjacent normal tissues. For example, a patient receiving a neoplastic drug for metastatic lesions in the intestinal nodes may have esophageal ulcerations due to the effect of the drug on epithelial tissue. Because all the drugs are cytotoxic, the drug regimen requires careful titration of dosage with the response of the patient. The margin between therapeutic dose and toxic dose (therapeutic index) is very narrow. Astute observation of the patient is necessary to provide maximum drug effect while protecting the patient from the toxic manifestations of therapy.

Drugs specifically used for their antineoplastic activity interfere with the production of cancer cells by interrupting the synthesis of proteins (Fig. 26-3). The drugs most frequently used for treatment of cancer are classified as antimetabolites and alkylating agents.

Antimetabolites. Drugs that are classified as antimetabolites act as antagonists to nucleic acid production by providing an abundant supply of an analog or close relative for a component necessary to DNA or RNA production. The cell is tricked into picking up the replacement analog in the race to meet building needs. The drug substitution is effective because of close similarity to normal cellular *purines, pyrimidines, vitamins,* and *amino acids.* The drugs prevent cancer cell development by breaking the genetic code for synthesis of proteins.

There are several analogs used clinically to mimic the natural purines and pyrimidines utilized by the cell for nucleic acid synthesis. Nu-

Cell proliferation 287

Table 26-1. Dosage range of antineoplastic agents

Nonproprietary name	Proprietary (trade) name	Daily adult dosage range	Nonproprietary name	Proprietary (trade) name	Daily adult dosage range
L-Asparaginase		I.V.: 200-1000 U./kg.	Mercaptopurine*	Purinethol	Oral: 2.5-5 mg./kg.
Azathioprine*	Imuran	Oral: 1-5 mg./kg.	Methotrexate*		Oral: 2.5-5 mg.
Busulfan†	Myleran	Oral: 2-6 mg.	Mithramycin‡	Mithracin	I.V.: 0.025-0.03 mg./kg.
Chlorambucil†	Leukeran	Oral: 0.1-0.2 mg./kg.	Mitotane	Lysodren	Oral: 2-16 Gm.
Cyclophosphamide†	Cytoxan, Endoxan	Oral: 1-5 mg./kg. I.V.: 3.5-5 mg./kg.	Pipobroman†	Vercyte	Oral: 0.1-3 mg./kg.
Cytarabine*	Cytosar	I.V.: 1-2 mg./kg. S.C.: 1-3 mg./kg.	Procarbazine hydrochloride	Matulane	Oral: 50-300 mg.
			Sodium iodide(I^{131})§	Iodotope, Oriodide, Theriodide	Oral: 30-200 mCi. I.V.: Same
Dactinomycin‡	Cosmegen	I.V.: 0.01 mg./kg.	Sodium phosphate (P^{32})§	Phosphotope	Oral: 0.04 mCi./kg. I.V.: Same
Daunomycin‡		I.V.: 1 mg./kg.	Thioguanine*		Oral: 2-3 mg./kg.
Floxuridine*	FUDR	I.V.: 0.5-1 mg./kg.	Thio-tepa†	Thio-TEPA	Oral: 5-10 mg. I.V.: 0.2 mg./kg.
Fluorouracil*		Oral: 3-15 mg./kg. I.V.: Same			
Gold(Au^{198})injection§	Aurcoloid, Auroscan, Aureotope	I.M.: 35-150 mCi.	Triethylenemelamine†		Oral: 2.5-5 mg. twice weekly
Hydroxyurea*	Hydrea	Oral: 20-30 mg./kg.	Uracil mustard†		Oral: 1-5 mg.
Mechlorethamine hydrochloride (nitrogen mustard)†	Caryolysine, Mustargen	Oral: 3 mg./kg. I.V.: 0.1-0.4 mg./kg.	Vinblastine sulfate‖	Velban	I.V.: 0.1-0.6 mg./kg.
			Vincristine sulfate‖	Oncovin	I.V.: 0.015-0.05 mg./kg. weekly
Melphalan†	Alkeran	Oral: 0.05-0.15 mg./kg.			

*Antimetabolite.
†Alkylating agent.
‡Antibiotic.
§Radioactive agent.
‖Plant alkaloid.

cleotides or letters of the genetic code combine to form organic bases in constructing DNA and RNA:

	PURINES	PYRIMIDIES
Deoxyribonucleic acid (DNA)	{ Guanine ← → Cytosine { Adenine ← → Thymine	
Ribonucleic acid (RNA)	{ Guanine ← → Cytosine { Adenine ← → Uracil	

Analogs of nucleotides necessary to both DNA and RNA synthesis will interrupt protein synthesis at more than one site in the DNA-RNA sequence.

Purine antagonists. Purine antagonists, acting as chemical analogs of the physiologic purines, inhibit utilization of the organic bases in the cell. Mercaptopurine (adenine analog) and thioguanine (guanine analog) are the primary representatives of the group of purine antagonists.

Azathioprine (adenine analog), in addition to purine antagonism, acts as an enzyme inhibitor by binding sulfhydryl groups. The combination of actions makes it useful as an immunosuppressive agent, and it is considered less effective as an antineoplastic agent than other members of the group. Each of the drugs is partially detoxified in the liver and excreted chiefly by the kidneys. Some of the drug products appear in the feces.

Pyrimidine antagonists. Exploitation of cellular need for pyrimidines in construction of long-chain nucleic acids has led to the development of pyrimidine antagonists. Fluorouracil and floxuridine (which is metabolized to fluorouracil in the body) are analogs of both thymine and uracil. Initially fluorouracil was administered only by intravenous infusion, but more recent clinical use has included oral administration (Table 26-1). Oral use of the liquid utilizes the physiologic pyrimidine transport system in the small intestine to deliver the drug to cancer sites. Prune juice or ginger ale is employed as a vehicle for the oral liquid. It is possible that the glucose content in each of the vehicles facilitates the uptake of the drug. Degradation of the drugs takes place in the liver where carbon dioxide is removed by catabolic metabolism. Liberated carbon dioxide is eliminated by the lungs. The remaining unchanged drug or its urea products are eliminated in the urine.

Cytarabine (cytosine analog) is also a pyrimidine antagonist. It crosses the blood-brain barrier and attacks malignant tissue in the central nervous system. The drug is deaminated rapidly in the liver and kidneys, and it is excreted in the urine.

Hydroxyurea (thymine analog) is a urea derivative. The drug is metabolized in the liver and excreted primarily in the urine as urea. Liver degradation releases carbon dioxide, which is eliminated by the lungs.

Folic acid antagonists. Methotrexate is the only folic acid antagonist in general clinical use. It acts by preventing the formation of folic acid reductase, which is necessary for conversion of the metabolically inactive folic acid to tetrahydrofolic acid, which in turn is essential to DNA- and RNA-directed red blood cell construction.

Recently the Food and Drug Administration expanded use of the drug to include treatment of psoriasis. The release included a recommendation that liver biopsy be done before treatment. Liver function is important in detoxification of the drug. A high incidence of hepatotoxicity has been reported with the use of methotrexate.

Undesirable systemic effects of methotrexate during intrathecal or organ perfusion are modified by concurrent administration of a folic acid metabolite, calcium leucovorin. The vitamin is readily metabolized to the tetrahydrofolic derivative necessary to cell construction, thus protecting normal cells during methotrexate therapy.

Alkylating agents. Drugs classified as alkylating agents act by transferring their side chains (alkyl groups) to molecules within the cells and reacting selectively with the phosphate groups of DNA. Because they cause chromatin disruptive effects similar to those of x-rays, they are called radiomimetic compounds.

Mechlorethamine hydrochloride, or nitrogen mustard, is the prototype of drugs in the group. Stimulation of the vomiting centers by the drug makes persistent emesis a frustrating problem. Because it is a powerful central nervous system stimulant, ataxia and intermittent convulsions occur during therapy. The drug is very irritating to tissues and causes blistering and injury when it is spilled. During therapy, fluid intake must be high enough to assure elimination of the toxic metabolites from the bladder. Accumulation of the metabolites causes hemorrhagic cystitis.

Drugs that are related to mechlorethamine hydrochloride are chlorambucil, cyclophosphamide, melphalan, and uracil mustard. Cyclophosphamide and carmustine, a new drug being tested in clinical trials, cross the blood-brain barrier and attack central nervous system tumors. Each of the agents is used as an alternate to the prototype in an attempt to maintain the therapeutic regimen with minimal adverse effects.

Busulfan, pipobroman, thio-tepa, and triethylenemelamine are alkylating drugs with pharmacodynamic effects similar to those of nitrogen mustard. Minor differences exist between drugs in the group (that is, cyclophosphamide, thio-tepa, and triethylenemelamine do not have the irritant effect on tissues that nitrogen mustard has).

Each of the drugs is available for oral use (Table 26-1). Preparation of the patient for self-adminstration of antineoplastic drugs should include careful instructions related to use of the particular drug he will be taking. He must be cautioned to keep the cytotoxic agents out of the reach of children.

Antibiotics. The antibiotics prescribed for treatment of cancer are highly toxic agents unsuited for use in treatment of infections. They interfere with cell division by binding with DNA to slow production of RNA. Antibiotics currently in use for cancer therapy include dactinomycin, daunomycin, and mithramycin. All the drugs are administered parenterally (Table 26-1). Intravenous administration sites must be observed carefully because leaking causes severe irritation in local tissues.

Distribution of the antibiotic in body tissues varies with the particular drug. Dactinomycin is found in high concentrations in the kidney, liver, and spleen. Mithramycin is distributed in the Kupffer cells of the liver, in renal tubular cells, and along bone surfaces. All the drugs are excreted in bile and urine.

Daunorubicin, adriamycin, and bleomycin are antibiotics currently being evaluated in clinical trials. Each of the drugs is reported to have an adverse effect on heart or lung tissue. Therapeutic dosage levels and effective routes of adminstration are being studied.

Plant alkaloids. Vinblastine sulfate and vincristine sulfate are plant alkaloids used for treatment of cancer. Although there is some specificity in phase interference, the drugs act on dividing cells by disorganization of the mitotic spindle to prevent cellular reproduction. Both drugs interfere with cellular glutamic acid utilization. Differences between the parent drug, vinblastine sulfate, and the derivative, vincristine sulfate, affect their clinical use. Vinblastine sulfate is used primarily for treatment of Hodgkin's disease or choriocarcinoma, and vincristine sulfate is effective in treatment of children with acute leukemia or Wilms' tumor. Both drugs cause constipation and diarrhea, as well as peripheral and central nervous system toxicity. During therapy the patient must be observed for evidence of ataxia, muscle weakness, and paresthesias. He should be asked to report any tingling, numbness, or tremor of his extremities.

Radioactive agents. The radionuclides emit beta particles that destroy tissue in the vicinity of drug placement sites. The radiopharmaceuticals continue to destroy cells by emission of beta particles until disintegration of the drug results in formation of a stable nucleus.

Use of nonencapsulated forms of radioactive materials is controlled by the radiologic protection unit in the agency using the drugs. Procedural guidelines are published, and consultation services are encouraged when problems arise. If the patient who has received a radioactive agent orally (i.e., sodium iodide or sodium phosphate) vomits soon after the drug is administered, the radiologic protection officer should be notified. He will want to know the specifics of the situation so that he can advise a plan of action. The most important factors are the relationship of time of emesis to time of administration, and the amount of the vomitus. All exposed materials will be handled according to his specific instructions, and the patient will be removed from the area after thorough bathing. Both radioactive sodium iodide and sodium phosphate are eliminated in the urine; therefore it will be necessary to review the agency guidelines for disposal and the specific precautionary measures to be used when caring for the patient receiving radioactive agents.

Gold (Au^{198}) injection emits both beta and gamma rays. It is administered intraperitoneally or intrapleurally to destroy cancer cells. Fibrosis at the cancer site and in the vessels feeding the tumor results in control of fluid accumulation in the body cavity. The drug has a biologic half-life of 217 days and remains in the cavity as a constituent of the phagocytic cells that pick up the radionuclide.

Sodium iodide (I^{131}) is taken up by the thyroid gland in the natural progression of iodides toward thyroid tissue. The emission of beta particles from gland sites may affect tissues within 2 to 3 mm. from the drug storage site. The drug is excreted primarily in the urine, but small amounts appear in the sweat, feces, and milk of lactating women. The biologic half-life of the radioactive drug is 8.08 days.

Sodium phosphate (P^{32}) is taken up by bone marrow, liver, and spleen cancer cells, which utilize phosphorus rapidly. Cellular demands for phosphorus speedily move the radionuclide to the site of action. Potassium is added to the drug to enhance gastrointestinal absorption. Calcium and aluminum salts (i.e., some antacids) form insoluble combinations with phosphates and prevent absorption from the gastrointestinal tract. Radioactive sodium phosphate has a biologic half-life of 8 days. Most of the drug (94%) is excreted in the urine within 24 hours after administration. Small amounts of the drug are found in the feces.

Other antineoplastic drugs. L-Asparaginase (Table 26-1) was recently tested in clinical trials, and it produced remission in patients with leukemia. The drug capitalizes on the biochemical differences between normal and cancer cells. The amino acid L-asparagine is synthesized by normal cells, but leukemic cells use the amino acid from body fluids to build proteins. The drug acts enzymatically to hydrolyze L-asparagine so that leukemic cells are deprived of the amino acid necessary for growth.

Mitotane (Table 26-1) acts specifically on neoplastic tissue in the adrenal medulla to suppress functional and nonfunctional tissue. Use of the drug decreases the biologic activity of high levels of glucocorticoids and 17-ketosteroids. The drug is distributed in all body tissues after oral administration, and it is stored in adipose tissue. The liver and kidneys metabolize the drug, and the products are excreted in bile and urine.

Procarbazine hydrochloride (Table 26-1) interferes with amino acid synthesis at many junctions in the protein building process. During therapy, care plans include observation of behavioral changes, sleep patterns, and peripheral neural function. The observations provide clues to central and peripheral neuropathy, which frequently necessitate discontinuance of therapy.

Drug administration. Antineoplastic drugs are available for administration by many routes. Parenteral administration is often the route used initially in an intensive effort to begin cancer cell control. Long-term therapy is facilitated by use of the oral drugs that the patient can manage himself (Table 26-1).

Concern with the potential physiologic problems inherent in systemically administered antineoplastic drugs has led to experiments with methods for delivering the drugs directly to the cancer site. Each of the techniques represents an attempt to provide high concentrations of the drug at the site of the tumor without incurring systemic toxicity. Leakage of drug during direct infusion can cause systemic toxicity, disruption of wound healing, and local tissue breakdown.

Intra-arterial infusion. Intra-arterial infusion is possible when cancer cells are confined to organs with a major blood supply (i.e., the liver). Introduction of a catheter into the artery supplying the organ allows continual bathing of the tissues with precalculated amounts of drug. A reservoir and regulating device are used for delivery of the drug. Tumor cells extrapolate most of the drug before extracellular fluids enter the venous circulation.

Isolation perfusion. Isolation perfusion is a technique for delivering the drug to an entire extremity. An involved part is shunted off from the circulation by occlusion of the arterial and venous contacts to the general circulation. Catheters from the vein and artery are connected to an external pump. In addition to moving the blood in the isolated area, the pump provides a mechanism to supply high concentrations of drug to the site and remove metabolic wastes. Provision is made for perfusion of tissues with oxygen and nutrients during the time of separation from the general circulation.

Intracavity instillation. Body cavities most frequently used for instillation of antineoplastic drugs are the pleural and peritoneal cavities. Cancer tissue may release large quantities of fluid into the cavity, and organ function is inhibited by the pressure. External needle puncture is done to remove excess fluid from the cavity before instillation of the drug. After the procedure the patient's position is changed frequently to assure distribution of the drug. Quinicrine hydrochloride injection (Atabrine) is one of the drugs used for the procedure. It inhibits fluid accumulation by inducing an inflammatory reaction on serous membranes. Cancer tissue sites and their blood vessels become fibrotic, and fluid release is hampered. The major problems after treatment with any agent used to cause fibrosis is the formation of organ-obstructing adhesions.

Patient care

Maximizing the effectiveness of the drug regimen is a challenge to all concerned with the patient's care. For the patient the drug regimen may be his only hope for remission, consolidation, or palliation of the malignant process. Each positive or negative sign is very important to him. To help him veiw his progess realistically, the nurse must know what constitutes progress for the particular patient. Cure is not yet a word that can be used when the patient has cancer, but he can be helped to maintain the holding process that helps him live fully each day.

Nursing guidelines. Careful definition and recording of the patient's base-line status provides a guide, or standard, against which to measure his progress during drug therapy. Organization of relevant data on a graphic record provides an easy reference grouping for use by all health team members. The graphic record should include current drug dosage, reports of hematologic and x-ray studies, weight profiles, fever, and vital sign notations, as well as specific references to the patient's functional or performance problems.

Several physiologic factors directly affect the patient's ability to tolerate large doses of antineoplastic drugs. Careful compilation of data for nursing care planning will assist team members in meeting the patient's needs. Changes in his nutritional status as determined by body weight, muscle tone, and skin turgor will be important throughout the therapeutic program.

It is particularly important to examine skin lesions, incisions, or wounds. The cell growth necessary to wound healing may be delayed by antineoplastic drugs. Infection places a burden on the metabolic activity of the body and affects the patient's tolerance to the drug regimen.

Each of the observations must be made with the knowledge that antineoplastic drugs constitute physiologic stressors, and tolerance to stressors is highly dependent on the physiologic status when a new stressor is introduced. Once base lines are established, it is possible to plan care and define progress based on the patient's current status.

Assessment of drug effect. All health team members are deeply concerned with the progress of the drug regimen, and each must plan appropriate measures based on the data reflecting the patient's progress. For example, x-ray and local evidence that there has been regression of brachial metastatic tissue, coupled with normal hematologic reports, are indications to the physician that the patient's therapeutic plan can be continued. The increased mobility of the patient's arm and freedom from constant pain are objective signs of progress that guide the nurse in planning modifications in the care plan. The nurse will encourage the patient to begin feeding himself without assistance because the patient will benefit nutritionally and psychologically from the new activity. Although physical readiness provides a basis for modification of care plans, the patient's tolerance to new activities must be tabulated carefully. Care of the patient during neoplastic drug therapy necessitates use of many skills in planning for his continually changing needs.

Assessment of drug adverse effect. Rapid lysis of cancer tissue liberates cellular components into the extracellular fluids. Electrolytes and glucose can be recycled to meet physiologic needs, and excess organic materials are eliminated by the kidneys. The level of organic nitrogen in the circulation is reflected by the blood urea nitrogen level (normal: 8 to 25 mg./100 ml.). The low energy level of the patient may be a result of hyperuricemia and decreased food intake (Fig. 26-4). Increasing the patient's fluid intake speeds the excretion of uric acid crystals and decreases the hazard of urate stone formation in the kidney pelvis.

Nausea, vomiting, and anorexia occur frequently during antineoplastic drug therapy. They are important problems because they are very frustrating to the patient and they affect his tolerance to food at a time when nutrient intake is necessary to maintaining cellular

292 Drugs used to control reproduction and fertility

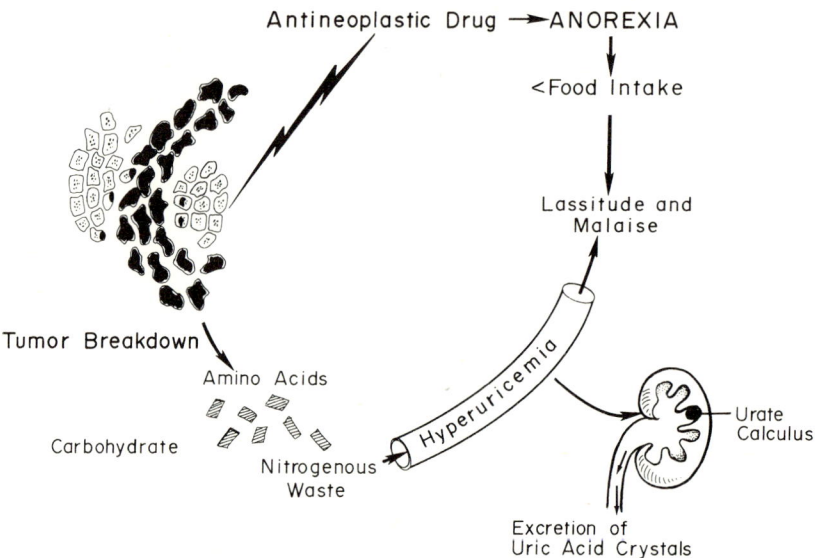

Fig. 26-4. Rapid tissue catabolism effected by antineoplastic drugs liberates nitrogenous products into the bloodstream. High concentrations of uric acid crystals in the kidneys may clump or form stones. Increased nitrogenous wastes and decreased food intake affect the energy levels of the patient.

function. Provision of small nutritious snacks and planning of meal schedules to meet the prime tolerance times of the patient may help modify the problems. Administration of oral drugs with meals or with a sedative at bedtime may also alleviate the problem. When tabulation of the patient's food intake indicates nutritional deficits, both the nutritionist and physician should be consulted. The nutritionist may have suggestions for additional modifications in foods that will raise the patient's caloric intake. The physician may order antiemetics, and intravenous or tube feedings if vomiting or food intolerance persists.

The destructive effect of antineoplastic drugs on normal epithelial and reticuloendothelial tissue may necessitate discontinuance of the drug. The tissues in the mouth facilitate assessment of epithelial tissue changes. Daily examination of the patient's mouth allows early identification of stomatitis and ulcerations, particularly at the inner margins of the lips. The patient may be the primary source of information, and he should be asked to report discomfort, bleeding from his gums, or a burning sensation when he drinks acid liquids.

Diarrhea or abdominal cramps may be indicators of hypermotility of the intestinal tract due to cellular damage. Both vomitus and stools should be tested for occult blood content. The frequency of episodes and test results are indicators of the extent of tissue destruction, and prompt reporting of observed changes both to nursing team members and the physician allows reconsideration of care plans.

Antineoplastic drug damage to the reticuloendothelial system affects the production of erythrocytes, platelets, granulocytes (neutrophils, eosinophils, basophils), and nongranular leukocytes (lymphocytes, monocytes) (Fig. 26-5). Destruction of blood cells disrupts the normal physiologic control of oxygen transport, bleeding, and infection.

Erythrocytes have a life-span of 120 days, and so their replacement rate is somewhat slower than that of other blood cells. The advantage is not great enough to protect them from destruction during prolonged antineoplastic drug therapy. A decrease in the hemoglobin normally available from mature erythrocytes affects the amount of oxygen available

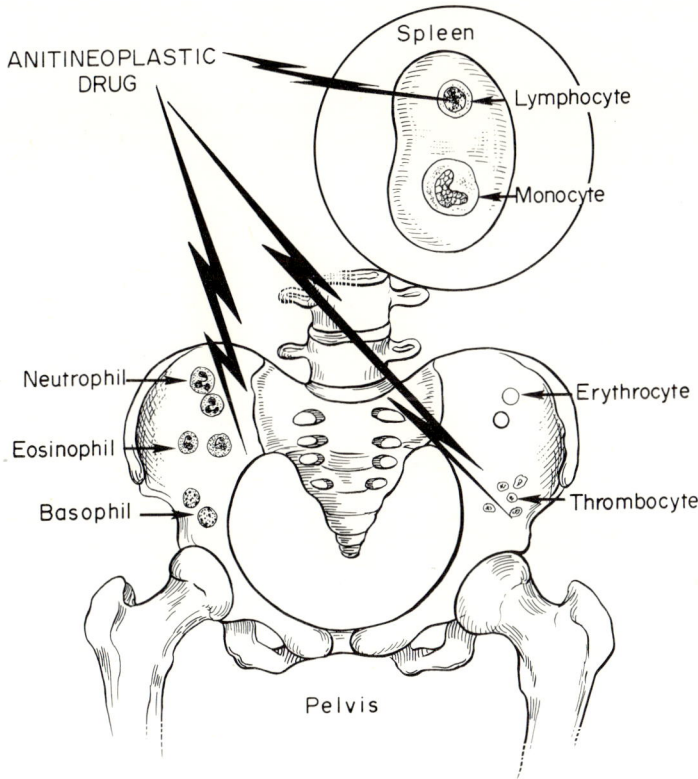

Fig. 26-5. Antineoplastic drugs affect rapidly proliferating blood cells. Leukocyte and platelet (thrombocyte) levels in the blood may drop precipitiously. The longer life-span of erythrocytes provides a slight margin of protection during therapy.

for cellular needs. Measures to conserve energy are indicated during the period when hemoglobin deficit exists.

Platelets are actively involved in the maintenance of clotting processes, and a decrease in the physiologic supply increases the bleeding potential from needle puncture sites, wounds, or tissue trauma. In addition to examination for surface bleeding sites, the stools, vomitus, and urine should be observed for changes. Tarry stools, dark-colored vomitus, or smoky colored urine provides evidence of organ bleeding sites, and they should be tested for red blood cell breakdown products (occult blood). Measures to protect the patient from tissue injury may include the use of a soft toothbrush and protective padding to bony prominences while the platelet count is low. When the platelet count falls below 100,000 mm.[3], platelet infusion may be planned to allow maintenance of blood levels and continuance of therapy.

Suppression of leukocyte production (leukopenia) decreases the physiologic response to invading pathogens. Antineoplastic drugs are used for patients with organ transplants to suppress the physiologic immune response that causes tissue rejection. During immunosuppressive therapy, antibiotics are administered to protect against infection, and the patient is placed in protective isolation to provide a germ-free environment. Daily blood studies and periodic aspiration of bone marrow from the sternum or iliac crest are planned to provide accurate profiles of the patient's hematologic status during intensive therapy. The same protection is indicated for the patient receiving the drugs for treatment of cancer when the leukocyte count falls below 2000 mm.[3].

Antineoplastic drugs also affect the epidermal cells responsible for production of hair and nails. When high doses of the drugs are used over prolonged periods of time, there may be loss of hair (alopecia). The patient should be forewarned of possible hair loss and told that it will regrow after the drug is discontinued.

REFERENCES

Allen, David W., and Cole, Phillip: Viruses and human cancer, The New England Journal of Medicine **286:**70, 1972.

Chalmers, Thomas C., Block, Jerome B., and Lee, Stephanie: Controlled studies in clinical cancer research, The New England Journal of Medicine **287:**75, 1972.

Dimitrov, Nikolay, and Ellegaard, Jørgen: Elevated lymphocyte adenosine triphosphatase activity in patients with gastrointestinal carcinoma, The New England Journal of Medicine **286:**353, 1972.

Dmochowski, Leon: Viruses and breast cancer, Cancer **28:**1404, 1971.

Dulbecco, Renato: The induction of cancer by viruses, Scientific American **216:**28, April, 1967.

Eisenhauer, Laurel A.: Drug-induced blood dyscrasias, Nursing Clinics of North America **7:**799, 1972.

Farber, S.: Chemotherapy in the treatment of leukemia and Wilms' tumor, The Journal of the American Medical Association **198:**826, 1966.

Frei, E., and Loo, T. L.: Pharmacologic basis for the chemotherapy of leukemias, Pharmacology for Physicians, **1:**1, 1967.

Gatti, R. A., Stutman, O., and Good, R. A.: The lymphoid system, Annual Review of Physiology **32:**529, 1970.

Gold, Phil: Tumor-specific antigen in GI cancer, Hospital Practice **7:**79, Feb., 1972.

Grant, Roald N.: The challenge of childhood cancer, Ca—A Cancer Journal for Clinicians **18:**35, 1968.

Gribbons, Carol A., and Aliapoulios, M. A.: Treatment for advanced breast carcinoma, American Journal of Nursing **72:**678, 1972.

Hersh, Evan M., Whitecar, John P., McCredie, Kenneth B., Bodey, Gerald P., Sr., and Freireich, Emil J.: Chemotherapy, immunocompetence, immunosuppression and prognosis in acute lukemia, The New England Journal of Medicine **285:**1211, 1971.

Hitchings, G. H.: A quarter century of chemotherapy, The Journal of the American Medical Association **209:**1339, 1969.

Holley, Robert W.: The nucleotide sequence of a nucleic acid, Scientific American **214:**30, Feb., 1966.

Karnofsky, David A.: Cancer chemotherapy agents, Ca—A Cancer Journal for Clinicians, **18:**72, 232, 1968.

Livingston, Barbara M., and Krakoff, Irwin H.: L-Asparaginase, American Journal of Nursing **70:**1910, 1970.

McKusick, Victor A.: The mapping of human chromosomes, Scientific American **224:**104, April, 1971.

Old, Lloyd, Boyse, Edward A., and Campbell, H. A.: L-Asparagine and leukemia, Scientific American **219:**34, Aug., 1968.

Orten, James M., and Neuhaus, Otto W.: Biochemistry, ed. 8, St. Louis, 1970, The C. V. Mosby Co.

Pisciotta, Anthony V.: Drug-induced leukopenia and aplastic anemia, Clinical pharmacology and therapeutics **12:**13, 1971.

Pochedly, Carl E.: The child with neuroblastoma, American Family Physician **5:**74, 1972.

Rapp, Fred, and Melnick, J. L.: The footprints of tumor viruses, Scientific American **214:**34, March, 1966.

Reilly, Mary Jo, editor: American hospital formulary service, vol. 1, sect. 10:00, Washington, D. C., 1973, American Society of Hospital Pharmacists.

Rosenthal, David S., and Moloney, William C.: Treatment of acute granulocytic leukemia in adults, The New England Journal of Medicine **286:**1176, 1972.

Rummerfield, Philip S., and Rummerfield, Marilyn J.: What you should know about radiation hazards, American Journal of Nursing **70:**780, 1970.

Santos, G. W.: The pharmacology of immunosuppressive drugs, Pharmacology for Physicians **2:**1, Aug., 1968.

Teitelbaum, Ann C.: Intra-arterial drug therapy, American Journal of Nursing **72:**1634, 1972.

Temin, Howard M.: RNA-directed DNA synthesis, Scientific American **226:**25, Jan., 1972.

Topor, Michele A.: Nursing the renal transplant patient, Nursing Clinics of North America **4:**461, 1969.

Vodopick, Helen, Rupp, Elizabeth M., Edwards, C. Lowell, Goswitz, Francis A., and Beauchamp, John J.: Cyclic leukocytosis and thrombocytosis in chronic granulocytic leukemia, The New England Journal of Medicine **286:**284, 1972.

Weiner, Leslie P., Herndon, Robert M., Narayan, Opendra, Johnson, Richard T., Shah, Keerti, Rubenstein, Lucien J., Preziosi, Thomas J., and Conley, Frances K.: Isolation of virus related to SV40 in patients with progressive multifocal leukoencephalopathy, The New England Journal of Medicine **286:**385, 1972.

Zamcheek, N., Moore, T. L., Dhar, P., and Kupchik, H.: Immunologic diagnosis and prognosis of human digestive-tract cancer: carcinoembryonic antigens, The New England Journal of Medicine **286:**83, 1972.

27

Gonadal function and fertility

Female sex cycle
    Pharmacodynamics
Conception control
    Conception inhibition
    Pharmacodynamics
Fertilization inhibition or cessation
    Pharmacodynamics
Conception enhancers
Labor induction
    Pharmacodynamics

The metamorphosis from child to adult occurs consequent to hypothalamus-stimulated anterior pituitary release of gonadotropic hormones. Emergence of secondary sex characteristics at puberty heralds the onset of changes in the sexual organs allowing participation in propagation of the species. Anterior pituitary release of gonadotropic hormones gradually establishes the appearance and reproductive potential of the male or female.

Follicle-stimulating hormone (FSH) and luteinizing hormone (LH) are the gonadotropic hormones of the pituitary gland that affect gonadal function in males and females. The basic steriod *androstenedione* is enzymatically converted to estrone or to testosterone in adrenals, testes, or ovaries. There are many intermediate steps in the biosynthesis of androstenedione, and some of the pathways of synthesis are preliminary to production of aldosterone and cortisone in the adrenal cortex. The simplified diagram below shows the major steps in biosynthesis of estrone, estradiol, and testosterone in the adrenal cortex. Estrogenic or androgenic hormone dominance is dependent on congenitally receptive tissues of the male or female.

In the male, luteinizing hormone stimulates the testicular Leydig cells to increase production of the androgenic hormone testosterone. Follicle-stimulating hormone begins the conversion of spermatogonia to sperm in the seminal vesicles, and testosterone acts concurrently to complete spermatozoa maturation.

Female sex cycle

In the female, follicle-stimulating hormone and luteinizing hormone act on the ovary to maintain the female sex cycle. The first menstrual cycle begins with the liberation of FSH from the anterior pituitary. Subsequent cycles are discussed as beginning on the first day of menstruation, since menses provide overt evidence of endogenous hormonal activity.

The developing follicle releases estrogens that begin proliferation of the endometrial lining of the uterus. Decreased plasma levels of estrogen provide feedback signals to the anterior pituitary gland that continues release of FSH and liberation of luteinizing hormone.

At the midpoint in the menstrual cycle, LH causes the ovarian follicle to rupture and release the mature ovum. Follicular corpus luteum continues to produce estrogen and progesterone, and the proliferative (estrogen-dominant) and secretory (progesterone dominant) development of the uterine lining progresses.

Hydrocholesterol ⟶ Androstenedione ⇌ Testosterone ⟶ Estradiol
                       ↳ Progesterone ↑   ↳ Estrone ⇌

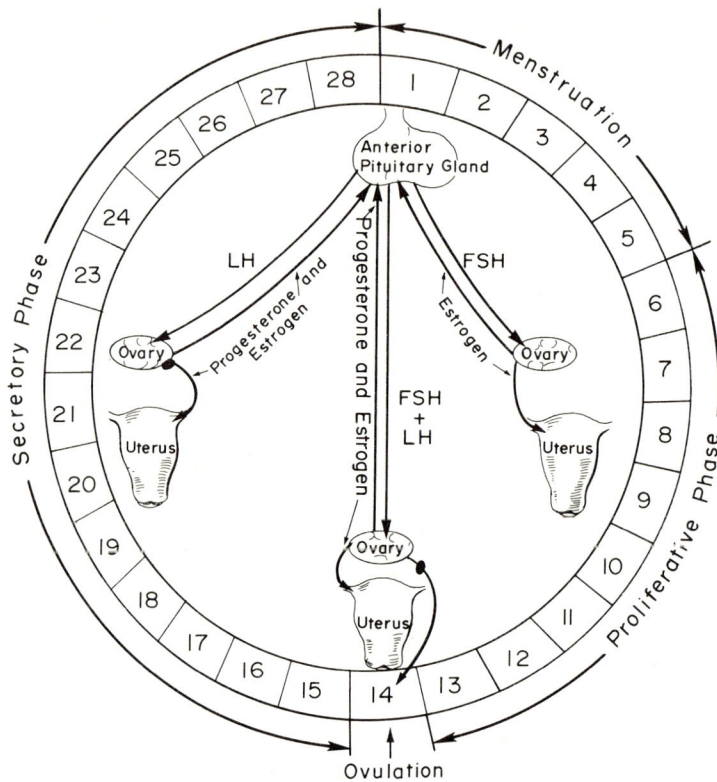

Fig. 27-1. The normal menstrual cycle maintains a feedback system for hormonal outflow to release the ovum, prepare the uterus for implantation, and remove the endometrial lining at the end of the female sex cycle.

Luteotropic hormone (LTH) is liberated from the anterior pituitary gland, and it is thought to intercede in producing secretions from the corpus luteum after LH has initiated its development. The combined activity of the three gonadotropic hormones maintains the endometrial lining in preparation for implantation of the fertilized ovum.

In the absence of fertilization, the uterine lining is shed during menstruation (Fig. 27-1). The cyclic development of follicles, ovulation, corpus luteum formation, and desquamation of the uterine lining reoccurs regularly.

The cycle is halted prior to uterine lining desquamation when there is fertilization of an ovum. The embedded *trophoblast* provides the tropic stimulus to maintenance of corpus luteum hormonal control. The tropic stimulus is liberated by the chorionic tissue formed from the trophoblast, and local ovarian control of estrogen and progesterone prevents ovulation by halting FSH and LH release. Menopause also terminates the female sex cycle.

Pharmacodynamics

Androgen therapy. Testosterone is the principal testicular hormone, and its presence is necessary for maintenance of male sex organ function and secondary sex characteristics. Androgens have an effect on congenitally receptive tissues that produces the typical male secondary sex characteristics. Androgens have varying pharmacodynamic intensity, but all the drugs promote a sense of well-being, weight gain, increased protein anabolism, and decreased amino acid catabolism. Anabolic androgens with minimal gonadal effects are presented in Chapter 23.

Commercially available forms of testosterone (Table 27-1) are prepared with additives that provide slow release of the hormone from depot sites. Prolonged hormonal effect is pro-

Table 27-1. Dosage range of androgens

Nonproprietary name	Proprietary (trade) name	Daily adult dosage range
Dromostanolone propionate	Drolban	I.M.: 100 mg. three times weekly
Fluoxymesterone	Halotestin, Ora-Testryl, Ultandren	Oral: 2.5-30 mg.
Methyltestosterone	Andrometh, Masenone, Metandren, Neo-Hombreol-M, Oreton-M, Synandrets, Synandrotabs	Oral: 30-150 mg. (÷3) S.L.: 15-25 mg.
Testolactone	Teslac	Oral: 150 mg.
Testosterone	Androlin, Andronaq, Andrusol, Aqua-Testerone, Diphasol testosterone, Malestrone, Mertestate, Neo-Hombreol-F, Oreton-F, Perandren, Synandrol-F, Testandrone, Testobase, Testosteroid, Testrone, Testryl	I.M.: 25 mg. Buccal: 10 mg.
Testosterone cypionate	Depo-testosterone cypionate	I.M.: 50-100 mg. weekly
Testosterone enanthate	Delatestryl	I.M: 200 mg. every 2 weeks
Testosterone propionate	Androlin in oil, Andronate, Andrusol-P, Masenate, Neo-Hombreol, Oreton, Sunandrol, Synerone, Testodet	I.M.: 25-75 mg.

vided by testosterone enanthate (2 weeks) and testosterone cypionate (1 week) after intramuscular injection.

The chief use of the drugs is to replace deficient hormones in the male after puberty and before the climacteric. Plans for androgen administration to improve development of secondary sex characteristics in adolescents necessitates close observation of the patient for bone development. Premature epiphyseal closure occurring as a result of drug therapy decreases the overall skeletal development and the height maximum of the adult male.

Androgens are used as hormonal antagonists in females. For example, an androgenic drug may be used to inhibit prolactin-induced lactogenic activity after delivery in the mother who plans to bottle-feed her baby.

Androgens also are used to cause regression of inoperable mammary cancer in women. The pharmacodynamic action of androgens converts the hormonal balance to protect congenitally receptive female tissues against the action of female hormones. The therapeutic goal is to cause malignant tissue regression. Masculinizing effects of the androgens present problems during prolonged administration at high dosage. Acne, facial hair, and deepening of the voice may gradually be reduced if therapy is terminated when they appear, but clitoris enlargement, hirsutism, and hypertrophy of muscles usually are irreversible. The prognosis of the patient affects evaluation of the problems and the decisions about modification of the pharmacotherapeutic plan. Therapy may be continued if the patient is receiving androgens for control of terminal cancer.

Estrogen-progesterone balance. Estrogen may be viewed as the key factor in the female sex cycle because it is required to stimulate the release of LH for progression of follicular development toward ovulation. Estrogen-mediated endometrial building initially begins preparation of the uterine stroma for trophoblast implantation. Progesterone release at the time of ovulation modifies estrogenic activity by preventing excessive proliferation of the endometrium.

Comparable synergistic activity between estrogen and progesterone occurs in development of breast tissue. Estrogen promotes development of ductal tissues, stroma, and fat accretion, and progesterone stimulates alveolar tissue and modifies excessive growth of ductal tissue.

The endocrine balance of the female is a complex interaction of the gonadal, thyroid, and adrenal hormones. Disturbance in function of the pituitary gland, ovaries, thyroid gland, or adrenal glands may disturb the normal cyclic occurrence of menstruation, and it is not unusual to find emotional responses to environmental stressors causing temporary cessation of menstruation (amenorrhea).

There are times when amenorrhea would seem to be a boon to the female, but the gonadal hormones are involved in many body processes, in addition to their effect on maintenance of the female sex cycle. Progesterone is a precursor to formation of adrenal and sexual steroids, and estrogen-progesterone levels act synergistically to control development of many body tissues.

Drugs with a pharmacodynamic action comparable to that of the natural pituitary or gonadal hormones are used to maintain or induce sexual function or secondary characteristics. In the past decade the widespread use of pituitary, chorionic, and female gonadal hormones for conception control has made the pharmacotherapeutic agents familiar to the entire population.

Estrogen therapy. The diverse effects of estrogen on congenitally receptive tissues in the female make it necessary to replace deficient hormone to maintain physiologic function. Estrogens may be used to maintain menses and fertility in females during the reproductive years, or they may be used to replace deficient hormones and control hormone balance in menopausal or postmenopausal women.

In addition to estrogenic effect on stimulation of reproductive organs and development of secondary sex characteristics, estrogen is involved in control of protein building, bone growth, and elasticity of the skin and vascular tissues. The natural physiologic effects of estrogen provide guidelines for observations when pharmacotherapeutic replacement is planned. Natural physiologic mechanisms control balanced estrogenic activity, but therapeutic replacement may exceed the physiologic limits or control mechanisms. Excesses in pharmacodynamic action during replacement therapy constitute adverse effects.

Anabolic activity in the female is enhanced by the action of estrogen on molding feminine body contour and promoting retention of the products necessary to tissue building. Estrogens are physiologically active in retaining salt, water, and nitrogen necessary to tissue building.

Bone growth is enhanced by the physiologic activity of estrogens. Osteoblastic activity gradually builds the skeleton. Increased estrogen levels at puberty speed deposition of calcium phosphate on the developing bone matrix. Epiphyseal changes after puberty and continued deposition of calcium phosphate after menopause are dependent on estrogenic activity. Excess estrogen administered to the adolescent female may speed epiphyseal closure and adversely affect skeletal development. Deficiency of estrogens in the female at menopause causes porosity of the bone (osteoporosis), and estrogenic replacement slows the process by changing the balance from osteoclastic to osteoblastic activity.

Peripheral tissue health is enhanced by the presence of physiologically active estrogen. Moisture, softness, and resilience of skin and the elasticity of the blood vessels are maintained by estrogen activity. Estrogenic effect is evident in the difference between the appearance of tissues in the young adult female with high estrogen levels and the elderly female with low endogenous estrogen levels. Estrogen lowers phospholipid and cholesterol levels, and the positive effect on vasculature is currently being considered as a rationale for maintenance of estrogen levels in the postmenopausal woman.

Historically there has been considerable controversy about hormonal replacement after surgical castration or physiologic menopause. Concern with estrogenic potentiation of cancer tissue in residual genital tissue has generally caused conservatism in hormonal replacement after hysterectomy or after menopause. Long-term studies indicate that elevated cholesterol levels and attendant predisposition to vascular changes may be lessened by administration of gonadal hormones to women after natural or surgical menopause. At low maintenance levels the hormones can maintain tissue effect without evidence of malignant growth above that occurring in untreated women.

The estrogenic drugs (Table 27-2) are pharmacologically differentiated into *steroidal* and *nonsteroidal* estrogenic substances. The nonsteroidal estrogens (chlorotrianisene, dienestrol, diethylstilbestrol, methallenestril) are

Table 27-2. Dosage range of estrogens

Nonproprietary name	Proprietary (trade) name	Daily adult dosage range	Nonproprietary name	Proprietary (trade) name	Daily adult dosage range
Chlorotrianisene	Tace	Oral: 12-48 mg. (÷1-4)	Estradiol dipropionate	Dimenformon dipropionate, Ovocylin dipropionate, Progynon-DP	I.M.: 2.5 mg.
Dienestrol	Restrol, Synestrol	Oral: 0.1-80 mg. (÷1-4) I.M.: 2.5-5 mg. twice weekly	Estradiol valerate	Atladiol, Delestrogen, Dura-estradiol, Duratrad, Estate, Estra-L, Estraval, Lastrogen, Valergen	I.M.: 20-40 mg. every 2 weeks
Diethylstilbestrol	Bio-des, DES, Stilbetin	Oral: 0.01-1 Gm. I.M.: 0.1-5 mg. three times weekly	Estrogenic substances, conjugated	Amnestrogen, Conestron, Estrifol, Hormesteral, Konogen, Premarin	Oral: 1.25-30 mg. I.V.: 20 mg./single dose
Diethylstilbestrol diphosphate	Stilphostrol	Oral: 150-600 mg. I.V.: 0.5-1 Gm. I.M.: 1-3 mg.	Estrone	Amniotin, Estrovarin, Estrugenone, Estrusol, Menformin (A), Theelin, Thelestrin, Wynestron	I.M.: 0.2-1 mg. weekly
Diethylstilbestrol dipropionate					
Estradiol	Aquadiol, Aquagen, Aquiol, Dimenformon, Diogyn, Diogynets, Estraldine, Ovocylin, Progynon	Oral: 0.3-0.6 mg. I.M.: 0.5-1.5 mg.	Ethinyl estradiol	Diogyn-E, Esteed, Estinyl, Ethinoral, Eticylol, Inestra, Lynoral, Menolyn, Novestrol, Oradiol, Orestralyn, Palonyl, Spanestrin, Ylestrol	Oral: 0.01-3 mg.
Estradiol benzoate	Dimenformon benzoate, Diogyn-B, Estrobev-E, Ovocylin benzoate, Progynon-B, Solestro	I.M.: 1-1.66 mg.	Methallenestril	Vallestril	Oral: 3-40 mg.
			Piperazine estrone sulfate	Ogen, Sulestrex piperazine	Oral: 1.5-22.5 mg. (÷5)
Estradiol cypionate	Depo-estradiol	I.M.: 1-5 mg.	Polyestradiol phosphate	Estradurin	I.M.: 40 mg. every 2 weeks

available in oral formulations. The differences between natural, semisynthetic, and nonsteroidal estrogens are related to chemical structure, but endogenous conversion produces comparable estrogenic effects during therapy. The wide range of dosage reflects the diversity of pharmacotherapeutic use of the drugs.

Low dosage may be used to support physiologic activity of endogenously available estrogen, but massive dosage may be used to convert the hormonal balance of a male with prostatic cancer from androgenic to estrogenic dominance in an attempt to decelerate proliferation of malignant cell growth. Postmenopausal women may receive massive doses of estrogens to halt mammary cancer growth. At about five years postmenopause the estrogenic level of the female is low. Intrusion on the natural level by using large estrogen doses constitutes a therapeutic change in hormonal dominance.

A single large dose of a nonsteroidal estrogen may be administered to retain the natural inhibition to milk production of the mother who does not plan to breast-feed her baby. Estrogen-progesterone levels act as natural inhibitors of milk production until delivery, when low hormonal levels allow milk production under prolactin control. Initial administration may be planned to correlate with 5 cm. dilation of the cervix, and subsequent administration is planned if additional control is required after delivery.

Estrone and estradiol are natural endogenous estrogens. Estradiol is the more potent of the two estrogens produced by the ovaries. The pharmacologic preparations available are natural and semisynthetic derivatives of the natural estrogens. A derivative of ethinyl estradiol known as mestranol is commonly used as the estrogen component in oral contraceptive formulations.

Degradation of the estrogens is accomplished by the liver. Catabolism involves hepatic–gastrointestinal tract recycling of free estrogens until the catabolic process is completed and metabolites are excreted in the urine. Nonsteroidal estrogens are more slowly metabolized than the natural estrogens. Prolonged effect of the natural estrogens has been accomplished by adding depot-inducers to the estrogenic component. Estrogenic depots slowly release the hormone and extend activity of estradiol benzoate (2 to 3 days), estradiol cypionate (14 to 28 days), estradiol dipropionate (7 to 14 days), and estradiol valerate (14 to 21 days).

Chlorotrianisene has a prolonged action period because the drug is stored in fatty tissues in the body and is released slowly from internal depot sites. For prolongation of effect, chlorotrianisene is available in capsules containing corn oil, which enhances adipose tissue storage.

Estrogens are natural physiologic hormones, and the pharmacotherapeutic plans for estrogenic use are predicated on the basis of deficiency in most instances. High dosage may cause extension of any of the planned pharmacodynamic actions of the drugs, but at average dosage the adverse effects occurring in a relatively large number of patients are anorexia, nausea, and vomiting. Individuals react differently to estrogen therapy, but patients receiving diethylstilbestrol more frequently have nausea and vomiting than patients receiving the other synthetic (nonsteroidal) compounds. The differences in reactions are related to structural variations in the drugs, and an alternate drug may be tolerated.

The natural effect of endogenous estrogens at the time of menstruation provides a useful frame of reference for consideration of the adverse effects of exogenous estrogen therapy. Females often note a weight gain of 3 to 5 pounds at the time of menstruation that is directly related to the effect of estrogens. The hormone has a salt and water-retaining effect that causes increased fluid accumulation in the pelvic organs or in peripheral tissues during menstruation. Estrogenic levels remain high during the desquamation of uterine lining, and increased interstitial fluid in the contracting uterus increases dysmenorrhea in some females. The same fluid accumulation may occur during therapy with estrogens.

Use of large dosage of estrogens for long-term control of malignant growth in males or postmenopausal females causes the emergence of secondary sex characteristics. In males there is decreased androgenic control, with consequent loss of male hair distribution and atrophy of the testicles concurrent with enlargement of breasts (gynecomastia). Most elderly men receiving the estrogens for control of prostatic cancer accept the changes as a small price to pay for palliative control of inoperable lesions. Regression of malignant tissue offers increased control of urination, decreased metastatic invasion of bone, and decreased pain. Improved function and mobility have a positive effect on the patient's receptivity to therapy.

Estrogen therapy for the postmenopausal woman provides palliative relief of inoperable malignant tissue invasion of the reproductive organs. Large dosage of estrogens in either sex may increase the accumulation of fluid in tissues. Periodic weighing of the patient, and examination of peripheral tissues may provide early evidence of emerging problems. Measures may be instituted for removal of excess tissue fluid (i.e., diuretics) to allow continuance of hormonal therapy.

Progesterone therapy. Progestogens (Table 27-3) have a pharmacodynamic effect comparable to that of the natural hormone. Desquama-

Table 27-3. Dosage range of progestogens

Nonproprietary name	Proprietary (trade) name	Adult dosage range
Dydrogesterone	Duphaston	Oral: 10-20 mg.
Ethisterone	Lutocylol, Ora-Lutin, Pranone, Progestoral, Proluton-C, Trosinone	Oral: 25-100 mg. S.L.: 10-50 mg.
Hydroxyprogesterone caproate	Delalutin	I.M.: 125-250 mg. every 4 weeks
Medroxyprogesterone acetate	Provera	Oral: 2.5-40 mg. I.M.: 50 mg.
Norethindrone	Norlutin	Oral: 5-40 mg.
Norethindrone acetate	Norlutate	Oral: 2.5-20 mg.
Progesterone	Lipo-Lutin, Lucorteum, Lutocylin, Lutromone, Migesterone, Progestin, Proluton	I.M.: 5-25 mg.

tion of the proliferative uterine lining is dependent on the presence of progesterone. Physiologic challenge of the postpuberty female with amenorrhea by administration of progesterone provides evidence of endogenous estrogenic activity. When estrogen has prepared the endometrial lining, administration of progesterone acts to cause desquamation, and menstruation ensues. The response indicates absence of endogenous progesterone, and replacement therapy is indicated.

The drugs are used extensively for conception control. Progesterone derivatives are part of a balanced plan for estrogen-progesterone control and duplication of the female fertility cycle.

The natural effect of progesterone in maintaining the uterine lining during pregnancy is the rationale for use of the drugs to prevent threatened abortion. Hydroxyprogesterone caproate and dydrogesterone are used for pregnancy maintenance because they have few estrogenic or androgenic properties. Selectivity in the use of "pure" hormones is necessary to prevent masculinization of the female fetus.

Initial use of progestogens for control of menstruation (i.e., metrorrhagia) may cause an initial period of profuse vaginal flow, for the drugs cause prompt shedding of estrogen-induced accumulations of endometrial tissue. Menstrual flow returns to normal levels after a short period of profuse bleeding.

Short-term use of the progestogens produces few adverse effects. Spotting and irregular bleeding, nausea, and lethargy are the only disturbing problems in most patients. Progestogen therapy may precipitate jaundice, the problem occurring more frequently in women who had low level icterus during pregnancies.

CONCEPTION CONTROL
Conception inhibition

The natural sequence of estrogen and progesterone activity consequent to follicle-stimulating hormone and luteinizing hormone release by the anterior pituitary gland is essential to preparing the endometrium to support development of the fertilized ovum. Oral contraceptives are used to provide the hormonal components in amounts that prevent feedback stimulation of the anterior pituitary gland.

Cessation of FSH and midcycle LH release occurs as the return message to pituitary sites indicates there is adequate hormone at gonadal sites. Hormonal activity continues proliferation of the uterine lining, but the absence of ovulation provides conception control.

Concurrent changes in the cervical mucus and in the endometrial lining support conception control by preventing activity of viable spermatozoa. The proliferative and secretory phases of endometrial development are shortened, and during the fourteenth to twenty-eighth day of the cycle a pseudodecidual lining is developed. The stromal tissue has sparse glands and is less vascular than that occurring with pituitary-controlled balance of hormonal activity. Oral contraceptives provide progestogen at the terminal days of the drug-controlled cycle, and progestogen-induced shedding of the endometrial lining leads to menstruation.

Pharmacodynamics

Exogenous administration of the hormones maintains an anovulatory cycle and allows estrogenic hormone maintenance of secondary sex characteristics. Inhibition of ovulation is planned by use of synthetic estrogen-progesterone combinations that provide exogenous hormone after menstruation and beyond the natural midcycle ovulatory time period.

Oral contraceptives provide varying quantities and combinations of estrogens and progestogens. Ethinyl estradiol and mestranol are the synthetic estrogens used in oral contraceptives. Dimethisterone, ethynodiol diacetate, norethindrone acetate, norethynodrel, or norgestrel are the progestogens used with the synthetic estrogens. *Fixed combinations* of an estrogen and a progestogen may be used throughout the 28-day control period, or a *sequential plan* for use of an estrogen and progestogen may provide conception control.

Fixed combination program. The estrogen component of the combination tablet suppresses the secretion of FSH, and the progestogen component inhibits the midcycle release of LH from the pituitary gland. Tablets are taken from the fifth to the twenty-fifth day. In the remaining seven days of the cycle, a placebo tablet may be taken. Plans for use of a placebo establish a ritualistic practice of taking the tablets every day. Oral contraceptives that are fixed combinations include the following:

Ethinyl estradiol and ethynodiol diacetate (Demulen)
Ethinyl estradiol and norethindrone acetate (Norlestrin)
Ethinyl estradiol and norgestrel (Ovral)
Mestranol and ethynodiol diacetate (Ovulen)
Mestranol and norethindrone (Norinyl; Ortho-Novum)
Mestranol and norethynodrel (Enovid)

Sequential program. Estrogen is administered daily for 14 to 16 days (fifth to eighteenth or twentieth day of the cycle), and a combination of estrogen and progestogen is used for 6 days. The plan provides estrogen for control of ovulation and progestogen to induce endometrial shedding. The amount of decidual endometrium produced is less than that occurring with fixed combination therapy. Estrogen-progestogen drugs used for sequential therapy include the following:

Ethinyl estradiol and dimethisterone (Oracon)
Mestranol and norethindrone (Norquen, Ortho-Novum SQ)

Scheduled use. Either fixed combination or sequential therapy has been found almost completely effective in conception control. Exogenous hormones are not required for conception control during menstruation, but most of the schedules for use of the oral contraceptives include a placebo to provide the patient with a consistent daily routine for taking tablets. Omission of the tablets prior to the predictable ovulation time in the established 28-day cycle decreases protection against conception. When tablets have been omitted for 3 days, the woman is instructed to use other conception control devices if sexual intercourse is planned during the remainder of the cycle.

Adverse effects. The chief adverse effect directly related to use of oral contraceptives is the occurrence of thrombosis. The cause-effect relationship is evident as a small number of individuals develop thrombophlebitis, pulmonary embolism, and cerebral or coronary thrombosis while taking the drugs. Studies are being conducted to delineate the specific factors that contribute to the incidence of thrombosis in some females. Estrogen content of oral contraceptives has been implicated in etiology of thrombophlebitis.

Maintenance of an anovulatory state is comparable to that occurring when ovum fertilization initiates pregnancy. In the pregnant female, the corpus luteum continues estrogen and progesterone production, with inhibition of the pituitary gonadotropic contribution to ovarian function. The discomforts of many females during the first 4 months of oral contraceptive therapy are similar to those of early pregnancy: headache, nausea and vomiting, breast fullness and tenderness, and depression and fatigue. Adverse effects may lessen with continued use of the drug, but in some instances the problems reappear cyclically during ensuing months. Discussion of the problems with the physician is encouraged because change to another oral contraceptive may alleviate persisting problems.

Brownish pigmentation of the face comparable to that occurring in pregnancy (chloasma gravidarum), fluid retention, and weight gain occurring during therapy may necessitate change to another method of conception control. Endometrial instability may cause intermenstrual spotting, but the problem usually lessens during subsequent cycles.

Cyclic control provides regularity of menstruation, decreases dysmenorrhea, and diminishes menstrual flow concurrent with providing conception control. The female usually describes a positive effect on libido. Periodic gynecologic evaluation with examination of cervical smears (Papanicolau smear) is an important aspect of prolonged therapy. Some physicians recommend annual rest periods from drug therapy to allow reinstitution of natural cyclic control. Many individuals interrupt the schedule voluntarily to allow conception and desired pregnancy. Withdrawal of the drugs usually leads to reestablishment of the normal sex cycle of the female without inordinate delay, although amenorrhea may persist for several cycles because of suppression of endogenous hormones during the conception control period.

FERTILIZATION INHIBITION OR CESSATION

Conception inhibition for the victim of sexual assault can be accomplished after careful analysis of the menstrual cycle to determine whether timing of the incident correlates with ovum availability. Calculations are based on the earliest and latest possible date of ovulation. Fertility is possible from the eighteenth day before onset of the earliest likely menstrual date through the eleventh day before the onset of the latest likely menstruation date because ovulation predictably occurs 14 days before menstruation. In a 28-day menstrual cycle, conception is possible if intercourse occurred between the eleventh through the eighteenth day from the beginning of the last menstrual period. Ova can be fertilized for about 24 hours after ovarian release, and spermatozoa are maximally available for fertilization of ova for 48 hours after sexual intercourse. The data aid in definition of probable conception and allow prompt drug-induced control of trophoblast development.

Pharmacodynamics

Administration of large doses of steroidal or nonsteroidal estrogen in the period after ovulation disrupts the estrogen-progesterone balance that maintains a dense endometrial nutrient bed for the fertilized ova. Estrogen-induced local inhibition of carbonic anhydrase with consequent excess of carbon dioxide at the implantation site is thought to raise the pH of tissues to a level incompatible with survival of the trophoblast.

Prostaglandins recently have been isolated from varying human tissues, including the amniotic fluid of pregnant women, and one of the prostaglandins (PGF_{22}) has an abortifacient effect. When injected intravaginally, the minute amounts of prostaglandins act to terminate the development of the early fetus without systemic adverse effects occurring with other abortion agents.

CONCEPTION ENHANCERS

Gonadotropic hormones can be introduced exogenously to stimulate ovarian function. Menotropins (Pergonal) is used to stimulate growth and maturation of ovarian follicles in women previously unable to become pregnant because of deficient ovum production. Menotropins acts pharmacodynamically to induce the same effect on ovarian follicle development and ovulation as that of the natural FSH and LH. Support of LH effect on ovulation is provided by concurrent administration of chorionic gonadotropin when follicle maturation has occurred. Chorionic gonadotropin has many different trade names (A.P.L., Almetropin, Antuitrin-S, Chorex, Chorigon, Follutein, Glucotropin-Forte, Khorion, Libigen, Luton, Pregnyl, Riogon, Stemutrolin). The combination of menotropins and chorionic gonadotropin has received wide publicity as the therapeutic plan causing multiple ovulations and consequent multiple births in previously infertile women. The high incidence of multiple births (20% of patients) makes it important for both husband and wife to be forewarned of the possibility.

The overall plan includes definition of follicular maturation by urinary estrogenic level increase, changes in cervical mucus production, and vaginal changes. After 9 to 12 days of intramuscular administration of menotropins, it is predictable that follicle maturation will occur. Chorionic gonadotropin is administered once intramuscularly at the termination of the menotropin dosage period. Daily sexual intercourse is necessary in the terminal days of menotropin administration through the period of chorionic gonadotropin stimulation of ovulation. Progesterone has a thermogenic property that causes the body temperature to rise 0.4° F. in the period after ovulation, and the female can determine prime conception time by assessing the rise in body temperature. Progesterone activity is high at the time of ovulation.

Multiple ovulation is partially controlled by evaluation of the urinary excretion of estrogen. When urinary levels of estrogen rise, hyperstimulation of the ovaries potentiates hyperovulation. To avoid multiple pregnancies, the drug is withdrawn in the presence of high urinary excretion of estrogens. Ovarian enlargement can become excessive, and the danger of rupture of ovarian cysts makes it necessary to refrain from intercourse. Cessation of therapy may be necessary, but repeat trials may be planned when ovarian size is reduced.

Chorionic gonadotropin is also used in males to stimulate testicular production of testosterone. In the male fetus, placental liberation of testosterone causes testicular descent, but in male infants with undescended testicles (cryptorchidism), chorionic gonadotropin administration may cause descent of testicles into the scrotum.

Clomiphene citrate (Clomid) is used orally (50 to 100 mg./24 hours) during the fifth to tenth day of the menstrual cycle to stimulate release of FSH and LH from the pituitary to increase the fertility of anovulatory women desiring pregnancy. It has both estrogenic and antiestrogenic properties, and its chief mode of action is to block estrogen at the anterior pituitary, thus increasing FSH-initiated follicle development so that smaller amounts of LH are effective and cause spontaneous ovulation. Successful therapy leads to pregnancy, but discontinuance of therapy returns the nonpregnant woman to an anovulatory state.

Multiple births have occurred when conception resulted from a period of drug therapy. The chief problems for the patient during drug therapy are visual changes (intensification and prolongation of afterimages) occurring in bright light. Dizziness or lightheadedness may make it necessary for the individual to limit driving of a motor vehicle or performing tasks requiring alertness and coordination during the short course of therapy.

LABOR INDUCTION

The drugs used to produce muscle contractions in the fetus-containing uterus simulate the actions of natural physiologic hormones produced concurrently with labor and delivery (Fig. 27-2). Physiologic readiness to move the fetus into the environment is heralded by the onset of uterine contractions. The clonic contraction cycles progressively become more frequent and stronger, and the predilated cervix opens more widely. The physical forces, aided by the compression on pelvic organs contributed by the mother, send the fetus out into the world. Umbilical detachment begins the life of an autonomous individual.

The placenta-containing uterus continues contraction to evacuate the remaining placental tissue. A combination of factors affects the continued contraction and expulsion of residual contents. The dilated cervix stimulates hypothalamic centers, and posterior pituitary sites release oxytocin to complete the removal of uterine products as preliminary preparation for reinstitution of the reproductive cycle.

Contraction of the uterine muscle decreases bleeding from exposed placental junction sites by direct pressure that closes capillary openings. The level of oxytocin production by cervical stimuli is insufficient to maintain the physiologic functions necessary to prevent hemorrhage, and additional hormone is needed. The stimulus of the infant nursing sends impulses to increase pituitary release of oxytocin. Additional hormone stimulates myoepithelial cells in the mammary glands to release milk. The cyclic effect of nursing–oxytocin release–milk expulsion concurrent with stimulation of uterine contractions is a physiologic survival mechanism of mammals.

Pharmacodynamics

Oxytocin (Table 27-4) mimics the action of the natural hormone during the delivery

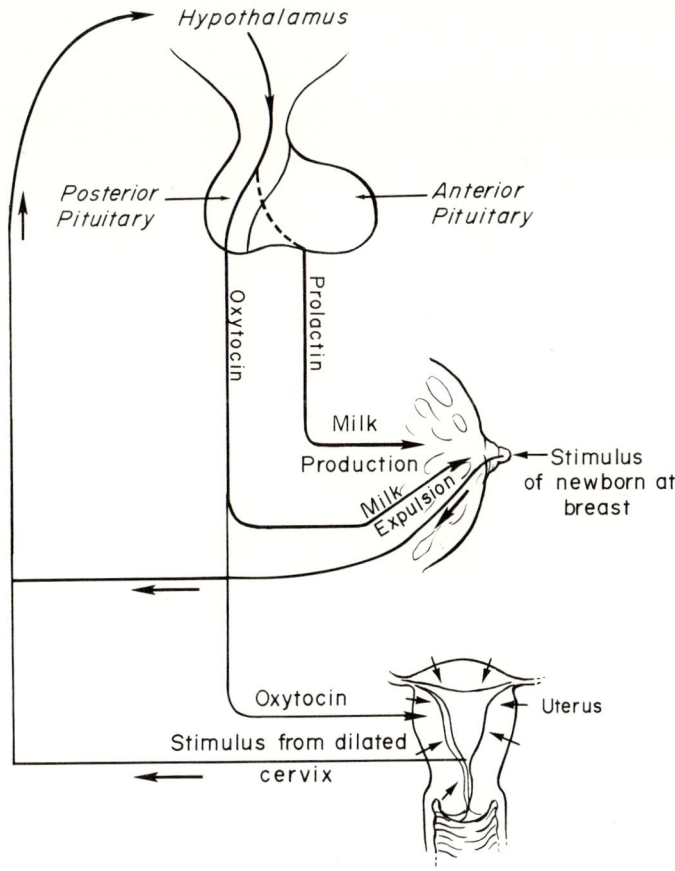

Fig. 27-2. Interrelated neural and hormonal factors control contraction of the uterus and availability of breast milk during the postpartum period.

process and stimulates the expulsion of milk from the mammary glands after delivery of the baby. The drug has a rapid onset of action when administered intramuscularly (3 to 7 minutes) or intravenously (1 minute). Timing of administration is correlated with emergence of the newborn in a planned approach to providing postpartum contractions of uterine muscle. Intramuscular injection is given after delivery of the anterior shoulder, and intravenous drug is given after delivery of the baby. The therapeutic plan is to provide uterine contractions in the immediate postpartum period that complete expulsion of uterine contents and decrease bleeding from endometrial sites. When the drug is given intramuscularly, it affects uterine muscle contraction for a 30- to 60-minute period.

Oxytocin reinforces the effect of endogenous hormone, and the time of administration is important to assure smooth continuance of the delivery process. Inadvertent early administration interrupts the contraction cycle of the uterus and causes rupture of the organ or asphyxia of the fetus.

The characteristic rhythmic contraction and relaxation (clonic) patterns of muscle contraction produced by oxytocin has expanded its use to therapeutic induction of labor at term. The drug is used when physiologic readiness is indicated by changes in the cervix. The practice is becoming increasingly more common and is called by young mothers delivery by appointment. Many factors have stimulated the present frequent practice of labor induction at full-term, but assurance that the mother has an opportunity for quality care before delivery is a primary

Table 27-4. Dosage range of drugs used in labor and delivery.

Nonproprietary name	Proprietary (trade) name	Daily adult dosage range
Ergonovine maleate	Ergotrate maleate	Oral: 0.4-2.4 mg. (÷2-6) I.V.: 0.2-0.4 mg./single dose
Methylergono-vine maleate	Methergine	I.M.: 0.2 mg./single dose I.V.: Same
Oxytocin	Pitocin, Syntocinon, Uteracon	I.M.: 0.5-2 U. single dose I.V.: 0.5-0.75 ml./min
Oxytocin citrate		Buccal: 200-600 U./single dose
Sparteine sulfate	Spartocin, Tocosamine	I.M.: 150-600 mg. (÷4)

concern. The drug is given by intramuscular, intravenous, subcutaneous, or buccal route to stimulate contractions, and the dosage is titrated with the onset of contractions. Local vasoconstriction sometimes occurs during use of buccal tablets, and absorption of the drug may become erratic. Induction of labor is only done under carefully controlled circumstances. The particular problems related to disruption of uterine dynamics and occlusion of the fetal route of exit make it necessary to have personnel and facilities prepared to protect both mother and baby during induction, labor, and delivery.

Sparteine sulfate (Table 27-4) is used for induction of labor at term, but it is an entirely different compound from oxytocin. The drug is used to stimulate uterine muscle contraction when inertia occurs during labor, and it produces a rhythmic pattern of contractions. Hypertonic contractions of the uterus have occurred during therapy. Sparteine sulfate lengthens the refractory period of myocardial tissue, and bradycardia may occur during labor-related administration.

Ergonovine maleate, and methylergonovine maleate (Table 27-4) increase the tone, rate, and amplitude of rhythmic uterine contractions during the postpartum period. The uterus is maintained in a slightly contracted state that makes the drugs useful to control bleeding from intrauterine sites. The drugs are administered intramuscularly at the end of delivery. They are used to promote involution of the uterus in the puerperium. Within 3 to 5 minutes after oral use of the drugs, patients are conscious of cramping sensations, indicating uterine contractions, and an increase in vaginal discharge.

Each of the drugs used for labor, delivery, or stimulation after delivery is a potent agent that is cautiously administered for the particular status or problems of the patient. The interrelatedness of the drugs and natural physical forces requires careful supervision of the progress of the patient throughout therapy.

A natural substance that has an effect on the stimulation of uterine contractions has been found. Prostaglandins (PGF_{22}) have been identified in the amniotic fluid and venous blood of women during the contractions of labor, and they play an important role in stimulating uterine muscle during parturition. When PGF_{22} is administered orally or intravenously, it facilitates labor, with completion of delivery in a few hours. Prostaglandins may be one of the substances eventually available commercially to facilitate labor and produce atraumatic therapeutic abortion in the early days of pregnancy.

REFERENCES

Backer, Matt H., Jr., and Cavanaugh, Denis: Secondary amenorrhea, Medical Clinics of North America 52:339, 1968.

Boyar, Robert, Finkelstein, Jordan, Roffwarg, Howard, Kapen, Sheldon, Weitzman, Elliot, and Hellman, Leon: Synchronization of augmented luteinizing hormone secretion with sleep during puberty, The New England Journal of Medicine 287:582, 1972.

Connell, Elizabeth B.: The pill and the problems, American Journal of Nursing 71:326, 1971.

Craver, Bradford N.: The treatment of the victim of rape with uses of the 'morning-after pill', The Medical Folio 4(2):1, 1971.

Daughaday, William H.: The diagnosis of hypersomatotropism in man, Medical Clinics of North America 52:371, 1968.

Donati, R. M., and Gallagher, N. I.: Hematologic

alteration associated with endocrine disease, Medical Clinics of North America **52:**231, 1968.

Federman, Daniel D.: Current concepts: the assessment of organ function—the testes, The New England Journal of Medicine **285:**901, 1971.

Goodman, Louis S., and Gilman, Arthur, editors: The pharmacological basis of therapeutics, ed. 4, New York, 1970, The Macmillian Co.

Kellie, A. E.: The pharmacology of estrogens, Annual Review of Pharmacology **11:**97, 1971.

Levine, Seymour.: Sex differences in the brain, Scientific American **214:**84, April, 1966.

McQuarrie, Howard G.: Oral contraception, Medical Clinics of North America **51:**1261, 1967.

Mountcastle, Vernon B., editor: Medical physiology, ed. 13, vol. 1, St. Louis, 1974, The C. V. Mosby Co.

Nilsson, Lennart, and Rybo, Goran: Treatment of menorrhagia, American Journal of Obstetrics and Gynecology **110:**713, 1971.

Odell, William D., and Moyer, Dean L.: Physiology of Reproduction, St. Louis, 1971, The C. V. Mosby Co.

Pike, John E.: Prostaglandins, Scientific American **225:**84, Nov., 1971.

Reilly, Mary Jo, editor: American hospital formulary service, vol. 2, sect. 68:00, Washington, D. C., 1973, American Society of Hospital Pharmacists.

Wilber, John F.: Alterations of endocrine function in pregnancy, Medical Clinics of North America **52:**253, 1968.

Young, Iven S., and Kupperman, Herbert S.: The management of the amenorrheic patient, The Medical Folio **2**(1):1, 1968.

INDEX

A

Abbocillin, dosage, 25
Acenocoumarol as anticoagulant
   discussion, 185
   dosage, 185
Acetaminophen for pain
   discussion, 249
   dosage, 248
Acetazolamide in fluid control, dosage, 100
Acetohexamide as hypoglycemic
   discussion, 274
   dosage, 274
Acetophenazine maleate as antipsychotic, dosage, 205
Acetophenetidin for pain
   discussion, 249
   dosage, 248
Acetosulfone sodium in leprosy, dosage, 37
Acetyldigitoxin
   discussion, 152
   dosage, 151
Acetylsalicylic acid for pain
   discussion, 248-249, 250-251
   dosage, 248
Achromycin; *see* Tetracycline
Acid-base shift, 83
Acidosis
   diabetic, 272
   metabolic, 272
Actase; *see* Fibrinolysin
ACTH
   administration, 74
   adverse effects, 74
   corticotropin-releasing center, 73
   corticotropin-releasing factor, 73
   as stimulus for adrenocorticoid release, 74
Actidil as antihistamine, dosage, 64
Acylanid; *see* Acetyldigitoxin
Adanon; *see* Methadone hydrochloride
Addiction
   addictive analgesics; *see* Analgesics, addictive
   amphetamine, 260-261
Addition, definition, 8
Ademol; *see* Flumethiazide
Adenosine phosphate for tissue fluid removal
   discussion, 119
   dosage, 118
ADH; *see* Antidiuretic hormone

Adiphenine hydrochloride
   discussion, 142
   dosage, 142
Ad-Nil as appetite suppressant, dosage, 258
Adrenalin; *see* Epinephrine hydrochloride
Adrenergic blocking, alpha, in hypertension, 175-176
Adrenergic drugs in bronchial constriction, 86-87
Adrenergic effectors to maintain peripheral blood pressure, 167-168
Adrenergic receptors and vascular tone, 164
Adrenocorticoid release, exogenous ACTH as stimulus for, 74
Adrenocorticotropic hormone; *see* ACTH
Adrenosem for antihemorrhagic effect, dosage, 188
Adrestat for antihemorrhagic effect, dosage, 188
Adriamycin in cancer, 289
Adrin; *see* Epinephrine hydrochloride
Adroyd in protein building, dosage, 261
Aerosporin; *see* Polymyxin B sulfate
Akineton in Parkinsonism, dosage, 220
Albamycin; *see* Novobiocin sodium
Albumin replacement, 103-104
Alcohol sensitizer, 133
Alcopara; *see* Bephenium hydroxynaphthoate
Aldactone in fluid control, 99
Aldinamide; *see* Pyrazinoic acid amide
Aldomet ester hydrochloride; *see* Methyldopa hydrochloride
Aldosterone
   antagonists, 99
   in fluid balance, 96-97
   replacement, 98
Alerin as antihistamine, dosage, 64
Alforone; *see* Fludrocortisone acetate
Alkajel, 137
Alkaloids
   plant, in cancer, 289
   Rauwolfia; *see* Rauwolfia alkaloids
Alkavervir in hypertension
   discussion, 175
   dosage, 173
Alkeran in cancer, dosage, 287
Alkylating agents in cancer, 288-289
Allergic reactions, 58-80
   to anti-infective drugs, 22-24
   delayed, 63
   to penicillin, 24-26
   to sulfonamides, 35

Allopurinol to remove tissue toxicants
  discussion, 115
  dosage, 113
Almefrin; see Phenylephrine hydrochloride
Almetropin as conception enhancer, 303-304
Alminate, 137
Aloin in constipation
  discussion, 123
  dosage, 122
Alophen; see Aloin
Alpen; see Ampicillin
Alpha adrenergic blocking in hypertension, 175-176
Alpha amylase for tissue fluid removal
  discussion, 119
  dosage, 118
Alphadrol, dosage, 76
Alphaprodine hydrochloride for pain
  discussion, 247
  dosage, 245
AlphaRedisol; see Hydroxocobalamin
Alseroxylon in hypertension
  discussion, 172-174
  dosage, 173
Althose; see Methadone hydrochloride
Al-U-Creme, 137
Aludrine; see Isoproterenol hydrochloride
Aludrox, 137
Aluminum carbonate gel, 137
Aluminum hydroxide gel, 137
Aluminum hydroxide with magnesium trisilicate, 137
Aluminum and magnesium hydroxides, 137
Aluminum nicotinate to lower blood lipid levels
  discussion, 183
  dosage, 183
Aluminum phosphate gel, 137
Alurate for sleep control, dosage, 231
Alverine citrate
  discussion, 142
  dosage, 142
Alzinox, 137
Amantadine hydrochloride, 67
Ambenonium chloride, dosage, 225
Amcil; see Ampicillin
Amebiasis, 47-50
  extraintestinal, 48
  intestinal, 47-48
  patient care in, 49-50
  pharmacodynamics in, 48-49
Amebicides
  dosage range of, 48
  extraintestinal, 48-49
  intestinal, 49
Amfetasul; see Dextroamphetamines
E-Amicar for antihemorrhagic effect, dosage, 188
Ami-CO; see Ampicillin
Amid-Sal for pain, dosage, 248
E-Aminocaproic acid for antihemorrhagic effect, dosage, 188
Aminophylline in bronchial constriction
  discussion, 85-86
  dosage, 86
Aminosalicylates in tuberculosis control
  discussion, 40-41
  dosages, 37
Aminosalicylic acid in tuberculosis control, dosage, 37

Amitriptyline hydrochloride in psychic depression
  discussion, 202-203
  dosage, 201
Ammonia removal, 115-117
Amnestrogen, 299
Amniotin; see Estrone
Amobarbital sodium for sleep control, dosage, 231
Amodiaquine hydrochloride in malaria
  discussion, 52
  dosage, 52
Amodril as appetite suppressant, dosage, 258
Amoebicon; see Glaucarubin
Am-Pen; see Ampicillin
Amphedrine; see Amphetamines
Amphedroxyn Desamine; see Methamphetamine hydrochloride
Amphetamine(s)
  abuse, 260-261
  administration schedules, 259
  adverse effects, 259-260
  in appetite suppression
    discussion, 258-260
    dosage, 258
  excretion control, 259
  formulations, 259
Amphex; see Dextroamphetamines
Amphojel, 137
Amphotericin B in fungal infection
  discussion, 45-46
  dosage, 45
Ampicillin
  dosages, 25
  microorganism susceptibility to, 20
Ampi-CO; see Ampicillin
Amplin; see Ampicillin
Amsustain; see Dextroamphetamines
A-M-T, 137
Amyl nitrite to dilate coronary arteries, 179
Amytal sodium for sleep control, dosage, 231
Anabolic steroids; see Steroids
Anadrol in protein building, dosage, 261
Analexin as muscle relaxant, dosage, 228
Analgesics
  addictive
    discussion, 245-248
    dosage range of, 245
    respiratory depression and, 247-248
    withdrawal signs, 247
  –anti-inflammatory drugs, 250-251
  –antipyretics, 248-250
    dosage range of, 248
  for pain
    discussion, 250
    dosage range of, 250
Ananase; see Bromelains
Anaphylaxis, 62
  anti-infective drugs and, 23
Anavar in protein building, dosage, 261
Ancobon; see Flucytosine
Androdiol in protein building, dosage, 261
Androgens
  discussion, 296-297
  dosage range of, 297
Androlin; see Testosterone
Andrometh, dosage, 297
Andronaq; see Testosterones

Andronate; see Testosterones
Androstenedione, 295
Andrusol; see Testosterones
Anectine and muscle contraction, 227
Anesthesia, 239-243
  hypersensitivity reactions, 243
  inhalation, 239-241
    agents used for, 240
    patient care in, 241
    pharmacodynamics in, 240-241
  local, 241-243
  stages, 239-240
  topical agents, 242-243
Angicap to dilate coronary arteries, dosage, 178
Angioedema, 62
  anti-infective drugs and, 23
Angiotensin, 96
Angiotensin amide to maintain peripheral blood pressure
  discussion, 168
  dosage, 167
Anhydron; see Cyclothiazide
Anileridine for pain
  discussion, 247
  dosage, 245
Anisindione as anticoagulant
  discussion, 185
  dosage, 185
Anisotropine methylbromide, 141
Anorexigenics, 258
  dosage range of, 258
Ansolysen; see Pentolinium tartrate
Antabuse; see Disulfiram
Antacids, gastric
  discussion, 137-138
  dosage range of, 137
Antepar; see Piperazine citrate
Anthiphen; see Dichlorophen
Antianxiety drugs; see Tranquilizers, minor
Antibiotic(s), 24-33
  in amebiasis, 49
  in cancer, 289
  chemotherapeutic drugs, 21
  definition, 21
  discussion, 30-32
  dosage limitations, 30-31
  dosage range of, 30
  reserve, 32-33
Antibody(ies)
  blocking, 61
  cell-fixed, 61
  formation, 17
Anticholinergics
  dosage range of, 141
  in gastric acidity and intestinal hypermotility, 139-143
  with local anesthetic activity, dosage range of, 142
Anticoagulant(s)
  dosage range of, 185
  food and, 187-188
  inactivators, dosage range of, 185
  progress of, graphic records, 186
Anticonvulsants
  discussion, 214-217
  dosage range of, 215
Antidepressants, dosage range of, 201
Antidiarrheal drugs, dosage, 125

Antidiuretic hormone
  fluid balance and, 97
  replacement, 98
Antiemetics
  action site, 130
  adverse effects, 130-131
  dosage range of, 130
Antifungal drugs, dosage range of, 45
Antigen
  lymphogranuloma venereum, in dermal reaction test, 60
  mumps skin test, 59-60
Antihelmintics, dosage range of, 55
Antihemophilic factor (human) for antihemorrhagic effect, dosage, 188
Antihemorrhagic effects, drugs for, 188
Antihistamine(s)
  discussion, 63-65
  dosage range of, 64
  suppressants, 90-91
Antihypertensives, dosage range of, 173
Anti-infective drugs
  adverse effects of, 21-22
  allergic reactions, 22-24
  discussion of term, 21
  dosage range, 21, 25
  microorganism susceptibility to, 20
Anti-inflammatory drugs, 250-251
Antimalarials, dosage range of, 52
Antimetabolites in cancer, 286-288
Antiminth; see Pyrantel pamoate
Antineoplastic agents
  administration of, 290-291
  discussion, 284-286
  dosage range of, 287
  effect of, 291
    adverse, 291-294
Antiparasitics, dosage range of
  amebicides, 48
  antihelmintics, 55
  antimalarials, 52
Antipsychotic drugs; see Tranquilizers, major
Antipyretics, 248-250
  dosage range of, 248
Antrenyl, 141
Antuitrin-S as conception enhancer, 303-304
Anturan; see Sulfinpyrazone
Anxiety states, 204-211
Apamide; see Acetaminophen
A.P.L. as conception enhancer, 303-304
Apodol; see Anileridine
Apomorphine hydrochloride in emesis induction
  discussion, 133
  dosage, 132
Appetite
  suppressants, 258
    dosage range of, 258
  suppression, 257-260
    pharmacodynamics in, 258-260
Apresoline; see Hydralazine hydrochloride
Aprobarbital for sleep control, dosage, 231
Aquadiol; see Estradiol
Aquagen; see Estradiol
Aqualin; see Theophylline
AquaMephyton as anticoagulant inactivator, dosage, 185

Aquatag; *see* Benzthiazide
Aqua-Testerone; *see* Testosterone
Aquatyl; *see* Dioctyl sodium sulfosuccinate
Aquiol; *see* Estradiol
Aralen; *see* Chloroquine
Aramine; *see* Metaraminol bitartrate
Arfonad; *see* Trimethaphan camsylate
Arginine glutamate in ammonia removal
    discussion, 116-117
    dosage, 113
Arginine hydrochloride in ammonia removal
    discussion, 116-117
    dosage, 113
Aristocort, dosage, 76
Arlidin; *see* Nylidrin hydrochloride
Armazid; *see* Isoniazid
Arrhythmias, 156-163
    drugs in
        dosage range of, 159
        effector site of, 157
    nursing guidelines, 162-163
    patient care in, 162-163
    patterns, periodic recordings of, 162
    pharmacodynamics in, 158-162
Arsenic chelation, 111
Artane in Parkinsonism, dosage, 220
Arteries
    arterial blood gases, 83
    chemoreceptors, 84
    coronary; *see* Coronary artery
    peripheral; *see* Peripheral artery
Arthropan for pain, dosage, 248
Arthus reaction, 63
A.S.A.; *see* Acetylsalicylic acid
L-Asparaginase in cancer
    discussion, 290
    dosage, 287
Aspidium oleoresin for tapeworms
    discussion, 55
    dosage, 55
Aspirin; *see* Acetylsalicylic acid
Asteric; *see* Acetylsalicylic acid
Atabrine; *see* Quinacrine hydrochloride
Atarax; *see* Hydroxyzine hydrochloride
Athrombin-K; *see* Warfarin
Atladio, 299
Atopic sensitization, 61
Atrial ectopic foci, 157
Atromid-S; *see* Clofibrate
Atropine sulfate
    in arrhythmias
        discussion, 158
        dosage, 159
    as gastrointestinal tract anticholinergic
        discussion, 140
        dosage, 141
Attapulgite in diarrhea, dosage, 125
Aurcoloid; *see* Gold injection
Aurcoscan; *see* Gold injection
Aureomycin, dosage, 29
Aureotope; *see* Gold injection
Aventyl; *see* Nortriptyline hydrochloride
Avlosulfon in leprosy control, dosage, 37
Azathioprine in cancer
    discussion, 287-288
    dosage, 287
Azulfidine, dosage, 34

B

Bacitracin, discussion, 33
Bacteria
    invading, 15-43
        drug classification, 21
        response assessment, 17
    replacement in diarrhea, 126
Bacterial infection, 15-24
    drug effect in, 42-43
    patient care, 41-43
    pharmacodynamics, 18-24
    process of, 16
Bacterial resistance to drugs, 19-20
Bacterial toxins, agents for active immunization against, 70-71
Bactericidal effect, 19
Bacteriostatic drugs, 19
BAL; *see* Dimercaprol
Banthine, 141
Barachlor as antihistamine, dosage, 64
Barbital for sleep control
    discussion, 235
    dosages, 231
Barbitone; *see* Barbital
Barbiturates in sleep control
    discussion, 234-235
    overdosage, 235-236
Basaljel, 137
BCG vaccine, 70, 72
Belladonna leaf, tincture, 141
Benactyzine hydrochloride in anxiety states
    discussion, 211
    dosage, 210
Benadryl; *see* Diphenhydramine hydrochloride
Bendroflumethiazide in fluid control
    discussion, 101-102
    dosage, 101
Benemid; *see* Probenecid
Bentyl; *see* Dicyclomine hydrochloride
Benuron; *see* Bendroflumethiazide
Benzapas in tuberculosis control, dosage, 37
Benzedrine sulfate as appetite suppressant, dosage, 258
Benzodiazepines, 210
Benzonatate as cough suppressant
    discussion, 91
    dosage, 90
Benzoylpas calcium in tuberculosis control, dosage, 37
Benzphetamine hydrochloride as appetite suppressant, dosage, 258
Benzthiazide in fluid control
    discussion, 101-102
    dosage, 101
Benztropine mesylate in Parkinsonism, dosage, 220
Bephenium hydroxynaphthoate in helminthiasis
    discussion, 56
    dosage, 55
Berubigen; *see* Cyanocobalamin
Beta-Chlor for sleep control, dosage, 231
Betalin
    S; *see* Thiamine hydrochloride
    12; *see* Cyanocobalamin
Betamethasone, dosage, 76
Betapar, dosage, 76
Betavine-12; *see* Cyanocobalamin
Betaxin; *see* Thiamine hydrochloride

Bethanechol chloride in intestinal hypomotility, 143-144
Bevidoral as hematopoietic, 192
Bevidox; *see* Cyanocobalamin
Bicillin, dosage, 25
Bidtinic as hematopoietic, dosage, 192
Bifacton as hematopoietic, dosage, 192
Bile salt removal, 117
Bio-des, 299
Bio-Heprin; *see* Heparin sodium
Biological agents to detect exposure-induced sensitivity, 60
Biopar; *see* Cyanocobalamin
Biperiden in Parkinsonism, dosage, 220
Bisacodyl in constipation
   discussion, 123
   dosage, 122
Bishydroxycoumarin as anticoagulant
   discussion, 184, 185
   dosage, 185
Bismuth subcarbonate in diarrhea, dosage, 125
Blastomycin in dermal reaction test, 60
Bleomycin in cancer, discussion, 289
Blocking
   alpha adrenergic, in hypertension, 175-176
   ganglionic, in hypertension, 175
Blood
   alkalinity decreasing calcium absorption, 268
   -brain barrier, 5-6
   cells, red blood cell deficiency, 191-195
   clotting; *see* Clotting
   coagulation; *see* Coagulation
   flow, renal, 102
   gases, arterial, 83
   lipid levels, drugs used to lower, dosage range, 183
   pressure
      differentials, 171
      peripheral, maintenance of, drug dosage range, 167
   supply, myocardial, 147
Bonine; *see* Meclizine hydrochloride
Brain, blood-brain barrier, 5-6
Bretylium tosylate in cardiac arrhythmias
   discussion, 159-160
   dosage, 159
Brevital in sleep control, discussion, 235
Bromelains for intravascular clot removal
   discussion, 117-118
   dosage, 118
Brompheniramine maleate as antihistamine, dosage, 64
Bronchial constriction, 85-87
   adrenergic drugs in, 86-87
   patient care in, 87
   pharmacodynamics in, 85-87
   theophyllines in, 85-86
Bronchodilators, 85-87
   adverse effects, 86-87
   dosage range, 86
Broxolin; *see* Glaucarubin
Brucella protein nucleate in dermal reaction test, 60
Bubartal sodium for sleep control, dosage, 231
Buclamase; *see* Alpha amylase
Buclizine hydrochloride in anxiety states
   discussion, 210-211
   dosage, 210
Busulfan in cancer
   discussion, 288-289
   dosage, 287
Butabarbital sodium for sleep control, dosage, 231
Butaperazine maleate as antipsychotic, dosage, 205
Butazolidin; *see* Phenylbutazone
Butisol sodium for sleep control, dosage, 231

C

Caffeine and sodium benzoate as respiratory stimulant
   discussion, 88
   dosage, 88
Calciferol to control calcium ion levels, dosage, 268
Calcium
   absorption, blood alkalinity decreasing, 268
   balance assessment, 268
   carbonate, precipitated, 137
   chelation, 110
   disodium edetate in lead poisoning
      discussion, 110
      dosage, 110
      Disodium Versenate; *see* disodium edetate *above*
   gluconate to control calcium ion levels, dosage, 268
   iodide in respiratory tract secretion removal
      discussion, 91
      dosage, 91
   ion balance, 266-269
   ion level regulation
      cation replacement and, 269
      drugs for, dosage, 268
      maintenance of, schematic presentation, 267
      pharmacodynamics in, 268-269
   lactate to control calcium ion levels, dosage, 268
   sources, 267
Calurin for pain, dosage, 248
Camoquin; *see* Amodiaquine hydrochloride
Campolon; *see* Liver injection
Cancer, 283-294
   nursing guidelines, 291
   patient care in, 291-294
   pharmacodynamics in, 284-291
Cantil, 141
Capastat in tuberculosis control, dosage, 37
Capla; *see* Mebutamate
Capreomycin sulfate in tuberculosis control, dosage, 37
Caprokol; *see* Hexylresorcinol
Capromycin in tuberculosis control, dosage, 37
Caraspirin calcium for pain, dosage, 248
Carbamazepine for pain
   discussion, 251-252
   dosage, 250
Carbazochrome salicylate for antihemorrhagic effect, dosage, 188
Carbenicillin disodium, dosage, 25
Carbetapentane citrate as cough suppressant
   discussion, 91
   dosage, 90
Carbinoxamine maleate as antihistamine, dosage, 64
Carbon dioxide pressures, 84
Carbonic anhydrase inhibitors, 99-100
   dosage range of, 100
Cardiac; *see* Heart
Cardigin; *see* Digitoxin

Cardilate; see Erythrityl tetranitrate
Cardiomone; see Adenosine phosphate
Cardrase in fluid control, dosage, 100
Care, patient, 9-12
Carisoprodol as muscle relaxant, dosage, 228
Carmustine in cancer, discussion, 288
Carphenazine maleate as antipsychotic, dosage, 205
Caryolysine; see Mechlorethamine hydrochloride
Cascara sagrada in constipation
    discussion, 123
    dosage, 122
Castor oil in constipation
    discussion, 123
    dosage, 122
Catecholamine
    depletion in hypertension, 172-174
    release and vascular tone, 164
Cathartics, dosage range of, 122
Cathomycin; see Novobiocin sodium
Cedilanid; see Lanatoside C
Cedilanid-D, 151
Celestone, dosages, 76
Cell(s)
    proliferation, 283-294
        patient care, 291-294
        pharmacodynamics, 284-291
    red blood cell deficiency, 191-195
Cellothyl; see Methylcellulose
Celontin; see Methsuximide
Cendex; see Dextroamphetamines
Cephalexin monohydrate, dosage, 27
Cephaloglycin, dosage, 27
Cephaloridine, dosage, 27
Cephalosporins, 27
    adverse effects, 27
    dosage range of, 27
Cephalothin sodium
    dosage, 27
    microorganism susceptibility to, 20
Cerebrocortical activity, 213-223
Cerespan to dilate peripheral arteries, 180
Cero-O-Cillin, dosage, 25
Chelates, 109
    dosage range of, 110
Chel-Iron as hematopoietic, dosage, 192
Chemipen; see Potassium, phenethicillin
Chemoreceptor(s)
    arterial, 84
    medullary, 83-84
    trigger zone, emetic, 128-129
        stimulation of, 133
Chemotherapeutic drugs, 21
Chemotherapy, 21
Chestamine as antihistamine, dosage, 64
Children, dosage determination, 4
Chiniofon in amebiasis
    discussion, 49
    dosage, 48
Chlo-Amine as antihistamine, dosage, 64
Chlophedianol hydrochloride as cough suppressant
    discussion, 91
    dosage, 90
Chloral betaine for sleep control, dosage, 231
Chloral hydrate for sleep control
    discussion, 232-233
    dosage, 231
Chloramate, dosage, 64

Chlorambucil in cancer, dosage, 287
Chloramphenicol
    discussion, 32
    microorganism susceptibility to, 20
Chlorcyclizine hydrochloride, dosage, 64
Chlordiazepoxide in anxiety states
    discussion, 210
    dosages, 210
Chlorisondamine chloride in hypertension
    discussion, 175
    dosage, 173
Chlormerodrin in fluid control
    discussion, 101
    dosage, 101
Chlormezanone as muscle relaxant, dosage, 228
Chloroguanide hydrochloride in malaria
    discussion, 52
    dosage, 52
Chloromycetin, 32-33
Chloroquine in malaria
    discussion, 52
    dosage, 52
Chlorothen citrate, dosage, 64
Chlorothiazides in fluid control
    discussion, 102
    dosage, 101
Chlorotrianisene
    discussion, 300
    dosage, 299
Chlorphenesin carbamate as muscle relaxant, dosage, 228
Chlorpheniramine maleate, dosage, 64
Chlorphenoxamine hydrochloride in Parkinsonism, dosage, 220
Chlorphentermine hydrochloride in appetite suppression
    discussion, 259
    dosage, 258
Chlorpromazines
    dosage, 205
    sensitivity to light and, 209
Chlorpropamide as hypoglycemic
    discussion, 274
    dosage, 274
Chlorprothixene as antipsychotic, dosage, 205
Chlortetracycline hydrochloride, dosage, 29
Chlorthalidone in fluid control
    discussion, 101-102
    dosage, 101
Chlor-Trimeton, dosage, 64
Chlorzoxazone as muscle relaxant, dosage, 228
Choledyl in bronchial constriction, dosage, 86
Cholera vaccine, 70
Cholestyramine resin in bile salt removal
    discussion, 117
    dosage, 113
Choline salicylate for pain, dosage, 248
Cholinesterase inhibitors, 225-226
    dosage range of, 225
    patient care, 226
    pharmacodynamics, 225-226
Choloxin; see Dextrothyroxine sodium
Chorex as conception enhancer, 303-304
Chorigon as conception enhancer, 303-304
Chorionic gonadotrophin as conception enhancer, 303-304
Chymar; see Chymotrypsin

Chymotrypsin for intravascular clot removal
    discussion, 117-118
    dosage, 118
Cilloral penicillin; see Penicillin, G potassium
Claysorb in diarrhea, dosage, 125
Cleocin, dosage, 28
Clindamycin hydrochloride, dosage, 28
Clistin as antihistamine, dosage, 64
Clofibrate to lower blood lipid levels
    discussion, 183
    dosage, 183
Clotting; see also Coagulation
    clot-producing factors, 182-183
    factor replacement, 189
    prophylaxis, 183-188
        patient care, 187-188
        pharmacodynamics, 184-187
    removal
Cloxacillin sodium
    dosage, 25
    microorganism susceptibility to, 20
CMC cellulose; see Sodium carboxymethylcellulose
Coagulation, 182-190; see also Clotting
    deficits, 188-189
        pharmacodynamics in, 189
    factor replacement, 189
Cobra venom extract for pain
    discussion, 250
    dosage, 250
Cobroxin; see Cobra venom extract
Coccidioidin in dermal reaction test, 60
Coco-Diazine; see Sulfadiazine
Codeine sulfate
    discussion, 245-246
    dosage, 245
Codone; see Hydrocordone bitartrate
Cohistine as antihistamine, dosage, 64
Co-Hydeltra, dosage, 76
Colace; see Dioctyl sodium sulfosuccinate
Colchicine for pain, 251
Colchine for pain, 251
Colistimethate sodium, dosage, 30
Colistin sulfate
    dosage, 30
    microorganism susceptibility to, 20
Cologel; see Methylcellulose
Colon irritants, 123
Coly-Mycin
    M, dosage, 30
    S; see Colistin sulfate
Compazine as antipsychotic, dosages, 205
Compocillin-V, dosage, 25
Compocillin-VK, dosage, 25
Conception
    control; see Contraceptives, oral
    enhancers, 303-304
Conestron, 299
Congentin in Parkinsonism, dosage, 220
Constipation, 121-125
    patient care in, 124-125
    pharmacodynamics in, 122-124
Contraceptives, oral, 301-303
    adverse effects of, 302-303
    fixed combination program, 302
    pharmacodynamics, 301-303
    scheduled use, 302
    sequential program, 302

Contraction, skeletal muscle, 224-229
Convul; see Diphenylhydantoin
Copper chelation, 111
Coramine; see Nikethamide
Corn oil to lower blood lipid levels
    discussion, 182-183
    dosage, 183
Coronary artery
    constriction, 177-179
        patient care in, 179
        pharmacodynamics in, 177-179
    dilation, drug dosage range, 178
Cort-Dome, dosage, 76
Cortef, dosage, 76
Corticosterone, 73
Corticotropin; see ACTH
Cortifan, dosage, 76
Cortinazin; see Isoniazid
Cortisol, dosage, 76
Cortisone, 73
    dosage, 76
Cortivite, dosage, 76
Cortogen, dosage, 76
Cortone, dosage, 76
Cortril, dosage, 76
Cosmegen; see Dactinomycin
Cough suppressants, 90-91
    antihistaminic, 90-91
    dosage range of, 90
    local anesthetic, 91
    narcotic, 90
Coumadin; see Warfarin
Creamalin, 137
Cremodiazine; see Sulfadiazine
Cremothalidine, dosage, 34
Cryptenamine in hypertension
    discussion, 175
    dosage, 173
Crystamin; see Cyanocobalamin
Crysticillin, dosage, 25
Crystodigin; see Digitoxin
Crystoids; see Hexylresorcinol
Cuemid; see Cholestyramine resin
Cupertin as antihistamine, dosage, 64
Cupric sulfate in emesis induction
    discussion, 133
    dosage, 132
Cuprimine as copper chelate, 110, 111
Curariform drugs, 227
Cyanocobalamin in red blood cell deficiency
    discussion, 192
    dosage, 192
Cyantin in urinary tract infection, 36
Cyclamycin, dosage, 28
Cyclandelate to dilate peripheral arteries
    discussion, 179-180
    dosage, 180
Cyclizine hydrochloride in motion sickness
    discussion, 131
    dosage, 130
Cyclizine lactate as antiemetic, dosage, 130
Cyclophosphamide in cancer
    discussion, 288
    dosage, 287
Cyclopropane, 240
Cycloserine in tuberculosis control, dosage, 37
Cyclospasmol; see Cyclandelate

Cyclothiazide in fluid control
  discussion, 101-102
  dosage, 101
Cycrimine hydrochloride in Parkinsonism, dosage, 220
Cydril in appetite suppression, dosage, 258
Cyproheptadine hydrochloride, dosage, 64
Cytarabine in cancer
  discussion, 288
  dosage, 287
Cytellin; see Sitosterols
Cytolav; see Chymotrypsin
Cytomel; see Liothyronine sodium
Cytosar; see Cytarabine
Cytoserpine; see Reserpine
Cytoxan; see Cyclophosphamide

D

Dactil; see Piperidolate hydrochloride
Dactinomycin in cancer
  discussion, 289
  dosage, 287
Dalmane; see Flurazepam hydrochloride
Danilone; see Phenindione
Danten; see Diphenylhydantoin
Danthron in constipation
  discussion, 123
  dosage, 122
Dapsone in leprosy control, dosage, 37
Daranide in fluid control, dosage, 100
Darbid, 141
Darcil; see Potassium, phenethicillin
Darenthin; see Bretylium tosylate
Daricon; see Oxyphencyclimine hydrochloride
Daro-Tab; see Dextroamphetamines
Dartal as antipsychotic, dosage, 205
Darvon; see Propoxyphene hydrochloride
Daserol as muscle relaxant, dosage, 228
Daunomycin in cancer
  discussion, 289
  dosage, 287
Davoxin; see Digoxin
DBI; see Phenformin hydrochloride
Debris; see Tissue, debris
Decadron, dosage, 76
Deca-Durabolin; see Nandrolone
Decamethonium bromide and muscle contraction, 227
Decapryn as antihistamine, dosage, 64
Declomycin, dosage, 29
Deferoxamine mesylate in iron poisoning
  discussion, 111
  dosage, 110
Delatestryl; see Testosterone
Delestrogen, 299
Delivery, dosage range of drugs used during, 306
Delta-Cortef, dosage, 76
Deltasone, dosage, 76
Deltra, dosage, 76
Delvinal for sleep control, dosage, 231
Demeclocycline hydrochloride, dosage, 29
Demerol; see Meperidine hydrochloride
Denyl; see Diphenylhydantoin
Deoxycorticosterones for aldosterone replacement, 98
Depo-estradiol, 299
Depo-Medrol, dosage, 76

Depo-testosterone cypionate, dosage, 297
Dermatitis, contact, 63
Deronil, dosage, 76
DES, 299
Desensitization, 61
Deserpidine in hypertension
  discussion, 172-174
  dosage, 173
Desferal; see Deferoxamine mesylate
Desipramine hydrochloride in psychic depression
  discussion, 202-203
  dosage, 201
Deslanoside, 151
Desoxyn; see Methamphetamine hydrochloride
Desyphed; see Methamphetamine hydrochloride
Dexameth, dosage, 76
Dexamethasone, dosage, 76
Dexbrompheniramine maleate, dosage, 64
Dexchlorpheniramine maleate, dosage, 64
Dexedrine sulfate; see Dextroamphetamines
Dexoval; see Methamphetamine hydrochloride
Dexstim; see Methamphetamine hydrochloride
Dextroamphetamines in appetite suppression
  discussion, 259
  dosage, 258
Dextromethorphan hydrobromide as cough suppressant
  discussion, 90
  dosage, 90
Dextromoramide tartrate for pain
  discussion, 246-247
  dosage, 245
Dextrose in fluid control, 103
Dextrothyroxine sodium to lower blood lipid levels
  discussion, 183
  dosage, 183
Diabetes mellitus, 271
  acidosis in, 272
Diabinese; see Chlorpropamide
Diafen as antihistamine, dosage, 64
Diamox in fluid control, dosage, 100
Dianabol in protein building, dosage, 261
Diapid for ADH replacement, 98
Diarrhea, 125-127
  drugs for, dosage range of, 125
  patient care in, 126-127
  pharmacodynamics in, 125-126
Diasone in leprosy control, dosage, 37
Diathesis, 213
Diazepam in anxiety states
  discussion, 210
  dosage, 210
Dibasic calcium phosphate to control calcium ion levels, dosage, 268
Dibenzyline; see Phenoxybenzamine hydrochloride
Dichlorophen in helminthiasis
  discussion, 55-56
  dosage, 55
Dichlorphenamide in fluid control, dosage, 100
Dicloxacillin sodium, dosage, 25
Dicodid; see Hydrocodone bitartrate
Dicumarol; see Bishydroxycoumarin
Dicyclomine hydrochloride
  discussion, 141-142
  dosage, 142
Didrex as appetite suppressant, dosage, 258
Dienestrol, 299

Diethyl oxide, 240
Diethylpropion hydrochloride in appetite suppression, dosage, 258
Diethylstilbestrol, 299
Digisidin; see Digitoxin
Digitaline Nativelle; see Digitoxin
Digitalis
  adverse effects of, 152-154
  discussion, 150-154
  dosages, 151
  nursing guidelines, 154-155
Digitalization, 151
Digitol; see Digitalis
Digitoxin
  discussion, 152
  dosage, 151
Digoxin
  discussion, 152
  dosage, 151
Dihycon; see Diphenylhydantoin
Dihydroxyaluminum aminoacetate as antacid, 137
Diiodohydroxyquin in amebiasis
  discussion, 49
  dosage, 48
Di-Lan; see Diphenylhydantoin
Dilantin; see Diphenylhydantoin
Dilaudid; see Hydromorphone hydrochloride
Dilor in bronchial constriction, dosage, 86
Diloxanide in amebiasis
  discussion, 49
  dosage, 48
Dimenformon; see Estradiol
Dimenhydrinate in motion sickness
  discussion, 131
  dosage, 130
Dimercaprol in arsenic, mercury and gold ingestion
  discussion, 111
  dosage, 110
Dimetane, dosage, 64
Dimethindene maleate, dosage, 64
Dimethone for pain, dosage, 248
Dimethyl tubocurarine iodide and muscle contraction, 227
Dimethylane as muscle relaxant, dosage, 228
Dimocillin-RT; see Methicillin sodium
Dimothyn, 137
Dinacrin; see Isoniazid
Dioctyl calcium sulfosuccinate in constipation
  discussion, 122-123
  dosage, 122
Dioctyl sodium sulfosuccinate in constipation
  discussion, 122-123
  dosage, 122
Diodoquin; see Diiodohydroxyquin
Diogyn; see Estradiol
Diogynets; see Estradiol
Diolandrone in protein building, dosage, 261
Dioloxol as muscle relaxant, dosage, 228
Diovac; see Dioctyl sodium sulfosuccinate
Dioxyline to dilate peripheral arteries
  discussion, 179-180
  dosage, 180
Di-Paralene, dosage, 64
Diphasol testosterone; see Testosterone
Diphemanil methylsulfate, 141
Diphenhydramine hydrochloride
  as antihistamine, dosage, 64

Diphenhydramine hydrochloride—cont'd
  as cough suppressant
    discussion, 91
    dosage, 90
Diphenidol hydrochloride in motion sickness
  discussion, 131
  dosage, 130
Diphenoxylate hydrochloride in diarrhea
  discussion, 126
  dosage, 125
Diphenylan sodium; see Diphenylhydantoin
Diphenylhydantoin
  in cardiac arrhythmias
    discussion, 160-161
    dosage, 159
  in seizure control
    discussion, 216-217
    dosage, 215
Diphenylpyraline hydrochloride, dosage, 64
Diphtheria toxin, 60
Diphtheria toxoid, 70
Diphylline in bronchial constriction, dosage, 86
Dipyridamole as anticoagulant
  discussion, 187
  dosage, 185
Dipyrone for pain, dosage, 248
Disipal in Parkinsonism, dosage, 220
Disodium edetate, 110
Disomer, dosage, 64
Disulfiram
  alcohol-containing medications and, 10
  in emesis induction
    discussion, 133
    dosage, 132
Ditubin; see Isoniazid
Diucardyn; see Mercaptomerin sodium
Diuretics, 99-103
  dosage range of, 100, 101
  osmotic, 102-103
  potassium-sparing, 99
Diuril; see Chlorothiazides
Diurnalpenicillin, dosage, 25
Divercillin; see Ampicillin
Divinyl oxide, 240
Docibin; see Cyanocobalamin
Dodecavite; see Cyanocobalamin
Dodekroid; see Cyanocobalamin
D-O-E; see Methamphetamine hydrochloride
Dolophine; see Methadone
L-Dopa; see Levodopa
Dopamine
  in peripheral blood pressure maintenance
    discussion, 168
    dosage, 167
  replacement in Parkinsonism, 220-221
Dopar; see Levodopa
Dopram; see Doxapram hydrochloride
Doraxamin, 137
Dorbane; see Danthron
Doriden; see Glutethimide
Dormethan; see Dextromethorphan hydrobromide
Dormin, dosage, 64
Dorsaphyllin in bronchial constriction, dosage, 86
Dosage
  determination based on body surface area, 4
  -response relationships, 3-4

Doxapram hydrochloride as respiratory stimulant
   discussion, 88
   dosage, 88
Doxepin hydrochloride in psychic depression
   discussion, 202-203
   dosage, 201
Doxical; see Dioctyl calcium sulfosuccinate
Doxinate; see Dioctyl sodium sulfosuccinate
Doxol; see Dioctyl sodium sulfosuccinate
Doxycycline hyelate, dosage, 29
Doxylamine succinate, dosage, 64
Doxyphed; see Methamphetamine hydrochloride
Dramamine; see Dimenhydrinate
Dramcillin; see Penicillin, G potassium
Dramcillin-S; see Potassium, phenethicillin
Drinalfa; see Methamphetamine hydrochloride
Drisdol to control calcium ion levels, dosage, 268
Drize, dosage, 64
Drodecavite; see Cyanocobalamin
Drolban, dosage, 297
Dromostanolone proprionate, dosage, 297
Dropcillin; see Penicillin, G potassium
Droperidol, dosage, 205
Drostene in protein building, dosage, 261
Drug(s)
   absorption of, 5
   abuse; see Addiction
   action summation, 8-9
   administration routes, 9-12
   antagonism, 8
   dependence; see Addiction
   distribution in body, 5-6
   distribution, legal regulation of, 2-3
   effects of
      adverse, 6-7
      cumulative, 6
   F.D.A. controls, 3
   individual responses to, 7
   interactions, 8-9
   protein binding, 5
   standards, official, 2
   therapy, 1-12
   trials, clinical, 1-2
Ducobee-Hy; see Hydroxocobalamin
Dulcolax; see Bisacodyl
Duphaston, 301
Durabolin; see Nandrolone
Duracillin, dosage, 25
Dura-estradiol, 299
Duratrad, 299
Dydrogesterone, 301
Dymelor; see Acetohexamide
Dynapen, dosage, 25
Dyrenium in fluid control, 99

E

Ecolid; see Chlorisondamine chloride
Ecotrin; see Acetylsalicylic acid
E.C.T. (enteric-coated tablet), 10
Edecrin in fluid control, dosage, 101
Edecrin sodium; see Ethacrynate sodium
Edrophonium chloride and muscle contraction, 227
Efedron; see Ephedrine hydrochloride
Efroxine; see Methamphetamine hydrochloride
EKKO; see Diphenylhydantoin
Elavil; see Amitriptyline hydrochloride
Eldofe as hematopoietic, dosage, 192

Electrolyte balance, kidney in, 94-96
Elixophyllin; see Theophylline
Elkosin, dosage, 34
Elorine, 141
Elpandryl as appetite suppressant, dosage, 258
Emesis, 128-134
   chemoreceptor trigger zone, 128-129
      stimulation of, 133
   induction, 132-134
      patient care in, 133-134
      pharmacodynamics in, 132-133
   patient care in, 131-132
   pharmacodynamics in, 130-131
   stimuli, 129-130
   vomiting center response, 128
   vomiting center stimulation, 133
Emetics, dosage range of, 132
Emetine in amebiasis
   discussion, 48-49
   dosage, 48
Emivan; see Ethamivan
Emotional responses, 199-212
E-Mycin; see Erythromycin
Emyclamate in anxiety states
   discussion, 209-210
   dosage, 210
Encephalitis, herpes simplex, idoxuridine in, 67
Endothyrin for thyroid hormone control, dosage, 266
Endotracheal tube in place, diagram, 88
Endoxan; see Cyclophosphamide
Endrate, 110
Enduron; see Methylclothiazide
Enkide; see Potassium iodide
EN-tabs, dosage, 34
Entamide; see Diloxanide
Enteric-coated tablet (E.C.T.), 10
Enteric elimination, 121-127
Enterogastric reflex, 137
Entero-Vioform; see Glycobiarsol
Environmental poisons, 108
Enzeon; see Chymotrypsin
Enzymes, microsomal liver enzyme system, 6
Ephedrine hydrochloride to maintain peripheral blood pressure
   discussion, 167-168
   dosage, 167
Ephetonin; see Ephedrine hydrochloride
Epinephrine hydrochloride
   in bronchial constriction, 86
   to maintain peripheral blood pressure
      discussion, 167
      dosage, 167
Episcorb; see Epinephrine hydrochloride
Equanil; see Meprobamate
Equilibrium; see Hemodynamic equilibrium
Ergonovine maleate for labor induction
   discussion, 306
   dosage, 306
Ergotrate maleate; see Ergonovine maleate
Erythrityl tetranitrate to dilate coronary arteries
   discussion, 178
   dosage, 178
Erythroblastosis fetalis, 69
Erythrocin; see Erythromycin
Erythrocyte deficiency, 191-195
Erythrol; see Erythrityl tetranitrate

Erythromycins, 27-28
    administration, 28
    adverse effects, 28
    dosages, 28
    elimination route, 27-28
    microorganism susceptibility to, 20
Erythropoiesis, 191-193
    pharmacodynamics in, 192-193
Esidrex; see Hydrochlorothiazide
Eskalith; see Lithium carbonate
Eskaserp; see Reserpine
Estate, 299
Esteed, 299
Estinyl, 299
Estradiol
    discussion, 300
    dosages, 299
Estradurin, 299
Estra-L, 299
Estraldine; see Estradiol
Estraval, 299
Estrifol, 299
Estrobev-E, 299
Estrogen(s)
    dosage range of, 299
    estrogenic substances, conjugated, 299
    -progesterone balance, 297-298
    therapy, 299-300
Estrone
    discussion, 300
    dosage, 299
Estrovarin; see Estrone
Estrugenone; see Estrone
Estrusol; see Estrone
Ethacrynate sodium in fluid control
    discussion, 102
    dosage, 101
Ethacrynic acid in fluid control, dosage, 101
Ethambutol hydrochloride in tuberculosis control
    discussion, 41
    dosage, 37
Ethamide in fluid control, dosage, 100
Ethamivan as respiratory stimulant
    discussion, 88
    dosage, 88
Ethchlorvynol for sleep control
    discussion, 234
    dosage, 231
Ether, 240
Ethinamate for sleep control
    discussion, 234
    dosage, 231
Ethinoral, 299
Ethinyl estradiol, 299
Ethionamide in tuberculosis control
    discussion, 41
    dosage, 37
Ethisterone, 301
Ethoheptazine citrate for pain
    discussion, 250
    dosage, 250
Ethopropazine hydrochloride in Parkinsonism, dosage, 220
Ethosuximide in seizure control
    discussion, 215
    dosage, 215
Ethotoin in seizure control, dosage, 215

Ethoxazene hydrochloride in urinary tract infection, 36
Ethoxzolamide in fluid control, dosage, 100
Ethyl chloride
    for inhalation anesthesia, 240
    for topical anesthesia, 242
Ethylene, 240
Ethylestrenol in protein building, dosage, 261
Eticylol, 299
Eutonyl; see Pargyline hydrochloride
Evronal; see Secobarbital sodium
Exna; see Benzthiazide
Expectorants, 91-92
    dosage range, 91

F

Factor IX complex (human) for antihemorrhagic effect, dosage, 188
F-Cortef; see Fludrocortisone acetate
F.D.A. controls on drugs, 3
Febrolin; see Acetaminophen
Fecal softeners, 122-123
    dosage range of, 122
Felsules; see Chloral hydrate
Female sex cycle, 295-296
Fendon; see Acetaminophen
Fentanyl citrate for pain
    discussion, 247
    dosage, 245
Feosol; see Ferrous sulfate
Fergon as hematopoietic, dosage, 192
Fer-in-Sol; see Ferrous sulfate
Ferralyn; see Ferrous sulfate
Ferro drops; see Ferrous lactate
Ferrocholinate as hematopoietic, dosage, 192
Ferrolip as hematopoietic, dosage, 192
Ferrous fumarate as hematopoietic, dosage, 192
Ferrous gluconate as hematopoietic, dosage, 192
Ferrous lactate
    as hematopoietic, dosage, 192
    in hemoglobin production, 193-194
Ferrous sulfate
    as hematopoietic, dosage, 192
    in hemoglobin production, 193
Fertility, 295-307
Fertilization
    cessation, 303
        pharmacodynamics in, 303
    inhibition, 303
        pharmacodynamics in, 303
Fibrinogen (human) for antihemorrhagic effect, dosage, 188
Fibrinolysin for intravascular clot removal
    discussion, 117-118
    dosage, 118
Firon as hematopoietic, dosage, 192
Flavoxate hydrochloride
    discussion, 142-143
    dosage, 142
Flaxedil and muscle contraction, 227
Florinef; see Fludrocortisone acetate
Floxuridine in cancer
    discussion, 288
    dosage, 287
Flucytosine in fungal infection
    discussion, 46
    dosage, 45

Fludrocortisone acetate
  administration, 75
  dosage, 76
Fluid
  adsorbents, 125-126
  balance, 94-107
    renal controls, 94-96
  control
    drugs in, effects of, 105-106
    nursing guidelines, 104-105
    patient care, 104-106
    pharmacodynamics, 98-104
  imbalance, 97-106
  tissue; see Tissue, fluid
Flumethiazide in fluid control
  discussion, 102
  dosage, 101
Fluorouracil in cancer
  discussion, 288
  dosage, 287
Fluoxymesterone, dosage, 297
Fluphenazine enanthate, dosage, 205
Fluphenazine hydrochloride, dosage, 205
Fluprednisolone, dosage, 76
Flurazepam hydrochloride in sleep control
  discussion, 234
  dosage, 231
Folate sodium as hematopoietic, dosage, 192
Folic acid
  antagonists, in cancer, 288
  as hematopoietic
    discussion, 192
    dosage, 192
Follutein as conception enhancer, 303-304
Folvite; see Folic acid
Folvite sodium as hematopoietic, dosage, 192
Foods
  anticoagulants and, 187-188
  monoamide oxidase inhibitors and, 202
Forhistal as antihistamine, dosage, 64
Fortizyme; see Alpha amylase
Fuadin; see Stibophen
FUDR; see Floxuridine
Fulvicin; see Griseofulvin
Fumasorb as hematopoietic, dosage, 192
Fumeron as hematopoietic, dosage, 192
Fungizone; see Amphotericin B
Fungus
  eradication, systemic, 45-47
  identification, 44
  invasion, 44-57
    patient care in, 47
    pharmacodynamics in, 44-47
Furachel in urinary tract infection, 36
Furadantin in urinary tract infection, 36
Furalan in urinary tract infection, 36
Furamide; see Diloxanide, furoate
Furosemide in fluid control
  discussion, 102
  dosage, 101

G

Gallamine triethiodide and muscle contraction, 227
Gamatrin; see Alverine citrate
Gammacorten, dosage, 76
Ganglionic blocking agents in hypertension, 175
Gantanol, dosage, 34

Gantrisin, dosages, 34
Garamycin; see Gentamicin sulfate
Gases, arterial blood, 83
Gastric
  acidity, 135-144
  antacids; see Antacids, gastric
  hyperacidity, 136-139
    patient care, 138-139
    pharmacodynamics in, 137-138
  secretion control, 139-143
    patient care in, 143
    pharmacodynamics in, 139-143
Gelusil, 137
Gemonil; see Metharbital
Genomes, 66
Gentamicin sulfate
  discussion, 32
  dosage, 30
Geopen, dosage, 25
Gitaligin; see Gitalin
Gitalin
  discussion, 152
  dosage, 151
Glarubin; see Emetine
Glaucarubin in amebiasis
  discussion, 49
  dosage, 48
Globulins
  animal serum, 68-69
  human serum, 69
Glucagon
  cardiac output and, 154
  hypoglycemia and, 273
Glucocorticoid(s)
  administration, 74-76
  biochemical actions of, 77
  dosage range of, 76
  levels, hypothalamic-pituitary-adrenal hormonal interaction and, 73
Glucokinase, 271
Glucose
  assimilation, 271-279
  insulin and, 273
Glucotropin-Forte as conception enhancer, 303-304
Glutavene; see Sodium glutamate
Glutethimide for sleep control
  discussion, 234
  dosage, 231
Glycerin in fluid control, 103
Glyceryl guaiacolate in respiratory tract secretion removal, dosage, 91
Glyceryl trinitrate to dilate coronary arteries
  discussion, 178-179
  dosage, 178
Glycobiarsol in amebiasis
  discussion, 49
  dosage, 48
Glycopyrrolate, 141
Glynazan in bronchial constriction, dosage, 86
Glyrol in fluid control, 103
Glysennid; see Sennosides A and B
Gold chelation, 111
Gold (AU[198]) injection in cancer
  discussion, 289
  dosage, 287
Gonadal function, 295-307
  pharmacodynamics in, 296-301

Gonadotrophin as conception enhancer, chorionic, 303-304
Grand mal seizures, 214
Grifulvin; see Griseofulvin
Grisactin; see Griseofulvin
Griseofulvin in fungus eradication
  discussion, 44-45
  dosages, 45
Guanethidine sulfate in hypertension
  discussion, 174
  dosage, 173

H

Haldol as antipsychotic, dosage, 205
Haldrone, dosage, 76
Haloperidol as antipsychotic, dosage, 205
Halotestin, dosage, 297
Halothane, 240
Harmonyl; see Deserpidine
Heart
  arrhythmias; see Arrhythmias
  chamber distention, 150-155
  conduction-contraction sequence, 156
  conduction pathway, 149
  contraction force, 149-150
  ectopic foci, 156-157
  output, 147-155
    glucagon and, 154
    maintenance, patient care in, 154-155
    maintenance, pharmacodynamics in, 150-154
Hedulin; see Phenindione
Helminthiasis, 54-57
  extraintestinal, 55
  intestinal, 54-55
  patient care in, 56-57
  pharmacodynamics in, 55-56
Hematopoietic agents, dosage range of, 192
Hemodynamic equilibrium, disrupted, 166-169
  compensatory mechanisms, 166-167
  patient care in, 168-169
  pharmacodynamics in, 167-168
Hemofil for antihemorrhagic effect, dosage, 188
Hemoglobin production, 193-194
  pharmacodynamics in, 193-194
Hemolysin, 18
Henle's loop transport mechanisms, 95
Heparin sodium as anticoagulant
  discussion, 184-186
  dosage, 185
Hepathrom; see Heparin sodium
Herpes simplex encephalitis, idoxuridine in, 67
Hetacillin, dosages, 25
Hexadrol, dosage, 76
Hexafluorenium bromide and muscle contraction, 227
Hexobarbital in sleep control
  discussion, 234
  dosage, 231
Hexocyclium methylsulfate, 141
Hexylresorcinol in helminthiasis
  discussion, 56
  dosage, 55
Hispril, dosage, 64
Histachlor, dosage, 64
Histadur, dosage, 64
Histadyl, dosage, 64

Histamine, 61-62
  inhibition, 63-66
    patient care, 65-66
    pharmacodynamics in, 63-65
Histaspan, dosage, 64
Histitrin, dosage, 64
Histoplasmin in dermal reaction test, 60
Histrey, dosage, 64
Homatropine methylbromide, 141
Hookworms, 54
Hormesteral, 299
Hormone(s)
  adrenocorticotropic; see ACTH
  antidiuretic; see Antidiuretic hormone
  in cancer, 284
  controls of fluid balance, 96-97
  parathyroid; see Parathyroid hormone
  pituitary; see Pituitary hormone
  thyroid; see Thyroid, hormone
Humatin, dosage, 30
Humoral immunity, 58-59
Hyaluronidase, 18
Hydeltra, dosages, 76
Hydeltrasol, dosage, 76
Hydralazine hydrochloride in hypertension
  discussion, 175
  dosage, 173
Hydrea; see Hydroxyurea
Hydriodic acid for removal of respiratory tract secretions
  discussion, 91
  dosage, 91
Hydrocalciferol to control calcium ion levels
  discussion, 269
  dosage, 268
Hydrochlorothiazide in fluid control
  discussion, 102
  dosage, 101
Hydrocodone bitartrate as cough suppressant
  discussion, 90
  dosage, 90
Hydrocortisone, dosage, 76
Hydrocortone, dosage, 76
Hydro-Diuril; see Hydrochlorothiazide
Hydroflumethiazide in fluid control
  discussion, 101-102
  dosage, 101
Hydrolose; see Methylcellulose
Hydromorphone hydrochloride for pain
  discussion, 246-247
  dosage, 245
Hydromox; see Quinethazone
Hydroxocobalamin as hematopoietic
  discussion, 192
  dosage, 192
Hydroxychloroquine sulfate in malaria
  discussion, 52
  dosage, 52
Hydroxyprogesterone caproate, 301
Hydroxyurea in cancer
  discussion, 288
  dosage, 287
Hydroxyzine hydrochloride in anxiety states
  discussion, 210-211
  dosage, 210
Hydroxyzine pamoate in anxiety states, dosage, 210
Hygroton; see Chlorthalidone

Hykinone, dosage, 185
Hypercalcemia, 267-268
Hyperpnea, 272
Hypersensitivity reactions to anesthetics, 243
Hypertensin; see Angiotensin amide
Hypertension, 172-177
  drugs in, dosage range, 173
  patient care in, 176-177
  pharmacodynamics in, 172-176
Hypertonicity; see Muscle, hypertonicity of
Hypnotics
  dosage range of, 231
  overdosage, 235-236
Hypocalcemia, 267
Hypoglycemia, epinephrine and glucagon release, 273
Hypoglycemic drugs, oral
  discussion, 274-275
  dosage range, 274
Hypoxia, myocardial, and coronary artery constriction, 178
Hytakerol; see Hydrocalciferol

I

Idoxuridine in herpes simplex encephalitis, 67
Ilosone, dosage, 28
Ilotycin; see Erythromycin
Imferon; see Iron dextran injection
Imipramine hydrochloride in psychic depression
  discussion, 202-203
  dosage, 201
Immune responses, 58-80
Immunity
  active, 69, 72-73
    relationship between passive immunity and, 67
  building, 66-67
  humoral, 58-59
  passive, 68-69
    relationship to active immunity, 67
  tissue, 59
Immunization, 67-73
  agents used for, 70-71
Imuran; see Azathioprine
Inapsine, dosage, 205
Inderal; see Propranolol hydrochloride
Indocin; see Indomethacin
Indomethacin for pain
  discussion, 251
  dosage, 250
Indon; see Phenindione
Inestra, 299
Infection; see Bacterial infection
Inflammatory response suppression, 73-79
  drug effect, assessment of, 77
    adverse effects, 77-79
  patient care in, 76-79
  pharmacodynamics in, 74-76
Influenza
  strain shift, concept of, 73
  vaccine, 70
INH; see Isoniazid
Inhalation anesthesia; see Anesthesia, inhalation
Inhiston as antihistamine, dosage, 64
Inositol hexanitrate to dilate coronary arteries, dosage, 178
Insulin
  deficiency, 271-272

Insulin—cont'd
  excess, 272-279
    patient care in, 277-279
    pharmacodynamics in, 274-277
  glucose and, 273
Interferons and viral resistance, 66
Intestine
  hypermotility, 139-143
    patient care in, 143
    pharmacodynamics in, 139-143
  hypomotility, 143-144
    patient care in, 144
    pharmacodynamics in, 143
  lubricant, 122
    dosage, 122
  motility, 135-144
Intrinase as hematopoietic, 192
Inversine; see Mecamylamine hydrochloride
Iodinated glycerol
  discussion, 91
  dosage, 91
Iodine solution, for thyroid hormone control, dosage, 266
Iodism, 91
Iodochlorhydroxyquin in amebiasis
  discussion, 49
  dosage, 48
Iodotope; see Sodium iodide
Ionamin as appetite suppressant, dosage, 258
Ioquin; see Diiodohydroxyquin
Iothiouracil sodium for thyroid hormone control
  discussion, 264-265
  dosage, 266
Ipecac in emesis induction
  discussion, 132-133
  dosage, 132
Iphyllin in bronchial constriction, dosage, 86
Ipral in sleep control, dosage, 231
Ircon as hematopoietic, dosage, 192
Iron chelation, 110-111
Iron dextran injection
  as hematopoietic, dosage, 192
  in hemoglobin production, 194
Iron sorbitex
  as hematopoietic, dosage, 192
  in hemoglobin production, 194
Ismelin; see Guanethidine sulfate
Isobarb; see Pentobarbital sodium
Isocarboxazid in psychic depression, dosage, 201
Isocrin; see Oxyphenisatin acetate
Isoject, dosage, 25
Isolyn; see Isoniazid
Isoniazid in tuberculosis control
  discussion, 39-40
  dosage, 37
Isopropamide, 141
Isoproterenol hydrochloride
  in bronchial constriction, 87
  in cardiac arrhythmias
    discussion, 159
    dosage, 159
  to maintain peripheral blood pressure
    discussion, 167-168
    dosage, 167
Isordil; see Isosorbide dinitrate

Isosorbide dinitrate to dilate coronary arteries
  discussion, 178
  dosage, 178
Isoxsuprine hydrochloride to dilate peripheral arteries
  discussion, 179-180
  dosage, 180
Istizin; *see* Danthron
Isuprel; *see* Isoproterenol hydrochloride
Itrumil; *see* Iothiouracil sodium
I.V., dosage, 28

J

Jacksonian seizures, 214
Jactofer; *see* Iron sorbitex

K

Kafocin, dosage, 25
Kanamycin sulfate
  discussion, 32
  dosage, 30
  microorganism susceptibility to, 20
Kantrex; *see* Kanamycin sulfate
Kaolin and pectin in diarrhea
  discussion, 125-126
  dosage, 125
Kaopectate; *see* Kaolin and pectin
Kappadione as anticoagulant inactivator, dosage, 185
Kappaxin as anticoagulant inactivator, dosage, 185
Kayexalate; *see* Polystyrene sodium sulfonate
Kayklot as anticoagulant inactivator, dosage, 185
Kayquinone as anticoagulant inactivator, dosage, 185
Keflex, dosage, 27
Keflin; *see* Cephalothin sodium
Kemadrin; *see* Procyclidine hydrochloride
Kenacort, dosage, 76
Kenalog, dosage, 76
Khorion as conception enhancer, 303-304
Kidney
  blood flow increase, 102
  role in fluid and electrolyte balance, 94-96
  -specific drugs, 36
Koglucoid; *see* Alseroxylon
Kolklot as anticoagulant inactivator, dosage, 185
Konakion as anticoagulant inactivator, dosage, 185
Konogen, 299
Konyne for antihemorrhagic effect, dosage, 188
Kynex, dosage, 34

L

Labor
  drugs used during, dosage range of, 306
  induction, 304-306
    pharmacodynamics in, 304-306
Lactobacillus acidophilus in diarrhea
  discussion, 126
  dosage, 125
Lactobacillus bulgaricus in diarrhea
  discussion, 126
  dosage, 125
Lanatoside C
  discussion, 152
  dosage, 151
Lanaxin; *see* Digoxin
Largon; *see* Propriomazine hydrochloride
Larodopa; *see* Levodopa
Lasix; *see* Furosemide
L-asparaginase; *see* Asparaginase
Lastrogen, 299
Lavema; *see* Oxyphenisatin acetate
L-dopa; *see* Levodopa
Lead chelation, 111
Ledercillin VK, dosage, 25
Legal regulation of drug distribution, 2-3
Leprosy, 37-39
  lepromatous-type, 37-38
  tuberculoid-type, 38
Leritine; *see* Anileridine
Lescopine, 141
Letter for thyroid hormone control, dosage, 266
Leukeran in cancer, dosage, 287
Leukocytosis-promoting factor, 16
Levallorphan tartrate in respiratory depression, 89
Levarterenol bitartrate to maintain peripheral blood pressure
  discussion, 168
  dosage, 167
Levodopa in Parkinsonism
  discussion, 220-221
  dosage, 220
Levo-Dromoran; *see* Levorphanol tartrate
Levoid for thyroid hormone control, dosage, 266
Levophed; *see* Levarterenol bitartrate
Levoprome; *see* Methotrimeprazine hydrochloride
Levopropoxyphene napsylate as cough suppressant
  discussion, 90
  dosage, 90
Levorphanol tartrate for pain
  discussion, 246-247
  dosage, 245
Levothyroxine sodium for thyroid hormone control, dosage, 266
Libigen as conception enhancer, 303-304
Libritabs; *see* Chlordiazepoxide
Librium; *see* Chlordiazepoxide
Lidocaine hydrochloride
  in cardiac arrhythmias
    discussion, 160, 161
    dosage, 159
  as topical anesthetic, 242-243
Linampheta as appetite suppressant, dosage, 258
Lincocin; *see* Lincomycin
Lincomycin hydrochloride
  dosage, 28
  microorganism susceptibility to, 20
Liothyronine sodium for thyroid hormone control
  discussion, 266
  dosage, 266
Lipid levels, blood, dosage range of drugs used to lower, 183
Lipo-Diazine; *see* Sulfadiazine
Lipo-Hepin; *see* Heparin sodium
Lipo-Lutin, 301
Liquaemin; *see* Heparin sodium
Liquamar; *see* Phenprocoumon
Liquiprin for pain, dosage, 248
Lithane; *see* Lithium carbonate
Lithium carbondate in psychic depression
  discussion, 203
  dosage, 201
Lithonate; *see* Lithium carbonate
Liver
  enzyme system, microsomal, 6

Liver—cont'd
  injection
    discussion, 192
    dosage, 192
Lomotil; see Diphenoxylate hydrochloride
Lorfan in respiratory depression, 89
Loridine, dosage, 27
Lorinal; see Chloral hydrate
Lotusate for sleep control, dosage, 231
Lubricants, intestinal, 122
  dosage range of, 122
Lucorteum, 301
Lugol's solution for thyroid hormone control, dosage, 266
Lullamin as antihistamine, dosage, 64
Luminal sodium in sleep control, dosage, 231
Lung ventilation, 83-93
Lutocylin, 301
Lutocylol, 301
Luton as conception enhancer, 303-304
Lutromone, 301
Lymphatic vessels and cancer tissue extension, 285
Lymphogranuloma venereum antigen in dermal reaction test, 60
Lynoral, 299
Lyovac; see Chlorothiazide
Lyovac sodium Edecrin; see Ethacrynate sodium
Lypressin for ADH replacement, 98
Lysodren; see Mitotane
Lyteca; see Acetaminophen

M

Maalox, 137
Macrodantin in urinary tract infection, 36
Macrophage activity during bacterial infection, 17
Madribon, dosage, 34
Madriqid, dosage, 34
Magaldrate
  discussion, 138
  dosage, 137
Magcyl; see Poloxalkol
Magmasil, 137
Magnesium carbonate as antacid, 137
Magnesium citrate in constipation
  discussion, 124
  dosage, 122
Magnesium hydroxide in constipation
  discussion, 124
  dosage, 122
Magnesium oxidase, 137
Magnesium sulfate
  in constipation
    discussion, 124
    dosage, 122
  in seizure control
    discussion, 215
    dosage, 215
Magnesium trisilicate, 137
Magsal, 137
Malaria, 50-54
  benign tertian, 50-51
  cure, 52
  patient care, 53-54
  pernicious malignant, 51
  pharmacodynamics in, 51-53
  prophylaxis, suppressive, 52
  therapy terminology, 51-52

Malestrone; see Testosterone
Malnutrition, 257-263
Manicole to dilate coronary arteries, dosage, 178
Mannitol in fluid control, 103
Mannitol hexanitrate, to dilate coronary arteries, dosage, 178
Maolate as muscle relaxant, dosage, 228
Marcumar; see Phenprocoumon
Marezine hydrochloride; see Cyclizine hydrochloride
Marezine lactate as antiemetic, dosage, 130
Marplan in psychic depression, dosage, 201
Masenate, dosage, 297
Masenone, dosage, 297
Matromycin; see Oleandomycin phosphate
Matulane; see Procarbazine hydrochloride
Maxibolin in protein building, dosage, 261
Maxipen; see Potassium phenethicillin
Maxitate to dilate coronary arteries, dosage, 178
Measles virus vaccine, 70
Mebaral; see Mephobarbital
Mebutamate in anxiety states
  discussion, 209-210
  dosage, 210
Mecamylamine hydrochloride in hypertension
  discussion, 175
  dosage, 173
Mechlorethamine hydrochloride in cancer
  discussion, 288
  dosage, 287
Meclizine hydrochloride in motion sickness
  discussion, 131
  dosage, 130
Mecostrin and muscle contraction, 227
Medinal; see Barbital
Medrol, dosage, 76
Medroxyprogesterone acetate, 301
Medullary chemoreceptors, 83-84
Mefenamic acid for pain
  discussion, 249-250
  dosage, 248
Mellaril as antipsychotic, dosage, 205
Melozets; see Methylcellulose
Melphalan in cancer, dosage, 287
Menadiol sodium diphosphate as anticoagulant inactivator, dosage, 185
Menadione as anticoagulant inactivator, dosage, 185
Menadione sodium bisulfite as anticoagulant, dosage, 185
Menformin (A); see Estrone
Menolyn, 299
Menotropins as conception enhancer, 303-304
Menpenzolate bromide, 141
Menstrual cycle, 295-296
Meperidine hydrochloride for pain
  discussion, 246-247
  dosage, 245
Mephenesin as muscle relaxant, dosage, 228
Mephentermine sulfate to maintain peripheral blood pressure
  discussion, 167-168
  dosage, 167
Mephenytoin in seizure control, dosage, 215
Mepherol as muscle relaxant, dosage, 228
Mephobarbital in seizure control
  discussion, 215
  dosage, 215
Mephson as muscle relaxant, dosage, 228

Index

Mephyton as anticoagulant inactivator, dosage, 185
Meprednisone, dosage, 76
Meprobamate in anxiety states
  discussion, 209-210
  dosage, 210
Mepropsan; *see* Meprobamate
Meprotabs; *see* Meprobamate
Meralluride in fluid control
  discussion, 101
  dosage, 101
Meratran; *see* Pipradol hydrochloride
Mercaptomerin sodium in fluid control
  discussion, 101
  dosage, 101
Mercaptopurine in cancer, dosage, 287
Mercuhydrin; *see* Meralluride
Mercurials, 100
Mercury chelation, 111
Merozoites, 50
Mertestate; *see* Testosterone
Mesantoin in seizure control, dosage, 215
Mesopin, 141
Mesoridazine, as antipsychotic, dosage, 205
Mestinon as cholinesterase inhibitor, dosage, 225
Metabolic acidosis, 272
Metabolic activity, 264-270
Metabolic products, retained, 112-117
  pharmacodynamics in, 113-117
Metal poisoning; *see* Poisoning
Metamine to dilate coronary arteries, dosage, 178
Metamucil; *see* Psyllium hydrophilic mucilloid
Metandren, dosage, 297
Metaraminol bitartrate to maintain peripheral blood pressure
  discussion, 168
  dosage, 167
Metaxalone as muscle relaxant, dosage, 228
Methacrycline hydrochloride, dosage, 29
Methadone hydrochloride for pain
  discussion, 246-247
  dosage, 245
Methadone maintenance, 247
Methahydrin; *see* Trichlormethiazide
Methallenestril, 299
Methamphetamine hydrochloride as appetite suppressant
  discussion, 259
  dosage, 258
Methandriol in protein building, dosage, 261
Methandrostenolone in protein building, dosage, 261
Methantheline bromide, 141
Methapyrilene hydrochloride as antihistamine, dosage, 64
Methaqualone for sleep control
  discussion, 234
  dosages, 231
Metharbital in seizure control
  discussion, 215
  dosage, 215
Methazolamide in fluid control, dosage, 100
Methdilazine hydrochloride as antihistamine, dosage, 64
Methedrine; *see* Methamphetamine hydrochloride
Methenamine in urinary tract infections, 36
Methergine; *see* Methylergonovine maleate
Methiacil; *see* Methylthiouracil
Methicillin sodium
  dosage, 25
  microorganism susceptibility to, 20
Methimazole for thyroid hormone control
  discussion, 264-265
  dosage, 266
Methixene hydrochloride
  discussion, 141-142
  dosage, 142
Methocarbamol as muscle relaxant, dosage, 228
Methohexital sodium in sleep control, discussion, 235
Methorate; *see* Dextromethorphan hydrobromide
Methostan in protein building, dosage, 261
Methotrexate in cancer
  discussion, 288
  dosage, 287
Methotrimeprazine hydrochloride in sleep control
  discussion, 233
  dosage, 231
Methoxamine hydrochloride to maintain peripheral blood pressure
  discussion, 168
  dosage, 167
Methoxyflurane, 240
Methoxylene as antihistamine, dosage, 64
Methoxyphenamine hydrochloride in bronchial constriction, dosage, 86
Methoxypromazine maleate, dosage, 205
Methscopolamine bromide, 141
Methsuximide in seizure control
  discussion, 215
  dosage, 215
Methyclothiazide in fluid control
  discussion, 101-102
  dosage, 101
Methylatropine nitrate, 141
Methylcellulose in constipation
  discussion, 123
  dosage, 122
Methyldopa in hypertension
  discussion, 174
  dosage, 173
Methyldopate hydrochloride in hypertension
  discussion, 174
  dosage, 183
Methylergonovine maleate for labor induction
  discussion, 306
  dosage, 306
Methylose; *see* Methylcellulose
Methylphenidate hydrochloride in psychic depression
  discussion, 203
  dosage, 201
Methylprednisolone, dosages, 76
Methylrosaniline chloride in helminthiasis
  discussion, 56
  dosage, 55
Methyltestosterone, dosage, 297
Methylthiouracil for thyroid hormone control
  discussion, 264-265
  dosage, 266
Methyprylon for sleep control
  discussion, 234
  dosage, 231
Meticortelone, dosages, 76
Meticorten, dosage, 76

Metropine, 141
Metubine and muscle contraction, 227
Microorganism
  characteristics, 17-18
  susceptibility to anti-infective drug action, 20
Microsomal liver enzyme system, 6
Microsul, dosage, 34
Midicel, dosage, 34
Migesterone, 301
Milibis; *see* Glaucarubin
Milk of Trinesium, 137
Milontin; *see* Phensuximide
Miltown; *see* Meprobamate
Mineral oil in constipation
  discussion, 122
  dosage, 122
Minocin, dosage, 29
Minocycline hydrochloride, dosage, 29
Mintezol; *see* Thiabendazole
Miradon; *see* Anisindione
Mithracin; *see* Mithramycin
Mithramycin in cancer
  discussion, 289
  dosage, 287
Mitotane in cancer
  discussion, 290
  dosage, 287
Moderil; *see* Rescinnamine
Modumate; *see* Arginine
Moebiquin; *see* Diiodohydroxyquin
Molofac; *see* Dioctyl sodium sulfosuccinate
Monitoring, prothrombin level, 186
Monoamine oxidase inhibitors, 201-202
Monodral, 141
MonoKay as anticoagulant inactivator, dosage, 185
Monotheamin in bronchial constriction, dosage, 86
Mornidine in emesis, dosage, 130
Morphine sulfate for pain
  discussion, 245-246
  dosage, 245
  respiratory depression due to, 247-248
Motility suppressants in diarrhea, 126
Motor end-plate inhibition, 226-227
  patient care in, 227
  pharmacodynamics in, 226-227
Motor end-plate transmission and muscle contraction, 224-225
Mucilose; *see* Psyllium hydrophilic mucilloid
Mucolytics, 91-92
  dosage range, 91
Multifuge; *see* Piperazine citrate
Mumps
  skin test antigen, 59-60
  virus vaccine, 70
Muracil; *see* Methylthiouracil
Muscle
  activity, effector sites of drugs used to modify, 225
  contraction, skeletal, 224-229
  hypertonicity of, 227-229
    patient care in, 229
    pharmacodynamics in, 228-229
  relaxants
    skeletal muscle, discussion, 228-229
    skeletal muscle, dosage range of, 228
    smooth muscle, discussion, 142-143
    smooth muscle, dosage range of, 142
  spasm, *see* hypertonicity of *above*

Mustard, black, in emesis induction
  discussion, 133
  dosage, 132
Mustargen; *see* Mechlorethamine hydrochloride
Myambutol; *see* Ethambutol hydrochloride
Myanesin as muscle relaxant, dosage, 228
My-B-Den; *see* Adenosine phosphate
Mycifradin; *see* Neomycin sulfate
Mycobacterium
  leprae, 37-39
    mycobacterial invasion in, 37-38
    sulfone therapy, discussion, 38-39
    sulfone therapy, dosage range, 37
  -specific drugs, 37-41
    dosage range of, 37
  tuberculosis; *see* Tuberculosis
Mycostatin; *see* Nystatin
Mylaxen and muscle contraction, 227
Myleran; *see* Busulfan
Myocardium
  blood supply, 147
  in hypoxia, and coronary artery constriction, 178
Myodigin; *see* Digitoxin
Myoxane as muscle relaxant, dosage, 228
Mysoline; *see* Primidone
Mytelase as cholinesterase inhibitor, dosage, 225

N

Nabadial in protein building, dosage, 261
Nacton, 141
Nafcillin sodium
  dosage, 25
  microorganism susceptibility to, 20
Nalidixic acid in urinary tract infection, 36
Nalline in respiratory depression, 89
Nalophine hydrochloride in respiratory depression, 89
Naloxone hydrochloride in respiratory depression, 89
Nandrolone in protein building
  discussion, 262
  dosages, 261
Napental; *see* Pentobarbital sodium
Naqua; *see* Trichlormethiazide
Narcan in respiratory depression, 89
Narcotic(s)
  antagonists, 8
    in respiratory depression, 89-90
  cough suppressants, 90
  interaction with narcotic antagonists, 8
  regulations, 3
Nardil in psychic depression, dosage, 201
Narone for pain, dosage, 248
Nartrate for pain, dosage, 248
Natorexic as appetite suppressant, dosage, 258
Naturetin; *see* Bendroflumethiazide
Navane as antipsychotic, dosage, 205
Nebs; *see* Acetaminophen
Necrosin, 16
Necrotic tissue removal, 118-119
Nectadon; *see* Noscapine
NegGram in urinary tract infection, 36
Nembutal; *see* Pentobarbital sodium
Neo-Antergan as antihistamine, dosage, 64
Neo-Hombreol, dosage, 297
Neo-Hombreol-F, dosage, 297
Neo-Hombreol-M, dosage, 297
Neohydrin; *see* Chlormerodrin

Neoloid; *see* Castor oil
Neomycin sulfate
 discussion, 31-32
 dosage, 30
Neopasalate-K in tuberculosis control, dosage, 37
Neostene in protein building, dosage, 261
Neostigmines, dosages, 225
Neo-Synephrine; *see* Phenylephrine hydrochloride
Neothylline in bronchial constriction, dosage, 86
Nephrons and fluid balance, 94-95
Neptazane in fluid control, dosage, 100
Niadrin in tuberculosis control, dosage, 37
Nialamide in psychic depression, dosage, 201
Niamid in psychic depression, dosage, 201
Nicalex; *see* Aluminum nicotinate
Niconyl; *see* Isoniazid
Nicotinyl alcohol to dilate peripheral arteries
 discussion, 179-180
 dosage, 180
Nicozide; *see* Isoniazid
Nikethamide as respiratory stimulant
 discussion, 88
 dosage, 88
Nionate as hematopoietic, dosage, 192
Nisentil; *see* Alphaprodine hydrochloride
Nitranitol to dilate coronary arteries, dosage, 178
Nitretamin to dilate coronary arteries, dosage, 178
Nitrofurantoin in urinary tract infection, 36
Nitrogen mustard; *see* Mechlorethamide hydrochloride
Nitroglycerin; *see* Glyceryl trinitrate
Nitrotalans to dilate coronary arteries, dosage, 178
Nitrous monoxide, 240
Nitrous oxide, 240
Noctec; *see* Chloral hydrate
Noludar; *see* Methyprylon
Norepinephrine
 blockers, 202-203
 release stimulators, in psychic depression, 203
 storage enhancer, in psychic depression, 203
 vascular tone and, 165
Norethindrones, 301
Norflex in Parkinsonism, dosages, 220
Norodrin; *see* Methamphetamine hydrochloride
Norlutate, 301
Norlutin, 301
Norpramin; *see* Desipramine hydrochloride
Nortriptyline hydrochloride in psychic depression
 discussion, 202-203
 dosage, 201
Noscapine as cough suppressant
 discussion, 90
 dosage, 90
Novaldin for pain, dosage, 248
Novatrin, 141
Novestrol, 299
Novobiocin
 discussion, 33
 microorganism susceptibility to, 20
Novrad; *see* Levopropoxyphene napsylate
N-Toin in urinary tract infection, 36
Numorphan; *see* Oxymorphone hydrochloride
Nursing guidelines
 in arrhythmias, 162-163
 in cancer, 291
 in cardiac output maintenance, 154-155
 in fluid control, 104-105

Nursing guidelines—cont'd
 in infection, 41-42
Nydrazid; *see* Isoniazid
Nylidrin hydrochloride to dilate peripheral arteries
 discussion, 180
 dosage, 180
Nyloxin; *see* Cobra venom extract
Nystatin in fungus eradication
 discussion, 44-45
 dosage, 45

O

Octrite to dilate peripheral arteries, 179
Octyl nitrite to dilate coronary arteries, 179
Ogen, 299
Oleandomycin phosphate
 dosage, 28
 microorganism susceptibility to, 20
Omnipen; *see* Ampicillin
Oncovin; *see* Vincristine sulfate
Ophthalgan in fluid control, 103
Opium (tincture) in diarrhea
 discussion, 126
 dosage, 125
Optiphyllin; *see* Theophylline
Oradiol, 299
Oral contraceptives; *see* Contraceptives
Ora-Lutin, 301
Oranixon as muscle relaxant, dosage, 228
Orapen; *see* Penicillin G potassium
Ora-Testryl, dosage, 297
Oratrol in fluid control, dosage, 100
Orestralyn, 299
Oretic; *see* Hydrochlorothiazide
Oreton; *see* Testosterone
Oreton-M, dosage, 297
Organidin; *see* Iodinated glycerol
Orinase; *see* Tolbutamide
Oriodide; *see* Sodium iodide
Orphenadrine citrate in Parkinsonism, dosage, 220
Orphenadrine hydrochloride in Parkinsonism, dosage, 220
Orthoxine in bronchial constriction, dosage, 86
Osmitrol in fluid control, 103
Osmōglyn in fluid control, 103
Osmotic diuretics, 102-103
Osmotic pressures, 96
Ouabain
 discussion, 152
 dosage, 151
Overdosage
 barbiturates, 235-236
 sedative-hypnotics, 235-236
Ovocylin; *see* Estradiol
Oxacillin sodium
 dosage, 25
 microorganism susceptibility to, 20
Oxamycin in tuberculosis control, dosage, 37
Oxandrolone in protein building, dosage, 261
Oxazepam in anxiety states
 discussion, 210
 dosage, 210
Oxtriphylline in bronchial constriction, dosage, 86
Oxucide; *see* Piperazine citrate
Oxycodone for pain
 discussion, 246-247
 dosage, 245

Oxygen pressure, 84-85
Oxymetholone in protein building, dosage, 261
Oxymorphone hydrochloride for pain
  discussion, 246-247
  dosage, 245
Oxyphenbutazone for pain
  discussion, 251
  dosage, 250
Oxyphencyclimine hydrochloride
  discussion, 141-142
  dosage, 142
Oxyphenisatin acetate in constipation
  discussion, 123
  dosage, 122
Oxyphenonium bromide, 141
Oxytetracycline hydrochloride, dosage, 29
Oxytocin for labor induction
  discussion, 304-306
  dosage, 306

P

Pagitane in Parkinsonism, dosage, 220
Pain, 244-253
  central pain control, 251-252
  patient care in, 252-253
  pharmacodynamics in, 245-252
Palfium; see Dextromoramide tartrate
Palonyl, 299
Paludrine; see Chloroguanide hydrochloride
Pamine, 141
Pamisyl in tuberculosis control, dosage, 37
Panheprin; see Heparin sodium
Panmycin; see Tetracycline hydrochloride
Pantopium for pain
  discussion, 246-247
  dosage, 245
Pantopon; see Pantopium
Panwarfin; see Warfarin
Papain for intravascular clot removal
  discussion, 117-118
  dosage, 118
Papase; see Papain
Papaverine hydrochloride to dilate peripheral arteries, 180
Paracort, dosage, 76
Paracortol, dosage, 76
Paradone; see Paramethadione
Paraflex as muscle relaxant, dosage, 228
Paraldehyde for sleep control
  discussion, 233
  dosage, 231
Paramethadione in seizure control
  discussion, 215-216
  dosage, 215
Paramethasone acetate, dosage, 76
Para-Pas in tuberculosis control, dosage, 37
Parasal in tuberculosis control, dosage, 37
Parathyroid hormone to control calcium ion levels
  discussion, 269
  dosage, 268
Paratyphoid vaccine, 71
Parazine; see Piperazine citrate
Parenogen for antihemorrhagic effect, dosage, 188
Parenzyme; see Trypsin
Parest; see Methaqualone
Pargyline hydrochloride in hypertension
  discussion, 174-175

Pargyline hydrochloride in hypertension—cont'd
  dosage, 173
Parkinsonism, 218-223
  drugs for, dosage range of, 220
  patient care in, 222-223
  pharmacodynamics in, 220-222
Parnate; see Tranylcypromine sulfate
Paroidin; see Parathyroid hormone
Paromomycin, dosage, 30
Parsidol in Parkinsonism, dosage, 220
Pasara; see Aminosalicylates
Pasca; see Aminosalicylates
Pasem in tuberculosis control, dosage, 37
Paskalium; see Aminosalicylates
Paskate; see Aminosalicylates
Pasmed; see Aminosalicylates
Pasna; see Aminosalicylates
Pathilon, 141
Pathocil, dosage, 25
Pathogen
  -drug spectra, 20-21
  elimination, 19
  identification, 19
  vulnerability, 18-19
Patient care, 9-12
Pava to dilate peripheral arteries, 180
Pavabid to dilate peripheral arteries, 180
Pavadel to dilate peripheral arteries, 180
Paveril; see Dioxyline
Pectin; see Kaolin and pectin
Pediamycin, dosage, 28
Peganone in seizure control, dosage, 215
Pemophyllin in bronchial constriction, dosage, 86
Penalev; see Penicillin G potassium
Penasoid; see Penicillin G potassium
Penbritin; see Ampicillin
Penicillamine as copper chelate, 110, 111
Penicillin, 24-27
  administration, 26-27
  adverse effects, 26
  allergic reactions, 24-26
  dosage range, 25
  endogenous penicillin inactivation, 26
  G
    benzathine, dosage, 25
    potassium, dosage, 25
    potassium, microorganism susceptibility to, 20
    procaine, dosage, 25
  O, potassium, dosage, 25
Pentaerythritol tetranitrate to dilate coronary arteries, dosage, 178
Pental; see Pentobarbital sodium
Pentapiperide methylsulfate, 141
Pentazocine for pain, dosages, 250
Penthienate bromide, 141
Pentids; see Penicillin G potassium
Pentobarbital sodium for sleep control
  discussion, 234
  dosage, 231
Pentolinium tartrate in hypertension
  discussion, 175
  dosage, 173
Pentothal for sleep control, 235
Pentritol to dilate coronary arteries, dosage, 178
Pen-Vee K, dosage, 25
Pen-Vee-L-A, dosage, 25
Perandren; see Testosterone

Perazil as antihistamine, dosage, 64
Performin hydrochloride as hypoglycemic, 274-275
Pergonal as conception enhancer, 303-304
Periactin as antihistamine, dosage, 64
Periclor for sleep control, dosage, 231
Peripheral artery constriction, 179-181
    drugs in, dosage range of, 180
    patient care in, 180-181
    pharmacodynamics in, 179-180
Peristaltin; see Cascara sagrada
Peristim; see Cascara sagrada
Peritrate to dilate coronary arteries, dosage, 178
Perke-One; see Dextroamphetamines
Permapen, dosage, 25
Permitil as antipsychotic, dosage, 205
Pernaemon; see Liver injection
Perphenazine as antipsychotic, dosage, 205
Persantin; see Dipyridamole
Pertussis vaccine, 70
Petit mal seizures, 214
PETN to dilate coronary arteries, dosage, 178
Petrichloral for sleep control, dosage, 231
Petrofrane; see Desipramine hydrochloride
Pharmacodynamics, 4-9
    definition, 4
Pharmacotherapeutics, definition, 4
Pharmasorb in diarrhea, dosage, 125
Phenacemide in seizure control, 216
Phenaglycodol in anxiety states
    discussion, 209-210
    dosage, 210
Phenazopyridine hydrochloride in urinary tract infection, 36
Phendimetrazine tartrate as appetite suppressant, dosage, 258
Phenegran; see Promethazine hydrochloride
Phenelzine sulfate in psychic depression, dosage, 201
Phenetron as antihistamine, dosage, 64
Phenformin hydrochloride as hypoglycemic
    discussion, 274-275
    dosage, 274
Phenindamine as antihistamine, dosage, 64
Phenindione as anticoagulant
    discussion, 185
    dosage, 185
Pheniramine maleate as antihistamine, dosage, 64
Phenmetrazine hydrochloride as appetite suppressant, dosage, 258
Phenobarbital sodium in sleep control, dosage, 231
Phenolax; see Phenolphthalein
Phenolphthalein in constipation
    discussion, 123
    dosage, 122
Phenothiazines
    producing Parkinsonian-like symptoms in elderly, 206
    subgroups of, 206
Phenoxene in Parkinsonism, dosage, 220
Phenoxybenzamine hydrochloride in hypertension
    discussion, 175-176
    dosage, 173
Phenoxymethyl penicillin, dosage, 25
Phenprocoumon as anticoagulant
    discussion, 185
    dosage, 185
Phensuximide in seizure control
    discussion, 215

Phensuximide in seizure control—cont'd
    dosage, 215
Phentermine as appetite suppressant, dosages, 258
Phenurone in seizure control, 216
Phenylbutazone for pain
    discussion, 251
    dosage, 250
Phenylephrine hydrochloride to maintain peripheral blood pressure
    discussion, 168
    dosage, 167
Phenylpropanolamine hydrochloride in bronchial constriction, dosage, 86
Pheny-PAS-Tebamin; see Aminosalicylates
Phenyramidol hydrochloride as muscle relaxant, dosage, 228
Phobex; see Benactyzine hydrochloride
Phosphaljel, 137
Phosphorylase, 273
Phosphotope; see Sodium phosphate
Phthalysulfathiazole, dosage, 34
Phyllicin; see Theophylline calcium salicylate
Phytonadione as anticoagulant inactivator, dosage, 185
Pill, the; see Contraceptives
Pinworms, 54-55
Pipamazine as antiemetic, dosage, 130
Pipanol in Parkinsonism, dosage, 220
Pipenzolate bromide, 141
Piperacetazine as antipsychotic, dosage, 205
Piperazine citrate in helminthiasis
    discussion, 56
    dosage, 55
Piperazine estrone sulfate, 299
Piperidolate hydrochloride
    discussion, 142
    dosage, 142
Pipizan; see Piperazine citrate
Pipobroman in cancer
    discussion, 288-289
    dosage, 287
Pipradrol hydrochloride in psychic depression
    discussion, 203
    dosage, 201
Piptal, 141
Pitocin; see Oxytocin
Pitressin for ADH replacement, 98
Pituitary hormone
    administration, 74
    adverse effects of, 74
Placental barrier, 6
Placidyl; see Ethchlorvynol
Plague vaccine, 70
Plant alkaloids in cancer, 289
Plaquenil; see Hydroxychloroquine sulfate
Plasma
    antihemophilic (human), for antihemorrhagic effect, dosage, 188
    expansion, 194-195
Plasmodia
    invasion, 50
    resistance, 52-53
Plasmodicidals, reserve, 53
Platelet aggregation effectors, 187
Plegine as appetite suppressant, dosage, 258
Poison control centers, 109

Poisoning
  arsenic, 111
  calcium, 110
  copper, 111
  environmental, 108
  gold, 111
  heavy metal, 108-112
  iron, 110-111
  lead, 110
  mercury, 111
  patient care in, 111-112
  pharmacodynamics in, 109-111
Polaramine as antihistamine, dosage, 64
Poldine methylsulfate, 141
Poliomyelitis vaccine, 71, 72
Poloxalkol in constipation
  discussion, 122-123
  dosage, 122
Polycillin; see Ampicillin
Polycycline; see Tetracycline hydrochloride
Polydipsia, 271
Polyestradiol phosphate, 299
Polykol; see Poloxalkol
Polymyxin B sulfate
  discussion, 32
  dosage, 30
  microorganism susceptibility to, 20
Polyphagia, 271
Polystyrene sodium sulfonate in potassium ion removal
  discussion, 113-114
  dosage, 113
Polythiazide in fluid control
  discussion, 101-102
  dosage, 101
Polyuria, 271
Ponstel; see Mefenamic acid
Postictal depression, 214
Potaba; see Aminosalicylates
Potassium
  chloride in potassium replacement, 106
  deficit, 105
  iodide as mucolytic
    discussion, 91
    dosage, 91
  ion removal, 113-114
  phenethicillin
    dosage, 25
    microorganism susceptibility to, 20
  phenoxymethyl penicillin, dosage, 25
  replacement, 106
  supplements, oral, 106
Potentiation, definition, 8-9
Povan in helminthiasis, dosage, 55
Pranone, 301
Prantal, 141
Prednis, dosage, 76
Prednisolone, dosage, 76
Prednisone, dosage, 76
Pregnyl as conception enhancer, 303-304
Preludin as appetite suppressant, dosage, 258
Premarin, 299
Premocel; see Methylcellulose
Pre-Sate; see Chlorphentermine hydrochloride
Pressonex; see Metaraminol bitartrate
Pressoreceptor effectors in hypertension, 175, 176

Pressure
  blood; see Blood, pressure
  carbon dioxide, 84
  differentials, 84-85
  osmotic, 96
  oxygen, 84-85
Primaquine phosphate in malaria
  discussion, 52
  dosage, 52
Primidone in seizure control
  discussion, 215
  dosage, 215
Principen; see Ampicillin
Pro-Banthine, 141
Probarbital sodium for sleep control, dosage, 231
Probenecid to remove urea
  discussion, 115
  dosage, 113
Procainamide hydrochloride in cardiac arrhythmias
  discussion, 160, 161
  dosage, 159
Procaine, 242
Procarbazine hydrochloride in cancer
  discussion, 290
  dosage, 287
Prochlorperazine, dosages, 205
Procyclidine hydrochloride in Parkinsonism
  discussion, 221-222
  dosage, 220
Profenil; see Alverine citrate
Progesterone
  dosage, 301
  estrogen balance, 297-298
  therapy, 300-301
Progestin, 301
Progestogens, dosage range of, 301
Progestoral, 301
Proguanil; see Chloroguanide hydrochloride
Progynon; see Estradiol
Proketazine as antipsychotic, dosage, 205
Prolax as muscle relaxant, dosage, 228
Prolixin as antipsychotic, dosages, 205
Proloid for thyroid hormone control, dosage, 266
Proluton, 301
Promacetin in leprosy control, dosage, 37
Promazine hydrochloride for sleep control
  discussion, 233
  dosage, 231
Promethazine hydrochloride as antiemetic
  discussion, 131
  dosage, 130
Promizole in leprosy control, dosage, 37
Promoxolane as muscle relaxant, dosage, 228
Pronestyl; see Procainamide hydrochloride
Propadrine in bronchial constriction, dosage, 86
Propanediol series, 210
Propantheline bromide, 141
Propiomazine hydrochloride for sleep control
  discussion, 233
  dosage, 231
Propoxyphene hydrochloride for pain
  discussion, 250
  dosage, 250
Propranolol hydrochloride in arrhythmias
  discussion, 159
  dosage, 159

Propylthiouracil for thyroid hormone control
  discussion, 264-265
  dosage, 266
Proscomide, 141
Prostaphlin; *see* Oxacillin sodium
Prostigmin as cholinesterase inhibitor, dosages, 225
Protalba; *see* Protoveratrines
Protamine sulfate as anticoagulant inactivator
  discussion, 184
  dosage, 185
Protein
  binding drugs, 5
  building, 261-262
    pharmacodynamics in, 261-262
  synthesis, factors in, schematic diagram, 283
Proternal; *see* Isoproterenol hydrochloride
Prothrombin
  inactivators, 185-187
  level monitoring, 186
Protoveratrines in hypertension
  discussion, 175
  dosage, 173
Protriptyline hydrochloride in psychic depression
  discussion, 202-203
  dosage, 201
Provell; *see* Protoveratrines
Provera, 301
Prulet; *see* Oxyphenisatin acetate
Pruritus, 271
Pseudoephedrine hydrochloride in bronchial constriction, dosage, 86
Psychic depression, 201-204
  drugs for, dosage range of, 201
  patient care in, 203-204
  pharmacodynamics in, 201-203
Psychic energizers, 201, 259
Psychomotor seizures, 214
Psychotropic drug therapy, 200-201
Psyllium hydrophilic mucilloid in constipation
  discussion, 123
  dosage, 122
Pulmonary ventilation, 83-93
Purine antagonists in cancer, 287-288
Purinethol in cancer, dosage, 287
Purodigin; *see* Digitoxin
Pydirone for pain, dosage, 248
Pyopen, dosage, 25
Pyral for pain, dosage, 248
Pyrantel pamoate in helminthiasis
  discussion, 56
  dosage, 55
Pyrathiazine hydrochloride as antiemetic, dosage, 130
Pyrazinamide; *see* Pyrazinoic acid amide
Pyrazinoic acid amide in tuberculosis control
  discussion, 41
  dosage, 37
Pyribenzamine; *see* Tripelennamine
Pyricidin; *see* Isoniazid
Pyridium in urinary tract infection, 36
Pyridostigmine bromide as cholinesterase inhibitor, dosage, 225
Pyrilamine maleate as antihistamine, dosage, 64
Pyrilgin for pain, dosage, 248
Pyrimethamine in malaria
  discussion, 52
  dosage, 52

Pyrimidine antagonists in cancer, 288
Pyronil as antihistamine, dosage, 64
Pyrrobutamine phosphate as antihistamine, dosage, 64
Pyrrolazote as antiemetic, dosage, 130
Pyrvinium pamoate in helminthiasis, dosage, 55

Q

Quaalude; *see* Methaqualone
Quelicin and muscle contraction, 227
Questran; *see* Cholestyramine resin
Quide as antipsychotic, dosage, 205
Quilene, 141
Quinacrine hydrochloride in malaria
  discussion, 53
  dosage, 52
Quinaglute in arrhythmias, 159
Quinethazone in fluid control
  discussion, 101-102
  dosage, 101
Quinicardine; *see* Quinidine sulfate
Quinidine gluconate in arrhythmias, dosage, 159
Quinidine sulfate in arrhythmias
  discussion, 160, 161-162
  dosage, 159
Quinine in malaria
  discussion, 53
  dosage, 52
Quinoxyl; *see* Chiniofon

R

Rabies vaccine, 71
Radioactive agents in cancer, 289-290
Raspberin for pain, dosage, 248
Raudixin; *see* Rauwolfia alkaloids
Rau-Sed; *see* Reserpine
RauTab; *see* Alseroxylon
Rautensin; *see* Alseroxylon
Rautina; *see* Rauwolfia alkaloids
Rautotal; *see* Rauwolfia alkaloids
Rauwiloid; *see* Alseroxylon
Rauwistan; *see* Rauwolfia alkaloids
Rauwoldin; *see* Rauwolfia alkaloids
Rauwolfia alkaloids in hypertension
  discussion, 172-174
  dosage range of, 173
Reflex, enterogastric, 137
Regulations, narcotic, 3
Regutol; *see* Dioctyl sodium sulfosuccinate
Rela as muscle relaxant, dosage, 228
Relaxar as muscle relaxant, dosage, 228
Remsed; *see* Promethazine hydrochloride
Renasul, dosage, 34
Rencal; *see* Sodium phytate
Renese; *see* Polythiazide
Renin, 96
Repoise as antipsychotic, dosage, 205
Rescinnamine in hypertension
  discussion, 172-174
  dosage, 173
Reserpine in hypertension
  discussion, 172-174
  dosage, 173
Reserpoid; *see* Reserpine
Residol; *see* Cyanocobalamin
Resistopen; *see* Oxacillin sodium

Respiratory depression, 87-90
  addictive analgesics and, 247-248
  narcotic antagonists in, 89-90
  pharmacodynamics in, 88-90
Respiratory stimulants, 88-89
  adverse effects, 89
  dosage range of, 88
Respiratory tract secretions, 90-92
  drugs to remove, dosage range, 91
Restrol, 299
Reticulogen; see Liver injection
Rezipas in tuberculosis control, dosage, 37
R-Gene; see Arginine hydrochloride
Rickettsia, agents for active immunization, 70-71
Rifadin; see Rifampin
Rifaldazine; see Rifampin
Rifampicin; see Rifampin
Rifampin in tuberculosis control
  discussion, 41
  dosage, 37
Rifamycin AMP; see Rifampin
Rimactane; see Rifampin
Rimifon; see Isoniazid
Riogon as conception enhancer, 303-304
Rlopan, 137
Ristocetin
  discussion, 33
  microorganism susceptibility to, 20
Ritalin; see Methylphenidate hydrochloride
Roampicillin; see Ampicillin
Robalate, 137
Robaxin as muscle relaxant, dosage, 228
Robinul, 141
Robitussin in respiratory tract secretion removal, dosage, 91
Ro-Cillin; see Potassium phenethicillin
Rocky Mountain spotted fever vaccine, 71
Rolitetracycline, dosage, 29
Rolsul as anti-infective, dosage, 34
Romilar; see Dextromethorphan hydrobromide
Rondomycin, dosage, 29
Roquine; see Chloroquine phosphate
Rothalid, dosage, 34
Rotoxamine tartrate as antihistamine, dosage, 64
Rubella virus vaccine, 71, 72
Rubramin; see Cyanocobalamin
Rubramin OH; see Hydroxocobalamin

S

Salamide for pain, dosage, 248
Salicim for pain, dosage, 248
Salicylamide for pain, dosage, 248
Salicylazosulfapyridine, dosage, 34
Saline cathartics, 123-124
  dosage, 122
Salrin for pain, dosage, 248
Salt, bile salt removal, 117
Saluron; see Hydroflumethiazide
Sandril; see Reserpine
Saroxin; see Digoxin
Schizonts, 50
Scopolamine hydrobromide
  discussion, 140
  dosage, 141
Secobarbital sodium in sleep control
  discussion, 234
  dosage, 231

Seconal sodium; see Secobarbital sodium
Sedatives
  dosage range of, 231
  overdosage, 235-236
Seizure(s), 213-218
  drugs for
    discussion, 214-217
    dosage range of, 215
  grand mal, 214
  Jacksonian, 214
  patient care in, 217-218
  petit mal, 214
  pharmacodynamics in, 214-217
  psychomotor, 214
Semikon as antihistamine, dosage, 64
Semopen; see Potassium, phenethicillin
Semoxydrine; see Methamphetamine hydrochloride
Senna in constipation
  discussion, 123
  dosage, 122
Sennosides A and B in constipation
  discussion, 123
  dosage, 122
Senokot; see Senna
Sensitivity
  acquired, 61-63
  exposure-induced, biological agents to detect, 60
  tests, 59-60
Sensitization, atopic, 61
Serax; see Oxazepam
Serenium in urinary tract infection, 36
Serentil as antipsychotic, dosage, 205
Serfin; see Reserpine
Seromycin in tuberculosis control, dosage, 37
Serpasil; see Reserpine
Serum sickness, 62-63
  anti-infective drugs and, 23-24
Serutan; see Psyllium hydrophilic mucilloid
Setrol; see Oxyphencyclimine hydrochloride
Sex cycle, female, 295-296
Sinan as muscle relaxant, dosage, 228
Sinaxar as muscle relaxant, dosage, 228
Sineguan; see Doxepin hydrochloride
Singoserp; see Syrosingopine
Sintrom; see Acenocoumarol
Sitosterols to lower blood lipid levels
  discussion, 183
  dosage, 183
Skelaxin as muscle relaxant, dosage, 228
Sleep
  control
    patient care in, 236-238
    pharmacodynamics in, 232-236
  cycles, 230
  disruption, 232
  drugs to control, dosage range of, 231
  induction, 232-235
  maintenance, 232-235
  patterns, 230-238
Smallpox vaccine, 71, 72
Sodium bicarbonate
  discussion, 137-138
  dosage, 137
Sodium biphosphate in constipation
  discussion, 124
  dosage, 122

Sodium bromide for sleep control
    discussion, 234
    dosage, 231
Sodium carboxymethylcellulose in constipation
    discussion, 123
    dosage, 122
Sodium deficit, 106
Sodium glutamate in ammonia removal
    discussion, 116-117
    dosage, 113
Sodium iodide in cancer
    discussion, 289
    dosage, 287
Sodium phosphate
    in cancer
        discussion, 290
        dosage, 287
    in constipation
        discussion, 124
        dosage, 122
Sodium phytate to control calcium ion levels
    discussion, 268
    dosage, 268
Sodium salicylate for pain, dosage, 248
Sodium transport inhibitors, 100-102
    dosage range of, 101
Sodizole, dosage, 34
Softran; see Buclizine hydrochloride
Solacen; see Tybamate
Solestro, 299
Solu-Cortef, dosage, 76
Solu-Medrol, dosage, 76
Soma as muscle relaxant, dosage, 228
Sombucaps; see Hexobarbital
Sombulex; see Hexobarbital
Somnafac; see Methaqualone
Somnicaps as antihistamine, dosage, 64
Somnos; see Chloral hydrate
Sonilyn, dosage, 34
Sopor; see Methaqualone
Sosol, dosage, 34
Spacolin; see Alverine citrate
Spanestrin, 299
Sparine; see Promazine hydrochloride
Sparteine sulfate for labor induction
    discussion, 306
    dosage, 306
Spartocin; see Sparteine sulfate
Spectinomycin dihydrochloride
    discussion, 32
    dosage, 30
Speed; see Methamphetamine hydrochloride
Spironolactone in fluid control, 99
Spontin; see Ristocetin
Stanozolol in protein building, dosage, 261
Stanzamine as antihistamine, dosage, 64
Staphcillin; see Methicillin, sodium
Steclin; see Tetracycline hydrochloride
Stelazine as antipsychotic, dosage, 205
Stemutrolin as conception enhancer, 303-304
Stenediol in protein building, dosage, 261
Sterane, dosage, 76
Sterile urea in fluid control, 103
Steroids, anabolic, 262
    adverse effects of, 262
    dosage range of, 262

Sterolone, dosage, 76
Stibophen in helminthiasis
    discussion, 56
    dosage, 55
Stilbetin, 299
Stilphostrol, 299
Stomach; see Gastric
Streptokinase
    for intravascular clot removal
        discussion, 117-118
        dosage, 118
    for necrotic tissue removal, 119
Streptomycin
    discussion, 30-32
    dosage, 30
    microorganism susceptibility to, 20
    in tuberculosis control, discussion, 40
Stressors and vascular tone, 164-166
Striatran; see Emyclamate
Strycin; see Streptomycin
Styramate as muscle relaxant, dosage, 228
Suavitil; see Benactyzine hydrochloride
Sublimaze; see Fentanyl citrate
Succinylcholine chloride and muscle contraction, 227
Succinylsulfathiazole, dosage, 34
Sucostrin and muscle contraction, 227
Sucraphen; see Phenylephrine hydrochloride
Sudafed in bronchial constriction, dosage, 86
Sugracillin; see Penicillin, G potassium
Sulamyd, dosage, 34
Sulestrex piperazine, 299
Sulfabid, dosage, 34
Sulfacetamide, dosage, 34
Sulfachlorpyridazine, dosage, 34
Sulfadiazine
    dosages, 34
    microorganism susceptibility to, 20
Sulfadimethoxine, dosage, 34
Sulfaethidole, dosage, 34
Sulfamerazine, dosage, 34
Sulfameter, dosage, 34
Sulfamethizole, dosage, 34
Sulfamethoxazole, dosage, 34
Sulfamethoxypyridazine, dosage, 34
Sulfaphenazole, dosage, 34
Sulfapyridine, dosage, 34
Sulfasol, dosage, 34
Sulfasuxidine, dosage, 34
Sulfathalidine, dosage, 34
Sulferous; see Ferrous sulfate
Sulfinpyrazone for urea removal
    discussion, 115
    dosage, 113
Sulfisomidine, dosage, 34
Sulfisoxazole, dosages, 34
Sulfonamides
    administration, 36
    adverse effects of, 35
    allergic reactions, 35
    discussion, 33-36
    distribution, 34
    dosage range, 34
    excretion, 34-35
Sulfones in Mycobacterium leprae control
    discussion, 38-39
    dosage range, 37

334 Index

Sulfoxone sodium in leprosy control, dosage, 37
Sulfstat, dosage, 34
Sulfurine, dosage, 34
Sulla, dosage, 34
Sul-Spansion dosage, 34
Sul-Spantab, dosage, 34
Sumadil as antihistamine, dosage, 64
Sumycin; see Tetracycline
Sunandrol, dosage, 297
Supen; see Ampicillin
Surfak; see Dioctyl calcium sulfosuccinate
Surital for sleep control, discussion, 235
Sus-Phrine; see Epinephrine hydrochloride
Symmetrel, 67
Synandrets, dosage, 297
Synandrol-F; see Testosterone
Synandrotabs, dosage, 297
Syncelose; see Methylcellulose
Syncillin; see Potassium phenethicillin
Syncurine and muscle contraction, 227
Syndrox; see Methamphetamine hydrochloride
Synergism, definition, 8
Synerone, dosage, 297
Synestrol, 299
Synkavite as anticoagulant inactivator, dosage, 185
Synophylate in bronchial constriction, dosage, 86
Syntetrin, dosage, 29
Synthroid for thyroid hormone control, dosage, 266
Syntocinon; see Oxytocin
Syraprim; see Trimethoprim
Syrosingopine in hypertension
    discussion, 172-174
    dosage, 173
Sytobex; see Cyanocobalamin
Sytobex-H; see Hydroxocobalamin

T

Tablets, enteric-coated (E.C.T.), 10
Tabocillin; see Ampicillin
Tacaryl as antihistamine, dosage, 64
Tace; see Chlorotrianisene
Tagathen as antihistamine, dosage, 64
Talbutal for sleep control, dosage, 231
Talwin for pain, dosages, 250
Tandearil for pain, dosage, 250
TAO, dosage, 28
Tapazole; see Methimazole
Tapeworms, 54
Taractan as antipsychotic, dosage, 205
Tebrazid; see Pyrazinoic acid amide
Tegopen; see Cloxacillin sodium
Tegretol; see Carbamazepine
Teldrin as antihistamine, dosage, 64
Temaril as antihistamine, dosage, 64
Tempra; see Acetaminophen
Tensilon and muscle contraction, 227
Tentone as antipsychotic, dosage, 205
Tenuate as appetite suppressant, dosage, 258
Tepanil as appetite suppressant, dosage, 258
Teratogenics during pregnancy, 6
Terpin hydrate elixir for removal of respiratory tract secretions
    discussion, 91
    dosage, 91

Terrabon, dosage, 29
Terramycin, dosage, 29
Teslac, dosage, 297
Tessalon; see Benzonatate
Testandrone; see Testosterone
Testobase; see Testosterone
Testodet, dosage, 297
Testolactone, dosage, 297
Testosteroid; see Testosterone
Testosterone
    discussion, 296-297
    dosages, 297
Testrone; see Testosterone
Testryl; see Testosterone
Tetanus toxoid, 71
Tetrabon; see Tetracycline hydrochloride
Tetracycline(s), 28-30
    administration, 29-30
    adverse effects, 28-29
    dosages, 29
Tetracycline hydrochloride
    dosage, 29
    microorganism susceptibility to, 20
Tetracyn; see Tetracycline hydrochloride
Tetrex; see Tetracycline hydrochloride
Theelin; see Estrone
Thelestrin; see Estrone
Thenylene as antihistamine, dosage, 64
Theobromine calcium salicylate in fluid control, 102
Theocalcin in fluid control, 102
Theocin in bronchial constriction, dosage, 86
Theoglycinate in bronchial constriction, dosage, 86
Theophylline(s)
    in bronchial constriction, 85-86
    dosages, 86
    in fluid control, 102
Thephorin as antihistamine, dosage, 64
Theriodide; see Sodium iodide
Thiabendazole in helminthiasis
    discussion, 56
    dosage, 55
Thiamine hydrochloride
    as hematopoietic, dosage, 192
    in hemoglobin production, 194
Thiamintol; see Thiamine hydrochloride
Thiamylal sodium for sleep control, 235
Thiazides in fluid control, 101-102
Thiazosulfone in leprosy control, dosage, 37
Thibex as hematopoietic, dosage, 192
Thiethylperazine maleate as antiemetic
    discussion, 131
    dosage, 130
Thioguanine in cancer, dosage, 287
Thiomerin; see Mercaptomerin sodium
Thiopental sodium for sleep control, 235
Thiopropazate hydrochloride as antipsychotic, dosage, 205
Thioridazine hydrochloride as antipsychotic, dosage, 205
Thiosulfil, dosage, 34
Thio-tepa in cancer
    discussion, 288-289
    dosage, 287
Thiothixene as antipsychotic, dosage, 205
Thiphenamil hydrochloride, 141-142
Thirst center, 97
Thorazine; see Chlorpromazines

Thoxidil as muscle relaxant, dosage, 228
Thrombin for antihemorrhagic effect, dosage, 188
Thrombolysin; see Fibrinolysin
Thylokay as anticoagulant inactivator, dosage, 185
Thyrar for thyroid hormone control, dosage, 266
Thyroglobulin for thyroid hormone control, dosage, 266
Thyroid
  dosage, 266
  glandular function, 264-266
    patient care in, 266
    pharmacodynamics in, 264-266
  hormone
    control, 264
    control, drugs for, dosage range, 266
    enhancers, 265-266
    inhibitors, 264-265
Thyrotropin for thyroid hormone control, dosage, 266
Thytropar for thyroid hormone control, dosage, 266
Tigan as antiemetic, dosage, 130
Tindal as antipsychotic, dosage, 205
Tiphenamil hydrochloride
  discussion, 141-142
  dosage, 142
Tisin; see Isoniazid
Tissue
  debris removal, 117-119
    drugs for, dosage range of, 118
    pharmacodynamics in, 117-119
  fluid removal, 117-119
    drugs for, dosage range of, 118
    pharmacodynamics in, 117-119
  immunity, 59
  necrotic, removal, 118-119
  toxicants, 108-120
    drugs to remove, dosage range of, 113
Titroid for thyroid hormone control, dosage, 266
Toclase; see Carbetapentane citrate
Tocosamine; see Sparteine sulfate
Tofranil; see Imipramine hydrochloride
Tolanate to dilate coronary arteries, dosage, 178
Tolazamide as hypoglycemic
  discussion, 274
  dosage, 274
Tolbutamide as hypoglycemic
  discussion, 274
  dosage, 274
Toleron as hematopoietic, dosage, 192
Tolferain as hematopoietic, dosage, 192
Tolhart as muscle relaxant, dosage, 228
Tolinase; see Tolazamide
Tolosate as muscle relaxant, dosage, 228
Tolseram as muscle relaxant, dosage, 228
Tolserol as muscle relaxant, dosage, 228
Tolulox as muscle relaxant, dosage, 228
Torecan; see Thiethylperazine maleate
Totacillin; see Ampicillin
Toxicants, tissue, 108-120
  drugs to remove, dosage range of, 113
Toxins, bacterial, agents for active immunization against, 70-71
Tral, 141
Trancopal as muscle relaxant, dosage, 228
Tranquilizers
  major, 206-209
    dosage range of, 205

Tranquilizers—cont'd
  major—cont'd
    patient care, 207-209
    pharmacodynamics, 206-207
  minor, 209-211
    patient care, 211
    pharmacodynamics, 209-211
Transinoculation, 69
Trantoin in urinary tract infection, 36
Tranylcypromine sulfate, 3
  in psychic depression
    discussion, 201
    dosage, 201
Trasentine; see Adiphenine hydrochloride
Trecator; see Ethionamide
Tremin in Parkinsonism, dosage, 220
Trest; see Methixene hydrochloride
Triamcinolones, dosage, 76
Triamterene in fluid control, 99
Trichinella extract in sensitivity test, 60
Trichlorethene, 240
Trichlorethylene, 240
Trichlormethiazide in fluid control
  discussion, 101-102
  dosage, 101
Triclofos sodium for sleep control
  discussion, 233
  dosage, 231
Triclos; see Triclofos sodium
Tricoloid, 141
Tri-Creamalate, 137
Tricyclamol chloride, 141
Tridihexethyl chloride, 141
Tridione; see Trimethadione
Triethylenemelamine in cancer
  discussion, 288-289
  dosage, 287
Trifluoperazine as antipsychotic, dosage, 205
Triflupromazine hydrochloride as antipsychotic, dosage, 205
Trihexyphenidyl hydrochloride in Parkinsonism, dosage, 220
Trilafon as antipsychotic, dosage, 205
Trimeprazine tartrate as antihistamine, dosage, 64
Trimethadione in seizure control
  discussion, 215-216
  dosage, 215
Trimethaphan camsylate in hypertension
  discussion, 175
  dosage, 173
Trimethobenzamide hydrochloride as antiemetic, dosage, 130
Trimethoprim in malaria
  discussion, 53
  dosage, 52
Trimethylene, 240
Trimeton as antihistamine, dosage, 64
Trinesium, 137
Tripelennamine citrate
  as antihistamine, dosage, 64
  in respiratory tract secretions removal
    discussion, 91
    dosage, 91
Tripelennamine hydrochloride as antihistamine, dosage, 64
Triprolidine hydrochloride as antihistamine, dosage, 64

Tri-Sil, 137
Trisogel, 137
Trobicin; see Spectinomycin dihydrochloride
Trocinate, 141-142
Troleandomycin, dosage, 28
Trolnitrate phosphate to dilate coronary arteries, dosage, 178
Trophozoites, 50
Trosinone, 301
Trypsin for intravascular clot removal
    discussion, 117-118
    dosage, 118
Tryptar; see Trypsin
Tube, endotracheal, in place, diagram, 88
Tuberculin skin test, 60
Tuberculosis, 39-41
    drugs for, 40-41
        dosage range, 37
    prophylaxis, 39-40
Twiston as antihistamine, dosage, 64
Tybamate in anxiety states
    discussion, 209-210
    dosage, 210
Tylahist as antihistamine, dosage, 64
Tylenol; see Acetaminophen
Typhoid vaccine, 71
Typhus vaccine, 71
Tyramine-containing foods and monoamide oxidase inhibitors, 202
Tyvin; see Isoniazid

U

Ulcerogenic agents, 137
Ulo; see Chlophedianol hydrochloride
Ultandren, dosage, 297
Ultran; see Phenaglycodol
Unipen; see Nafcillin sodium
Unisulf, dosage, 34
Unitensen; see Cryptenamine
Uracil mustard in cancer, dosage, 287
Urea
    removal, 114-115
    sterile, in fluid control, 103
Ureaphil in fluid control, 103
Urecholine in intestinal hypomotility, 143-144
Urevert in fluid control, 103
Uricosuric agents, 102, 115
Urispas; see Flavoxate hydrochloride
Urosulfin, dosage, 34
Urosulfon, dosage, 34
Urticaria, 62
    anti-infective drugs and, 23
Uteracon; see Oxytocin
Utrasul, dosage, 34

V

Vaccines, 70-71
Valergen, 299
Valium; see Diazepam
Vallestril, 299
Valmid; see Ethinamate
Valpin, 141
Vancocin; see Vancomycin
Vancomycin
    discussion, 32
    dosage, 30
    microorganism susceptibility to, 20

Vanogel, 137
Vasal to dilate peripheral arteries, 180
Vasodilan; see Isoxsuprine hydrochloride
Vasodilator, direct-acting, in hypertension, 175
Vasodrine; see Epinephrine hydrochloride
Vasopressin for ADH replacement, 98
Vasoxyl; see Methoxamine hydrochloride
V-Cillin, dosage, 25
V-Cillin K, dosage, 25
Velacycline, dosage, 29
Velban; see Vinblastine sulfate
Ventilation, pulmonary, 83-93
Ventricular ectopic foci, 157-158
Veracillin, dosage, 25
Veralba; see Protoveratrines
Vercyte; see Pipobroman
Veriloid; see Alkavervir
Veronal; see Barbital
Versapen, dosages, 25
Vesprin as antipsychotic, dosage, 205
Vessel(s)
    constriction, 171-181
    lymphatic, and cancer tissue extension, 285
    tone, 164-170
Vestibular stimulus depression, 131
Vibazine; see Buclizine hydrochloride
Vibramycin, dosage, 29
Vinactane in tuberculosis control, dosage, 37
Vinbarbital for sleep control, dosage, 231
Vinblastine sulfate in cancer
    discussion, 289
    dosage, 287
Vincristine sulfate in cancer
    discussion, 289
    dosage, 287
Vinyl ether, 240
Viocin in tuberculosis control, dosage, 37
Vioform; see Glycobiarsol
Viomycin sulfate in tuberculosis control, dosage, 37
Vio-Thene; see Oxyphencyclimine hydrochloride
Viruses
    agents for active immunization against, 70-71
    invasion, 66-67
    resistance, and interferons, 66
Vistaril; see Hydroxyzine pamoate
Vitamin B_{12}, 192-193
Vitamin D to control calcium ion levels, 268
Vitamin E to lower blood lipid levels
    discussion, 183
    dosage, 183
Vitamin K_1 as anticoagulant inactivator, dosage, 185
Vivactil; see Protriptyline hydrochloride
Vomiting; see Emesis
Vontrol; see Diphenidol hydrochloride

W

Warcoumin; see Warfarin
Warfarin as anticoagulant
    discussion, 185
    dosage, 185
Water output with normal metabolic rate, 41
Wilpo as appetite suppressant, dosage, 258
Winstrol in protein building, dosage, 261
Wyacort, dosage, 76
Wyamine; see Mephentermine sulfate
Wycillin, dosage, 25
Wynestron; see Estrone

X

Xanthines, 102
Xylocaine; *see* Lidocaine hydrochloride

Y

Yellow fever vaccine, 71
Ylestrol, 299
Yodoxin; *see* Diiodohydroxyquin

Z

Zactane; *see* Ethoheptazine citrate
Zamitan; *see* Dextroamphetamines
Zarontin; *see* Ethosuximide
Zyloprim; *see* Allopurinol